CW00829475

TRANSPORT OF THE CRITICAL CARE PATIENT

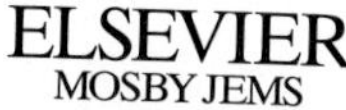

3251 Riverport Lane
St. Louis, MO 63043

TRANSPORT OF THE CRITICAL CARE PATIENT ISBN: 978-0-323-08272-3

The Publisher International Standard Book Number: 978-0-323-08272-3

Publisher: Michael Ledbetter
Managing Editor: Laura Bayless
Publishing Services Manager: Julie Eddy
Project Manager: Richard Barber
Design Direction: Karen Pauls

Printed in United States

Last digit is the print number: 9 8 7 6 5 4 3 2 1

TRANSPORT OF THE CRITICAL CARE PATIENT

Rosemary Adam, RN, EMT-P
Nurse Instructor
Emergency Medical Services Learning Resources Center
The University of Iowa Hospitals and Clinics
Iowa City, Iowa

Chris Cebollero, CCEMT-CCP
Chief
Emergency Medical Services
Christian Hospital
St. Louis, Missouri

ELSEVIER
MOSBY JEMS

*Dedicated to those who have had to put up with me…
Especially my family, who made me who I am: Bill and Mary Hester, my wonderful parents, and to my children, Amy and Chris, who are my pride and joy. Truly they represent generations of love. Thanks.*

ROSEMARY ADAM

While reading dedications in other publications, I always wondered what this person meant to the author and how did he or she get such an honor of having that book named after them. I have had such a great and successful EMS career. As I sit and wonder who gave me the greatest opportunity in attaining this great milestone of being an author, there are a number of people who come to mind. My children: Zachery, Kristen, Lauren, and Angela, the support you shared in understanding how much time this took away from yelling at you to clean your room, do your chores, and not being around to give you all my money was like a mini vacation for all of us. My wife, Lee; your understanding about the countless number of books on the kitchen table, the hours away from honey do's and missing many a date night, defines your support, love, and friendship that makes you my pickle nanny. The foundation, however, of my EMS career would not have even been possible without the guidance, support, and love of two people: This book is dedicated to Chip and Diane.

CHRIS CEBOLLERO

Author Acknowledgments

The educational curriculum entitled "Critical Care Paramedic" is owned and offered through the University of Iowa Hospitals and Clinics' EMS Learning Resources Center (EMSLRC). Our thanks to that prestigious organization and its director, Douglas K. York, for the encouragement and support for this project.

We would like to take this opportunity to send a special thank you to two women who took us through the sometimes scary world of first-edition book development. Kathy Sartori and Krissy Prysmiki were on our initial development team as developmental editors and taught us just how much we did not know about writing a book. Their patience, knowledge, professionalism, and humor allowed us to develop a fantastic end product. Thank you both for being part of this project and ensuring its success.

ROSEMARY ADAM

CHRIS CEBOLLERO

Publisher Acknowledgments

CONTRIBUTORS

Azeemuddin Ahmed, MD, FACEP, MBA
Interim Vice Chair and Clinical Associate Professor
Medical Director, University of Iowa *AirCare* and EMSLRC
University of Iowa Department of Emergency Medicine
Iowa City, Iowa

Jimmy Aycox, LP, CCEMP-T, NREMP-T
Paramedic
MedStar EMS
Forth Worth, Texas

Lisa Bennett, LP, CCEMTP
Arlington Fire Department
Arlington, Texas

Chris Bennett, BS, LP, CCP
Primary Paramedic
MedStar EMS
Fort Worth, Texas

Laura Denton, BSRC, RRT, CPFT, RCP
Manager, Respiratory Care
Baylor Health Care System
Fort Worth, Texas

Anna M. Lorence, MD
Department of Emergency Medicine
Mercy Medical Center
Dubuque, Iowa

Eric Endahl, BS, RRT-NPS
Pediatric Services Supervisor, Respiratory Care
The University of Iowa Hospitals and Clinics
Iowa City, Iowa

Harold Etheridge, Lic-P, NREMT-P, CCEMT-P
Field Training Officer
MedStar EMS
Forth Worth, Texas

Mark A. Graber, MD, FACEP
Professor of Emergency and Family Medicine
University of Iowa Carver College of Medicine
Iowa City, Iowa

Daniel Hallam
Intensive Care Fellow
The University of Iowa Hospitals and Clinics
Iowa City, Iowa

Ryan Hobbs, BS, Pharm
Clinical Pharmacy Specialist, Cardiology
Department of Pharmaceutical Care
The University of Iowa Hospitals and Clinics
Iowa City, Iowa

Paul Hudson, MHA, FACHE, MBA
Chief Operating Officer
Acute Care, Inc.
Ames, Iowa

Charles Jennissen, MD
Clinical Associate Professor, Pediatric Emergency Medicine
The University of Iowa Hospitals and Clinics
Iowa City, Iowa

Michael Kaiser, RN, CPT-C
Organ Clinical Specialist
Iowa Donor Network
North Liberty, Iowa

Richard E. Klabunde, PhD
Associate Professor of Physiology
Department of Biomedical Science
Ohio University College of Osteopathic Medicine
Athens, Ohio

Sundar Krischnan
Associate, Department of Anesthesia
The University of Iowa Hospitals and Clinics
Iowa City, Iowa

Mark Miksch, RN, BSN, MS
Educational Media Coordinator, ICU Nurse
The University of Iowa Hospitals and Clinics
Iowa City, Iowa

Pam Normandin, RN, MSN, CCRC
Clinical Nurse Specialist, Clinical Research Coordinator
Clinical Trials Office
Iowa Health Systems
Des Moines, Iowa

Tim Penic, NREMT-P, CCP
Paramedic
MedStar EMS
Forth Worth, Texas

Mary J. Potratz, RN, MEd, MSN, CCRN
Critical Care Educator, Patient Care Coordinator
Iowa Methodist Medical Center
Des Moines, Iowa

Lee Ridge, EMT-P
EMS Instructor, EMS Learning Resources Center
Director, EMS Center & Mobile Emergency Treatment Center
Department of Emergency Medicine
The University of Iowa Hospitals and Clinics
Iowa City, Iowa

Sudarshan Setty, MD, DNB
Department of Anesthesia
Montefiore Medical Center
Bronx, New York

Jonathan S. Simmons, DO, MS, FCCP
Clinical Associate Professor
Co-Director, Critical Care Fellowship Program
Chair of Emergency Management
Medical Director, Admission and Transfer Center
Co-Director, Extracorporeal Life Support Program
Departments of Anesthesia, Internal Medicine and Emergency Medicine
Surgical Intensive Care Unit
The University of Iowa Hospitals and Clinics
Iowa City, Iowa

Suzanne Witte, LISW
Social Work Specialist II, Supervisor
Family Support Program Coordinator
The University of Iowa Hospitals and Clinics
Iowa City, Iowa

REVIEWERS

Azeemuddin Ahmed, MD, FACEP, MBA
Interim Vice Chair and Clinical Associate Professor
Medical Director, University of Iowa *AirCare* and EMSLRC
University of Iowa Department of Emergency Medicine
Iowa, City, Iowa

Robert P. Breese, EMT-P, MICP, CCEMT-P, FP-C
Associate Paramedic Program Coordinator
Monroe Community College
Rochester, New York

John S. Cole, MD, FACEP, EMT-P
Medical Director
STAT MedEvac
Pittsburgh, Pennsylvania

William Black, NREMT-P/CCEMT-P
STAT Critical Care Transport Team, Westchester Medical Center, Transcare
Valhalla, New York

Kevin T. Collopy, BA, CCEMT-P, NREMT-P, WEMT
Flight Paramedic, Lead Instructor
Spirit Ministry Transportation Service, Wilderness Medical Associates
Marshfield, Wisconsin

T. Kevin Crump, NREMT-P, CCEMT-P
Paramedic
Fort Worth, Texas

Steve Dralle, MBA, LP
San Antonio, Texas

Hunter Elliott
Paramedic
Center for Emergency Health Services, Richmond Ambulance Authority
Richmond, Virginia

Harold Etheridge, Lic-P, NREMT-P, CCEMT-P
Field Training Officer
MedStar EMS
Fort Worth, Texas

Thomas E. Ezell III, NREMT-P, CCEMT-P
James City County Fire Department
Williamsburg, Virginia

Michael Fisher, BHS, NREMT-P, CCEMT-P
Professor, Director of Human Patient Simulation
Greenville Technical College
Greenville, South Carolina

Rudy Garrett, AS, NREMT-P, CCEMT-P
Flight Paramedic
Air Methods
Somerset, Kentucky

Chuck Gipson, AAS NREMT-P, CCP
Quality, Education Manager
MEDIC EMS
Davenport, Iowa

Thomas James Gottschalk, CCEMT-P Educator
Platnum Educational Group LLC
Jenison, Michigan

Lynn Peirzchalski-Goldstein, RPh, BSP, PharmD
Pharmacy Clinical Coordinator
Penrose St. Francis Health System, and, University Colorado
Colorado Springs, Colorado

Brandon J. Gregozeski, CCEMT-P
Bell Ambulance
Milwaukee, Wisconsin

Brian Helland, AS, CCEMT-P
Clive Fire Department
Clive, Iowa

Gary Hoertz, NREMT-P, CCEMT-P
EMS Division Chief
Kootenai County Fire & Rescue
Post Falls, Idaho

Cathryn A. Holstein, CCEMT-P
Clinical Manager
Rural/Metro Ambulance
Seattle, Washington

Paul J. Honeywell, NREMT-P
Training Director
Southwest Ambulance
Phoenix, Arizona

Rob Jackson, NREMT-P, CCEMT-P, BA, MAPS, MAR
Paramedic
University of Missouri EMS
Columbia, Missouri
Cole County EMS
Jefferson City, Missouri

Ryan Jacobsen, MD
Truman Medical Centers
Kansas City, Missouri

Don Kimlicka, NREMT-P CCEMT-P
EMS Coordinator
Saint Clare's Hospital
Weston, Wisconsin

Richard R. Moskalski Jr., NREMT-P, CICP, EMS-I
The Cleveland Clinic EMS Academy
Cleveland, Ohio

Larry Richmond, AS, NREMT-P, CCEMT-P
EMS Coordinator
Rapid City IHS Hospital
Rapid City, South Dakota

Rob Jackson, BA, MAPS, MAR, NREMT-P, CCEMT-P
Paramedic
University of Missouri Health Care
Columbia, Missouri

David Stamey, CCEMT-P
Flight Paramedic, EMS Educator
STAT MedEvac—University of Pittsburgh Medical Center,
University of Maryland Fire & Rescue Institute
Pittsburgh, Pennsylvania

James Steffen, REMT-P, AAS
Henry County Health Center
Mount Pleasant, Iowa

Douglas R. Stevenson, BA, NREMT-P, EMS-C
Alvin Community College
Alvin, Texas

David M. Tauber, NREMT-P, CCEMT-P, FP-C, I/C
Education Coordinator
New Haven Sponsor Hospital Program
New Haven, Connecticut

A. Laura Torrez, CCLP, A.A.S
EMS Education Coordinator
Methodist Health Systems
Dallas, Texas

Robert S. Wales, BS, NREMT-P, CCEMT-P
Paramedic, Training Officer
Pickens County EMS
Pickens, South Carolina

Brian Williams, BS, NREMT-P, CCEMT-P
EMS Captain
Glacier County EMS
Cut Bank, Montana

Preface

Being a prehospital provider is one of the best jobs in the world. We are asked to deal with life, death, challenges, and uncertainty every day. One of the key components for delivering the highest care possible is our knowledge, skills, and experience. Education is the cornerstone to gaining that experience. We wanted to develop a reference that would give you the knowledge necessary to achieve, refresh, and continue your education in the critical care specialty. This reference was designed with the University of Iowa Hospitals' EMSLRC Critical Care Paramedic curriculum as a template. Each chapter begins with a case study designed to challenge your critical thinking skills and ask key questions that will be answered in the ensuing chapter. Your core knowledge will be enhanced by each chapter defining key points, explaining disease processes, and necessary treatments. Along with detailed chapters, you will also find step-by-step procedures taking you through the skills essential to the critical care specialty. Each chapter has a number of "Did You Know?" boxes that share interesting tidbits of information about that specific paragraph, medication, or general knowledge. At the end of each chapter we re-examine the case studies from the beginning of the chapter and tie it all together.

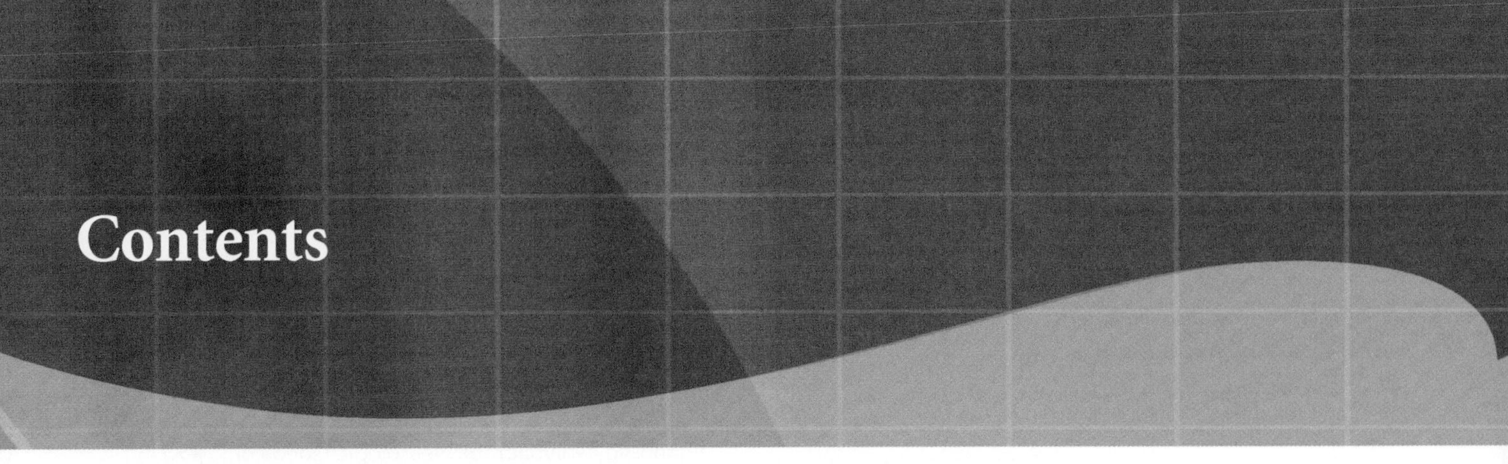

Contents

CHAPTER 1

Foundations of Critical Care Transport

OBJECTIVES

1. Recall pertinent laws regarding out-of-hospital medical control, communications, medical practice acts, standards of care, and protocol use.
2. Summarize regulations established by the Consolidated Omnibus Reconciliation Act of 1986 (COBRA) and the Emergency Medical Treatment and Active Labor Act (EMTALA) as they relate to the transfer of patients from one hospital to another hospital, including stabilization, communication, documentation, hand-off reports, equipment and personnel needs, standards of care, and responsibilities.
3. Recognize current payers and legislative trends pertaining to reimbursement for emergency medical services and the way reimbursement affects the delivery of critical care in the prehospital environment.

Scenario

As an emergency medical services (EMS) provider, you are faced with a personal and professional decision today that has you feeling a lot of stress. You have been suspicious of your best friend and partner for several months. You are worried that he is using, and possibly stealing, controlled drugs. This is not the partner and eventual best friend you met 5 years ago. He was ambitious, smart, and an excellent EMS provider. You have never actually witnessed him taking drugs, nor has he confided in you. However, his behavior has been erratic, and he displays sudden signs of slurring, uncoordinated walking, and poor eye-hand coordination while at work. You have been helping him with patient care by making decisions and correcting his errors in judgment, dosages, and treatment before he completes them.

You confronted him at work last night between calls, and he became defensive and angry and now refuses to speak to you. The department's rumor mill is telling of unaccounted for controlled substances.

Your personal challenge is that he is a friend, and you'd like to get him some help without jeopardizing his job, his family, and your friendship. Your professional challenge is that you think you could be placing your own career in peril by not notifying your employer and the licensing/certification board about your strong suspicions. The third real dilemma is that you are worried about your partner's decision making and ability to take good care of patients.

This chapter introduces the foundations for providing professional critical care transport. Some of the content on ethics and medical-legal issues may be a review from your initial curriculum. Some of the content is an introduction to understanding the federal rules of legal transfer. As you ponder the case study, ask yourself: Do ethical, moral, and legal issues arise in the decisions that must be made?

ETHICAL AND LEGAL DECISION MAKING

Ethical Decision Making

Healthcare professionals must adhere to professional ethics specific to their role in the delivery of health care. The healthcare professional has an obligation to facilitate patient care, placing the welfare and rights of the patient above all other considerations. These professional ethics exist within the context of morality, values, and duty:

Morality is composed of guidelines to preserve society.

Ethics are a systematic reflection on morality.

Values are a language with which people talk about things they hold dear.

Duty is a language for describing actions imposed on us by ourselves or others.

As you consider the concept of morality, you usually hear two words together: morally right. This speaks to individual consideration of right and wrong. This is

- directed by your conscience
- decided by you
- a matter of our "hearts"
- considered right, wrong, and fair

Ethics is considered the science, and *morality* is the conduct or behavior. Our family teaches us the morality of life. Our litmus test is the old Golden Rule, that we should do unto others as we would have others do unto us. Box 1-1 lists the principles of ethics.

Box 1-1 Principles of Ethics

Nonmaleficence: The ethical principle of doing no harm.
Beneficence: I am in a position to benefit others.
Fidelity: I have made a promise.
Autonomy: I have the opportunity to exercise my freedom.
Veracity: I am in a position to tell the truth.
Justice: I am in a position to distribute benefits and burdens.

To refresh your memory, log on to the National Association of Emergency Medical Technicians website (www.naemt.org) and reread the EMT oath and Code of Ethics.

Professional ethics are integrated into a critical care transport team's decision-making process when the team systematically approaches a challenging situation using a five-step process:

1. *Clarify*—Determine what must be decided
2. *Gather*—Assemble all relevant information
3. *Decide*—Evaluate options and make a judgment
4. *Implement*—Enact a plan
5. *Evaluate*—Assess the effectiveness of the plan enacted; reevaluation may be required

Legal Decision Making

To make good professional decisions, you must have a sound ethical and moral foundation, so that you are worthy of the trust placed in your service by the people of your community. You are bound by your profession to meet these responsibilities to your patients. Along with ethical considerations, you must consider the legal and financial aspects of critical care transport.

Legal Considerations

Legal Basis for Prehospital Care

The critical care transport team is expected to demonstrate competency in assessment, decision making, communication, and treatment. Team members are provided with the training, guidelines, guidance, and support to meet these responsibilities. However, it is important to remember that the sophisticated care that characterizes the critical care paramedic's performance is governed by the state's medical practice statutes and the **delegation of authority** that emanates from a licensed physician. In practical terms, the skills and privileges of the critical care transport team are codified in policies and protocols that are compatible with the state statutes on scope of practice for the nurse, paramedic, or respiratory therapist and are approved and supported by the service's medical director. Understanding and abiding by these policies and protocols and using medical control as instructed in those documents constitute the concise, correct approach to ensuring compliance with the legal requirements for a healthcare provider. To ensure that you are compliant with the legal requirements of performance, you must understand several fundamental aspects of the judicial system, including types of law (Box 1-2).

Box 1-2 Purpose of Laws

In general, the purpose of laws and their adjudication in the legal system is to:

- Ensure *peace* (to provide a substitute mechanism for retaliation)
- Determine **culpability** (to find fault if a wrong has been committed)
- Establish **deterrence** (to specify unpleasant consequences for violating society's norms)
- Provide *compensation* (to indemnify the injured individual for the harm suffered)

Types of Law

Criminal Law

Criminal law codifies conduct that is prohibited because it is deemed injurious to the public. The aim of criminal law is to prevent harm to society by making clear what is not allowed and by imposing penalties for violating those rules.

Violation of criminal law is exceedingly rare in professional circumstances. However, the critical care transport team must always remember that they often are involved in situations in which judgments must be made about patients' self-determination and freedom. Accusations of assault, battery, or kidnapping (all criminal complaints) may be leveled at a healthcare professional who, though well intentioned, is thought to have violated the laws governing these behaviors.

Civil Law

Civil law deals with noncriminal actions between two parties and is designed to protect individuals' rights. An aspect of civil law particularly pertinent to the practice of medicine is the determination of *tort liability.* A **tort** is a civil wrong, other than a breach of contract, committed against a person or property for which a court provides a remedy in the form of an action for **damages**.

An often contentious interface between the legal and medical professions is the matter of *medical malpractice liability*. This form of tort liability is based on the prospect for a judgment pertaining to a civil wrong that provides compensation for the patient (or his or her survivors), serves as a deterrent for providers, and ensures protection for society (Box 1-3). The court proceedings are the mechanism for assigning judgment and establishing resolution. As a means to ensure their continued ability to practice medicine, medical providers must maintain resources to support themselves if they are accused of medical malpractice.

Access to affordable professional liability insurance (i.e., medical malpractice insurance) has become one of the nation's key healthcare issues and a source of rising healthcare costs for the consumer. Medical professionals contend that excessive awards are driving up the cost of insurance. Patients' attorneys contend that instances of malpractice actually are rarely reported. Healthcare policy experts observe that fear of malpractice leads to the practice of **defensive medicine**, which involves the allocation of time and resources that could have

Box 1-3 Elements of a Course of Action

If an accusation that a legal wrong has occurred is to be valid, the elements for a course of action must be present.

1. A *duty* must exist. A duty is a moral or legal obligation. Critical care paramedics have a duty to care for the patient, a "duty to act."
2. A **breach** of duty must have occurred. A breach of duty is failure to meet the standard of care. Members of the team would be considered in breach if they did not perform in the manner that could be expected of a reasonable person with the same level of training in similar circumstances.
3. *Damages* must have occurred. Actual or noneconomic (intangible) losses (or both) must be associated with the harm done by the action of the healthcare professional.
4. **Proximate causation** must exist. There must be proof that the healthcare professional's actions were the immediate cause of the damage, that the injuries or other damages did not occur for a different reason.

been more rationally applied to other healthcare priorities. Meanwhile, the increasing cost of and limited access to professional liability insurance has reduced the supply, recruitment, and retention of physicians in key medical specialties and geographic locales.

Damages

In the case of medical providers, damages are a sum of money the law or jury imposes for a breach of duty. The judge or jury may elect to impose **compensatory** (economic) damages. The money awarded is intended to compensate the aggrieved party (the plaintiff) for past, present, and future harm caused by loss or injury and to attempt to place the person in the same position as before the defendant's negligent act. *Economic damages* include compensation for medical expenses and lost wages or earning potential. *Noneconomic damages* are intended to compensate the plaintiff for physical and mental pain and suffering, loss of consortium (business associations), and loss of chance. The judge or jury also may decide to levy **punitive** (exemplary) damages to punish the defendant and to set an example ("send a message") that would dissuade others from engaging in the same behavior.

Negligence

Healthcare professionals' dedication to their duties and legal obligations includes steering clear of actual or perceived **negligence**. Medical malpractice is negligence, because generally there is no intent to do harm. **Ordinary negligence** is the failure to do what a reasonable person would do or not do under the circumstances. **Gross negligence** is to intentionally or wantonly omit care that would be proper to provide or to do that which would be improper to do. Negligence does not require intent. It is based on failure to use reasonable care under specific circumstances.

A determination of negligence is based on a judgment of whether the team member followed the applicable **standard of care**. Standards of care are guided by state statutes pertaining to the prescribing requirements critical care paramedics must follow and by protocols and policies developed to comply with state and local law. Adjudication of an accusation of negligence also may include testimony about standards as exemplified by medical textbooks and journals, and statements from EMS medical directors directly involved in establishing standards of care. Other expert witnesses, including other critical care paramedics, nurses, or respiratory therapists, may be called on to interpret the protocols and apply them to the facts of the case.

Minimizing Risk

Members of the critical care transport team can ensure proper risk management in their careers and protect themselves from accusations of malpractice by knowing their scope of practice, maintaining skill competency in the specialized care associated with that scope of practice, and limiting their care to those skills and techniques. They must always keep in mind that accurate, complete documentation is the essential record of the care they provide, and they must make sure they respect **patient confidentiality** by discussing patient information only with those with a demonstrated professional need to know. A consistent professional demeanor is more than expected courtesy and an attribute of exemplary behavior; it is a key asset in reducing patient dissatisfaction and the prospect of legal action.

Consent and the Patient's Rights

The professional relationship between the healthcare provider and the patient is governed by **consent**. Permission to initiate and carry out assessment and treatment is based on consent, which is defined as voluntary agreement by a competent person. Consent can be expressed through verbal or written means and is implied by silence.

Consent is a fundamental patient right. It is codified in the Patient Self-Determination Act of 1990, and is part of the Medicare and Medicaid Conditions of Participation. The intent of these provisions is to ensure that patients are aware of and empowered to make decisions about their medical care, including the right to accept or refuse medical or surgical care. As a matter of public policy, we have decided that an adult, possessed of a sound mind, has the right to decide what is done with his or her body. This consent must be fully informed. Patients have a right to know the potential risks and benefits of and the alternatives to any proposed procedure. The critical care transport team must always attempt to obtain informed consent. Complying with the obligation of **informed consent** takes into account the fact that any medical procedure is associated with a chance of complications without fault, even if the procedure is performed perfectly. To comply with informed consent, the team members must provide information that would ordinarily be provided to a patient under like circumstances by healthcare providers engaged in a similar practice.

Who gives the consent? When **competent**, the patient gives consent. If the patient is incompetent or unable to consent, others may substitute their judgment and consent for that of the patient. As noted previously, *implied consent* is a central tenet of emergency care; it is invoked when silence, caused by illness or injury, is interpreted as consent to perform lifesaving care. When the decision must be made for less emergent patient needs and the patient is unable to consent personally, someone else can give consent, provided this delegated judgment is clear, legal, and fair. Examples of substituted judgment include guardianship, durable power of attorney, and parental consent for minors. Whoever authorizes for another person must have sufficient information to make an intelligent judgment on behalf of the patient. A specialized case of substituted judgment is **involuntary consent**, which is used for individuals who are a threat to themselves or the community. Involuntary consent usually involves collaboration with law enforcement officials.

Treatment of Minors

The treatment of minors presents specific challenges for compliance with the rules of consent. As mentioned, the authorization of a parent or legal guardian *usually* is necessary before medical care can be provided to a minor. However, the care of minors is complex and involves access and liability issues, including considerations of confidentiality, economic constraints, and constitutional interests. In particular, medical conditions associated with possible physical and sexual abuse lead to complicated considerations of parental involvement. Many states have established an emergency exception, under which care can be provided to a minor when any condition requires prompt treatment and/or urgent attention, or if a condition is causing a child pain or fear, and no parent is reasonably available.

Confidentiality

In the course of evaluation and treatment of patients, the critical care transport team gains access to, uses, and communicates confidential medical information. The release of any patient information to anyone outside the team's organization and the personnel of other organizations directly involved in the patient's care is prohibited unless it is necessary for treatment, payment, or healthcare operations. The Health Insurance Portability and Accountability Act of 1996 (HIPAA) specifically addresses the matter of privacy and provides a definition of protected health information (PHI). Under HIPAA, protected health information includes any *individually identifiable* health information. *Identifiable* refers not only to data that are explicitly linked to a particular individual (i.e., *identified* information), but also to health information with data items that reasonably could be expected to allow individual identification.

Discussions of PHI within your organization and between providers should be limited. Acceptable uses of PHI within your organization include but are not limited to the exchange of patient information needed for the treatment of the patient, essential healthcare operations, and quality assurance activities.

Abandonment

Having established a relationship by gaining consent and having initiated the assessment and treatment of the patient, the critical care transport team should take care not to engage in **abandonment**. The team may terminate the medical relationship without fear of being held liable for abandonment if:

- The patient does not require medical assistance.
- The patient terminates the relationship.
- The patient's care is transferred to another, similarly qualified medical professional.

The last point deserves examination, because one of the distinguishing roles of the critical care transport team is the continuation of sophisticated medical care during an interfacility transport. Providing a report and transfer of care to the professionals at the end point of that transport is an essential component of your time with and responsibility for your patient. Failure to complete this step, particularly by relinquishing the patient's care to a member of the receiving facility's team who does not have equivalent or more extensive training than your team, interrupts the continuity of care; this places the patient at risk and could lead to an accusation of abandonment.

State law and the transferring physician play key roles in determining the correct crew mix for transporting a patient and avoiding issues of abandonment. Each hospital must examine the laws and rules in its state and instruct its physicians and nurses as to who may safely and legally transport patients to other acute care facilities. State law may mandate who can attend a patient in a ground or aeromedical transport company. These individuals may be required to have special training over and above a certification or license, which eliminates the possibility of "taking along" a nurse from the transferring hospital. Under EMTALA, the transferring and receiving physicians ultimately are responsible for specifying the mode of transport and level of attendant care, but factors such as weather may sway the decision.

Slander

By respecting patient confidentiality, consistently engaging in professional conduct, and demonstrating respect both for patients and for fellow professionals, the critical care transport team can minimize the chance of an accusation of defamation or slander. Generally speaking, **defamation** is the issuance of a false statement about another person that causes the person to suffer harm. **Slander** is the making of defamatory statements by a transitory (nonfixed) representation, usually an oral (spoken) representation. Team members must take care to avoid the use of slang or labels in discussions with or about patients and to remember that unconscious patients often can hear, recall, and recount what is being discussed and by whom.

Mandatory Reporter

Some but not all states assign **mandatory reporter** requirements and responsibilities to those who examine and attend to children and dependent adults. Mandatory reporters are required to exercise reasonable and good faith in reporting circumstances in which they believe it is possible a child or dependent adult has suffered abuse or has otherwise been exploited. They are required to cooperate with and assist in the investigation, and in doing so they receive civil and criminal immunity. If a mandatory reporter *knowingly* and *willfully* fails to report such circumstances, he or she is guilty of a simple misdemeanor and potentially liable for damages proximately caused by the failure to report. Initial training is required, as is periodic review and renewal training.

FEDERAL RULES IN HEALTH CARE AND TRANSPORT

Medicare

The federal government provides payment for medical care for our oldest adults and the poor through the Centers for Medicare and Medicaid Services (CMS). With this guaranteed payment comes many rules and regulations that also affect the practice of and decision making in critical care transport.

Rules Against Kickbacks

The federal **anti-kickback law** imposes criminal and civil monetary penalties on any entity or individual who knowingly and willfully pays or offers to pay, solicits, or receives any remuneration in exchange for referral of patients for any item or service covered by a federal healthcare program. Medicare and Medicaid both are considered federal healthcare programs for purposes of the anti-kickback law. The anti-kickback law also prohibits a person from arranging for or recommending the purchase of goods or services for which payment may be made under a federal healthcare program in exchange for remuneration.

Ambulance Restocking

Some time ago, the practice of ambulance restocking by hospitals came under scrutiny, because although it is a courtesy, it could be construed as an inducement to bring patients to a particular hospital. On December 4, 2001, the Office of Inspector General (OIG) issued a final rule (effective January 3, 2002) that established an ambulance restocking "safe harbor" under the federal anti-kickback law; this safe harbor rule protects certain arrangements involving hospitals or other receiving facilities that replenish drugs and medical supplies used by ambulance providers when transporting patients to the hospital or receiving facility. In addition to several statutory exemptions to the anti-kickback law, the OIG established a number of safe harbors, outlining various payment and business practices that the OIG does not treat as violations of the anti-kickback law.

Safe harbors are established for transactions or arrangements that technically may be capable of inducing prohibited referrals but that improve the quality of healthcare services for needy patients and are lawful in the vast majority of cases. As mentioned, ambulance restocking is the practice by hospitals and other receiving facilities of restocking medications or supplies used by ambulance providers during transport of a patient to the hospital or receiving facility. The purpose of restocking is to ensure that the ambulance is fully stocked with appropriate supplies and medicine and ready to respond to emergencies at all times.

Ambulance restocking arrangements technically implicate the anti-kickback law because the receiving hospital gives something of value (e.g., drugs or medical supplies) to a potential source of federal healthcare program business (e.g., ambulance providers). Recognizing that in the vast majority of cases, ambulance restocking arrangements are lawful and serve a significant public interest, the OIG promulgated the ambulance restocking safe harbor to the anti-kickback law. The safe harbor covers the restocking of medications and supplies used on both emergency and nonemergency transports, provided the ambulance is used to respond to emergencies an average of three times a week measured over any reasonable time period.

The final regulations address three categories of restocking: (1) general restocking (whether for free or for a charge); (2) fair market value restocking; and (3) government-mandated restocking. Parties unsure whether their restocking is at fair market value or is mandated by a government authority may look to the general restocking category. To qualify for safe harbor protection, a restocking arrangement must satisfy four conditions, which apply to all three types of restocking arrangements.

1. *Appropriate billing of federal healthcare programs:* The ambulance provider and the hospital may not both bill for the same restocked drug or supply.
2. *Documentation requirements:* Either the hospital or the ambulance provider may generate the necessary documentation, so long as the other party receives and maintains a copy of it for 5 years. If certain requirements are satisfied, the prehospital care report (including a trip sheet, patient care report, or patient encounter report), typically prepared by the ambulance service provider and filed with the receiving facility, is sufficient to meet the documentation requirements.
3. *Absence of ties to referrals:* The regulations prohibit any restocking arrangement that is conditioned on or otherwise takes into account the volume or value of any referrals or other business generated between the parties for which payment may be made by a federal healthcare program.
4. *Compliance with all other applicable laws:* Both the receiving facility and the ambulance provider must comply with all federal, state and local laws regulating ambulance services, such as laws relating to the handling of controlled substances.

Critical care transport services are bound to comply with all CMS rules for all patient care and system processes. CMS also defines the levels of care and those things for which the service can bill. CMS's rules include many definitions that the members of the critical care transport team must understand.

Types of Transport

Medicare covers the following levels of ambulance service:

- Basic life support (BLS) (emergency and nonemergency)
- Advanced life support, level 1 (ALS1) (emergency and nonemergency)
- Advanced life support, level 2 (ALS2)
- Specialty care transport (SCT)
- Paramedic ALS intercept (PI)
- Fixed wing air ambulance (FW)
- Rotary wing air ambulance (RW)

These levels of service are defined in Box 1-4.

Medical Necessity

As a general rule, Medicare covers medically necessary ambulance services only if the services are furnished to a beneficiary whose medical condition is such that other means of transportation are contraindicated. The patient's condition must require both the ambulance transportation itself and the level of service provided for the billed service to be considered medically necessary (see Box 1-4).

Nonemergency transportation by ambulance is appropriate if (1) the patient is **bed confined** and his or her condition has been documented to be such that other methods of transportation are contraindicated; or (2) the patient's medical condition, regardless of bed confinement, is such that transportation by ambulance is medically required. Bed confinement, therefore, is not the sole criterion for the medical necessity of ambulance transportation; it is one factor that is considered in medical necessity determinations.

Did You Know?

For a Medicare beneficiary to be considered bed confined, three criteria must be met: (1) the patient must be unable to get up from bed without assistance; (2) the patient must be unable to ambulate; and (3) the patient must be unable to sit in a chair or wheelchair.

Box 1-4 Federal Designation of Ambulance Service Levels

- Basic Life Support (BLS)
  - When medically necessary, the provision of basic life support (BLS) services as defined in the National Emergency Medicine Services (EMS) Education and Practice Blueprint for the Emergency Medical Technician (EMT), including the establishment of a peripheral intravenous (IV) line.
- Advanced Life Support, Level 1 (ALS1)
  - When medically necessary, the provision of an assessment by an advanced life support (ALS) ambulance provider or supplier and the furnishing of one or more ALS interventions. An ALS assessment is performed by an ALS crew and results in the determination that the patient's condition requires an ALS level of care, even if no other ALS intervention is performed. An ALS provider or supplier is defined as a provider trained to the level of the advanced EMT or paramedic as defined in the National EMS Education and Practice Blueprint. An ALS intervention is defined as a procedure beyond the scope of an EMT as defined in the National EMS Education and Practice Blueprint.
- Advanced Life Support, Level 2 (ALS2)
  - When medically necessary, the administration of at least three different medications or the provision of one or more of the following ALS procedures:
    - Manual defibrillation/cardioversion
    - Endotracheal intubation
    - Central venous line
    - Cardiac pacing
    - Chest decompression
    - Surgical airway
    - Intraosseous line
- Specialty Care Transport (SCT)
  - When medically necessary, for a critically injured or ill beneficiary, a level of interhospital service furnished beyond the scope of the paramedic as defined in the National EMS Education and Practice Blueprint. This is necessary when a beneficiary's condition requires ongoing care that must be furnished by one or more health professionals in an appropriate specialty area (e.g., nursing, emergency medicine, respiratory care, cardiovascular care, or a paramedic with additional training).
- Paramedic ALS Intercept (PI)
  - These services are defined in Sec. 410.40(c), Paramedic ALS Intercept Services. These are ALS services furnished by an entity that does not provide the ambulance transport. Under limited circumstances, Medicare payment may be made for these services. (For additional information about paramedic ALS intercept services, please refer to the March 15, 2000 final rule [65 FR 13911]).
- Fixed Wing Air Ambulance (FW)
  - Fixed wing air ambulance services are covered when the point from which the beneficiary is transported to the nearest hospital with appropriate facilities is inaccessible by land vehicle, or great distances or other obstacles exist (e.g., heavy traffic), and the beneficiary's medical condition is not appropriate for transport by either BLS or ALS ground ambulance.
- Rotary Wing Air Ambulance (RW)
  - Rotary wing (helicopter) air ambulance services are covered when the point from which the beneficiary is transported to the nearest hospital with appropriate facilities is inaccessible by ground vehicle, or great distances or other obstacles exist (e.g., heavy traffic), and the beneficiary's medical condition is not appropriate for transport by either BLS or ALS ground ambulance.

FEDERAL RULES OF TRANSFER

Emergency Medical Treatment and Active Labor Act (EMTALA)

EMTALA establishes specific responsibilities for physicians attending an Emergency Department (ED) patient. "Emergency department" actually is an inexact term, because the provisions of the law apply to patients who present on *hospital property* for the purposes of examination and treatment of a medical complaint. Note that "hospital property" includes circumstances in which patients are attended to by the staff of hospital-based ambulance services. It also includes the arrival of an ambulance in the ED's entry with a patient who was not expected or diverted to another facility by direct radio contact.

Consolidated Omnibus Budget Reconciliation Act of 1986

EMTALA was passed as part of the Consolidated Omnibus Budget Reconciliation Act of 1986, which sometimes is referred to as the "COBRA law" or, simply, COBRA. In fact, a number of different laws come under that general name. A familiar provision, also referred to under COBRA, is the law that governs the continuation of medical insurance benefits after termination of employment. EMTALA was passed by Congress amid growing concern over the availability of emergency healthcare services for the poor and uninsured. The law was designed principally to address the problem of "patient dumping," a practice by which hospital emergency departments deny uninsured patients the same treatment provided paying patients either by refusing care outright or by transferring uninsured patients to other facilities.

Emergency Medical Condition

Under EMTALA, each patient must be examined to determine whether the person has an "emergency medical condition." An *emergency medical condition* is defined as a medical condition that manifests itself by symptoms so severe that the absence of immediate medical attention could reasonably be expected to (1) place the health of the individual (or, for a pregnant woman, the health of the woman or her unborn child) in serious jeopardy; (2) result in serious impairment of bodily functions; or (3) result in serious dysfunction of any bodily organ or part.

"Active labor" also is defined. A pregnant woman who is having contractions is said to be in *true labor* unless a physician certifies that, after a reasonable period of observation, the woman is in *false labor.*

Under EMTALA, stabilizing treatment must be provided for all patients with an emergency medical condition. The physician is held to this standard of care in making decisions about treatment.

EMTALA Investigations

A large number of EMTALA investigations arise because on-call physicians refuse to come in to see the patient, come in late, or order the patient transferred without coming in to stabilize the patient's condition. The law is specific in its application to on-call physicians. Generally, on-call physicians are expected to attend the patient physically. If the on-call physician refuses to attend to the patient or fails to appear within a reasonable time, this fact must be reflected in the patient's record and the transfer materials. Furthermore, the hospital's records must reflect quality assurance and disciplinary records regarding the incident.

EMTALA also addresses the patient's decisions during the ED visit. Documentation is required for each of the following circumstances:

- *Refusal to consent to treatment:* The record must reflect the examination and/or treatment refused by the patient.
- *Refusal to consent to transfer:* Documentation must reflect whether the patient refused a transfer recommended by the physician after being informed of the risks and benefits of that transfer. The medical record must include notation of that refusal, the details of the proposed transfer, and the risk/benefit ratio as described to the patient.
- *Request for transfer:* If the patient or the person's delegate requests a transfer, the record must include that request, its rationale, and the fact that the individual was informed of the risks and benefits of the transfer.

Hospital Transfer Regulations

Transfer of the ED patient to another facility falls under EMTALA regulations. The law imposes restrictions on how and when a patient may be transferred. The hospital is obligated to ensure (and document) that the patient has been informed of the hospital's obligation to examine and treat the person and the risk/benefit ratio of the proposed transfer. The transfer is considered appropriate only if qualified staff members with adequate equipment provide "necessary life support measures" en route to the receiving facility and that facility has agreed to accept the patient.

EMTALA itself does not address the question of whether a patient transported by ambulance is considered to have "presented" to the hospital. However, the regulations that have evolved from the law specify that a patient in a non-hospital-owned ambulance in transit is not considered to have "come to the Emergency Department" even if the ambulance is in contact with the hospital by telephone or radiotelemetry. Also, the hospital may deny access to the patient in transit if it is in **diversionary status**; that is, if it does not have the staff or facilities to accept additional patients.

Under previous regulations, an ambulance owned by a hospital was obligated to transport the patient to that hospital, even if another or a more suitable facility were closer. The 2003 regulations removed that obligation for hospital-owned ambulances if they are "integrated" with EMS services. The net effect is that these ambulances may transport patients to a suitable hospital and are not required to transport patients automatically to the hospital that owns them.

Complete documentation is delivered to the receiving facility, including consent forms and records of the medical examination and treatment of the patient.

Penalties for EMTALA Violations

Violations of EMTALA's regulations can result in significant penalties. If a hospital knowingly, willingly, or negligently violates EMTALA rules, its provider agreement may be terminated. Also, hospitals may be fined $25,000 to $50,000 per violation. The physician responsible for examining, treating, or transferring the patient may be fined $50,000 per violation. This provision also applies to on-call physician violations. The physician involved can be excluded from Medicare and Medicaid programs, and a patient can sue the hospital for personal injury in civil court. A receiving facility that suffers a financial loss as a result of another hospital's violation of EMTALA can sue to recover those damages.

EMTALA provides a structure for the proper examination, treatment, and transfer of patents in the Emergency Department. Healthcare providers abide by the law by attending to those who present for care on hospital property, by providing life-sustaining care, and by ensuring informed patient transfer. Documentation of each aspect of care and communication is central to compliance with the law.

Physician and Nurse Reports to Receiving Hospitals

While transporting patients from one acute care facility to another, the critical care transport team becomes under the jurisdiction of the EMTALA regulations and therefore must understand them. Before transfer, the hospital and physician have obligations that must be met (described previously). The physician (or clinician, nurse practitioner, or physician's assistant) must obtain consent from the physician who will continue care for the patient at the receiving facility. This physician-to-physician communication is one of the first steps. The critical care transport team must obtain the name of the physician that has accepted care.

Next, the hospital must perform a nurse-to-nurse report as a standard "hand off" according to the rules and guidelines of The Joint Commission (formerly known as The Joint Commission on the Accreditation of Healthcare Organizations) and CMS. The nurse from the referring hospital must relay the patient information to the appropriate nurse at the receiving hospital in a timely fashion. For nurses serving as members of the critical care transport team, delivering the nurse-to-nurse report on arrival at the receiving hospital creates problems both for the team and for the patient.

If your transport crew is a hospital-based service that originates from the receiving hospital, crew members must be careful that the referring hospital does not assume that a hand-off report to the crew meets the requirements of the nurse-to-nurse report. The nurse-to-nurse report has two purposes: (1) It relays important patient information to the nurse in the department where the patient is to be delivered; and (2) by accepting the information, the receiving nurse technically confirms that the hospital has an available bed and is obligated to take the patient. Even though, according to CMS, your transport team is a part of that receiving hospital, having the nurse from the referring hospital hand off the patient only to you is a shortcut that may cause problems, and it does not fulfill the second requirement of the nurse-to-nurse report.

The hand-off report is a transfer of care guided by an explanation of the patient's condition and details of the assessment and treatment provided before and during transport. It is crucial, and its format has been spelled out by various regulatory agencies. The members of the critical care transport team must make sure they know the name of the receiving hospital and the name of the physician who has accepted care, and they must ensure that a nursing report is made to a nurse on the unit to which the patient is going.

Hand-Off Report

When a very sick patient is moved from hospital to hospital, unit to unit, or caregiver to caregiver, important information may be left behind. Each person who takes care of a patient must have up-to-date information on the patient's status, current treatment, critical diagnostic results, and recent changes. In 2006 The Joint Commission established the National Patient Safety Goal and instructed hospitals to develop a standardized approach to patient hand-offs. This has implications for critical care transport.

A critical care transport event has all the elements that can result in miscommunication, which may lead to a patient care mistake. First, hospital personnel and caregivers are quickly trying to resuscitate and stabilize a sick patient whose condition may have just deteriorated or who may have arrived in the ED quite ill and beyond the facility's capabilities. These healthcare providers are distracted and hurrying to get the patient out the door before the person's condition worsens. Second, the caregivers usually do not know the members of the critical care transport team as well as their own colleagues. Third, the primary nurse often has been operating by verbal or stat orders, has been working with several people in the department to comply with those orders, and may not have had time to document everything. The nurse may know some of the information associated with the patient's care but may lack documentation of the rest of the patient's assessment and treatment.

SBAR Hand-Off Reports

The healthcare system has many tools for standardizing the hand-off report, but one type seems to be most commonly used: the situation-background-assessment-recommendation (SBAR) style. Some advocate the addition of an "I" (ISBAR) to denote "introduction." Because the transport crew members work with many healthcare providers they do not know, an introduction should begin the process. Introductions clarify the roles and capabilities of each team member.

An SBAR (or ISBAR) hand-off report might proceed as follows: The team members and primary nurse introduce themselves. The primary nurse (or healthcare provider) summarizes what happened to the patient and then gives the patient's background (i.e., past and recent history, medications, and so on). The assessment is summarized with the pertinent findings. The primary nurse or healthcare provider then concludes the hand-off report by relaying the local healthcare team's recommendations (i.e., treatments instituted before transport or started en route and those that need to be continued).

Documentation

Each patient encounter generates a patient care record (PCR), which is critical for good patient care. The importance of good verbal communication as part of the patient hand-off is clear, but the written document also is a key piece of the process. Wolfberg and Wirth[1] outlined five reasons the PCR must be scrupulously prepared.

1. *Clinical applications:* The PCR from the critical care transport team is integrated into the patient's medical record at the receiving hospital. Because it is the written part of the patient hand-off, timely completion of the report is important and may be required by law. If you have electronic PCR software but no laptop with you, complete your report as soon as possible and fax it directly to the correct department in the receiving hospital. The report serves as a record of the assessments you made and the care you provided. To ensure continuity of care, it is essential that the PCR be made available to the next "link" in the chain of healthcare providers caring for the patient to ensure that they understand and can act on information about your care.
2. *Legal applications:* Documentation of the event provides evidence that you and the rest of the transport crew acted within the standards of care for the patient. This is your "substituted memory" of the transport; it should be accurate, detailed, and timely.
3. *Operational applications:* The times of transports, skills of crew members, procedures performed, medications administered, and even patients' locations all are included in the documentation, which your service director or a regional planner can use to determine needs and prove quality. For example, if an annual review shows that you and your partner have not transported a patient with a balloon pump, education on balloon pumps should be planned for you.
4. *Financial applications:* Information that facilitates billing and reimbursement are part of any PCR. Accuracy, timeliness, and completeness all are important. Critical care transports are regarded as specialized transports and are reimbursed according to the complexity of the undertaking. Therefore, documentation of that care plays an important role in establishing a rationale for reimbursement.
5. *Compliance applications: Compliance* is a legal term that means that you and your employer are operating according to all contracts, laws, and performance requirements or standards. This includes compliance with your state's rules on minimum staffing or equipment standards and compliance with EMTALA rules on scope of practice during the transfer of a patient.

If a critical care paramedic is teamed with a nurse or respiratory therapist, a policy must be in place that specifies who completes the documentation and whether all members of the professional team must sign off on the PCR. Each team member who provided care is responsible for helping to prepare the PCR, read the draft, and edit and approve the report, even if he or she is not the person who ultimately signs the document.

Scenario Conclusion

You call your partner and arrange for a face-to-face meeting today. You've rehearsed what you're going to say. You confront the facts and tell him what you have to do. You keep repeating that you are acting on behalf of good patient care. You provide him with some good options for in-patient drug and alcohol rehabilitation in the area, along with information on the employee assistance program at work.

SUMMARY

The fundamentals of critical care transport are grounded in the ethical, legal, and organizational issues associated with your role and responsibilities as a critical care paramedic, your role in your organization, and your interaction with other healthcare professionals. The chapters that follow provide more detailed information about the clinical aspects of the care you will provide.

KEY TERMS

abandonment The abandoning of a patient needing further medical care by the person responsible for that care without adequate warning.

anti-kickback law A federal law that imposes criminal and civil monetary penalties on any entity or individual who knowingly and willfully pays or offers to pay, solicits, or receives any remuneration in exchange for referral of patients for any item or service covered by a federal healthcare program. Medicare and Medicaid both are considered federal healthcare programs for purposes of the anti-kickback law. The anti-kickback law also prohibits a person from arranging for or recommending the purchase of goods or services for which payment may be made under a federal healthcare program in exchange for remuneration.

autonomy The state of functioning independently, without extraneous influence.

bed confined A defined Medicare condition that must meet three criteria: (1) the patient must be unable to get up from bed without assistance; (2) the patient must be unable to ambulate; and (3) the patient must be unable to sit in a chair or wheelchair.

beneficence The quality of being kind, helpful, or generous.

breach Failure to perform some promised act or obligation; to act in disregard of laws, rules, contracts, or promises.

civil law The body of laws established by a state or nation for its own regulation; the branch of law that deals with disputes between individuals and/or organizations.

compensatory That which makes up for the loss or a lack of some capability or for an injury.

competent Properly or sufficiently qualified, capable, or efficient.

consent To assent to or approve; to grant permission.

criminal law Any of various bodies of rules in different jurisdictions for which the common characteristic is the potential for unique and often severe impositions; also called *penal law.*

culpability The state of being at fault if a wrong has been committed.

damages A sum of money paid in compensation for loss or injury.

defamation A false accusation of an offense or a malicious misrepresentation of a person's words or actions.

defensive medicine The practice of diagnostic or therapeutic measures that are performed primarily not to ensure the patient's health, but as a safeguard against possible malpractice liability.

delegation of authority A statement from the medical director that is given to the provider to delegate authority and assign responsibility. The delegation of authority can include objectives, priorities, expectations, constraints, and other considerations or guidelines.

deterrence An act or process that discourages actions or prevents occurrences by instilling fear, doubt, or anxiety.

diversionary status Circumstances in which a hospital may divert individuals (patients) because it does not have the staff or facilities to accept any additional emergency patients at that time.

duty The social force that binds a person to the courses of action demanded by that force; work that a person is obliged to perform for moral or legal reasons.

ethics The rules or principles that govern right conduct. *Clinical ethics* is the application of ethical analysis to decision making in the care of individual patients. *Medical ethics* defines the values and guidelines that should govern decisions in medicine.

fidelity The principle that forbids misleading or deceiving any creature capable of being misled or deceived.

gross negligence Fault characterized by extreme carelessness showing willful or reckless disregard for the consequences to the safety or property of another.

informed consent Voluntary permission given by a subject or guardian for participation in a study or investigation, or for medical care, after having been informed of the purpose, methods, procedures, benefits, and risks.

involuntary consent A term that applies to a patient who is unable to give consent because of a physical or mental impairment. The source of consent varies among the states but generally follows this order: (1) spouse (legally married); (2) spouse (common law); (3) parent; (4) adult child; (5) adult sibling; (6) adult uncle, aunt, or grandparents; (7) court system. In some special situations, involuntary consents are initiated, such as treatment rendered in an abuse situation, treatment needed for a prisoner, or any consent obtained from the court system.

justice The quality of being just or fair; judgment involved in the determination of rights and the assignment of rewards and punishments.

mandatory reporter A professional who, in the ordinary course of his or her work and because the professional has regular contact with children, disabled persons, senior citizens, or other identified vulnerable groups of people, is required to report (or cause a report to be made) whenever financial, physical, sexual, or other types of abuse have been observed or are suspected or when there is evidence of neglect, knowledge of an incident, or an imminent risk of serious harm.

morality Concern with the distinction between good and evil or right and wrong; right or good conduct.

negligence Failure to act as a reasonably prudent person with the same knowledge, experience, and background would under similar circumstances, resulting in injury or damage to a person.

nonmaleficence The ethical principle of doing no harm, which is based on the Hippocratic maxim, *primum non nocere* (first, do no harm).

ordinary negligence Failure to do what a reasonable person would do or would not do under the circumstances.

patient confidentiality In medical ethics, the principle that the information a patient reveals to a healthcare provider is private and is protected by limits on how and when it can be disclosed to a third party; usually the provider must obtain permission from the patient to make such a disclosure.

proximate causation An event that is closest, or immediately responsible, for causing some observed result.

punitive Inflicting punishment (e.g., punitive justice, punitive damages).

slander Words falsely spoken that damage the reputation of another.

standard of care In medicine, treatment that experts agree is appropriate, accepted, and widely used. Healthcare providers are obligated to provide patients with the standard of care. Also called standard therapy or best practice.

tort (law) Any wrongdoing for which an action for damages may be brought.

values Beliefs of a person or social group in which they have an emotional investment (either for or against something). A language to talk about things held dear.

veracity Unwillingness to tell lies.

REFERENCE

1. Wolfberg DM, Wirth SR: *Five good reasons for better EMS documentation*, *Emerg Med Serv* 34:51-52, 54, 56, 2005.

Bibliography

Bitterman RA: *Providing emergency care under federal law: EMTALA*, Washington, DC, 2004, American College of Emergency Physicians.

Centers for Medicare and Medicaid Services (CMS): *Ambulance services center (website)*. www.cms.hhs.gov/center/ambulance.asp. Accessed January 28, 2010.

Commission on Accreditation of Medical Transport Systems (CAMTS): *Accreditation standards (website)*. www.camts.org. Accessed January 28, 2010.

Connolly JV, Fetcho S, Hageman JR: Education of personnel involved in the transport program, *Crit Care Clin* 8:481-490, 1992.

Department of Health and Human Services: IV. Centers for Medicare and Medicaid Services, *Federal Register* 42 CFR Parts 410 and 414, 2-27-02.

Emergency Nurses Association (ENA) and National Flight Nurses Association (NFNA): *Joint position statement: role of the registered nurse in the prehospital environment,* 1987

Gillespie C: *EMT oath and code of ethics*. National Association of Emergency Medical Technicians (website). www.naemt.org/about_us/emtoath.aspx. Accessed January 28, 2010.

Harris DM: *Healthcare law and ethics*, Chicago, 2003, Foundation of the American College of Healthcare Executives.

High K, Demmons LL, Stevens L, et al: *Transport nurse safety in the transport environment—position paper*, Greenwood Village, Colorado, 2006, Air and Surface Transport Nurses Association (ASTNA).

Hill D: General overview of ethics. Lecture and notes presented for the Des Moines University Masters in Healthcare Administration program, Des Moines, Iowa, February 27, 2004.

Hill D: The law of tort liability. Lecture and notes presented for the Des Moines University Masters in Healthcare Administration program, Des Moines, Iowa, February 27, 2004.

Hill D: What is law and how does it work? Lecture and notes presented for the Des Moines University Masters in Healthcare Administration program, Des Moines, Iowa, January 23, 2004.

Kaiser Permanente of Colorado: *SBAR technique for communication: a situational briefing model* (website). www.ihi.org/IHI/Topics/PatientSafety/SafetyGeneral/Tools/SBARTechniqueforCommunicationASituationalBriefingModel.htm. Accessed January 28, 2010.

Lynn J, Colson E: *Emergency medical services sourcebook*, Detroit, 2002, Omnigraphics.

McNew R: *Emergency department compliance manual*, ed 4, 2001, Aspen Health Law & Compliance Center.

Merck P: Fraud and abuse. Lecture and notes presented for the Des Moines University Masters in Healthcare Administration program, Des Moines, Iowa, February 28, 2004.

Merck P: Legal and ethical obligations to provide care. Lecture and notes presented for the Des Moines University Masters in Healthcare Administration program, Des Moines, Iowa, February 28, 2004.

National Highway Traffic Safety Administration (NHTSA) and Health Resources & Services Administration: *A leadership guide to quality improvement for emergency medical services (website)*. www.nhtsa.dot.gov/people/injury/ems/leaderguide/index.html. Accessed January 28, 2010.

Runy LA: *Patient handoffs*, 2008, Hospital and Health Networks.

Strategies for Nurse Managers: *ISBAR: Adding an extra step in handoff communication (website)*. www.strategiesfornursemanagers.com/ce_detail/222773.cfm. Accessed January 28, 2010.

Warren J, Robert E. Jr, Orr RA, et al: Guidelines for the inter- and intrahospital transport of critically ill patients, *Crit Care Med* 32:256-262, 2004.

Suggested Resource

Gillespie CB: *EMT Oath and code of conduct: National Association of Emergency Medical Technicians (website)*. www.naemt.org/about_us/emtoath.aspx. Accessed February 5, 2010.

REVIEW QUESTIONS

1. In the case study at the beginning of the chapter, you, as an EMS provider, believe that you are morally correct to notify your employer and the certifying board of your partner's behavior. In this decision, you are considering:
   A. The dictates of your conscience and heart
   B. The bylaws of your employer
   C. The expectations of your medical director
   D. What your partner would want if he were thinking clearly

2. You are about to transport a 19-month-old child to another facility. The parents arrive and insist that they want to give you cash so that you "take good care of him." What is your correct course of action?
   A. Take the cash; it is easier than having to work your way through a long discussion.
   B. Respectfully state, "Thank you so much, but you do not need to pay me to take good care of your son."
   C. Refuse and suggest that the couple give the cash to a local charity of their choice.
   D. Accept the cash and tell the parents it will be given to the ambulance service to pay the bill.

3. The local hospital is evaluating a patient who presented with severe back pain. The physician on call refuses to come to see the patient, and the patient requests a transfer. When you arrive, the nurses are very upset about transferring the patient without the physician present. Under EMTALA, what must the hospital do?
   A. Call in the chief of staff to see the patient.
   B. Transfer the patient and notify Medicare immediately.
   C. Comply with the rest of the EMTALA rules of transfer, transfer the patient, and then investigate (and document) the incident in the hospital.
   D. Hold the patient locally until the physician on call comes in.
4. A man has arrived at your company's business office and is having quite an argument with your office manager. He wants the bill for his neighbor's recent ambulance transport so that he can take up a collection to pay for it. The office manager insists that he cannot release this information because of HIPAA restrictions. What should be done?
   A. The man should be shown the standard charges for a 9-1-1 call so that his group has a goal.
   B. Because the request is for a charitable cause, the man should be asked that his group mention the ambulance service when taking up the collection (i.e., free advertising). If he agrees, he should be shown the bill.
   C. The HIPAA regulations should be calmly explained again.
   D. Because what he wants to see is just a bill (and not the PCR), it should be shown to him.
5. Your fire service employs mostly nationally registered Advanced Emergency Medical Technicians (AEMTs). Your chief wants you to begin transporting some of the critical care transfers that occur from the local hospital, because he has heard that these pay more than 9-1-1 calls. You have found that a need exists for this service; can you provide it with your current staffing configuration?
   A. Yes, as long as the medical director approves it.
   B. Yes, as long as the service director approves it.
   C. If the local hospital agrees to send properly trained nurses on the transfer.
   D. No, and you should notify the state certification/licensing board right away about your chief's plan.
6. Your shift is operating today without the Critical Care Paramedic (CCP), and the local Emergency Department needs an emergency transfer of a critically ill patient. Your boss wants one of the nurses from the ED to go with you to replace the missing staff person. Your service has never done this. Choose the correct plan for this dilemma.
   A. Insist that the licensed nurse delegated by the hospital must be oriented to the ambulance (work environment, protocols) and approved by medical control before departure.
   B. Go ahead; just let her ride along. What can happen?
   C. Refuse to transport the patient.
   D. Because nurses are not allowed to do ambulance transports unless they have EMS certification, notify the medical director of the service.
7. You have just landed at a small airport with your critical care team (CCP and nurse) and a critically ill patient who is to be admitted to the intensive care unit (ICU). An ambulance from the local service arrives to take the patient to the hospital; the ambulance is staffed with a paramedic and an EMT-Basic. The pilot is worried about incoming weather and wants you to just have the ambulance crew take the patient on to the hospital so that you can quickly take off for home. Choose the best decision for this situation.
   A. Insist that standard safety guidelines must be followed; then accompany the patient to the hospital according to those guidelines.
   B. Explain the situation to the ambulance crew; they will do fine for 10 to 15 minutes with the patient without your team.
   C. Halt the transfer; have the pilot fly the crew and patient back to the referring hospital.
   D. Ask the pilot to wait; then accompany the patient to the hospital and quickly hand the person off to the ED.
8. Your helicopter program has an agreement with several local hospitals for an exchange of supplies. When you bring a patient to a hospital, you are replenished with all supplies used free of charge to your program. You know that both the hospital and your program bill the patient for these supplies. Choose the best explanation of this situation.
   A. This is a kickback.
   B. This exchange program is acceptable under "safe harbor" practices.
   C. This is illegal and should be reported to the local county attorney.
   D. This practice is common and acceptable under common law.

9. You are transporting an elderly trauma patient to a local hospital (your service is based in a different county). The patient, who lives with her family in a private residence, shows signs of physical abuse. The hospital intends to report the incident as elder abuse to the local social services office. Choose your best course of action.
   A. You do not need to report the case, because the local hospital will do it; too many reports just confuse the system.
   B. You do not need to report the case, because you are not a physician.
   C. Because you are from a different county, you cannot report this incident.
   D. Everyone who assesses or treats a patient who is dependent on others and in whom abuse is suspected must report such cases. You must follow your state's abuse reporting procedures.
10. You are giving a deposition in a case in which you, your partner, the service, and the medical director are being sued for negligence. The case involved an unbelted, drunk driver who was ejected from his car in a single-vehicle accident and suffered fatal facial and head injuries. The attorney representing the man's family is asking detailed questions about the airway management of the patient. You remember that this was a difficult intubation, and both you and your partner made attempts. What point is the attorney trying to prove to make a case of negligence?
    A. Duty to act
    B. Tort liability
    C. HIPAA requirements
    D. Proximate cause
11. Which statement is true about the nurse-to-nurse report from the referring hospital during a transfer? (Assume that you work on the critical care transport team at a large hospital.)
    A. The local nurse can give you the hand-off report, because you represent your hospital; the nurse does not need to report by phone to the ICU or to the floor nurse.
    B. One hand-off report is sufficient, from the referring physician to the receiving physician.
    C. A hand-written report must be delivered to the receiving hospital (written reports are always better than oral reports).
    D. The nurse-to-nurse report provides patient information and confirms that the receiving hospital has a bed for the patient.
12. Choose the best explanation of the clinician-to-clinician report, one of the steps in a legal transfer.
    A. The receiving physician gives consent for the hospital where he or she practices.
    B. The receiving physician must be consulted for advice on stabilizing the patient's condition before transfer and not just to ensure acceptance of the patient's care.
    C. This report must take place between two physicians; it cannot be performed by midlevel practitioners such as nurse practitioners or physician assistants.
    D. The clinician providing care at the referral hospital reports to the receiving physician, who consents to take care of the patient.
13. In determining whether you, as an EMS provider, have been negligent, the law:
    A. Compares your actions with those of the physician community in your area
    B. Compares your actions with your protocols and the actions of your peers
    C. Determines whether your actions were "gross"
    D. Must prove the patient had a right to refuse your care
14. Your service's billing department has requested that you add "intravenous (IV) fluid intake" at the conclusion of your PCR so that the service can obtain higher reimbursement for completed orders. Choose the best statement about this situation.
    A. This is illegal; you cannot add nonessential documentation for billing purposes.
    B. You will comply with the template for a PCR that you learned in your initial training.
    C. This is acceptable and worth adding to your documentation.
    D. Billers have no business looking at the PCR; this is a HIPAA violation.
15. Which statement correctly describes CMS reimbursement issues for rotary wing (RW) transport?
    A. The service must document transport to the nearest appropriate facility and provide a detailed explanation of why several hospitals were bypassed to get to the destination.
    B. The PCR must show that the patient required an ICU bed on arrival.
    C. The patient cannot have a "do not resuscitate" (DNR) document on file, or rotary wing transport is not allowed.
    D. Rotary wing transport is very expensive and is not allowed by CMS.

16. A local hospital has requested your adult critical care transport team for the transport and management of a 2-year-old with severe sepsis. The child has been intubated, is on a ventilator, and has an arterial line with three vascular access sites through which three medications are being infused. The receiving pediatric hospital wants to send its own team, but the team will not arrive for 90 minutes. Choose the best plan.
    A. Your team does not have the training or equipment for necessary pediatric life support measures. Performing this transfer may be poor patient care and an EMTALA violation.
    B. This child requires rapid transport; you should not wait for the pediatric specialty crew.
    C. You may take this transfer as long as the ED physician accompanies you.
    D. You may take this transfer as long as the ED nurse accompanies you.
17. Your partner on the critical care team has a moral dilemma. The team has been asked to transport a young woman who has sepsis and disseminated intravascular coagulation (DIC) to a tertiary care center. The condition developed after a surgical abortion. Your partner is a pro-life activist and refuses to be involved in the transfer. You are now stuck at the referral hospital by yourself. Choose the best course of action.
    A. Halt the transfer; you must allow your partner to stick to his convictions.
    B. Attempt to find someone at the referral hospital to accompany you.
    C. Call your supervisor and arrange for another crew to come and pick up the patient.
    D. Explain the duty to act to your partner privately and call your supervisor.
18. You are calling in a patient report by cell phone 10 minutes before you are due to arrive at the resource hospital on a transfer. The charge nurse reports that they know nothing about this patient, and they have no beds. You forgot to get the name of the physician who accepted care from the referral hospital. In fact, you forgot all the documentation from the referral hospital. Choose the best course of action for this situation.
    A. Drop the patient off in the ED; they have to take care of the patient.
    B. Continue to transport the patient to the hospital area assigned; they might change their mind.
    C. Call the referral hospital and explain the situation. Obtain the name of the accepting physician and ask that a referral hospital staff member fax the PCR to the resource hospital.
    D. Halt the transfer, turn around, and take the patient back to the referral hospital.
19. The transport service's education coordinator has organized classes for the crew that involve "run reviews." Interesting cases will be presented and discussed with the medical director so that everyone learns. Your partner thinks this is a HIPAA violation. Which statement about this issue is correct?
    A. As long as this is part of an organized quality assurance activity, it is allowed.
    B. Your partner is correct; this should not be allowed.
    C. As long as you do not present patients' names, it is acceptable.
    D. This sounds like a "witch hunt," and you should protest the activity.
20. Which statement best explains a principle of ethics?
    A. I can cause harm in health care but have promised not to do so.
    B. I am never afforded autonomy in my decisions.
    C. I must tell the truth.
    D. I will dress and act appropriately.

CHAPTER 2

Pharmacology

OBJECTIVES

1. Discuss the critical care paramedic's responsibilities and scope of management in the administration of medications.
2. Use a knowledge of anatomy and physiology in pharmacologic decision making.
3. Calculate the correct dose for administration when given a medication order.
4. Identify the correct route of administration for a particular medication.
5. Discuss the components of a drug profile indexing system.
6. For a case scenario involving a patient receiving multiple medications, discuss the compatibility and interactions of the medications.
7. For a case scenario involving a patient being prepared for transport, discuss considerations in selecting alternative administration procedures to accommodate the required equipment.
8. Identify specific drugs and toxins that are major causes of cardiopulmonary emergencies.

Scenario

You are asked by a small hospital to transport a patient who is described as a "stable man with a small dissection of an aneurysm in the thoracic aorta." On arrival, you find the 78-year-old patient conscious, alert, and oriented in a bed in the intensive care unit (ICU). He states that he came to the hospital 3 hours ago with throat and neck pain and weakness. A diagnostic workup revealed a small aortic dissection, which needs to be evaluated by a thoracic surgeon. A 12-lead electrocardiogram shows no new developments, and early enzyme levels are unremarkable.

The monitor shows the sinus rhythm at 62 beats/min. The blood pressure (BP) is 140/82 mm Hg (mean arterial pressure [MAP], 101 mm Hg). Work of breathing is not increased; the lungs are clear; and the respiratory rate is 13 breaths/min. The patient is receiving 2 L of oxygen by nasal cannula. He has peripheral intravenous (IV) lines with 18-gauge catheters in both arms.

Two IV lines with medication are in place on the hospital's pumps. No. 1 is nitroglycerin, mixed 50 mg in 250 mL of D_5W, running at 6 mL/hour; no. 2 is labetalol, mixed 500 mg in 100 mL, running at 60 mL/hour; both of these lines were started just about 15 minutes earlier. You calculate the same numbers into your IV pumps and switch from the ICU's pumps to yours.

A thorough understanding of critical care pharmacology is crucial for emergency medical services (EMS) providers. Critical care practitioners must know not only the pharmacokinetics, but also the pharmacodynamics, of the medications they carry and of the drugs used in their patients. During transport, critical care patients frequently have several intravenous (IV) drips running off not only IV pumps, but also syringe pumps. EMS providers must apply their knowledge of these medications to the individual circumstances to ensure that the patient receives the optimum treatment.

This chapter reviews the principles of anatomy and physiology as they relate to pharmacology and touches on the processes of pharmacokinetics and pharmacodynamics. It also discusses some common critical care medications, reviews formulas for calculating the dosage of a drug, and looks at various devices for administering medications.

ANATOMY AND PHYSIOLOGY RELATED TO PHARMACOLOGY

Integration of the activities of the nervous system and the endocrine system determines the way the body functions. These systems achieve their responses using distinct mechanisms. The endocrine system releases chemicals into the blood, and the nervous system uses nerve fibers and chemicals between the nerve fibers to influence the body's actions.

The nervous system is made up of two major subdivisions, the *autonomic nervous system* and the *somatic nervous system.*

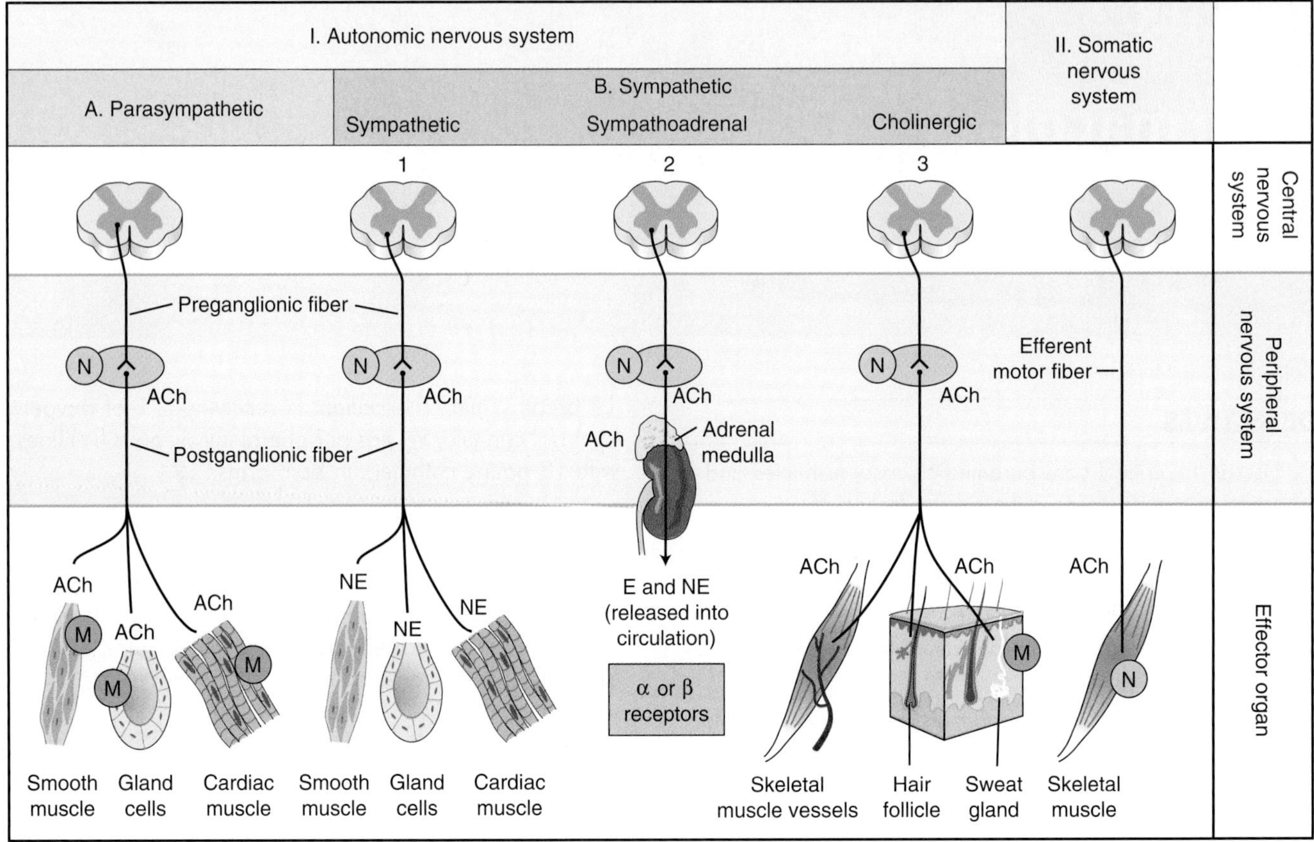

Figure 2-1

Receptor sites for neurohumoral transmission. A, Autonomic nervous system, where the preganglionic fibers of both the parasympathetic and sympathetic nerves synapse in the ganglia. B, Somatic motor nervous system. *Ach,* Acetylcholine; *E,* epinephrine; *M,* muscarinic receptors; *NE,* norepinephrine; *N,* nicotinic receptors. (From McKenry L, Tessier E, Hogan MA: *Mosby's pharmacology in nursing,* ed 22, St Louis, 2006, Mosby.)

The somatic nervous system is primarily responsible for the consciously controlled functions of the body, such as movement. From a critical care standpoint, the functions of the somatic nervous system are not as important as the core body functions regulated by the autonomic nervous system, which we will explore in further detail.

Autonomic Nervous System

The autonomic nervous system is primarily responsible for the automatic functions of the body, such as cardiac output. It consists of two subdivisions: the *sympathetic* (or *adrenergic*) *nervous system* (SNS) and the *parasympathetic* (or *cholinergic*) *nervous system* (PNS). The sympathetic and parasympathetic nervous systems function continuously and simultaneously. The SNS is predominant during times of stress, or "fight or flight," and the PNS predominates during calm states.

The SNS and PNS use two neuron links to transmit their impulses from the central nervous system (CNS) to the target organ. Both systems have **preganglionic** fibers, which exit from the central nervous system and extend to the ganglia, and **postganglionic** fibers, which extend from the ganglia to the effector organ. Many of the SNS ganglia are located close to the spinal cord, and the PNS ganglia are located closer to the effector organs. The junction between the neurons is called the *synapse* (Figure 2-1).

Neurotransmitters

Neurotransmitters are chemicals that are released at the neuron terminus and that cross the synapse to activate another neuron or effector organ. The neurotransmitter for the PNS at both the preganglionic and postganglionic synapse is acetylcholine (ACh). In the SNS, the preganglionic synaptic neurotransmitter is acetylcholine, and the postganglionic neurotransmitter is predominantly norepinephrine.

Acetylcholine binds to two possible cholinergic receptors after presynaptic release from vesicles: **muscarinic receptors** and nicotinic receptors. Muscarinic receptors are found in cardiac and smooth muscle, the exocrine glands, and the brain. **Nicotinic receptors** are found at the skeletal muscle neuromuscular end plate and the spinal cord. Nicotinic receptor binding by acetylcholine results in excitation, whereas muscarinic receptor binding may result in either excitation or inhibition. After receptor binding, **acetylcholinesterase (AChE)** breaks down acetylcholine into choline and acetate, which are taken back up into the nerve terminus and reform into acetylcholine, to be stored in the vesicles for repeated use.

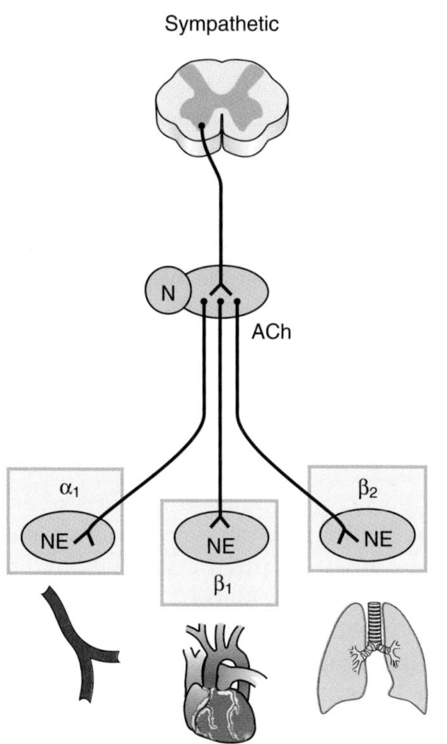

Figure 2-2

Site of action of adrenergic drugs. *ACh,* Acetylcholine; *N,* nicotinic receptors; *NE,* norepinephrine. (From McKenry L, Tessier E, Hogan MA: *Mosby's pharmacology in nursing,* ed 22, St Louis, 2006, Mosby.)

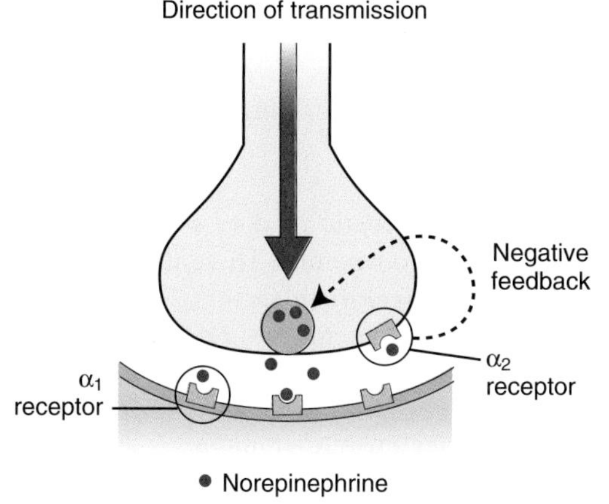

Figure 2-3

Site of action of alpha and beta receptors. (From McKenry L, Tessier E, Hogan MA: *Mosby's pharmacology in nursing,* ed 22, St Louis, 2006, Mosby.)

Norepinephrine is released across the adrenergic postganglionic synapse. It binds to two distinct adrenergic receptors in the tissue of the effector organs: alpha receptors and beta receptors (Figures 2-2 and 2-3). These adrenoreceptors are further grouped into four subtypes: $alpha_1$, $alpha_2$, $beta_1$, and $beta_2$. Stimulation of $alpha_1$ receptors results in vasoconstriction of the arterioles, with subsequent shunting of blood to the heart and brain, relaxation of the gut, and pupil dilation.

Table 2-1 Autonomic Receptors

Type	Site
Cholinergic Receptors	
Nicotinic	Skeletal muscle neuromuscular end plate and spinal cord
Muscarinic	Cardiac and smooth muscle, exocrine glands, and brain
Adrenergic Receptors	
$Alpha_1$	Vascular smooth muscle, gut, and pupils
$Alpha_2$	Presynaptic
$Beta_1$	Heart
$Beta_2$	Lungs, arterioles, pancreas, and uterus

Stimulation of $alpha_2$ receptors, which are **presynaptic**, inhibits the release of norepinephrine. $Beta_1$ receptors are located primarily in the heart. Stimulation of these receptors causes an increase in the heart rate (positive chronotropy), an increased force of contraction (positive inotropy), and increased automaticity. $Beta_2$ receptors are located in the lungs, arterioles, pancreas, and uterus. Stimulation of $beta_2$ receptors results in bronchodilation, vasodilation, glycogenolysis, and relaxation of the uterus (Table 2-1).

Adrenoreceptor Agonists

Norepinephrine predominantly stimulates $alpha_1$ receptors and has a lesser effect on beta receptors. Epinephrine, an endogenous catecholamine excreted by the adrenal medulla, stimulates both alpha and beta receptors to varying degrees, depending on the site of action and concentration. Dopamine, a precursor of epinephrine and norepinephrine, stimulates the dopaminergic receptors; it also stimulates the alpha and beta receptors to varying degrees, depending on the concentration. **Phenylephrine** and isoproterenol are exogenous chemicals that are pure adrenergic agonists; they stimulate only alpha receptors and beta receptors, respectively.

Adrenoreceptor Antagonists

Adrenoreceptor antagonists are exogenous chemicals that bind to specific receptors and prevent stimulation of the receptor or elicit the opposite effect of stimulation. Selective $beta_1$ receptor antagonists slow the heart rate, reduce the force of contraction, and decrease automaticity. Nonselective $beta_1$ and $beta_2$ blockers prevent stimulation (or elicit the opposite effect) in $beta_1$ receptors and also cause bronchoconstriction and a small degree of arteriole vasoconstriction. $Alpha_1$ blockers cause vasodilation and lower the blood pressure.

PHARMACOKINETICS

Pharmacokinetics is the study of the ways medications move through the body and are eliminated. Five main processes determine a drug's pharmacokinetics: absorption, distribution, metabolism, and excretion.

Absorption

Absorption indicates the amount of a drug that enters the bloodstream after administration. The rate and extent of absorption may be altered by food or other factors. Depending on the medication and absorption factors, the rate and extent of absorption may be increased or decreased, and these two elements are not dependent on each other.

Rate and extent also determine a medication's **bioavailability**. *Bioavailability* describes the percentage of a drug that is active and available in the circulation after initial administration. For IV medications, the bioavailability frequently is 100%. The bioavailability of oral medications may be close to 100% or it may be significantly lower, depending on factors that can reduce the available amount.

Distribution

Distribution refers to the transport of a drug in body fluids from the bloodstream to the various tissues of the body and ultimately to its site of action. Distribution expresses the overall amount of medication in the body as a proportion (percentage) of the serum concentration of the medication if it were to be distributed equally. Major factors that affect a medication's volume of distribution include lipid solubility and protein binding. Lipid-soluble drugs can easily cross capillary membranes and enter most tissues; water-soluble drugs, on the other hand, require more time to arrive at their point of action. The more highly protein bound a medication is, the more likely it is to have a lower volume of distribution, because most of the medication remains bound to proteins in the blood.

Metabolism

Metabolism is the process by which a medication is converted to a *metabolite,* or a modified version of the original chemical. This process usually converts the chemical to a form that is less toxic and more easily eliminated by the body. **Clopidogrel**, an antiplatelet medication used in acute coronary syndromes, must be converted to its active form in the liver.

Occasionally the body may convert a chemical to a more toxic or active form of the medication. For example, the analgesic acetaminophen, if taken in excessive doses, can form a toxic metabolite that may cause severe liver dysfunction, leading to liver failure.

Chemicals or medications may undergo further metabolism to aid in their elimination. Many medications are metabolized in the liver. Other sites of metabolism include the kidneys, blood, lungs, and gastrointestinal tract.

Excretion

Excretion is the process by which substances are eliminated from the body. The predominant site for excretion is the kidney. The three main mechanisms involved in the excretion of medications by the kidney are **glomerular filtration,** reabsorption, and **tubular secretion.** Substances that are not protein bound and are water soluble are the primary entities excreted through this filtration process. Lipid-soluble medications are reabsorbed in the tubules and enter the circulation; water-soluble substances cannot be reabsorbed. Tubular secretion is the process by which unbound substances cross from the blood through the tubules into the urine via a concentration gradient.

If metabolites are not excreted by the kidneys, they may be transported by the bile and removed in the feces. Some substances undergo recycling in the bile and are returned to the circulation. Other organs involved in the elimination of substances from the body are the intestines, lungs, and salivary, sweat, and mammary glands.

PHARMACODYNAMICS

Pharmacodynamics is the study of the effect of a medication on the body. Many factors can alter the normal pharmacodynamics of a drug. It is crucial that healthcare providers be knowledgeable about the normal pharmacodynamics of a drug and also about specific factors that can alter a medication's actions. A drug's pharmacodynamics can be affected by age, genetics, body mass, disease state, and environmental factors (also see Drug Action later in the chapter). The mechanism of action is included in pharmacodynamics; this may include the drug-receptor or drug-enzyme interaction.

Age

Elderly and young patients frequently are more sensitive to the pharmacodynamic effects of medications. Renal and hepatic function may be immature, or it may be failing because of advanced age. For example, a reduced dose of morphine must be used for elderly patients to achieve analgesia without causing excessive adverse reactions.

Genetics

Patients may have a genetic predisposition that can alter a medication's pharmacodynamics. These alterations frequently are caused by **pharmacokinetic factors.** For example, an isoenzyme in the liver, **cytochrome P450 2D6 (CYP2D6)**, is responsible for the metabolism of many medications; but almost 10% of Caucasians do not carry significant amounts of this isoenzyme. CYP2D6 is required to metabolize codeine to its active form; if this conversion does not occur, the pharmacodynamic effect of codeine is virtually nonexistent.

Body Mass

Body mass may play a major role in the pharmacodynamics of a medication. Patients at the extremes of body size usually are the most affected. Obese patients may require larger doses of medications that distribute to adipose tissue, but dose increases may be unnecessary with medications that do not distribute to adipose tissue. Dosing for children is almost always based on body size.

Disease State

Specific diseases can alter the pharmacodynamic effect of a medication. Malnourished individuals with a low serum albumin level may show pronounced effects of highly protein-bound medications, such as phenytoin. This excessive pharmacodynamic response occurs because of the increased free amount of medication available in the circulation; this can result in significant toxicity, even if the total amount of drug in the serum appears normal. The unbound, or free, portion of the drug may be near a toxic level, and the free drug level, rather than the total drug level, may need to be followed to prevent toxicity.

Environmental Factors

Environmental factors can enhance or diminish the pharmacodynamic effects of medications. Smoking can dramatically increase the clearance of certain medications. For example, theophylline is a bronchodilator occasionally used for asthma or chronic obstructive pulmonary disease. Patients who smoke or inhale secondhand smoke frequently require larger doses of theophylline to achieve adequate serum levels and obtain the desired pharmacodynamic response.

Alcohol is another significant factor in pharmacodynamics. Of the 100 most commonly prescribed drugs, about 50 contain at least one ingredient known to interact adversely with ingested alcohol.

Mechanism of Action

The *mechanism of action* refers to the way or the reason a drug affects its target. The three mechanisms of action for drugs are drug-receptor interactions, drug-enzyme interactions, and nonspecific interactions.

Drug-Receptor Interactions

Each drug has a complex chemical shape that enables it to fit into a receptor site and produce an effect. With reversible binding, the drug can be separated from its receptor site, which stops the interaction and halts the drug's effects. With irreversible binding, the drug cannot be separated from its receptor site.

Agonists and Antagonists

An *agonist* is a drug that stimulates the target receptor once bound to it. Epinephrine, for example, is an alpha and beta agonist. An *antagonist* is a drug that prevents activation of the targeted receptor. Metoprolol is a beta antagonist (beta blocker). There are two types of antagonists:

- *Competitive antagonists,* which compete with agonists to bind to the receptor.
- *Noncompetitive antagonists,* which bind to the site near the receptor and change the receptor's structure, thereby making it inactive. This type of antagonism is less reversible.

Affinity, Efficacy, and Potency

Drugs and their receptors have a chemical attraction, known as *affinity.* An example of this pharmacodynamic is the attraction between an antigen and the antibody created to destroy it. *Efficacy* is the ability of a drug or treatment to have the desired effect; an opioid is efficacious for pain control. *Potency* compares the drug dosages required to produce the same effect. For example, both morphine and fentanyl can produce analgesia; however, 0.10 mg of fentanyl has the same potency as 10 mg of morphine. Fentanyl, therefore, is more potent.

Drug-Enzyme Interactions

Enzymes are catalysts that mediate chemical reactions. Many enzymes work by binding to the drug. An interaction occurs when a drug and an enzyme are similar in appearance. Either stimulation or blockade of the enzyme follows this interaction. For example, if ciprofloxin is given to a patient who is receiving theophylline, the enzyme that breaks down theophylline is blocked, thereby allowing it to accumulate and possibly cause toxicity to the patient.

Nonspecific Drug Interaction

There are medications with no structural or chemical makeup that bind or produce an enzyme for a mechanism of action to occur. Thereby labeled nonspecific, these drugs have a general effect directly on cells and their processes. Examples of these types of drugs are anesthetics, which act directly on the cell membrane.

DRUG ACTION

A clinician prescribes a medication to achieve an effect that diminishes or eliminates a disease or its symptoms. However, medications have side effects; some are minor, whereas others can be dangerous. Reducing the medication dose or discontinuing the drug may eliminate the side effects. Some adverse effects are *idiosyncratic;* that is, they are considered rare and could not be predicted. Allergic reactions and anaphylaxis are examples of immunologic reactions (Table 2-2).

Factors that can affect the action of a drug include:

- Intestinal absorption
- Renal excretion
- Drug metabolism
- Action at the receptor site
- Alteration of electrolyte balance
- Interactions with other drugs
- Competition for plasma protein binding
- Drug incompatibilities
- Drug-induced malabsorption of food and nutrients
- Food-induced malabsorption of drugs
- Alteration of enzymes
- Alcohol consumption
- Cigarette smoking
- Alterations in drug excretion caused by food

Plasma Level Profile

The *plasma level profile* is a description of a drug's activity. Blood tests are used to determine and measure the concentration of a drug (e.g., digoxin) in the plasma, and drug dosages are adjusted according to these levels.

Biologic Half-Life

The *biologic half-life* is the amount of time the body needs to eliminate half of a drug. This is important information for

Table 2-2 Adverse Drug Responses

Type	Description	Explanation
Predictable	Desired action	The intended benefit of the drug
	Side effect	An effect of a drug other than the one for which it was given
Iatrogenic	Iatrogenic drug response	An unintentional disease or drug effect produced by a treatment
Unpredictable	Additive effect	The combined effect of two different drugs given at the same time, resulting in an increase in the observed effect
	Adverse reaction	An unintentional and often undesirable effect of a drug
	Anaphylactic reaction	An allergic reaction, often exaggerated, to a foreign substance
	Cross-tolerance	Decreasing responsiveness to the effects of a drug in a drug class and the likelihood of development of decreased responsiveness to another drug in the same class
	Cumulative action	Increased intensity of a drug's action after administration of several doses
	Delayed reaction	A delay between exposure and the onset of action
	Drug allergy	A reaction to a medication; an immunologic reaction to a drug
	Drug antagonism	An interaction between two drugs in which one partly or completely inhibits the effects of the other
	Drug dependence	A physical need or adaptation to a drug with or without the psychological need to take the drug
	Drug interaction	The way in which drugs interact with each other or with food
	Hypersensitivity	Altered reactivity to a medication that occurs after sensitization; the response has nothing to do with the dose
	Idiosyncrasy	An unexpected and usually individual adverse response to a drug
	Interference	The ability of one drug to limit the function of another drug
	Potentiation	A prolongation or increase in the effect of a drug caused by another drug
	Summation	The combined effects of two or more drugs that equal the sum of their individual effects
	Synergism	The interaction of drugs so that the total effect is greater than the sum of the individual effects
	Tachyphylaxis	A rapid decrease in response to a drug or physiologically active agent after administration of a few doses; rapid cross-tolerance
	Tolerance	Decreased responsiveness to the effects of a drug; increasing doses in amount and frequency are required to achieve the desired effect.

Modified from Aehlert B: *Paramedic practice today,* St Louis, 2010, Mosby.

determining how often the medication should be administered. A drug with a half-life of 3 hours should be given more often throughout the day than a drug with a half-life of 12 hours.

The half-life also determines how long the drug's effect lasts. Drugs with a short half-life clear the body quickly. This is an important factor in the administration of long-acting drugs for which a prolonged effect may have an undesired consequence.

Therapeutic Threshold

The *therapeutic threshold* is also known as the *minimum effective concentration.* It is the drug concentration needed to obtain the desired effect.

Therapeutic Index

The *therapeutic index* (TI) is the safe dosing range for a drug. It is calculated by using the effective dose and the lethal dose at a 50:50 ratio. The closer the index is to 1, the more harmful the drug is to the patient. For example, digoxin has a very low TI. Dosing is based on the patient's weight, and digoxin toxicity is easily created.

Drug Effect

A drug's effect can be categorized into various groups based on the type of drug, the receptor site, and the tissues or organs affected. This chapter reviews these general categories; the specific drugs are described in the appropriate clinical chapters. The drug profiles of commonly used medications are featured in the Drug Guide on the Evolve site for *Transport of the Critical Care Patient.*

CARDIOVASCULAR MEDICATIONS

Antiarrhythmics

Antiarrhythmic drugs have been categorized into four classes (Table 2-3). Two other cardiac antiarrhythmic drugs, adenosine and digitalis, are not included in the list because they are unique. Adenosine is a **nucleoside** that is used to control supraventricular tachycardia; digitalis is a cardiac glycoside that slows and strengthens the heart.

Did You Know?

Atropine works by holding back acetylcholine and increasing conduction through the sinoatrial (SA) node.

Did You Know?

Cardiac glycosides have both a negative chronotropic effect and a positive inotropic effect, allowing the heart to pump slower but more efficiently.

Table 2-3 Classes of Antiarrhythmics

Class	Major Action
IA	Block fast sodium channels in cardiac muscle, resulting in decreased excitability; prolong repolarization (e.g., quinidine, procainamide, disopyramide)
IB	Block fast sodium channels in cardiac muscle, resulting in decreased excitability; shorten repolarization or have little effect (e.g., lidocaine, tocainide, mexiletine)
IC	Profoundly slow conduction (e.g., flecainide, propafenone)
II	Beta blockers; suppress automaticity and rate of impulse conduction (e.g., propranolol, esmolol, atenolol)
III	Markedly prolong repolarization, usually by interfering with outflow of potassium through potassium channels (e.g., amiodarone, sotalol)
IV	Calcium channel blockers; block inward movement of calcium to slow impulse conduction (particularly through the atrioventricular node) and vascular smooth muscle contraction (e.g., verapamil, diltiazem)

From Aehlert B: *Paramedic practice today,* St Louis, 2010, Mosby.

Did You Know?

Lidocaine cannot be given orally, because the first-pass effect removes the active drug, preventing a therapeutic effect.

Sympathomimetics

Adrenergic drugs are designed to mimic the effects of the sympathetic nervous system and therefore are called *sympathomimetics* (Table 2-4). Because these are stimulatory drugs, their effects include increased cardiac output, vasoconstriction, and bronchial dilation.

Antihypertensives

Some drugs are designed to reduce the blood pressure by working directly on the renal or vascular system. The goal is to reduce the workload of the heart while maintaining adequate blood pressure for tissue perfusion, in addition to preventing undesirable side effects and allowing long-term administration (Table 2-5).

Did You Know?

Loop diuretics block the reabsorption of sodium, allowing it to be excreted with water in the urine.

Table 2-4 Sympathomimetics

Organs Affected	Receptor Type	Adrenergic Response
Heart	$Beta_1$	Increased force of contraction, increased heart rate, increased automaticity, increased conduction velocity
Lungs		
Bronchial smooth muscles	$Beta_2$	Bronchodilation
Bronchial glands	$Alpha_1$, $beta_2$	Inhibition
Blood vessels		
Coronary arterioles	$Alpha_1$	Constriction
Cerebral arterioles	$Alpha_1$	Constriction
Liver	$Beta_2$	Glycogenolysis
Pancreas (insulin secretion)	$Alpha_2$	Decreased
Kidney		
Secretion of renin	$Beta_1$	Increased

Modified from McKenry L, Tessier E, Hogan MA: *Mosby's pharmacology in nursing,* ed 22, St Louis, 2006, Mosby.

Table 2-5 Antihypertensive Medications

Drug Type	Action
Diuretics	
Loop	Reduce the circulating volume by promoting urine production (e.g., furosemide [Lasix])
Thiazide	Increase the excretion of sodium, chloride, and water at the tubules (e.g., hydrochlorothiazide [HCTZ])
Potassium sparing	Increase sodium and water excretion in the distal tubules while allowing reabsorption of potassium (e.g., spironolactone)
Osmotic	Mannitol diffuse solvent across membranes in response to a concentration gradient
Adrenergic Blocking Agents	
Beta blockers	Occupy beta receptor sites, reducing cardiac output and the heart rate (e.g., the "olol" drugs: metoprolol, esmolol)
Centrally acting adrenergic inhibitors	Block sympathetic stimulation from the central nervous system (e.g., methyldopa [Aldomet] and clonidine [Catapres])
Peripherally acting adrenergic inhibitors	Reduce blood pressure by reducing effect of the peripheral blood vessels (e.g., guanethidine sulfate [Ismelin], prazosin hydrochloride [Minipress], phentolamine [Regitine])
Angiotensin-converting enzyme (ACE) inhibitors	Block renal effect of angiotensin and aldosterone on vessel dilation and reabsorption of water (e.g., the "pril" drugs: lisinopril [Prinivil], enalapril [Vasotec])
Calcium channel blockers	Prevent vasoconstriction of vascular smooth muscle; may also be included as a dysrhythmic (e.g., diltiazem [Cardizem], verapamil [Calan])
Vasodilators	Allow dilation of peripheral vessel walls, inhibiting circulation (e.g., diazoxide [Hyperstat], hydralazine [Apresoline], minoxidil [Loniten], nitroglycerin, isosorbide)

Antiplatelet Agents, Anticoagulants, and Fibrinolytics

When a blood clot forms in a vessel, blood flow is obstructed, creating an infarction or other serious medical condition. Drugs that prevent clot formation or help degrade clots that have formed are categorized as antiplatelet agents, anticoagulants, or fibrinolytics.

Antiplatelet Agents

When platelets stick together, they facilitate clot formation and obstruction of blood flow. Some of the agents that prevent this clumping are aspirin, clopidogrel (Plavix), dipyridamole (Persantine), ticlopidine (Ticlid), and abciximab (ReoPro).

Anticoagulants

Anticoagulants usually are prescribed when a thrombus already exists. These drugs do not break up a clot, but they help prevent extension of the clot or the formation of a new clot. Warfarin (Coumadin) and enoxaparin (Lovenox) are examples of anticoagulants.

Fibrinolytics

Fibrinolytics are used to reestablish blood flow through blocked blood vessels, because these drugs break up existing clots. Major side effects of fibrinolytics include intracerebral or gastrointestinal hemorrhage. This group of drugs includes tissue plasminogen activator (t-PA; Alteplase), reteplase (Retavase), and tenecteplase (TNKase).

Antihemophilic Agents

Hemophilia, a hereditary disorder caused by the absence of one or more clotting factors from the plasma, can lead to uncontrollable hemorrhage even with minor injuries. Hemophilia has several subcategories. For example, hemophilia A is the classic Factor VIII deficiency. A patient with hemophilia B (Christmas disease) lacks Factor IX. Specific factor replacement therapy now is available for many of these disorders, and these drugs may even be administered at home by the patient's family. Factor VIII preparations may include Koate-HP, Recombinate, or Kogenate-FS. Desmopressin (DDAVP), Factor VIIa (NovoSeven), Factor VIII (Advate), and Factor IX (BeneFix) are other commercially available agents.

Electrolytes

The administration of electrolytes is discussed in Chapters 4 and 6. More detailed drug information also is available in the Drug Guide on the Evolve site for *Transport of the Critical Care Patient.*

RESPIRATORY MEDICATIONS

Medications that have a specific action on the mechanisms of respiration are commonly used in emergency medical transport. These same drugs are continued during critical care transport (Table 2-6).

GASTROINTESTINAL MEDICATIONS

Various drugs, especially antiemetics, that can prevent aspiration of gastric contents play an important role during the transport of ill or injured patients. Some H_2 receptor drugs also are used as antinausea agents.

Table 2-6 Respiratory Medications

Drug Type	Action
Antihistamines	Compete for receptor sites; affect vessels, bronchi, and gastrointestinal tract (e.g., diphenhydramine [Benadryl])
Bronchodilators	
Sympathomimetics	Function as beta agonists at $beta_2$ receptor sites (e.g., albuterol [Proventil], terbutaline [Brethine])
Anticholinergics	Block acetylcholine, relaxing bronchial smooth muscles (e.g., ipratropium bromide [Atrovent])
Xanthine derivatives	Relax smooth muscles (e.g., theophylline [Theo-Dur])
Leukotriene antagonists	Stabilize cells' response to inflammation (montelukast [Singulair])

Table 2-7 Antiemetics

Drug Name	Class	Mechanism of Action
Chlorpromazine (Thorazine) Prochlorperazine (Compazine) Promethazine (Phenergan) Thiethylperazine (Torecan)	Phenothiazine	Dopamine blockade; extrapyramidal effects possible
Droperidol (Inapsine) Haloperidol (Haldol)	Butyrophenone	Prolonged Q-T interval with droperidol, haloperidol
Metoclopramide (Reglan)	Prokinetic gastrointestinal agent	$Dopamine_2$ blockade, 5-HT3 antagonist
Diphenhydramine (Benadryl) Dimenhydrinate (Dramamine)	Antihistamine	H_1 blockade, antimuscarinic effects
Dolasetron (Anzemet) Granisetron (Kytril) Ondansetron (Zofran) Palonosetron (Aloxi)	Selective serotonin receptor antagonist	5-HT3 receptor antagonists (used primarily for chemotherapy-induced and postoperative nausea)

Modified from McKenry L, Tessier E, Hogan MA: *Mosby's pharmacology in nursing*, ed 22, St Louis, 2006, Mosby.

Antiemetics

The medulla of the brain controls the act of vomiting. The signs and symptoms of nausea and vomiting have various causes, but common antiemetics block acetylcholine, dopamine, and histamine receptors (Table 2-7).

ENDOCRINE MEDICATIONS

In the United States, as many as 25% of all hospitalized patients are treated for hyperglycemia and diabetes, regardless of their original diagnosis. Diabetes mellitus is the sixth leading cause of death, and it is estimated that 6% of the population is affected by this disease.[1] In addition, it is associated with serious complications.

Many critical care transport patients will have an endocrine disease and the related complications. It is crucial that critical care transport providers keep up-to-date on the endocrine medications and the indications for their use (Table 2-8); they also must be knowledgeable about the different types and effects of insulin preparations (Table 2-9).

IMMUNE SYSTEM AGENTS

Immune system drugs defend the body against antigens. In patients who have received an organ transplant, these medications suppress the normal immune response to prevent organ rejection. Such drugs may include corticosteroids (methylprednisolone), azathioprine (Imuran), cyclophosphamide (cytoxan), and cyclosporine.

Antibiotics and Antiviral and Antifungal Agents

Antibiotics kill or suppress the growth of microorganisms by disrupting the cell wall or general cell function. They are classified into many different categories, including penicillins, cephalosporins, macrolides, tetracyclines, fluoroquinolones, and other agents. The type used depends on the tissues infected and whether the organism grows with oxygen (aerobic) or without it (anaerobic).

Many of the patients you will transport will have been prescribed antibiotic, antiviral, or antifungal medications, to be given at routine intervals. Life-saving antibiotics are administered before transport in patients who are septic; however, it is important that you follow the schedule of the IV antibiotic prescribed, even during transport. Many of these drugs have strict guidelines for IV administration.

Antiretroviral Agents

The Retroviridae family of viruses causes B- and T-cell pathologic conditions in the immune system. The most common of these viruses, the human immunodeficiency virus (HIV), causes acquired immunodeficiency syndrome (AIDS). HIV type 1 (HIV-1) is the worldwide viral agent; HIV type 2 (HIV-2) generally is confined to western Africa.

Since the mid-1990s and the advent of highly active antiretroviral therapy (HAART), the mortality rate for early retroviral disease has fallen by 42%.

Table 2-8 Endocrine Medications

Location	Drug	Indications
Pituitary gland	Octreotide (Sandostatin)	Growth hormone inhibitor
	Corticotropin (Acthar, ACTH)	Diagnostic testing
	Somatrem (Protropin)	Growth hormone deficiency in children
	Somatropin (Humatrope)	Prader-Willi syndrome
	Sermorelin (Geref)	Growth hormone deficiency
	Vasopressin (Pitressin)	Diabetes insipidus, acute massive hemorrhage
	Lypressin (Diapid)	Diabetes insipidus
	Desmopressin (DDAVP)	Diabetes insipidus
Parathyroid gland	Calcifediol (Calderol)	Hypocalcemia
	Calcitonin-salmon	Hypercalcemia
	Plicamycin (Mithracin)	Hypercalcemia, bone resorption inhibitor
Thyroid gland	Levothyroxine (Synthroid)	Synthetic thyroid hormone replacement
	Liotrix (Euthroid)	Synthetic thyroid hormone replacement
	Potassium iodide (Lugol's iodine)	Antithyroid preparation (hyperthyroidism)

From Aehlert B: *Paramedic practice today*, St Louis, 2010, Mosby.

NEUROLOGIC MEDICATIONS

Medications used for patients with primary neurologic conditions usually include those that can reduce cerebral edema and those that stop or prevent seizures. Chapter 5 presents more detailed descriptions of these drugs with their associated disease process.

Benzodiazepines

Benzodiazepines (BZ) exert a wide range of effects that may include, depending on the drug, muscle relaxation, antianxiety, antiseizure, or antihypnotic effects. BZ-1 receptors in the cerebellum mediate anxiety and sedation. BZ-2 receptors are associated with muscle relaxation and memory and sensory functions in the basal ganglion. Alprazolam (Xanax), diazepam (Valium), midazolam (Versed), and lorazepam (Ativan) are examples of benzodiazepines.

Anticonvulsants

Anticonvulsant medications are used to treat seizure disorders (Tables 2-10 and 2-11). Most of these drugs depress the excitability of neurons while terminating abnormal neuronal discharges.

Analgesics and Sedatives

Analgesics are medications that relieve pain. (Chapter 10 presents a complete description of the physiology of receptors and pain medication.) The critical care team must pay particular attention to good pain control during transport. Examples of analgesic drugs include morphine sulfate, fentanyl citrate (Sublimaze), meperidine (Demerol), butorphanol (Stadol), and ketorolac (Toradol).

Antipsychotic Agents

Antipsychotic agents affect the chemical neurotransmitters in specific areas of the CNS. These psychotropic medications affect mental processes, emotions, or behaviors. The four classes of psychotropic drugs are CNS stimulants, antidepressants, anxiolytics, and antipsychotics. Although many patients

Table 2-9 Insulin Preparations

Action	Type	Onset	Peak Effect	Duration of Action
Rapid acting	Lispro (Humalog)	15-30 min	30 min to 2.5 hours	3-5 hours
	Aspart (Novolog)	10-20 min	1-3 hours	3-5 hours
Short acting	Regular	30 min to 1 hour	2-5 hours	5-8 hours
Intermediate acting	NPH	2 hours	4-12 hours	18-24 hours
	Lente	1-2.5 hours	3-10 hours	18-24 hours
Long acting	Lantus	1-1.5 hours	Given once daily; no peak; delivered steadily for 20-24 hours	20-24 hours
Combinations	Humulin 50/50	30 min	3 hours	22-24 hours
	Humulin 70/30, Novolin 70/30	30 min	4-8 hours	24 hours

Modified from Aehlert B: *Paramedic practice today*, St Louis, 2010, Mosby.

Table 2-10 Parenteral Antiseizure Medications

Drug	Use
Barbiturates	Eclampsia; status epilepticus; severe, recurrent seizures; antiepileptic drug toxicity; other convulsive states
Phenytoin	Status epilepticus, seizure during neurosurgery
Magnesium sulfate	Severe toxemias of pregnancy
Benzodiazepines	Status epilepticus; severe, recurrent seizures; alcohol withdrawal seizures
Levetiracetam (Keppra)	Prevention of seizures in neurologic pathologic conditions; seizure states

Modified from McKenry L, Tessier E, Hogan MA: *Mosby's pharmacology in nursing,* ed 22, St Louis, 2006, Mosby.

Table 2-11 Anticonvulsants: Indications for Parenteral Use of Antiepileptic Medications

Parenteral Drug	Use
Barbiturates, especially phenobarbital, also amobarbital	Eclampsia; status epilepticus; severe, recurrent seizures
Pentobarbital sodium and secobarbital sodium	Tetanus, antiepileptic drug toxicity, other convulsive states
Phenytoin	Status epilepticus, seizure during neurosurgery
Magnesium sulfate	Severe toxemias of pregnancy (preeclampsia and eclampsia)
Benzodiazepines (e.g., diazepam, lorazepam, clonazepam)	Status epilepticus; severe, recurrent seizures; alcohol withdrawal seizures

From McKenry L, Tessier E, Hogan MA: *Mosby's pharmacology in nursing,* ed 22, St Louis, 2006, Mosby.

take these medications, they are rarely used as antipsychotic agents during a critical care transport.

Neuromuscular Blocking Agents

Neuromuscular blocking agents (NMBAs) are subclassified into two types of paralytic drugs, depolarizing and nondepolarizing. (These drugs are described in detail in Chapter 3.)

Depolarizing Paralytic Drugs

Succinylcholine is the only depolarizing paralytic drug. It is similar to acetylcholine and competes with ACh for the receptor site, rendering the muscles paralyzed for a short period.

Nondepolarizing Paralytic Drugs

Nondepolarizing paralytic drugs bind to ACh receptor sites, preventing muscle contraction. These drugs, which are grouped according to their duration of action, include vecuronium (Norcuron) and rocuronium (Zemuron).

DRUG CALCULATIONS

The critical care practitioner must have a clear understanding of drug math and drug calculations. In today's critical care field, the use of IV pumps has made the job of calculating drug dosages a snap; however, the practitioner must be able to perform these calculations manually in the event of equipment failure. This section presents a brief overview of a few methods of performing drug math. The intent is not to enforce rules, but rather to offer options on some of the simpler drug calculation formulas.

Calculating the Appropriate Volume Dose

Formula:

$$\text{Volume to be administered} = \frac{\text{Volume on hand} \times \text{Desired dose}}{\text{Dose on hand}}$$

Example:
According to the protocol, you should give 5 mg of Valium. Your carpujet contains 10 mg in 2 mL. What is your delivered dose?

$$\frac{(2\ \text{mL} \times 5\ \text{mg})}{10\ \text{mg}}$$

$$10 \div 10 = 1\ \text{mL}$$

Calculating Medication Infusions

Formula:

$$\text{Drops per minute} = \frac{\text{Volume on hand} \times \text{Drops per milliliter in set} \times \text{Desired dose}}{\text{Dose on hand}}$$

Example:
According to the cardiac arrest protocol, you should administer 3 mg/min of lidocaine after the appropriate bolus. You have 1 g of lidocaine in a vial to mix in 250 mL of D_5W. How many drops per minute (gtt) would you administer?

$$\text{Drops/min} = \frac{250\ \text{mL} \times 60\ \text{gtt/mL} \times 3\ \text{mg/min}}{1000\ \text{mg}}$$

$$45{,}000 \div 1000 = 45\ \text{drops}$$

Calculating a Fluid Infusion Over Time

Formula:

$$\text{Drops per minute} = \frac{\text{Volume to be infused} \times \text{Drops per milliliter per set}}{\text{Time (min)}}$$

Example:
You need to administer 250 mL of normal saline over 1 hour. How many drops per minute would you administer with a 10 drop/mL set?

$$\frac{250\text{ mL} \times 10\text{ drops/mL/set}}{60}$$
$$= 42\text{ drops}$$

Time Constant Method

The time constant method of calculating a fluid infusion is a very easy way to figure out how much fluid to administer. This method is based on the drip set used divided by the fluid to be infused per hour. The time constant number is found by using the drip set on hand and multiplying it by x to equal 60.
Example:

$$\text{Drip set} \times x = 60$$

Drip set	Equation	Time constant
10	$10 \times x = 60$ $x = 6$	6
15	$15 \times x = 60$ $x = 4$	4
20	$20 \times x = 60$ $x = 3$	3

The time constant then is divided by the amount of fluid to be administered per hour.
Example:
A 10-drop set will be used to administer 200 mL/hour. The time constant is 6 ($10 \times 6 = 60$), which is divided by 200 mL:

$$200 \div 6 = 33\text{ drops/min}$$

For infusions to be given over several hours, the amount of fluid per hour must be calculated.
Example:
The physician instructs you to administer 1000 mL of normal saline over 4 hours ($1000 \div 4 = 250$ mL/hour). The amount per hour then is divided by the time constant (e.g., 4) to obtain the drops per minute:

$$250 \div 4 = 63\text{ drops/min}$$

Medicated Intravenous Infusions Set Up in Micrograms

For many, calculating the infusion of high-risk IV medications is especially frustrating. First, the units must be converted from micrograms (mcg) to milligrams (mg). Then, the amount of drug that should be present in each milliliter of the IV bag must be determined.

The following practical shortcut for calculating these infusions has been taught for years, with no clear citation of origin.

Step 1: Determine how many milligrams of the drug you are putting in the IV bag (or, if the bag was prefilled by the company, how many milligrams were put in it).

Step 2: Determine how many milliliters of fluid are in the IV bag.

Step 3: Use the following formula to calculate how many micrograms/milliliter (mcg/mL) you have on hand:

IV total ml in the bag x = 1000 mL

The number of milligrams added to the IV bag is multiplied by that multiplier to find the micrograms per milliliter. For example:
800 mg of dopamine is added to 500 mL of NS
500 mL × 2 = 1000
2 × 800 mg of dopamine = 1600 mcg/mL

Remember, if you mix grams into a fluid, the drug is administered as milligrams; if you mix milligrams into a fluid, the drug is administered as micrograms. Because the 800 mg of dopamine is added to fluid, it will be administered in micrograms.

Now you know what you have on hand. Next, calculate how much dopamine you need.

Step 4: How many micrograms per kilogram were ordered (or, how many micrograms per minute were ordered)?

If the dopamine order was for 10 mcg/kg/min and the patient weighs 100 kg, the desired dose would be 1000 mcg/min.

Step 5: How should you set your pump for milliliters per hour? The formula is:

$$\frac{\text{Desired dose} \times 60}{\text{Dose on hand}}$$

From the example, the desired dose is 1000 mcg/min and the dose on hand is 1600 mcg/mL:

$$\frac{1000 \times 60}{1600}$$
$$= 37.5$$

Your pump should be set to deliver 37.5 mL/hour.

Let's try another example. You are ordered to administer 10 mcg/min of epinephrine via IV infusion. You will add 5 mg of the drug to 250 mL of NS. How should the pump be?

1. 5 mg
2. 250 mL
3. 4 × 250 mL = 1000 mL; therefore, 4 × 5 mg = 20 mcg/mL in this mix
4. 10 mcg/min was ordered (10 ÷ 20 = 0.5 × 60)
   20 mcg/mL on hand
5. The pump should be set at 30 mL/hour.

DRUG ADMINISTRATION TECHNIQUES

Intravenous Lines

Most of the IV lines the critical care transport team will deal with will be standard peripheral access lines. Central access lines include single-, double-, or triple-lumen devices (Figure 2-4) with specially colored distal connections that denote whether the line is distal, medial, or proximal.

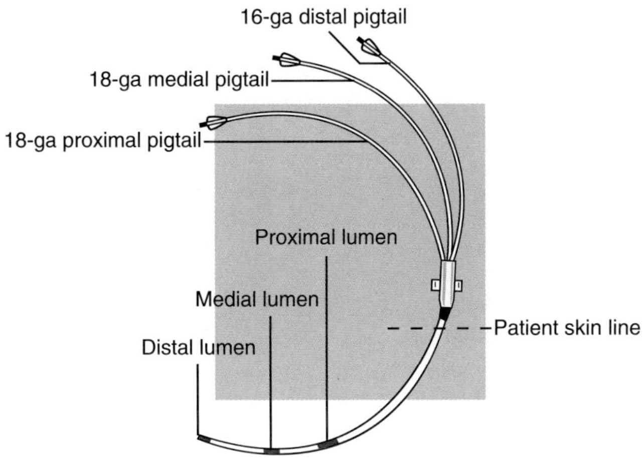

Figure 2-4

Triple-lumen catheter. (From Macklin D, Chernecky C: *Real world nursing survival guide: IV therapy*, St Louis, 2004, Saunders.)

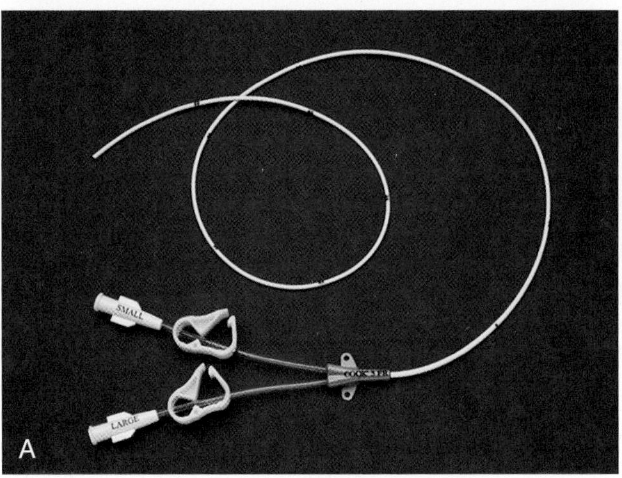

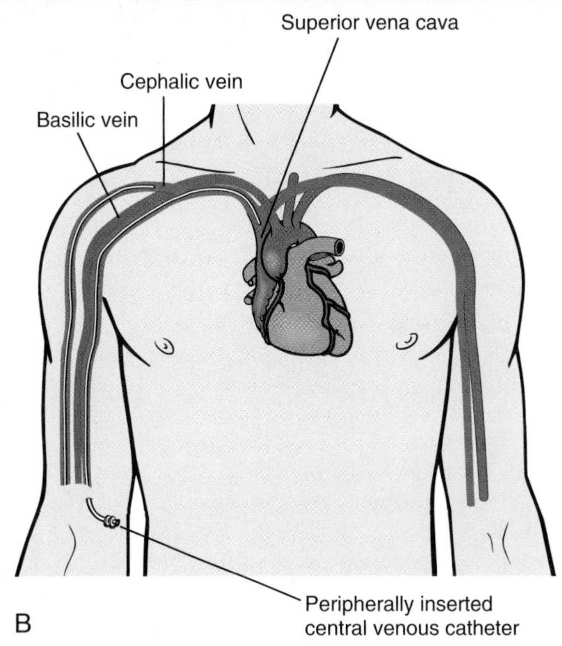

Figure 2-5

A, Peripherally inserted central catheter (PICC) line. **B,** Placement of a PICC line. (**A** from Aehlert B: *Mosby's comprehensive pediatric emergency care*, St Louis, 2007, Mosby; **B** from Perry AG, Potter PA: *Clinical nursing skills and techniques*, ed 6, St Louis, 2006, Mosby.)

Central Venous Access Devices

The two broad categories of central venous access devices (CVADs) are tunneled catheters and nontunneled catheters. To implant a tunneled catheter, the surgeon directs a needle into the subclavian or internal jugular vein and then directs a trocar from the subclavian vein down the chest wall, tunneling toward the nipple level. This leaves a durable silicone catheter well secured into chest tissue. Tunneled catheters are designed for long-term use and can remain in place for years. Hickman, Broviac, Groshong, Hohn, and Leonard catheters are examples of these types of catheters. Some of these catheters are implanted entirely under the skin (e.g., Portacath), whereas others have access ports on the chest wall.

Nontunneled central venous catheters are large-bore catheters that are inserted into the internal jugular, subclavian, or femoral vein. They have one to four lumens and are meant to provide access for several days to 1 to 2 weeks. The life span of the line depends on how well it is maintained.

With any central access device, meticulous attention must be paid to infection control procedures when the device is accessed, and care must be taken not to dislodge the line when the patient is moved.

Peripherally inserted central catheters (PICCs) are common long-term venous access devices. This type of catheter is peripherally inserted (nontunneled) into the medial vessel of the antecubital fossae. The Seldinger technique is used to thread the long catheter to the vena cava, near the right atrium (Figure 2-5).

A Hickman catheter is commonly used for long-term therapy, including drug or fluid therapy, blood sampling, or hyperalimentation. Single-, double-, or triple-lumen catheters are tunneled through the chest wall, and the tip of the catheter usually extends through a central vein and into or near the right atrium. The distal ports have an intermittent infusion port attached. Routine maintenance with saline or low-dose heparin keeps the catheter patent.

Implanted devices also are used for special long-term therapeutic needs, such as chemotherapy (e.g., MediPort and Portacath). A small pocket is created surgically in the subcutaneous tissue of the upper chest or arm, and a central catheter is tunneled into position. A special noncoring needle, called a Huber needle (Figure 2-6), must be used to gain access to these implanted devices.

The care of patients with CVADs during transport can be complex. The critical care team must be trained in the use of these devices (Skill 2-1), and treatment protocols must be established; in addition, ongoing education programs are crucial to the team's skill maintenance.

Skill 2-1

CENTRAL VENOUS ACCESS DEVICES (CVADs): OBTAINING VASCULAR ACCESS

INDICATIONS

Deliver medications, IV solutions, and blood products

Obtain blood samples

CONTRAINDICATIONS

Nonpatent device

Signs of inflammation around device

PREPROCEDURE

Position the patient supine.

Evaluate the access device; if it is an implanted type, palpate the borders and center of the device.

Evaluate for redness, fever, induration, and other signs of infection.

If it is a tunneled, cuffed device, make sure all bulldog clamps are on.

Remove all dressings.

Have a physician verify correct line placement through radiographic confirmation.

EQUIPMENT

- Skin cleansing agent (2% chlorhexidine gluconate [CHG])
- 90-degree, noncoring needle (Huber needle)
- 5-10 mL Luer-Lok syringes (syringes should not be smaller than 5 mL)
- Sterile 2 × 2 gauze sponges
- Tape
- Alcohol pledgets
- 5-10 mL normal saline (NS) flush in prefilled syringes
- Heparin (optional; check device instructions): 100 units/mL concentration
- Luer-Lok cap
- Skin protective agent
- Transparent dressing
- Sterile gloves

Procedure for Implanted Port

1. Perform good hand hygiene before touching any part of the CVAD.
2. Practice standard precautions. Use a sterile field and don sterile gloves to access the device.
3. Open the CVAD access kit and establish a sterile field. Open the sterile supplies onto the sterile field. Prime all tubing and lock devices with NS.
4. Cleanse the device site and surrounding tissue with 2% CHG, scrubbing in a side-to-side fashion for at least 30 seconds.
5. While the tissues air dry, attach the primed tubing to the noncoring needle and flush.
6. Use the nondominant hand to palpate the borders of the implanted device and to stabilize it in the tissues while the dominant hand maneuvers the noncoring needle.
7. Hold the vertical fin of the noncoring needle between the thumb and middle finger of the dominant hand. Press down firmly with the index finger and puncture the skin, penetrating the center of the port at a 90-degree angle.

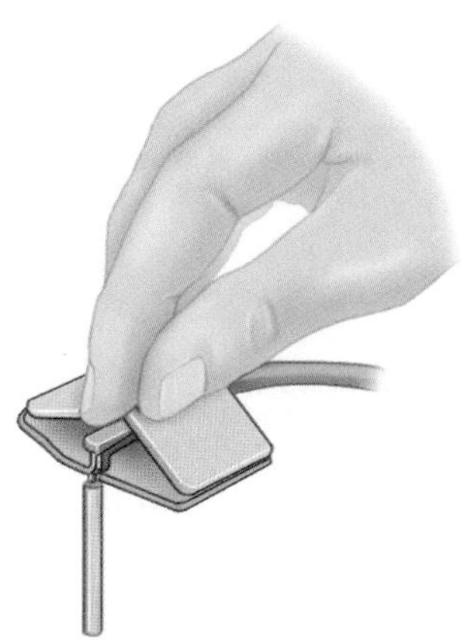

8. Push the noncoring needle firmly through the skin and septum until the back of the port is felt.
9. Attach pre-filled NS syringe to needle connection. Aspirate blood to verify patency. Flush with the attached NS syringe and then clamp the device.
10. While flushing, observe for resistance, pain, or swelling at the site. If any of these is noted, the noncoring needle may not be fully inserted. Readjust the needle and reattempt flushing.
11. Place folded 2 × 2 gauze sponges under needle wings and secure with thin adhesive strips (e.g., Steri-Strips) if needed. Apply a transparent dressing and secure the tubing with tape.
12. Attach the primed IV tubing and begin the infusion by opening the clamp.
13. When the infusion is complete, reestablish the heparin lock on the clamped port by unclamping the port and flushing it with 5 mL of heparin (follow the manufacturer's or institution's instructions for the use of heparin).
14. Close the clamp and remove the noncoring needle by grasping the outer wing edges with the thumb and finger and squeezing the wings together.

Procedure for Tunneled, Cuffed Device

1. Perform good hand hygiene before touching any part of the CVAD.

2. Practice standard precautions. Use a sterile field and don sterile gloves to access the device.
3. Open the CVAD access kit and establish a sterile field. Open the sterile supplies onto the sterile field. Prime all tubing and lock devices with NS.
4. Identify the infusion port. Remove the Luer-Lok cap with the clamp engaged.
5. Vigorously cleanse the port with alcohol or an approved cleansing agent and allow it to air dry.
6. Attach a 5-10 mL, prefilled Luer-Lok syringe, open the clamp, and attempt to aspirate blood. This device should allow easy aspiration and flow; do not use it if resistance is felt.
7. Flush the catheter with NS before use. To prevent the back flow of blood, engage the bulldog clamp while flushing the catheter. Cleanse the port as in step 5.
8. Attach the primed IV tubing and begin the infusion by opening the clamp.
9. When the infusion is complete, follow the manufacturer's or institution's policy for heparin lock or saline lock. Cleanse the port, allow it to air dry, instill a flush solution, and apply the clamp as the solution nears the end of the syringe.

MAINTENANCE

1. Always strictly observe medical aseptic technique to prevent sepsis.
2. Clamp the catheter before entering to prevent air entry or the back flow of blood.
3. Place bulldog clamps on the catheter only for an emergency break and only if the device does not already have a clamp.
4. Groshong catheters: Flush with 10 mL NS after each use. If the catheter is not being used, the device is flushed weekly with NS. Heparin is not necessary for Groshong catheters.

TROUBLESHOOTING

Central lines should allow easy aspiration and flow. If problems occur, rule out catheter obstruction.

1. Check for a mechanical obstruction.
   a. Look for kinks in the tubing and clamp malfunction.
   b. Inspect the exit site for sutures that are too tight.
   c. Make sure the device is not kinked, twisted, or out of place.
2. Change the patient's position.
   a. Have the patient raise the arms forward or above the head.
   b. Position the bed in the Trendelenburg position.

   If the device then flushes, notify the physician that it may be kinked.
3. If allowed, have the patient perform the Valsalva maneuver or take a deep breath and cough as you attempt to irrigate and withdraw blood.
4. If all maneuvers fail, notify the physician.

POSTPROCEDURE

Document the type and amount of medications and fluids infused. Note whether heparin was used for a lock after the infusion was complete and if so, specify its concentration.

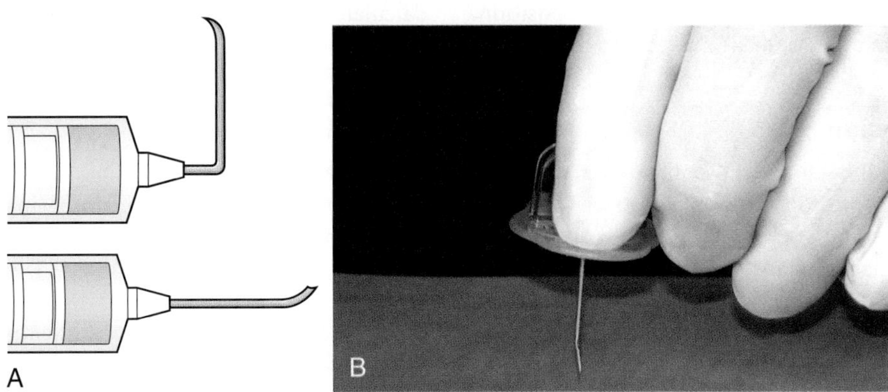

Figure 2-6

Huber needles used to access an implantable device, such as a MediPort or Portacath. **A**, Two types of Huber needles used to enter an implanted port. **B**, Insertion of a Huber needle. (From Perry AG, Potter PA: *Clinical nursing skills and techniques,* ed 6, St Louis, 2006, Mosby.)

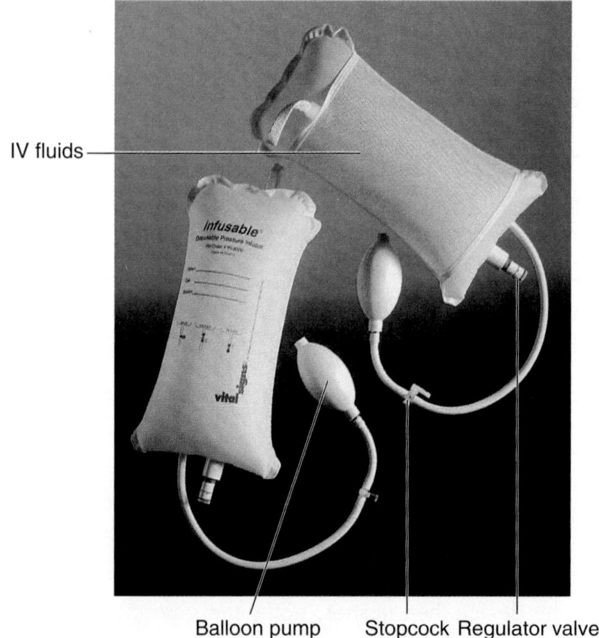

Figure 2-7

A 1000 mL pressure bag. (Courtesy Vital Signs, Totowa, New Jersey.)

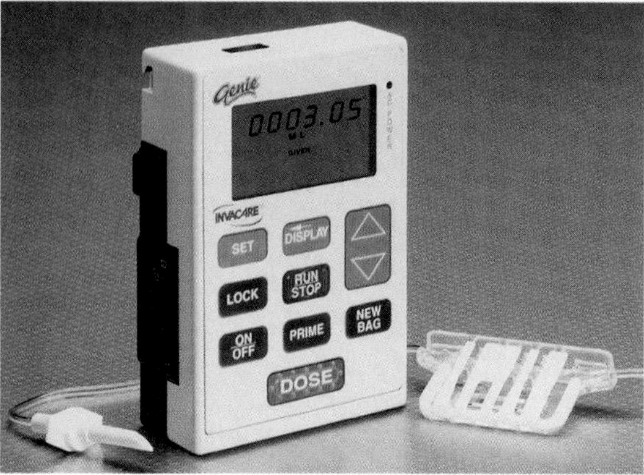

Figure 2-8

External infusion pump. (From Monahan F: *Phipps' medical-surgical nursing: health and illness perspectives,* ed 8, St Louis, 2007, Mosby.)

Intravenous Pressure Bags

Various devices can be used to force fluid out of an IV bag, but the most reliable one is the inflatable IV pressure bag. These bags, available as 500 and 1000 mL pressure bags, can increase the volume through a gravity-flow system. An IV bag sleeve, valve regulator, and stopcock are located in the pressure-inflation tubing. The stopcock must be in the lateral position to inflate the bag. The desired pressure noted on the valve regulator is 300 mm Hg. Once this pressure level has been achieved, the stopcock is turned to the upward position. Deflation occurs when the stopcock is turned downward (Figure 2-7).

Intravenous Infusion Sets

Vented infusion sets allow air to flow into the glass bottle (vacuum), facilitating infusion. Nonvented sets are designed for closed plastic infusion bags.

Volume control chambers are designed for pediatric IV maintenance infusions to prevent an accidental overdose of fluids. The calibrated chamber is prefilled with the timed amount according to the orders given or the patient's weight, and the roller clamp between the chamber and the IV bag is then closed. This device should *not* be used for administration of an IV fluid bolus.

Pump Systems

IV pumps are standard equipment in critical care ambulances. Critical care patients usually have multiple drips running at the same time, and each drug must be managed during transport. Several types of IV pumps are commercially available, and each service should evaluate several makes and models to determine which product best suits their patients' needs. MedStar EMS in Fort Worth, Texas, currently uses the Alaris Ivac Medsystem III 2863 triple chamber pump, which allows crew members to manage up to three drips administered from the same device. Several manufacturers produce IV pumps appropriate for use with critical care patients, such as Alaris, Baxter, Abbott, and IMED, to name a few.

Infusion controllers or pumps provide an accurate means of delivering medications and fluid to the critically ill patient. The critical care team must invest in and maintain its own IV pumps. However, as a team member, you will encounter many different types during the transport of patients from all over your response area. Various pumps have many different modes of set-up (e.g., volumetric [common], infusion controllers, and artificial pancreas; Figures 2-8 and 2-9.) Some pumps calculate rates at less than 1 mL/hour (pediatric use), and others have limited parameters for high rates.

Alternative Routes of Medication Administration

Epidural Route

An epidural catheter is inserted into the epidural space of the vertebral column to deliver regional analgesia or anesthesia.

Patient-Controlled Analgesia or Patient-Controlled Epidural Analgesia

Patient-controlled analgesia (PCA) systems use both venous and epidural sites for pain control. Limits are locked into the system by the practitioner, but the patient controls when the analgesic is given. These systems use syringe pumps, and critical care transport teams may continue their use en route if pump drives are compatible. The major hurdle is leaving a hospital with a syringe loaded with opioids signed out on tracking systems unique to the hospital. If the team transports patients who need these systems, prearrangements

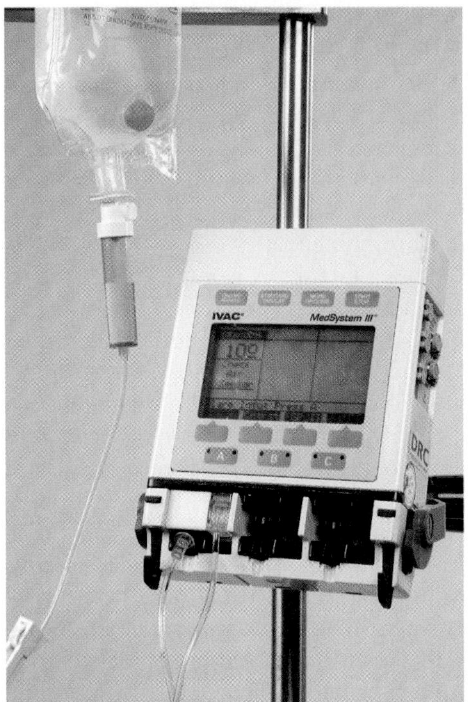

Figure 2-9

Intravenous infusion pump. (From Aehlert B: *Paramedic practice today: above and beyond,* St Louis, 2009, Mosby.)

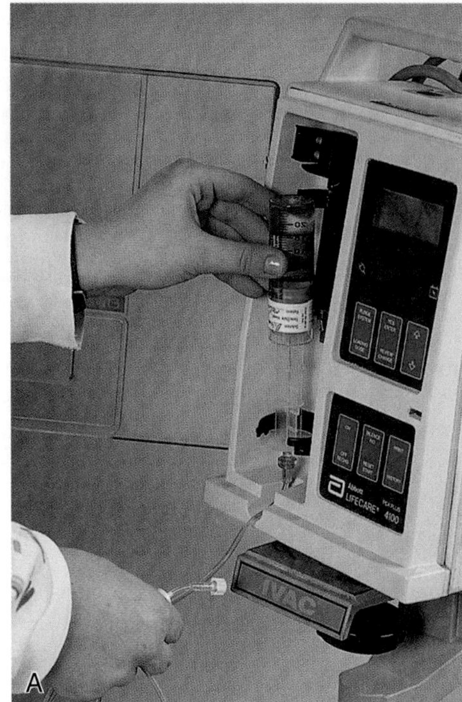

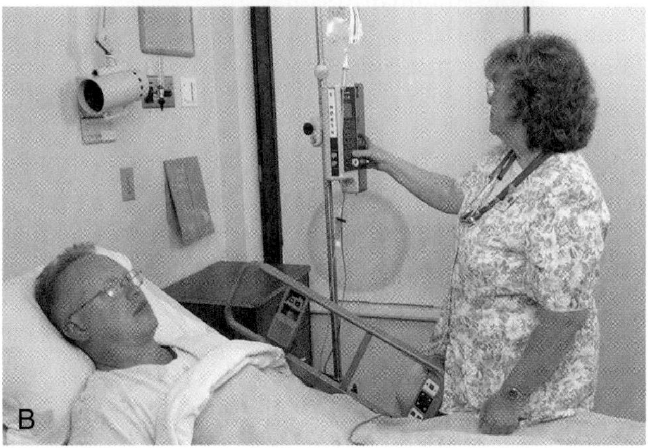

Figure 2-10

A, Patient-controlled analgesia (PCA) pump with syringe chamber, designed for patient- or clinician-activated medication delivery. **B,** The nurse sets the pump to deliver an ordered dose, which the patient can administer by pushing buttons on the handheld device at the bedside. (**A** from Christensen B: *Foundations of nursing,* ed 6, St Louis, 2011, Mosby; **B** from Edmunds M: *Introduction to clinical pharmacology,* St Louis, 2009, Mosby.)

must be made with the hospital, or the team must have special protocols in place (Figure 2-10).

Scenario Conclusion

In the scenario, you had a patient whose heart rate and blood pressure began dropping rapidly right after you started your IV pump with two drugs: nitroglycerin, mixed 50 mg in 250 mL, running at 6 mL/hour; and labetalol, mixed 500 mg in 100 mL, running at 60 mL/hour.

Your partner reaches over and quickly stops both IV infusions on the pump. She then reevaluates the patient. An IV fluid bolus of 250 mL is quickly infused, and the patient's vital signs return to pretransport levels within 5 minutes. The IV drugs are recalculated, and the infusion pump setting is corrected. The rest of the transport is uneventful.

SUMMARY

Critical care is a high-stakes arena in which healthcare providers must apply their knowledge of medications and their uses, often quickly and under emergency conditions. Medications should be administered with confidence and with a clear knowledge of the intended outcome. Therefore, a thorough understanding of critical care pharmacology is vital for each member of the critical care transport team.

KEY TERMS

acetylcholinesterase (AChE) An enzyme of the hydrolase class that catalyzes the cleavage of acetylcholine to choline and acetate. AChE is found in the central nervous system, particularly in the gray matter of nerve tissue; in red blood cells; and in the motor end plates of skeletal muscle.

activated partial thromboplastin time (aPTT, APTT) The partial thromboplastin time (PTT) or activated partial thromboplastin time is a performance indicator that measures the efficacy of both the "intrinsic" pathway (now referred to as the *contact activation pathway*) and the common coagulation pathway. It detects blood clotting abnormalities and also is used to monitor the treatment effects of heparin, a major anticoagulant.

Adams syndrome A condition of episodic cardiac arrest and syncope caused by the failure of normal and escape pacemakers, with or without ventricular fibrillation; it is the principal clinical manifestation of severe heart block.

antithrombin III An alpha$_2$ globulin of the serpin family that is synthesized in the liver and found in plasma and various extravascular sites. It inactivates thrombin in a time-dependent, irreversible reaction. It also inhibits certain other proteinases with serine active sites, including coagulation Factors Xa, XIIa, XIa, and IXa, and kallikrein. An inherited deficiency of the protein, a rare autosomal dominant disorder, is associated with recurrent deep vein thrombosis and pulmonary emboli. The complications are prevented and (in conjunction with heparin) treated with a preparation of antithrombin III from pooled human plasma that is administered intravenously.

Bioavailability The degree to which a drug or other substance becomes available to the target tissue after administration.

catecholomethyltransferase (COMT) An intracellular enzyme located in the postsynaptic neuron that is involved in the inactivation of the catecholamine neurotransmitters (dopamine, epinephrine, and norepinephrine). COMT introduces a methyl group, donated by S-adenosylmethionine (SAM), to the catecholamine. Any compound with a catechol structure (e.g., catecholestrogens and catechol-containing flavonoids) is a substrate of COMT.

clopidogrel A platelet aggregation inhibitor that is administered orally and used as an antithrombotic to prevent myocardial infarction, stroke, and vascular death in patients with atherosclerosis.

cytochrome P450 2D6 (CYP2D6) A member of the cytochrome P450 mixed-function oxidase system and an important enzyme involved in the metabolism of xenobiotics. CYP2D6 is involved in the oxidation of a wide range of substrates of all the cytochrome P450 enzymes (CYPs), but its expression in the liver varies considerably. The gene is located near two cytochrome P450 pseudogenes on chromosome 22q13.1. Alternatively spliced transcript variants encoding different isoforms have been found for this gene.

erythematous A descriptive term for redness of the skin caused by capillary congestion (i.e., erythema). The condition can be caused by infection, massage, electrical treatments, acne medications, allergies, exercise, solar radiation (sunburn), or waxing and plucking of hairs; all of these can cause capillary dilation, resulting in redness. Erythema is a common side effect of radiotherapy treatment, because the patient is exposed to ionizing radiation.

Factor II (prothrombin) A plasma protein that is converted to the active form, thrombin (Factor IIa) by cleavage by activated Factor X (Xa) in the common pathway of blood coagulation. Thrombin cleaves fibrinogen to its active form, fibrin. Deficiency of Factor II leads to hypoprothrombinemia.

Factor X (Stuart factor) A storage-stable factor that participates in both the intrinsic and extrinsic pathways of blood coagulation, uniting them to begin the common pathway of coagulation. Once activated, it forms a complex with calcium, phospholipid, and Factor V; the complex (prothrombinase) can cleave and activate prothrombin to thrombin. Deficiency of this factor may cause a systemic coagulation disorder. It also is called *autoprothrombin C, Prower factor,* and *Stuart-Prower factor.* The activated form is also called *thrombokinase.*

G protein Any of a family of similar heterotrimeric proteins of the intracellular portion of the plasma membrane that bind activated receptor complexes and, through conformational changes and cyclic binding and hydrolysis of GTP, directly or indirectly effect alterations in channel gating, thereby coupling cell surface receptors to intracellular responses. Some G proteins are named for their activities (e.g., G_s stimulates and G_i inhibits enzyme activity).

glomerular filtration rate (GFR) The amount of glomerular filtrate formed per unit of time in all nephrons of both kidneys, equal to the inulin clearance; usually measured clinically by the endogenous creatinine clearance.

implanted port A catheter that is tunneled beneath the skin that has a subcutaneous port attached to a reservoir with a self-sealing septum. It is accessed with a noncoring needle.

monamine oxidase (MAO) A mitochondrial enzyme present in many tissues that plays a vital role in the regulation of catecholamines in nerve endings of the peripheral sympathetic nervous system.

muscarinic receptors A term denoting the effects of muscarine or acetylcholine at muscarinic receptors. G protein-coupled acetylcholine receptors are found in the plasma of certain neurons. They act as the end-receptor stimulated by acetylcholine, released by the parasympathetic nervous system.

myasthenia gravis A disorder of neuromuscular function caused by the presence of antibodies to acetylcholine receptors at the neuromuscular junction; characteristics include muscle fatigue and exhaustion (which tend to fluctuate in severity) without sensory disturbance or atrophy. The manifestations may be restricted to one muscle group or may become generalized, marked by severe weakness and sometimes ventilatory insufficiency. The disease may affect any muscle of the body, but the muscles most frequently involved are those of the eye, face, lips, tongue, throat, and neck. Also called

Erb-Goldflam disease, Goldflam's disease, or *Goldflam-Erb disease.*

nicotinic receptors Cholinergic receptors that are stimulated initially and blocked at high doses by the alkaloid nicotine and blocked by tubocurarine; they are found on autonomic ganglion cells, on striated muscle, and on spinal central neurons.

nontunneled central venous catheters Noncuffed catheters that are placed by a cutdown or percutaneous approach and secured by sutures or an intact dressing.

nucleoside A heterocyclic nitrogenous base, particularly a purine or pyrimidine, in N-glycosidic linkage with a sugar, particularly a pentose; it often is used specifically to denote a compound obtained by hydrolysis of nucleic acids, a purine or pyrimidine linked to ribose or deoxyribose (e.g., adenosine or cytidine).

pharmacokinetic factors The activity or fate of drugs in the body over a period of time, including the processes of absorption, distribution, localization in tissues, biotransformation, and excretion.

phenylephrine A direct-acting sympathomimetic amine that stimulates alpha-adrenergic receptors and is a powerful vasoconstrictor.

pheochromocytoma A usually benign, well-encapsulated, lobular, vascular tumor of chromaffin tissue of the adrenal medulla or sympathetic paraganglia. Because of increased secretion of epinephrine and norepinephrine, intermittent or persistent hypertension is a cardinal symptom of this tumor. During severe attacks, the individual may have headache, sweating, palpitations and tremors, pallor or flushing of the face, nausea and vomiting, pain in the chest and abdomen, and paresthesias of the extremities. Also called a medullary chromaffinoma, medullary paraganglioma, chromaffin cell tumor, and pheochromoblastoma.

postganglionic Situated posterior or distal to a ganglion; said especially of autonomic nerve fibers so located.

preganglionic Situated anterior or proximal to a ganglion; said especially of autonomic nerve fibers so located.

presynaptic A term that means "before the synapse." The synapse is the site of functional apposition between neurons, the point where an impulse is transmitted from one neuron to another.

thiocyanate A salt produced in the metabolism of cysteine and the detoxification of cyanide; it is excreted in the urine.

tunneled, cuffed catheters Catheters implanted in the subclavian, internal jugular, or femoral vein that have a cuff to prevent the migration of organisms into the tract.

REFERENCE

1. Ekoé J-M et al: *The epidemiology of diabetes mellitus: an international perspective*, Chichester, England, 2001, John Wiley & Sons.

Bibliography

American Diabetes Association website at www.diabetes.org.

Baselt RC: *Disposition of toxic drugs and chemicals in man*, ed 3, St Louis, 1989, Year Book Medical.

Bauer LA: *Applied clinical pharmacokinetics*, New York, 2001, McGraw-Hill.

Brunton LL et al, editors: *Goodman and Gilman's the pharmacological basis of therapeutics*, ed 11, New York, 2006, McGraw-Hill.

Burton ME et al, editors: *Applied pharmacokinetics and pharmacodynamics*, ed 4, Philadelphia, 2006, Lippincott Williams & Wilkins.

Clarke TC et al: The metabolism of clopidogrel is catalyzed by human cytochrome P450 3A and is inhibited by atorvastatin, *Drug Metab Dispos* 31:53-59, 2003.

McKenry L, Tessier E, Hogan MA: *Mosby's pharmacology in nursing*, ed 22, St Louis, 2006, Mosby.

Rogers JF et al: Pharmacogenetics effects, dosing, efficacy, and toxicity of cytochrome P450–metabolized drugs, *Am J Med* 113:746-750, 2002.

Sanders MJ: *Mosby's paramedic textbook*, St Louis, 1994, Mosby.

Viera-Negron E: *Diabetes in the hospital: epidemiology*. Arizona Diabetes Association (website). www.azdiabetes.org/meetings/azdin_060105/vensor.ppt. Accessed March 2007.

REVIEW QUESTIONS

1. In the opening scenario, the patient is receiving IV nitroglycerin and labetalol: nitroglycerin, 200 mcg/mL, at 20 mcg/min and labetalol, 5 mcg/mL, at 10 mcg/hour. (To check the correct dosage of these two drugs, please refer to the Drug Guide on the Evolve site for *Transport of the Critical Care Patient.*) What is the normal dose for nitroglycerin and labetalol and to what setting should the IV pumps have been dialed to achieve those doses?
   A. The nitroglycerin was in the correct dosing range, but the labetalol dose was too high. The pump for the labetalol should have been set to 12 to 36 mL/hour.
   B. The nitroglycerin dose was incorrect. The pump should have been dialed to 60 mL/hour; the labetalol was administered correctly.
   C. Both drugs were being given correctly. The patient's response was exaggerated because of heart disease.
   D. Both drugs were being administered in incorrect dosages. The nitroglycerin should have been given at 100 mL/hour and the labetalol at 2 mL/hour.
2. In the opening scenario, what procedure should the critical care transport team have performed before transport that would have prevented this medication error?
   A. They should have called medical control for approval to continue administration of the medications at those dosages.
   B. They should have reviewed the patient's history and physical examination findings.
   C. They should have recalculated the drug mix, the amount per milliliter, and the normal dosage range before administering the drugs via the transport team's pumps.
   D. They should have scolded the local hospital's nursing staff for inappropriate care, called the hospital's pharmacy for consultation, and reported them all to the state authorities.
3. The team is about to administer a drug that affects cardiac and smooth muscle. The cholinergic receptor responsible for action in this tissue is the:
   A. ACh receptor
   B. Exocrine receptor
   C. Muscarinic receptor
   D. Nicotinic receptor
4. A $beta_2$ antagonist may be used to relax or reduce activity in the:
   A. Brain
   B. Heart
   C. Stomach
   D. Uterus
5. $Alpha_1$ antagonism would cause the patient to experience:
   A. An increase in the heart rate
   B. Constriction of the bronchi
   C. A drop in blood pressure
   D. Gut dilation
6. The dose of a medication should be adjusted for an obese patient if:
   A. The drug is filtered through the liver.
   B. The drug is distributed to adipose tissues.
   C. The patient has kidney stones.
   D. Opiates are being used.
7. An emaciated patient is started on phenytoin to prevent seizures. Within 1 week, the patient has symptoms of phenytoin toxicity, even though the serum levels are within normal limits. What may be causing this?
   A. The loss of skeletal muscle has caused the drug to become too easily available in the liver.
   B. The patient obviously has liver disease.
   C. The drug dose must be too high, and the laboratory results are incorrect.
   D. This protein-bound medication has too few albumin and is readily available in the bloodstream.
8. The drug reference states that a drug's half-life is 1 hour. This indicates that:
   A. The therapeutic plasma level is achieved in 1 hour.
   B. Half of the drug will be eliminated within 1 hour.
   C. The drug should be given every hour.
   D. The therapeutic plasma level will be gone in 1 hour.
9. Which statement is correct about anticoagulation, antiplatelet, and fibrinolytic therapy?
   A. Antiplatelet medications reduce the number of platelets.
   B. Anticoagulation therapy prevents clot formation.
   C. Fibrinolytics prevent clots from forming in the bloodstream.
   D. These three medications thin the blood.
10. The transport team performs the procedure for accessing a tunneled, cuffed CVAD, but initial aspiration produces no blood return. The team can find no mechanical obstruction. What troubleshooting methods might they use to facilitate flow?
   A. Have the patient cough or perform the Valsalva maneuver during aspiration.
   B. Elevate the head of the patient's bed while aspirating.
   C. Escort the patient to fluoroscopy for direct visualization.
   D. Dilute the blood by irrigating with 1 L of saline and then aspirate.

CHAPTER 3

Respiratory System

OBJECTIVES

1. Apply the principles of respiratory anatomy, physiology, and pathophysiology to the assessment and management of a critically ill patient.
2. Identify a patient in need of airway and ventilatory support.
3. Formulate a plan for airway and ventilatory support.
4. Discuss the special problems associated with patients who have artificial airways or are dependent on a ventilator.

Scenario

Your team is dispatched to a 150-bed hospital with a five-bed adult intensive care unit (ICU). The hospital has a 19-year-old patient with pneumonia who is on a ventilator, and the staff is having difficulty oxygenating him. The hospital official tells the dispatcher that the pulmonary specialist is going on vacation, and no one is available to take care of this patient.

On arrival, you find the patient, who is 74 inches tall and weighs 200 pounds (90 kg), in a supine position. He has an 8-mm tracheal tube, which is connected to a ventilator that is sounding the alarm for high pressure. You attach your capnography device and note that the carbon dioxide level (CO_2) is 45 mm Hg; you also note incomplete exhalation. Pulse oximetry shows 90%. When you auscultate the patient's lung fields, you hear diffuse crackles, and a recent chest radiograph shows patchy white areas in both lungs.

You also learn the following facts about the patient:

- The most recent arterial blood gas (ABG) results are: pH, 7.36; arterial carbon dioxide pressure ($PaCO_2$), 48 mm Hg; base excess (BE), 0; bicarbonate (HCO_3), 22 mEq/L; arterial oxygen pressure (PaO_2), 60 mm Hg.
- The ventilator settings are: assist-control (A/C) mode; 100% oxygen; tidal volume (V_T), 900 mL; rate, 18/min; positive end-expiratory pressure (PEEP), 12 cm H_2O. You note that the sensitivity settings are very low; therefore, the machine does not count the patient's spontaneous respirations.
- One chest tube has been placed in the right axillary line. The pleural drainage system is fluctuating and has no air leaks, and there is a small amount of serosanguinous fluid in the collection chamber.
- The patient has two peripheral intravenous (IV) lines in place. Dopamine is running at 20 mcg/kg/min (800 mg in 250 mL; 34 mL/hour/pump), and the 2nd IV has normal saline running at 100 mL/hour. The patient's pulse is 110 beats/min, and his blood pressure (BP) is 100/70 mm Hg.
- The patient has been receiving intermittent doses of midazolam for restlessness, and he makes attempts at spontaneous respiration.
- Five days ago, the patient developed influenza A; on day 3, he developed pneumonia with respiratory failure. He has had intermittent periods of hypotension and developed a pneumothorax on day 4. Oxygenating him has become increasingly difficult, even with administration of 100% oxygen and the addition of therapeutic PEEP.

You organize your equipment and begin to switch him to your preset ventilator. However, as soon as you disconnect him from the hospital's ventilator, he desaturates and his heart rate drops significantly. You quickly reconnect him to the hospital's ventilator, and he stabilizes within a few seconds.

This chapter reviews the respiratory system, first the airways and then the breathing aspects of critical care. It addresses the relevant anatomy and physiology, some of the major disease processes encountered in critical care and the treatment of airway compromise, medication-assisted intubation, and ventilation assistance with supporting diagnostics.

The respiratory system performs several functions. For example, the main purpose of the lungs is to bring oxygen inside the body and exchange it for carbon dioxide. The respiratory system also aids in acid-base balance, metabolism, speech, and defense of the lungs. To understand how all these functions are accomplished, you must know what resources the respiratory system has to use, the mechanisms by which those resources are used, and ways the respiratory system can be manipulated when problems arise.

RESPIRATION AND VENTILATION

Two terms commonly used in discussions of the respiratory system are *respiration* and *ventilation*. **Ventilation** is the cyclic process of moving air into and out of the lungs. The first part of this cycle is *inspiration* (or, the **inspiratory time [I time, T_I]**); the second part is *expiration* (or, the **expiratory time [E time, T_E]**), which lasts twice as long as the T_I. **Respiration** is the process of gas exchange. To understand how ventilation and respiration work interdependently, critical care students must understand both basic anatomy, which is involved with ventilation, and physiology, which is more closely associated with respiration.

ANATOMY AND PHYSIOLOGY

Airway and Airway Patency

Airway assessment is crucial in patients with respiratory problems, because they must depend on the airway not only for the passage of air into and out of the lungs, but also for defense of the lung through coughing and mucociliary transport. As with any assessment, both the objective and subjective components must be considered.

The Airway

The structures of the respiratory system are divided into the upper and lower **airways.** These divisions indicate the structures' location relative to the vocal cords. For the purpose of this section, all airway structures above the glottis are considered the upper airway, and those below the glottis are considered the lower airway (Figure 3-1).

Upper Airway

The upper part of the respiratory system, or upper airway, includes the nose, mouth, laryngopharynx, and larynx. The floor of the nasal cavity is composed of the hard palate, and the lateral walls are formed by bony ridges coated with respiratory mucosa. The sinuses are cavities in the bones of the skull that connect to the nasal cavities by small channels. The back of each nasal cavity opens into the nasopharynx, which is the superior part of the pharynx. The nasopharynx extends from the internal nares to the level of the uvula. As is the nasal cavity, the nasopharynx is lined with mucous membrane. At the level of the uvula, the nasopharynx ends and the oropharynx begins. The oropharynx extends down to the level of the epiglottis; this oral cavity is made up of the lips, cheeks, teeth, tongue (which is attached to the mandible), and hard and soft palates.

The laryngopharynx, which extends from the tip of the epiglottis to the glottis and the esophagus, is lined with mucous membrane, which protects the internal surfaces from abrasion.

The larynx (Figure 3-2) has three main roles: It serves as the air passageway between the pharynx and the lungs; it acts as a protective sphincter that prevents solids and liquids from passing into the respiratory tree; and it is involved in the production of speech. The most inferior cartilage of the larynx is the unpaired cricoid cartilage, the only complete cartilaginous ring in the larynx.

Did You Know?

The lungs stay inflated because the pressure surrounding them (*intrapleural* pressure) is always lower than the pressure within them (*intrapulmonary* pressure). Why?

The intrapleural pressure is always lower than the intrapulmonary pressure and the atmospheric pressure; it is considered negative because of the "pull" of the two pleural membranes in opposite directions. The parietal pleura, which is attached to the chest wall, is pulled outward because the elastic fibers in the intercostal muscles exert outward pressure on the ribs. These fibers are in a relaxed state when the rib cage is fully expanded (e.g., during a deep inhalation). The visceral pleura, which is attached to the lungs, is pulled inward because the elastic fibers in the lungs, which are responsible for elastic recoil, exert pressure to make the lungs smaller. Elastic fibers in the lungs are relaxed only when the lung is at its smallest configuration (e.g., during maximal exhalation).

Therefore, because of the opposite pull of the chest wall and the lungs and because the pleural membranes are attached to these structures, the two membranes constantly pull in opposite directions. The subatmospheric pressure that results within the pleural space, plus the higher than atmospheric intrapulmonary pressure within the lungs, allows the lungs to remain inflated. If for some reason (open chest wall) the pressure within the pleural space rises to atmospheric pressure or higher, one or both lungs collapse, a condition known as *pneumothorax.*

Lower Airway

The chest wall is made up of the rib cage, the skeletal muscles, and the pleurae. The ribs provide a flexible cage capable of expanding with the pull of the muscles of the chest. The pleurae are two membranes that arise from the mediastinum and wrap around the lungs, providing a lining inside the chest wall. The pleura reduces friction between the lungs

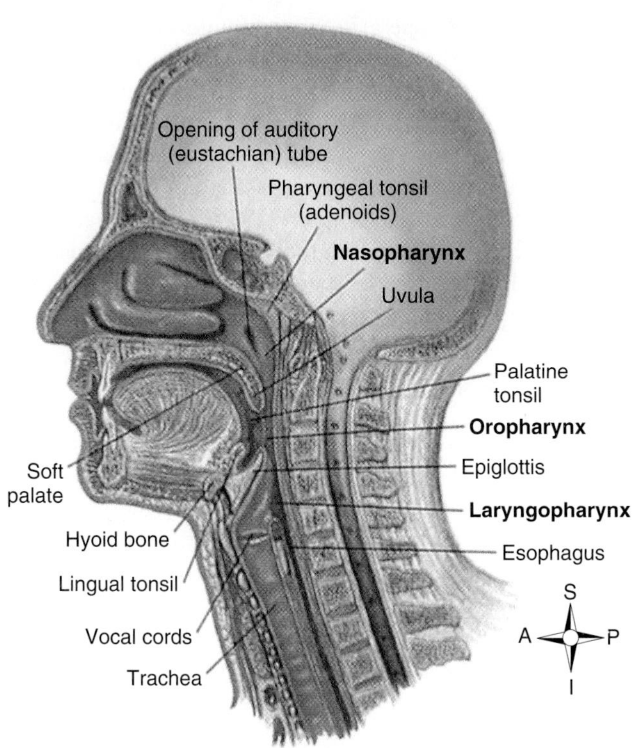

Figure 3-1

Airway structures. (From Sanders M: *Mosby's paramedic textbook,* ed 3, St Louis, 2007, Mosby.)

and the chest wall as the lungs inflate and deflate. The primary muscle of ventilation is the diaphragm.

The use of skeletal muscles around the thoracic cage produces a bellows action as the lungs inflate and deflate. These muscles are considered accessory, or secondary, muscles of respiration. They include the sternocleidomastoids, scalenes, pectorals, and serratus on inspiration and the internal and external obliques and rectus abdominis on expiration. A normal patient at rest does not need to use these muscles. An increase in the work of breathing, which often is defined as use of the accessory muscles of respiration, is an indicator of respiratory muscle fatigue and impending ventilatory failure.

The lung consists of three basic units: the upper airway, the bronchial tree, and the lung parenchyma. The upper airway is composed of the nasal passages, oral cavity, nasopharynx, oropharynx, and glottis, and the larynx, which houses the vocal cords. The airways, both the upper and lower bronchial tree, are divided into two categories: the **conducting airways,** which do not contribute to gas exchange, and the **functional airways,** which are capable of gas exchange. These functional or respiratory airways are referred to in this chapter as *terminal* or *respiratory* bronchioles and are considered part of the lung parenchyma.

The terminal bronchioles branch into respiratory bronchioles, which are smaller in diameter and contain tissue capable of gas exchange. The lung **parenchyma** is made up of respiratory bronchioles and alveoli, which are tiny, thin-walled air sacs that are the primary sites of gas exchange. The alveoli are

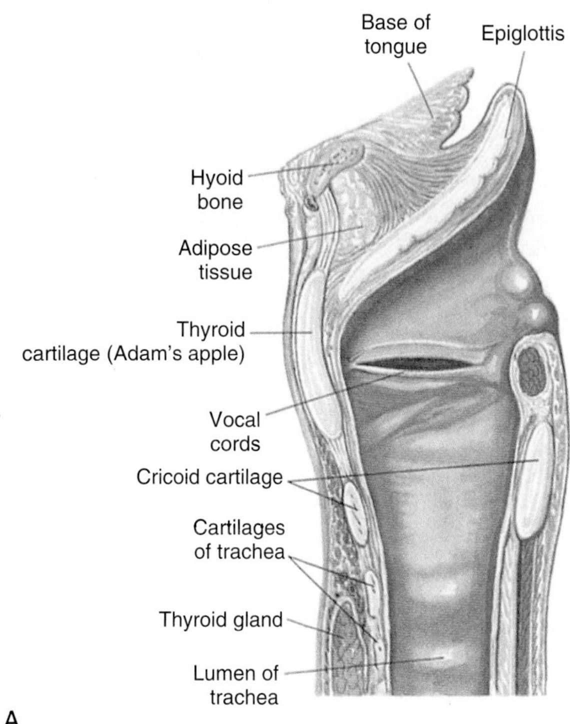

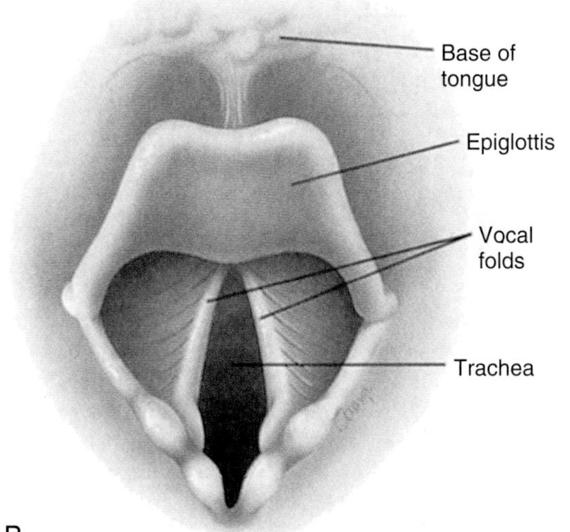

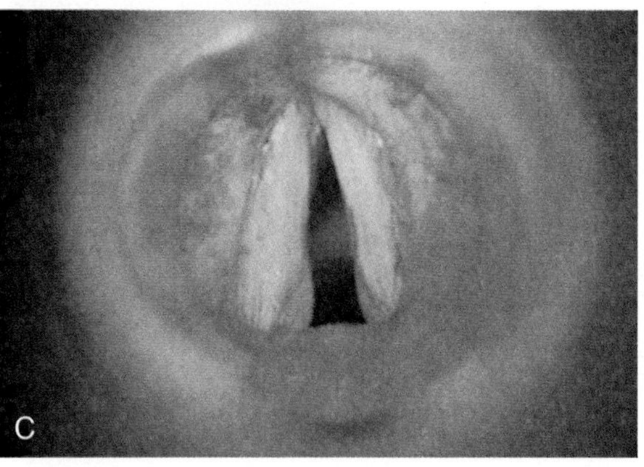

Figure 3-2

Larynx. **A,** Sagittal section. **B,** Superior view. **C,** Endoscopic image. (From Sanders M: *Mosby's paramedic textbook,* ed 3, St Louis, 2007, Mosby.)

lined with surfactant, which reduces surface tension inside the air sac and prevents their collapse during exhalation. The alveoli are surrounded by a network of pulmonary capillaries. The lung tissue itself has a spongy texture and is lightweight because of the air in the alveoli. It also is extremely elastic; this allows the lungs to stretch and enlarge during inhalation and then passively recoil, while maintaining their shape, during exhalation (Figures 3-3 to 3-5).

Perfusion of the lung naturally follows gravity, and the development of pulmonary capillaries increases in the lower lobes. Ventilation follows perfusion, but many things can alter either of these two factors, including the patient's position, level of consciousness, degree of pain, and any disease processes.

The term **dead space ventilation** refers to areas of the lung that are underventilated. Two types of dead space may be seen in the lung, anatomic dead space and physiologic dead space. **Anatomic dead space** refers to the conducting airways, including artificial airway devices. **Physiologic dead space** includes both the anatomic dead space and the areas of the lung parenchyma that do not contribute to gas exchange. Physiologic dead space occurs either because of an inability to ventilate the area or because perfusion of the area is impaired.

The relationship between ventilation and perfusion is expressed as a ratio **(V/Q)**; it is approximately matched in a normal lung (V/Q = 0.8 to 1). Matching of ventilation and perfusion maintains normal gas exchange in the lung.

V/Q mismatch refers to an anatomic or a physiologic diversion of ventilation and perfusion away from airways (shunt) and it is an indicator of impaired gas exchange. When a disease process causes V/Q mismatch, critical care management efforts must include methods to dilate the vessels around the alveoli and recruit gas exchange airways (these methods are discussed later in the chapter). The goal is to match ventilation with perfusion without producing systemic vasodilation. Most disease processes that alter pulmonary function do so by causing varying degrees of V/Q mismatch.

ASSESSMENT

Textbooks and instructors make it sound so simple: "You should assess and manage the ABCs." You know that airway assessment and management are important. The steps of the process may be easy to read and easy to write, but often they are very difficult to accomplish.

Assessment of the Airway

The three assessment parameters—look, listen, and feel—do not really have much to do with airway assessment; they are best saved for the breathing assessment. Assessment of the airway begins with your across-the-room (or across-the-scene) evaluation of the patient. From across the room, the patient should look up at you and should have no unusual airway noises. If this is not the case, a quick primary

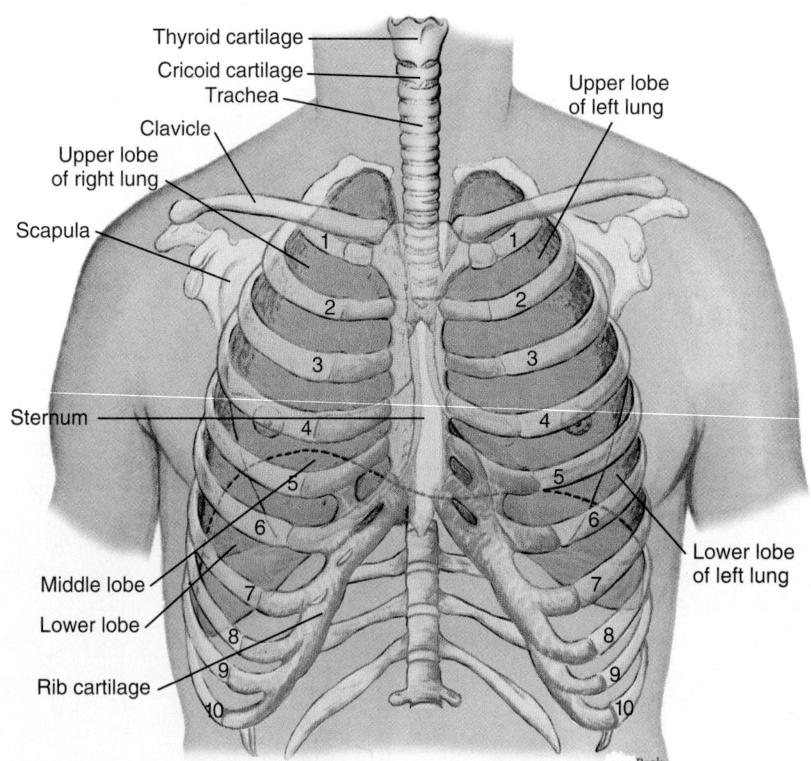

Figure 3-3

Ventilatory structures of the chest wall and lungs, including the ribs (numbered) and the lobes of the lungs. Each intercostal space takes the number of the rib above it. The dotted line indicates the location of the diaphragm at inhalation and exhalation. Note the apex of each lung rising above the clavicle. (From Thibodeau GA: *Anthony's textbook of anatomy and physiology*, ed 18, St Louis, 2009, Mosby.)

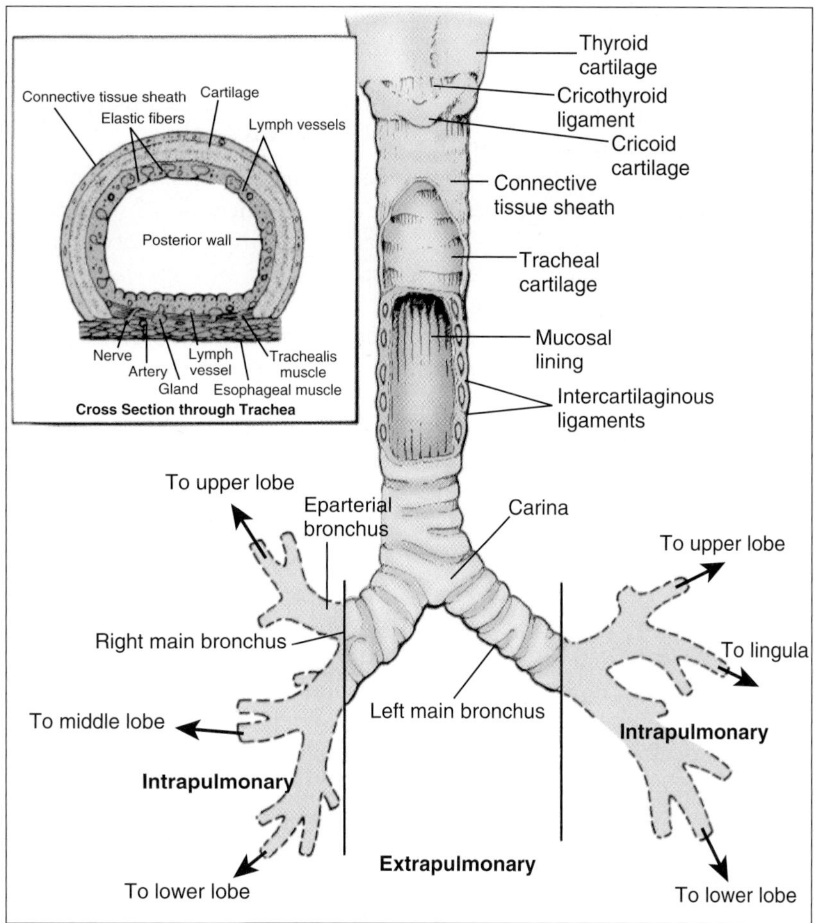

Figure 3-4

Anterior view of the trachea and primary bronchi and a cross section through part of the trachea, including a C-shaped cartilaginous element. (From Martin DE: *Respiratory anatomy and physiology,* St Louis, 1988, Mosby.)

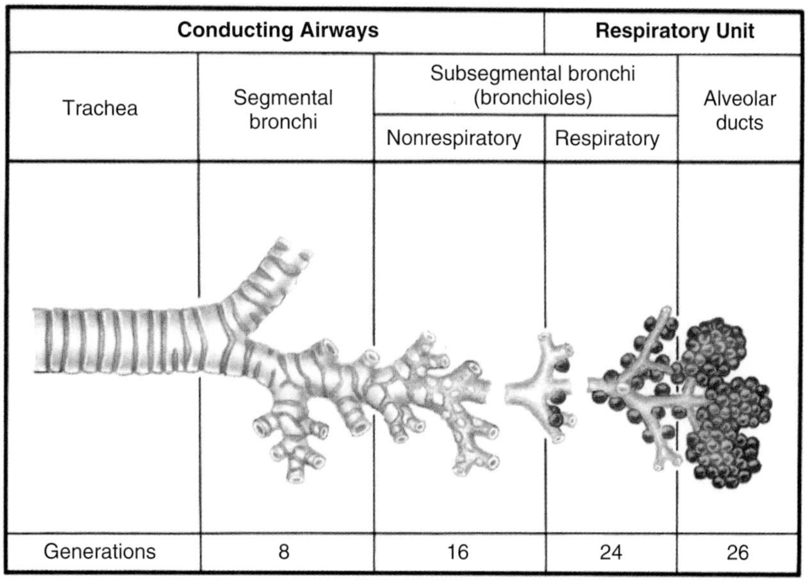

Conducting Airways			Respiratory Unit	
Trachea	Segmental bronchi	Subsegmental bronchi (bronchioles)		Alveolar ducts
		Nonrespiratory	Respiratory	
Generations	8	16	24	26

Figure 3-5

Conducting and functional airways. Note the branching with increasing generations. (From Thompson JM et al: *Mosby's clinical nursing,* ed 5, St Louis, 2002, Mosby.)

assessment must be performed at the patient's side, for two reasons: airway patency and airway protection (level of consciousness).

For the airway assessment in the primary survey, you must determine the patient's level of consciousness. Is he awake now? Can he protect his airway? Will I need to perform airway maneuvers on the patient now or in the next few minutes to protect the airway?

To determine airway patency, look inside the mouth. Are secretions, blood, vomitus, loose teeth, or other debris present in the orifice that need to be suctioned? The most important airway tools you have are your gloved hands and a good suction device.

In many critical care transport patients, airway devices already have been inserted. Once you have assessed the mouth for debris, check any foreign devices in the upper airway. If the patient already has an adjunct in place, evaluate that device for patency and effectiveness. Will you need to upgrade this device? Keep in mind the old adage, "If it ain't broke, don't fix it." (The decision whether to change from one airway device to another is discussed later in the chapter.)

Remember: During airway management in a trauma patient, always keep the patient in a neutral spine position. Make sure the patient's ear canal is in a straight line with the sternal notch. Provide neutral, in-line immobilization devices according to your protocols. Spine boards may be applied before transport.

Cough and Airway Assessment

The presence of sputum with cough complicates the patient's ability to maintain a patent airway. Pneumonia, cystic fibrosis, bronchiectasis, pulmonary abscess, and pulmonary carcinoma all produce purulent sputum. The volume and texture of the sputum may affect airway clearance. The thicker the secretions, the more difficult they are to clear. If the patient's ability to cough is impaired, an alternative plan must be made to maintain a patent airway. A means of suctioning to clear the airway, especially an artificial airway, should be available. Oxygen and a bag-valve-mask device also should be available in the event of respiratory compromise.

If the patient is unable to produce a spontaneous cough or to clear the airway of secretions, airway maintenance becomes a mechanical procedure and requires the use of an aseptic suctioning technique (patients who are not intubated) or a sterile suctioning technique (intubated patients and those with a tracheotomy). In patients who are not intubated, suctioning of the lower airway is best accomplished by the nasotracheal route. Care should be taken with a blind suctioning technique, because it may cause laryngospasm and surface trauma to the tracheal mucosa.

Suctioning of an intubated patient is more easily accomplished but still requires caution. Hitting the surface of the carina and lower trachea with the tip of the suction catheter can leave "pock marks" on the carina and remove portions of the mucosal wall, interfering with the lungs' natural defense mechanism. The use of closed system suction catheters has greatly reduced the incidence of infection of the lower respiratory tract during ventilation and also helps maintain constant levels of PEEP.

Assessment of the Respiratory System—Look, Listen, and Feel

Look, listen, and feel, mentioned earlier, are the general steps in the assessment of the respiratory system (typically the "B" part of the circulation, airway, and breathing [CAB] primary examination).

Look: Symmetry and Breathing Patterns

On arrival at the bedside, you should be able to look at the thorax for chest **excursion** and the respiratory pattern (Table 3-1). Excursion should be bilateral and evenly distributed side to side. Uneven excursion suggests uneven distribution of ventilation. Common causes of uneven excursion are trauma (e.g., flail chest), tension pneumothorax, neuromuscular impairment, and intubation of the right mainstem bronchus. An abnormal respiratory pattern suggests that the **work of breathing (WOB),** or the amount of energy expended to accomplish ventilation, is increasing. Everyone expends energy in breathing, but this work usually is not noticeable.

Stable, normal respiratory efforts consume approximately 5% to 10% of cardiac output. With a severe, underlying illness (e.g., septic shock or acute respiratory distress syndrome [ARDS]), this can increase to 50% of total cardiac output, which severely impairs the body's ability to protect other vital organs.

Use of the accessory muscles (i.e., the sternocleidomastoids and scalenes) is another indicator of chronic obstructive disease, failure of the respiratory pump, and chronic muscle fatigue. *A paradoxical breathing pattern indicates severe acute respiratory muscle fatigue and almost certainly signals impending ventilatory failure.* A patient with paradoxical respirations requires immediate intervention either by intubation or the use of noninvasive ventilation.

A paradoxical breathing pattern in an intubated patient indicates a condition called **asynchronous ventilation** (also called *dyssynchrony*) and requires immediate attention. This usually is a sign that the patient is fighting the endotracheal tube and the ventilator. Sedation and/or the use of paralytic drugs may be the first step in managing this situation. If the patient is already medicated, inadequate flow from the ventilator may be the cause of the problem. Asynchronous ventilation, which can lead to tension pneumothorax, often can be resolved by adjusting the volume-controlled ventilator settings. If the patient has not been chemically paralyzed, a temporary switch to pressure support modes can ease the problem while the underlying factors (e.g., sedation, mandatory ventilator settings) are investigated and adjusted.

Tachypnea is easily recognized; this condition may be tolerated in a patient with chronic respiratory disease if the patient is able to maintain adequate acid-base balance and is not at risk for hypoxia. Quiet tachypnea (i.e., no increase in the WOB) may be a sign of acidosis and various other pathophysiologic conditions.

Table 3-1 Respiratory Patterns

Pattern	Manifestation	Disease
Eupnea	Normal respiratory rate: 12-20/min, slower during sleep	None
Tachypnea	Increased rate: >24/min	Pain, acidosis, sepsis, pneumonia, pulmonary edema
Bradypnea	Decreased rate: <10/min	Drug overdose, increased intracranial pressure
Apnea	No respirations	Death
Hyperpnea	Increased depth of respiration	Head injury
Hypopnea	Decreased rate and depth of respiration	Central apnea
Hyperventilation	Increased rate and depth of respiration	Asthma, chronic respiratory failure, acute head injury, anxiety
Kussmaul's respirations	Increased effort and depth of respiration	Diabetic ketoacidosis
Biot's respirations	Short, shallow respirations followed by pauses	Stroke, head trauma
Cheyne-Stokes respirations	Apnea, followed by a series of breaths waxing and waning in depth, followed by apnea	Encephalopathy, stroke, head trauma, cardiac disease, carbon monoxide poisoning; also seen just before death
Ataxic or agonal respirations	Unregulated, disconcordant breaths with pauses of varying lengths	Extreme hypoxia; often seen during cardiac arrest

Remember that observing the cycle of respirations should be divided into two parts: the work of breathing and the rate of breathing.

Listen: Breath Sounds

Auscultation of breath sounds is the most frequently performed part of an assessment for respiratory disease. To perform auscultation properly, a few good practices are imperative: (1) Use the diaphragm of the stethoscope; (2) place it on the patient's skin if possible; and (3) do not allow the tubing to touch anything during auscultation. These practices eliminate outside interference.

When listening, always compare and move with purpose: superior to inferior, side to side, and site to site. If you hear something different, stop, move the stethoscope to a new site, and listen again. Following these simple rules repeatedly hardwires good auscultation practices into the brain.

Breath sounds can be categorized simply as normal or abnormal. Normal sounds may be heard in one area and abnormal sounds in another. Abnormal, or **adventitious,** breath sounds can be heard in any lung area, and several sounds are associated with particular respiratory diseases (Table 3-2). Breath sounds are reviewed briefly here and addressed in relation to disease processes later in the chapter.

Wheezing

The wheeze is the classic sound of airway obstruction or airway hyperreactivity. Usually heard on expiration, wheezing can have a musical quality, or it may be quite harsh. The pitch varies with the size of the airway. Expiratory wheezes are heard in asthma, bronchitis, and chronic obstructive lung disease. Wheezes associated with other diseases, such as pneumonia or heart failure, are considered signs of a reactive airway. The area is inflamed, and the bronchi are edematous.

Crackles (Rales)

Crackles (also called *rales*) on inspiration are associated with fluid accumulation in the smaller airways and may not clear with coughing. Because the smaller airways are best examined through the patient's back (i.e., the lung bases), auscultation must always include a thorough examination of both the back and the front of the thorax. Crackles have a fine, high-pitched, harsh quality. They are most likely to be heard in patients with pneumonia, congestive heart failure, and pulmonary edema.

Rhonchi

Rhonchi indicate the accumulation of secretions in the larger airways. These sounds, the result of air passing through the secretions, are heard on expiration and often are described as "bubbly" or "slurpy." Patients with bronchiectasis, cystic fibrosis, and aspiration pneumonitis are likely to have rhonchi when the underlying disease is severe.

Pleural Friction Rub

Pleural fluid reduces friction between the two layers of the pleura as the lungs expand and contract during normal respiration. A pleural friction rub results when this fluid buffer is lost. A pleural friction rub can develop as a result of pneumonia, pleurisy, or contusion of the lung, and it is associated with chest wall pain. Auscultation is limited to the area adjacent to the pain.

Table 3-2 Breath Sounds and Diseases

Location	Sound	Phase	Disease Process
Upper airway	Stridor	Inspiration	Viral croup, epiglottitis, foreign body aspiration
	Rhonchi	Expiration	Frank aspiration, bronchitis, cystic fibrosis
Lower airway	Wheeze	Either inspiration or expiration or both	Reactive airways disease, asthma, congestive heart failure, chronic bronchitis, emphysema, endobronchial obstruction
	Rales (crackles)	End inspiration	Pneumonia, exacerbation of congestive heart failure, pulmonary edema
	Diminished breath sounds	Either inspiration or expiration or both	Emphysema, atelectasis, tension pneumothorax, flail chest, neuromuscular disease, pleural effusion
Chest wall	Pleural rub	Either inspiration or expiration or both	Pleuritis, pleurisy, pleural effusion

Diminished Breath Sounds

Diminished (or distant) breath sounds are noted in patients with respiratory disorders that lead to increases in the functional residual capacity (an increase in the resting volume of gas in the lung). The classic disorder in this group is emphysema, in which destruction of the alveolar walls results in less surface area for gas exchange; in addition, gas flow becomes less turbulent and produces a softer sound. Other disorders marked by diminished breath sounds are atelectasis, pneumothorax, and neuromuscular disorders that limit the inspiratory volume.

Stridor

Stridor is a sound limited to the upper airway. It is the product of large airway obstruction or inflammation and is heard only on inspiration. Viral croup and epiglottitis are two disorders in which stridor is heard. In the critical care field, angioedema, postextubation swelling, and trauma are commonly associated with stridor.

Feel: Palpation and Percussion

Palpation of the neck and chest wall is always recommended for trauma patients, but it also can be helpful for patients with medical problems. Palpation is performed to detect pain or deformities. The assessment should include the position of the trachea, thoracic chest wall expansion, and the quality of **fremitus** (a palpable vibration). The trachea should be midline, without a deviation that might indicate a change in thoracic pressure. The chest wall should move symmetrically; inadequate lung expansion or asymmetric movement indicates a disease process that is interfering with expansion of the lungs.

To assess for fremitus, palpate both the trachea and around the chest wall as the patient repeatedly says "ninety-nine." Vibration should be palpated in the trachea but not very well in the thorax. The vibration is decreased with disorders such as pleural effusion, pneumothorax, and emphysema; increased fremitus is noted with pneumonia and pulmonary fibrosis.

Percussion of the thorax can provide good information about certain abnormalities, but it usually is not performed by transport crews. This form of physical assessment can help determine the location of an underlying lung structure and also the movement of the diaphragm. Areas of air, solid, and liquid can be distinguished by tapping methodically over the chest wall.

DIAGNOSTICS

By applying their knowledge of anatomy and physiology, in addition to the techniques for assessing the patient's airway and respiratory status, the members of the transport team create a list of differential diagnoses that can be whittled down through the use of diagnostic techniques. Various types of radiographic images, testing of respiratory functions, and laboratory and monitoring parameters can help the team in the overall care of the patient.

Imaging

The chest radiograph is among the most common radiologic examinations performed on critically ill patients. However, it is not the only imaging modality used in the ICU; some conditions are better identified with other radiologic tools, such as ultrasonography, computed tomography (CT), magnetic resonance imaging (MRI), and fluoroscopy.

Chest Radiograph

The chest radiograph is the essential imaging device for diagnosis and follow-up. It provides supporting evidence of proper placement of invasive catheters, endotracheal tubes, chest drainage tubes, and nasogastric or orogastric tubes. Because critical care patients require constant attention and repositioning, daily follow-up on tube placement is necessary, and daily chest radiographs are a staple. The chest radiograph allows the clinician not only to verify tube placement, but also to provide treatment for cardiopulmonary changes. Chest radiographs can detect pneumothorax and other air-fluid disturbances.

However, the portable chest radiograph is not without limitations; the structures on the portable film are not as well defined, and the patient's condition may cause the angle and density of the film to vary from day to day. Serial comparison, therefore, may not be as reliable as it is for standing posterior-anterior (PA) films done in the radiology department. At the very least, the critical care transport team should verify the interpretation of the latest chest radiograph before transporting the patient to ensure proper positioning of support devices.

Ultrasonography

Ultrasonography, which is the use of ultrasound techniques to image soft tissues, can be used for diagnostic purposes and also as part of the treatment of some disease processes. Trained clinicians use ultrasound to aid biopsy of soft tissues or drainage of fluid collections, such as pleural effusion. Traditionally, ultrasonography has provided a two-dimensional view of soft tissues, and newer technology provides a three-dimensional view.

In critical care, the diagnostic use of ultrasound usually is associated with cardiovascular studies (e.g., echocardiography, carotid artery studies) and other vascular studies to rule out the presence of clots, tumors, or congenital disease.

Ultrasonography also has its limitations. Small or deep vessels are difficult to image, and blood flow may appear falsely obstructed or reduced. In addition, because of patient positioning and other characteristics, clear ultrasound images frequently are difficult to obtain.

Computed Tomography

Currently, portable CT scans are not possible, and this imaging study requires in-hospital transport. Advances in technology have greatly reduced the scanning time and improved the images obtained. Soft tissue images are much sharper than with traditional radiographs, and three-dimensional scanning now is available. CT scans are useful for the diagnosis of chest trauma, chest masses, and interstitial diseases (e.g., pulmonary fibrosis). Spiral CT is very useful for identifying pulmonary embolus. Much like ultrasonography, CT also can be used to aid therapeutic procedures. The limitations of CT scanning include the patient's size, the need to transport a critically ill patient to the scanner, and the possible need for IV contrast, which has the potential to cause renal injury.

Magnetic Resonance Imaging

MRI also requires in-hospital transport. Because the technique uses a very strong magnetic field, it provides much sharper images than are possible with CT. However, because of the magnetic field, many patients are unable to undergo MRI. Many ventilators are incompatible with the magnetic field, as are pacemakers and some other implantable metallic devices (usually orthopedic replacements).

Fluoroscopy

Fluoroscopy uses ionizing radiation to capture real-time images of internal structures. Advances in fluoroscopy equipment have made bedside studies possible, but serious concerns arise about increased exposure to radiation. In respiratory patients, fluoroscopic guidance aids tissue biopsy through a flexible bronchoscope. This can be helpful in the diagnosis of lung masses and for identifying the source of a respiratory infection (although fluoroscopy frequently is not necessary for these indications, because CT scans and a knowledge of respiratory anatomy usually are sufficient). Other uses of fluoroscopy include heart catheterization, placement of a peripheral intravenous central catheter (PICC) for long-term IV access, carotid angiography, and orthopedic surgery. Limitations of fluoroscopy include the aforementioned radiation risk; also, space may be a limiting factor because of the size of the portable fluoroscopy machinery.

Pulmonary Function Testing

Spirometry

Spirometry, which is the measurement of airflow, comprises several tests. The basic test is measurement of the **forced vital capacity.** Patients with obstructive disease (asthma, chronic obstructive pulmonary disease [COPD]) require more time to exhale the vital capacity than patients with normal lung function. Vital capacity is one of the weaning parameters, which are measurements that help assess a patient's readiness to be removed from mechanical ventilation.

The use of spirometry and determination of lung volumes can be very helpful in the diagnosis of lung disease. Normal values vary and are based on height, age, and gender. Use of these values is somewhat limited in critical care, primarily because acquiring them depends on patient effort. Critically ill respiratory patients are unable to participate in most testing maneuvers.

Plotted against time, spirometric measurements demonstrate airflow. Measurement of the expiratory flow is a good diagnostic tool for determining the degree of obstructive disease. Two studies commonly performed in the Emergency Department (ED) are the peak expiratory flow rate (PEFR), which is the maximum flow generated on expiration, and the forced expiratory volume in 1 second (FEV_1), or the amount of air forcibly exhaled in 1 second. Patients with asthma have a reduced PEFR. Peak flow meters can be used to monitor functional improvement with treatment. The FEV_1 also improves with treatment but much more slowly. Other measured flow rates can be used to determine airway resistance, which is a clinical manifestation of obstructive defects. A decreased vital capacity usually indicates restrictive defects, but it also can be seen with obstructive defects when other volumes are increased.

Bronchoscopy

Bronchoscopy (discussed later in the chapter) is an invasive procedure for visualizing the upper and lower respiratory tracts. It allows diagnosis and management of a spectrum of inflammatory, infectious, and malignant diseases of the airways and lungs.

Laboratory Assessment

Oxygenation and ventilation can be assessed simply and efficiently with the technology currently available. Pulse oximetry, capnography, and point of care laboratory equipment can bring arterial blood gas measurement to the bedside.

Pulse Oximetry

Pulse oximetry (which measures the functional oxygen saturation, or Spo_2) now is routinely considered a basic vital sign. The monitor uses a light emitter with red and infrared light-emitting diodes (LEDs) that shine through a reasonably translucent site with good blood flow. Sites typically used in adults and children are the finger, toe, and pinna (top) or lobe of the ear. Sites in infants include the foot, big toe, palm, or thumb. Newer probes are available for the forehead.

Pulse oximetry may be limited by poor signal strength in patients with cardiovascular compromise, the presence of carbon monoxide on the hemoglobin (smoke inhalation), and interference caused by other electrical devices, nail polish (particularly red), and ambient light. The temperature of the measuring site also may affect the reliability of oximetry.

It is important to note that oximetry values below 90% correlate with a significantly reduced Pao_2. With few exceptions, maintaining the Spo_2 above 90% is adequate during critical care transport.

Advances in technology have significantly improved the ability of pulse oximeters to function during periods of motion and low perfusion, making pulse oximetry much more reliable than in the past. Handheld units have made monitoring portable. They also can now provide estimations of other hemoglobinemias, such as carboxyhemoglobin and methemoglobin; however, the overall usefulness of these values is limited to a handful of clinical situations.

Capnometry and Capnography

Qualitative carbon dioxide monitors are better known as *CO2 detectors*. Disposable CO_2 detectors are commonly used in the ED and ICU, because they are reliable, less expensive, and require less storage space. Colorimetric detectors use a litmus paper sensor and are attached directly to the manual resuscitator or endotracheal tube (ETT). They do not measure the gas level directly; rather they provide qualitative measurements, giving a range of percentages based on the color change in the litmus sensor. These devices are effective only for 12 to 24 hours because of exposure of the sensor to room air.

End-exhalation CO_2 levels in a perfusing patient also can be determined by two other methods: **capnometry,** which provides only a numeric value, and **capnography,** which provides the CO_2 level plotted against time. Skill 3-1 presents step-by-step instructions for monitoring the end-tidal carbon dioxide level (**$PETco_2$**), and Table 3-3 lists some of the possible causes of a change in the $PETco_2$.

Table 3-3 Causes of Change in End-Tidal Carbon Dioxide ($PETco_2$) Level

Increases $PETco_2$	Decreases $PETco_2$
Equipment-Related Causes	***Equipment-Related Causes***
• Added dead space (tubing, attachments, devices) • External sources of CO_2 • Defective CO_2 absorber	• Water blocking the sampling line or sensor • High positive end-expiratory pressure (PEEP) • Air entrainment during sampling
Patient-Related Causes	***Patient-Related Causes***
• Rebreathing • Decreased respiratory rate • Decreased tidal volume • Hyperthermia • Hypercatabolic state, resulting in muscle weakness and acidosis • Acute respiratory failure • Hypertension	• Pulmonary embolism • Decreased cardiac output • Increased respiratory rate • Increased tidal volume • Hypothermia • Hyperventilation • Hypovolemia • Cardiac arrest

Skill 3-1

CONTINUOUS END-TIDAL CARBON DIOXIDE ($PETco_2$) MONITORING

To properly evaluate a patient's ventilatory status, the carbon dioxide (CO_2) level must be measured, because it is the end result of effective respiration. Perfusion is required to view the CO_2 level; therefore, both ventilation and blood flow in the lungs may be measured.

Traditionally, the measurement of blood gases has been the gold standard for evaluating ventilation status; however, acquiring blood samples is not so easy. New technology and equipment allow continuous monitoring of the patient's spontaneous respiratory effort and positive pressure ventilations. Because the result is measured at the end of exhalation, the term *end tidal* is used. Two means of measurement can be used:

- A *capnometer* (used for *capnometry*) measures the amount of CO_2 and projects a number. This measurement is not placed on a graph.
- A *capnograph* (used for *capnography*) expresses the CO_2 measurement as a waveform that is recorded over time; this measurement is considered more valuable to the critical care provider.

The exhaled gas is measured by infrared gas analysis, usually through an exhalation port. The information relayed to the provider may include an estimation of the partial pressure of arterial carbon dioxide ($Paco_2$), ventilation-perfusion (V/Q) abnormalities, pulmonary blood flow, and confirmation of correct tracheal tube placement.

A review of the physiology of CO_2 exhalation can help explain the other terminology related to this valuable measurement. When venous blood is returned to the lungs, the carbon dioxide (measured in the venous blood as the partial pressure of CO_2 [$P\text{v}CO_2$]) diffuses from the capillaries into the alveoli (the partial pressure of CO_2 in the alveoli [i.e., arterial blood] is expressed as the $PaCO_2$). The normal $P\text{v}CO_2$ is 45 mm Hg, and normal $PaCO_2$ is 40 mm Hg. The pressure difference of 5 mm Hg causes the CO_2 to diffuse out of the capillaries into the alveoli for elimination. As the blood passes through the capillaries, the pressures are equal. The pressure of CO_2 near the end of exhalation ($PETCO_2$) is the end-tidal CO_2. With normal perfusion, the $PETCO_2$ is approximately 1 to 5 mm Hg lower than the $PaCO_2$.

INDICATIONS

Baseline and continuous end-tidal CO_2 levels and waveform ($PETCO_2$)

Continuous monitoring of airway patency and ventilation status

Early detection of abnormal patterns in ventilation, perfusion, or CO_2 production

Guide for hyperventilation therapy

Measurement of perfusion

WAVEFORM CHARACTERISTICS

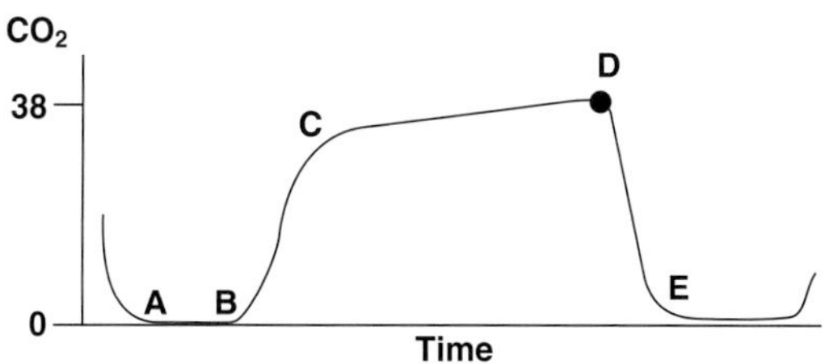

Essentials of a normal capnographic waveform. (Nellcor Puritan Bennett [Covidien], Boulder, Colo.)

1. *Section A-B* shows the waveform at zero baseline on the graph. The zero baseline occurs at the end of inspiration, just before exhalation.
2. As exhalation begins, an upstroke waveform appears (*section B-C*), which is positively deflected as the device begins to quickly detect CO_2.
3. *Section C-D* shows a slowing of the velocity of the exhalation.
4. *Part D* indicates the maximum of exhaled CO_2 at the end of exhalation.
5. *Section D-E* reflects the rapid inhalation as the next breath begins. This would be negatively deflected, because very little CO_2 would be detected in this part of the respiratory cycle.

PROCEDURE

1. Follow your medical director's protocols for the use of capnometry and capnography. Use standard precautions.
2. Assess for proper functioning of the capnograph, including the airway adapter, sensor, and display monitor; make sure all connections are secure.
3. Turn on the device and allow it to calibrate. If prolonged monitoring is expected, make sure the battery life is adequate or plug the unit into a grounded source.
4. Follow the manufacturer's recommendations for inserting the airway adapter and sensor. Plug the cable into the monitor. In general, the closer the sensor is to the patient, the better.

NOTE: This connection adds a fairly significant weight to the end of the tracheal tube. Place padding on the patient's lower anterior neck or chest and allow the sensor and connection to lie on the padding. Allowing the heavy connection to lie to the side of the mouth may cause extubation.

5. Set the alarms on the monitor according to the protocol and the manufacturer's recommendations (common limits are 5% above and below the standards).
6. Check the quality of the waveform; a poor waveform means that the $PETCO_2$ reading may be inaccurate.

RISING $PETCO_2$ LEVELS

Increases greater than 10% from the baseline measurements must be investigated. Common causes include a hypermetabolic state, sepsis, fever, hypoventilation, a partial airway obstruction, inadequate minute ventilation, use of respiratory depressant drugs or neuromuscular blockade, and metabolic alkalosis or malfunction of the ventilator.

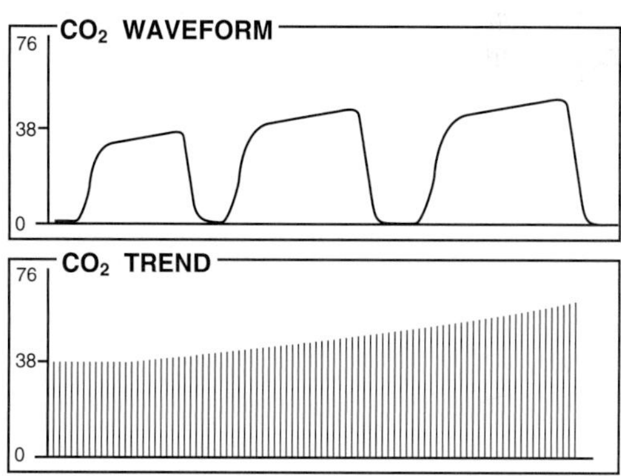

Gradually increasing $PETCO_2$. (Nellcor Puritan Bennett [Covidien], Boulder, Colo.)

FALLING $PETCO_2$ LEVELS

A decrease by 10% from the baseline reading also must be investigated, because this reflects increasing dead space ventilation. Common causes include a decrease in or loss of perfusion (shock, cardiac arrest), a high minute volume, hypothermia, metabolic acidosis, or an airway leak or obstruction. The following figure illustrates an exponential fall in the $PETCO_2$ waveform caused by a sudden increase in dead space ventilation, which may be seen in cardiac arrest, pulmonary embolism, or a decrease in blood flow to the lungs.

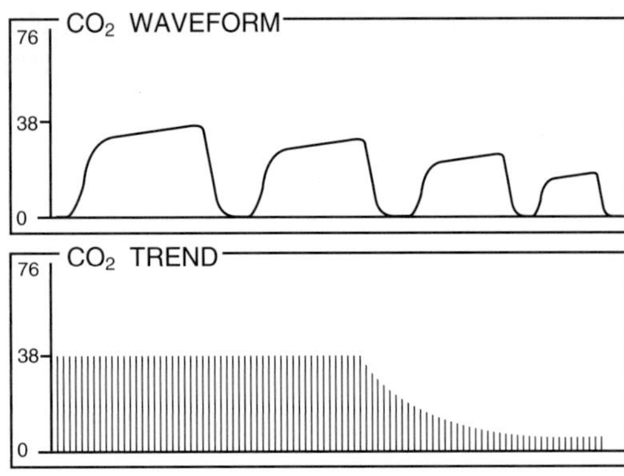

Exponential fall in PETCO_2. (Nellcor Puritan Bennett [Covidien], Boulder, Colo.)

The following figure illustrates a sudden decrease in the PETCO_2 values, possibly caused by a poor sample, leakage in the system (partial disconnection), partial airway obstruction, or ventilator malfunction.

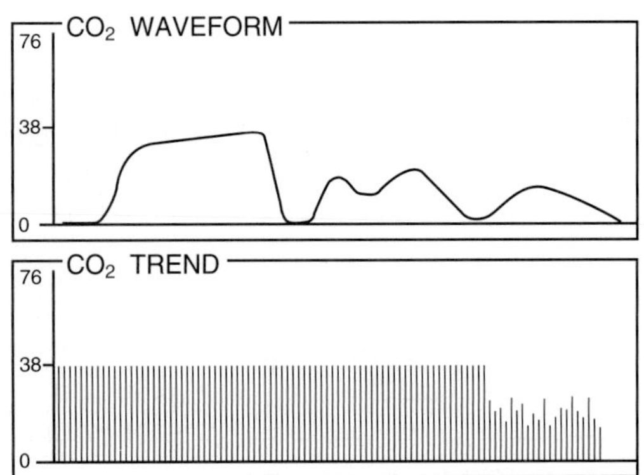

Sudden decrease in PETCO_2. (Nellcor Puritan Bennett [Covidien], Boulder, Colo.)

LOW PETCO_2 LEVELS

Sustained low PETCO_2 levels indicate poor ventilation. This may be caused by airway obstruction (a kink in the airway), bronchospasm, a mucous plug, or inadequate expiration time on the ventilator. Listen to the breath sounds, check the airway and connections for obstructions and, if necessary, suction the tracheal tube. The following figure illustrates a low PETCO_2 level, possibly caused by shock or decreased production of CO_2 as a result of high minute volumes, hypothermia, or acidosis.

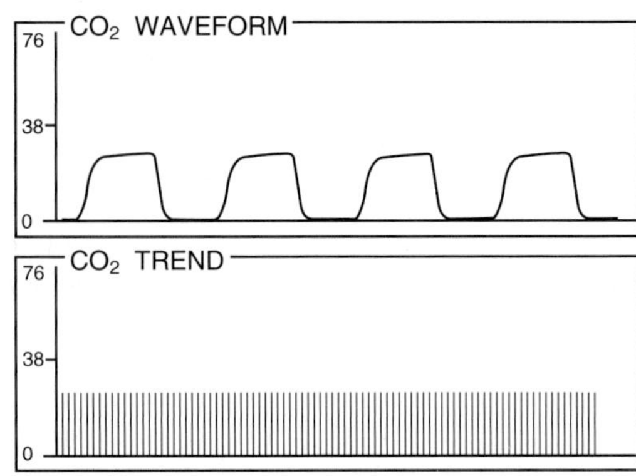

Decreased PETCO_2. (Nellcor Puritan Bennett [Covidien], Boulder, Colo.)

The following figure illustrates the low CO_2 levels and lack of an alveolar plateau that result from poor alveolar emptying (possibly caused by a kinked endotracheal tube, bronchospasm, or mucous plug) or from an incomplete expiratory time on the ventilator.

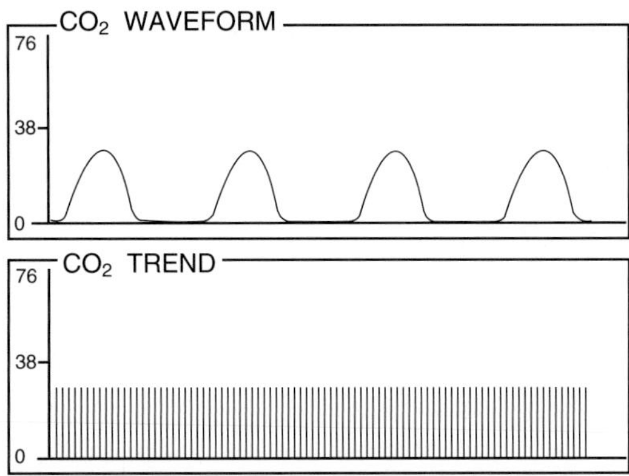

Low PETCO_2 without alveolar plateau. (Nellcor Puritan Bennett [Covidien], Boulder, Colo.)

COMPARISON OF PETCO_2 AND PaCO_2

As mentioned earlier, in patients with normal cardiopulmonary status, the PETCO_2 is 1 to 5 mm Hg less than the PaCO_2. In patients with poor perfusion or respiratory impairment, the difference between the PETCO_2 and the PaCO_2 is greater than 5 mm Hg; this is called *dead space,* which is an indicator of areas of the lungs of little or no perfusion and therefore no gas exchange.

NONINVASIVE CAPNOMETRY

Sublingual devices used to measure the PETCO_2 not only provide an assessment of the patient's ventilatory status, but also indicate the overall perfusion status. These devices accurately measure blood flow in the gastrointestinal (GI) system. The GI system is very sensitive to low flow states and is 90% sensitive for measurement of the true CO_2 level. Recent studies have shown that this measurement can identify patients at risk for poor perfusion and multisystem organ dysfunction syndrome (MODS).

Point of Care Testing

Advances also are occurring in laboratory analysis at the bedside, known as *point of care testing.* Arterial blood gases, chemistry, and blood glucose now can be measured from a single sample at the patient's bedside. These tests are valuable aids in rapid assessment, and the results are comparable to those obtained with conventional testing and analysis. Point of care analyzers are portable, durable, and easily calibrated; therefore, they can be easily adapted to emergency medical needs and for use in critical care, surgery, and transport.

Did You Know?

When it comes to your equipment, remember: *no numbers are better than wrong numbers.* To ensure the technical accuracy and reliability of measurements, always follow the equipment manufacturer's instructions for sensor placement, calibration, and maintenance. Always inspect the quality and shape of the waveform before accepting any numeric value from a monitoring device.[1]

Laboratory Values

Respiratory illnesses would be very difficult to manage without chemistry, microbiology, and hematology studies. A good clinician understands the need for these tests and uses them appropriately to refine treatment. The ABGs and their interpretation are important for managing respiratory diseases, and these values may prove the most valuable test results available to the critical care paramedic.

Interpretation of Arterial Blood Gas Values

Blood gas analysis frequently is confusing to healthcare providers. Nevertheless, the critical care transport team must have a basic understanding of these findings and how they influence the treatment of a patient, particularly with regard to proper mechanical ventilation. You cannot just turn on a ventilator and hope it works. The settings you choose must be based on numerous clinical findings, including the ABG results (Table 3-4).

When the pH is low (a condition called *acidosis*), you must determine whether the cause is respiratory or metabolic. In respiratory acidosis, the $Paco_2$ increases (carbon dioxide is an acid), causing the pH to fall. In metabolic acidosis, HCO_3 falls; bicarbonate is a buffer and binds to acid, causing the pH to fall with it. Although acidosis is more common in the critical care setting, alkalosis also can occur. In respiratory alkalosis (an abnormally increased minute ventilation, induced by either the patient or the caregiver), the pH rises as the $Paco_2$ falls. In metabolic alkalosis, HCO_3 rises as the pH rises.

Although normal values are useful for determining an underlying disorder, remember that you cannot interpret normal values correctly unless you also understand the clinical situation. For example, a "normal" $Paco_2$ in the setting of hyperventilation should not be considered normal without further, careful consideration of the entire clinical scenario.

Table 3-4 Key Blood Gas Results

		Abnormal Findings	
	Normal Range	**Acidosis**	**Alkalosis**
pH	7.35-7.45	↓	↑
Partial pressure of carbon dioxide ($Paco_2$)	35-45 mm Hg	↑	↓
Base excess	−2 to +2 mEq/L	↓	↑
Bicarbonate (HCO_3)	22-26 mEq/L	↓	↑

A quick notation can help guide you to the correct interpretation of ABG results: Put an up arrow or a down arrow next to the result. Is the result higher than normal range? If so, put an up arrow next to it. Is the result below the normal range? If so, put a down arrow next to it. Compare your notes to the table above.

For example, the ABG results for your patient read:

pH: 7.20
$Paco_2$: 78 mm Hg
BE: −2 mEq/L
HCO_3: 22 mm Hg

You note that the pH is down, the $Paco_2$, is up, and the base excess and bicarbonate levels are normal; this indicates respiratory acidosis. (Remember, all laboratory results must correlate with the patient's clinical condition.) You know that in this case, you can correct the respiratory acidosis by increasing the **minute volume.** If the patient were mechanically ventilated, you would adjust the minute volume by increasing the rate (frequency *[f]*) or the V_T or both (Table 3-5).

All of the body's processes are intended to be in balance, a condition called *homeostasis.* The mechanisms that adjust for acid base abnormalities work first and quickest through the buffer system; second and more slowly through the respiratory system; and third, days later, through the renal system.

An example of a compensating patient is an individual in early hemorrhagic shock with these ABG results: pH, 7.38; $Paco_2$, 25 mm Hg; BE, −8 mEq/L; HCO_3, 15 mm Hg. Clinically, the patient demonstrates tachypnea (an early sign of shock) and is blowing off CO_2 to minimize the availability of carbonic acid. In fact, the respiratory system has done so well that the pH remains normal. This is called *complete compensation,* which means that the metabolic acidosis is fully compensated.

Using ABG Values to Manage Ventilation

Consider the following equation:

$$(Paco_2 \times f \times V_T) \div \text{Target } Paco_2 = \text{Target } V_E$$

Where Target V_E is the target minute ventilation.

Table 3-5 Blood Gas Abnormalities

Abnormality	pH	$PaCO_2$	HCO_3
Uncompensated metabolic acidosis	Low	Normal	Low
Uncompensated respiratory acidosis	Low	High	Normal
Compensated metabolic acidosis	Low normal	Low	Low
Compensated respiratory acidosis	Low normal	High	High
Mixed metabolic and respiratory acidosis	Low	High	Low
Uncompensated metabolic alkalosis	High	Normal	High
Uncompensated respiratory alkalosis	High	Low	Normal
Compensated metabolic alkalosis	High normal	Low	High
Compensated respiratory alkalosis	High normal	Low	Low
Mixed metabolic and respiratory alkalosis	High	Low	High

HCO_3, Bicarbonate; *$PaCO_2$*, partial pressure of carbon dioxide.

According to this equation, the same number of CO_2 molecules are eliminated by high ventilation at a low $PaCO_2$ as by low ventilation at a high $PaCO_2$. The target ventilation is calculated by dividing by the target $PaCO_2$. This is a reliable means of arriving at the desired $PaCO_2$, but the data and the time to calculate it may not be available in an emergency situation.

A simpler idea may be to look at the problem from a practical standpoint:

1. The $PaCO_2$ is largely a function of *f* and V_T.
   - To increase the $PaCO_2$: Increase *f* (× 2 to 5) *or* V_T (× 50 to 100 mL).
   - To decrease the $PaCO_2$: Decrease *f* (× 2 to 5) *or* V_T (× 50 to 100 mL).
2. Acute changes in the SpO_2 require adjustment of the fraction of inspired oxygen (FiO_2) and PEEP. Changes in PEEP must be made cautiously, especially when the PEEP level is higher than 7 to 10 cm H_2O.
   - If the SpO_2 rises above 95%: Reduce the FiO_2 in increments of 5% to maintain the SpO_2 at 90% to 92%.

Skill 3-2 presents step-by-step instructions for obtaining an arterial blood sample.

Table 3-6 Comparison of Arterial and Venous Blood Gas Values

	ABGs	VBGs
pH	7.38-7.42	7.35-7.38
$PaCO_2$	38-42 mm Hg	44-48 mm Hg
PaO_2	90-100 mm Hg	40 mm Hg
HCO_3	24 mEq/L	22-22 mEq/L

ABG, Arterial blood gas; *$PaCO_2$*, partial pressure of carbon dioxide; *PaO_2*, partial pressure of oxygen; *HCO_3*, bicarbonate; *VBG*, venous blood gas.

Venous Blood Gas Analysis

Some emergency medicine departments have begun to rely on venous blood gas (VBG) values in certain clinical circumstances. This practice has obvious clinical advantages: It reduces the number of high-risk arterial punctures required to obtain laboratory samples; it provides clinicians with enough data to detect some metabolic disorders; and it eliminates a painful experience for the patient. Except for the venous oxygen pressure (PvO_2,), the VBG values can serve as predictors of arterial values. Venous blood samples drawn from an upper body central line (PICC or internal jugular or subclavian line) may be used to determine the central venous oxygen saturation ($ScvO_2$). This is a useful surrogate marker for cardiac output, and it is being used more often during resuscitation from most shock states.

VBG testing has some disadvantages. ABG samples must be drawn if the venous values do not correlate with the patient's clinical condition. The absence of a reliable PO_2 is another drawback, although pulse oximetry may be used as an adjunct screening tool with VBG sampling. Table 3-6 presents a comparison of ABG and VBG values.

Skill 3-2

OBTAINING A RADIAL ARTERY BLOOD SAMPLE

Blood may be obtained from an artery at any easily accessible site for the purpose of measuring blood gas or carboxyhemoglobin levels. You must follow the scope of practice guidelines and your employer's credentialing criteria. Possible complications also must be considered when you choose a site.

- The radial artery is the preferred site; it involves the least amount of risk and is the most accessible. Most individuals have collateral circulation to the hand from the ulnar artery. The ulnar artery is deeper and poses more problems for applying direct pressure.
- The brachial artery is larger than the radial artery and is easily compressed against bone, as long as the puncture site is not more than a few centimeters superior to the antecubital fossa. Most experts consider this the second-choice site for obtaining an arterial blood sample.
- Use of the femoral artery is preferred if the patient has poor perfusion. However, this site is difficult to compress, and it is located in an area that poses an increased risk of infection and limb ischemia.
- The dorsalis pedis artery in the top of the foot may be used, because it is fairly easily accessed and

compressible. However, because of the potential for clot formation in the lower extremities, it should not be the first-choice site.

ALTERNATIVES TO ARTERIAL BLOOD GAS ANALYSIS

Capillary blood gas (CBG) and venous blood gas (VBG) sampling may be acceptable alternatives to the more invasive arterial blood gas (ABG) techniques. Several studies have shown a fairly consistent correlation among the results of all three methods. CBG sampling is frequently done in children, and VBG sampling is done in adults for various other laboratory analysis in the healthcare setting. Good correlation is seen in the pH, partial pressure of carbon dioxide (PCO_2), partial pressure of oxygen (PaO_2), Base Excess or base (BE), and bicarbonate (HCO_3) levels among ABG, VBG, and CBG values. However, if hypotension is a factor, PaO_2 values are suspect in anything but an ABG sample. Most clinicians do not recommend CBG or VBG sampling to determine the PaO_2 of blood gas results.

INDICATIONS

Measurement of the PaO_2, $PaCO_2$, pH, oxygen saturation, HCO_3, and base levels

Evaluation of the acid-base balance, oxygen and carbon dioxide levels, and ventilation status

Additional laboratory testing as needed (e.g., ammonia, lactate, carboxyhemoglobin)

CONTRAINDICATIONS

Contraindications to use of a site may include occlusion, infection, inability to compress the site, and signs of lack of collateral circulation to the distal tissues.

PROCEDURE

1. Wash your hands and follow standard precautions.
2. Obtain an order for ABG analysis and perform patient identification procedures as described by your employer. Label all tubes and orders appropriately.
3. Perform the modified Allen test.
4. Obtain a heparinized syringe and needle. If only a nonheparinized syringe is available, add heparin as follows:
   a. Attach a 22-gauge needle to a 1 to 3 mL syringe.
   b. Aspirate 1 mL of heparin (standard concentration) into the syringe; move the plunger back and forth to coat the inside of the syringe with heparin.
   c. Expel all heparin from the barrel of the syringe.
   d. Make sure the plunger is tight against the proximal tip of the barrel.
5. Assemble all equipment and supplies within reach. Obtain a 2 × 2 sterile, dry gauze sponge; a 2 × 2 skin prep, a cap for the syringe, the appropriate patient ID label, and a laboratory specimen transport device with crushed ice inside.
6. Explain the procedure to the patient.
7. Prepare the skin with a 2% chlorhexidine–based antiseptic solution. To reduce the chance of infection, rub the site back and forth with some friction for at least 30 seconds. Allow the site to air dry (do not blow on the site).
8. Follow your employer's policies for intradermal injection of a local anesthetic at the site. Injection of a local anesthetic may make palpation of the pulse more difficult and often unnecessary, particularly if the patient is already receiving sedative and pain control drugs.
9. Place the patient's forearm and hand in a supinated position with some slight dorsiflexion of wrist (this may be enhanced with a small towel or cloth roll under the patient's wrist).
10. With your gloved, nondominant fingers, palpate the radial artery to locate the point of maximum intensity. Hold two fingers to the site to identify the location and stabilize the tissues.
11. Hold the assembled needle and syringe in your dominant hand. Place your hand in a position that is comfortable for you but that also puts the medial aspect of your rotated hand and wrist on the patient's forearm or hand (depending on your position); this stabilizes your hand and prevents inadvertent movement and tiring.
12. With the bevel of the needle up, puncture the skin at the identified site at an angle of approximately 30 to 50 degrees. Insert the needle slowly until a flash of blood appears; hold the needle at that point.
13. Allow the syringe to fill passively from the arterial pressure. Note the pulsation and the color of the blood as it enters the syringe.
14. Collect at least 1 mL of blood.
15. Withdraw the needle and immediately apply the sterile, dry 2 × 2 gauze sponge to the site. Apply firm pressure for at least 5 minutes or until no bleeding into the subcutaneous tissues or from the puncture site is seen.

NOTE: Patients taking anticoagulant drugs may need compression on the site for longer than 5 minutes.

16. While you maintain compression on the puncture site, have an assistant push all excess air carefully out of the syringe and then apply the cap and the patient label. Place the syringe on ice and transport it to the laboratory with the requisition.
17. Document the procedure. Check the puncture site frequently for bleeding. Apply a dressing to the site once compression is complete. Check the patient's distal perfusion frequently.
18. *If difficulty arises in obtaining blood:* With the needle inserted toward the palpated artery, withdraw the needle slightly and change the angle toward the point of maximum pulse intensity. Readvance the needle until blood appears in the tip of the syringe. Do not attempt to continue a difficult acquisition by prolonged movement of the needle; this may damage vessels and tissue and is painful for the patient.

Respiratory Monitoring Compared with Blood Gas Analysis

Transport teams can perform some laboratory testing and blood gas determinations, but the equipment must be calibrated, and team members must be well trained in its use (skills compliance must be verified annually). Pulse oximetry and capnography are becoming routine measurements; therefore, critical care teams must rely on the portable critical care monitoring systems to guide respiratory management. As must other equipment, pulse oximeters and capnographers must be calibrated regularly. After applying these external or in-line devices, team members should compare the arterial oxygen saturation (SaO_2) and the $PETCO_2$ to recent blood gas results.

DISORDERS OF THE AIRWAY AND RESPIRATORY SYSTEM

Threat to the Airway or Airway Compromise

Once the patient has been assessed, the critical care team may need to make some decisions. Does the patient have a patent airway right now? Can the patient maintain the airway unaided throughout the transport? If the patient has an artificial airway, is it working properly or should it be upgraded to a different device?

Management of the respiratory system and airway is a crucial skill in emergency and critical care situations. The critical care transport team must not only maintain the patient's airway and respiratory status, but also anticipate any changes that may occur during transport. Transport team members must support the patient for a much longer period than is required in an acute emergency setting. For this reason, team members must have excellent airway and ventilatory management skills.

Airway Tools: The Basics

If a patient is unable to maintain the airway (decreased level of consciousness) or has (or may develop) an airway obstruction, a definitive airway should be placed by the local healthcare team or the critical care crew. All agree that a definitive airway is the tracheal tube. One percent to 3% of your patients will have what is called a "difficult airway," which means that placing the tracheal tube will be difficult, if not impossible.[2] Whether you place other airway adjuncts as a bridge (temporary device) to intubation or as a rescue from a failed intubation attempt, all these devices may become important to your success. The organization of these adjuncts is based on their position above or below the glottis.

A good worker uses tools to manage problems. The tools of a critical care transport team include knowledge, good decision-making skills, and the equipment required for the job. At times this job is difficult. The more tools and skills you have, the better you will be able to manage the patient's airway.

Simple Positioning

The head-tilt/chin-lift and head-neutral/jaw-thrust maneuvers are easy to perform, and these positions generally are reliable. However, positioning a patient with an unprotected airway flat on the back poses the risk of aspiration. In medical patients, the recovery position (side lying) also is good for maintaining airway patency and preventing aspiration.

The problem with relying on position only is that there is no subglottic protection vs. aspiration in the patient with altered mental status, and one person usually is occupied with airway management only. If one of the two crew members is totally engrossed with manual airway management, the other important patient care skills might be impeded. (Figures 3-6 to 3-8).

Did You Know?

***Supraglottic airways* are a relatively new airway category. A supraglottic airway is a properly positioned airway adjunct that rests above the glottis in its final position. Many new devices on the market fall into this category.**

Nasal and Oral Airways

Nasal airways are designed for use in a conscious or semiconscious patient with an intact gag reflex. They have limited use in critical care situations. They are considered among the best devices for use just after extubation and for patients having a generalized seizure. The airway is passed gently along the floor of a lubricated nostril with the **distal,** slanted opening positioned medially, if possible (Figure 3-9). This generally means that, because of its design, the device should be inserted into the right naris. If the right naris is obstructed, the left

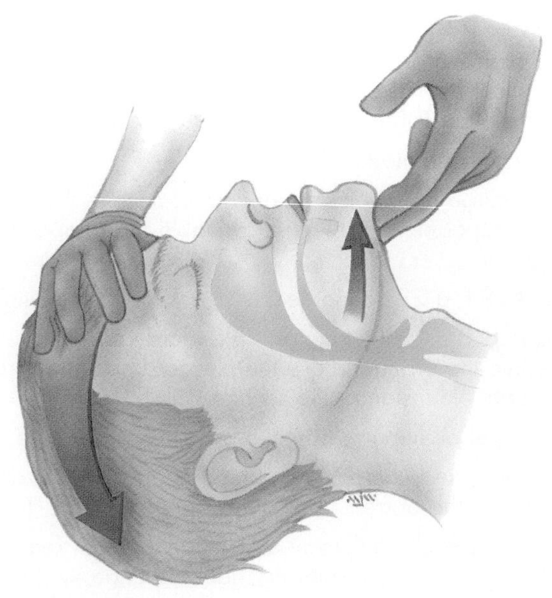

Figure 3-6

Head-tilt/chin-lift maneuver. (From Sanders M: *Mosby's paramedic textbook*, ed 3, St Louis, 2007, Mosby.)

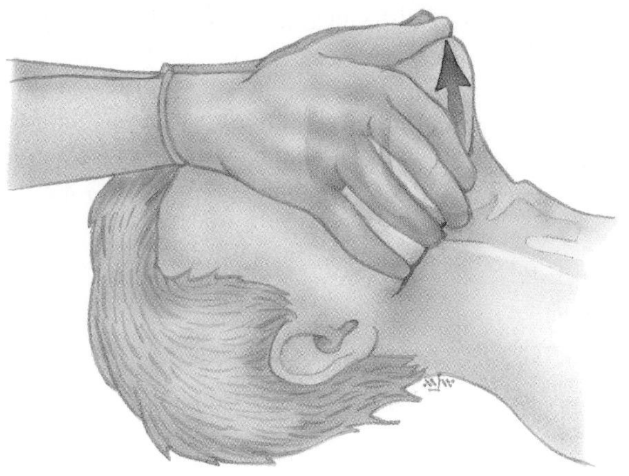

Figure 3-7

Jaw-thrust maneuver. (From Sanders M: *Mosby's paramedic textbook*, ed 3, St Louis, 2007, Mosby.)

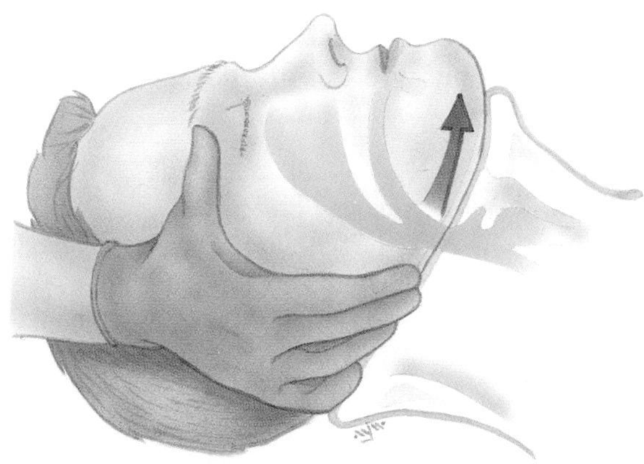

Figure 3-8

Jaw-thrust maneuver without head tilt. (From Sanders M: *Mosby's paramedic textbook*, ed 3, St Louis, 2007, Mosby.)

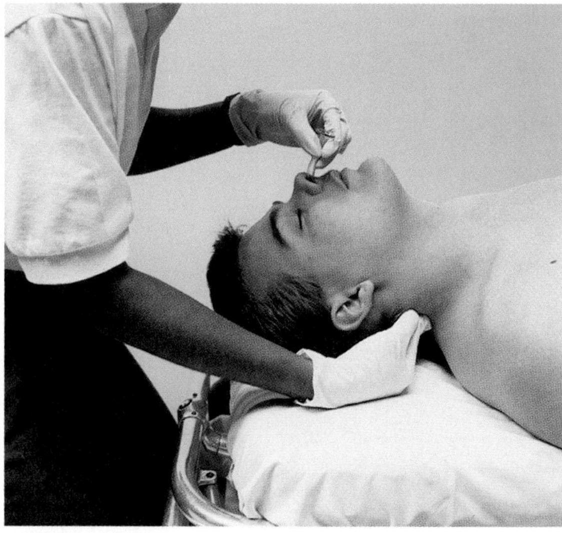

Figure 3-9

Insertion of a nasal airway. (From Sanders M: *Mosby's paramedic textbook*, ed 3, St Louis, 2007, Mosby.)

naris may be used; however, the device should be inserted upside down and that orientation should be maintained until the distal tip is past the **nasal turbinates.** Nasal bleeding, laryngospasm, and vomiting may occur with insertion of a nasal airway, especially if the airway chosen is too large or too long for the patient.

An oral airway is designed to displace the tongue forward in the pharynx, and this positioning usually stimulates the gag reflex. Before attempting to insert an oral airway, you should assess for the presence of a gag reflex and measure for the correct-sized airway. The distal flange should rest at the level of the central incisors with the bite block parallel to the hard palate. Two insertion techniques are used (Figure 3-10), and

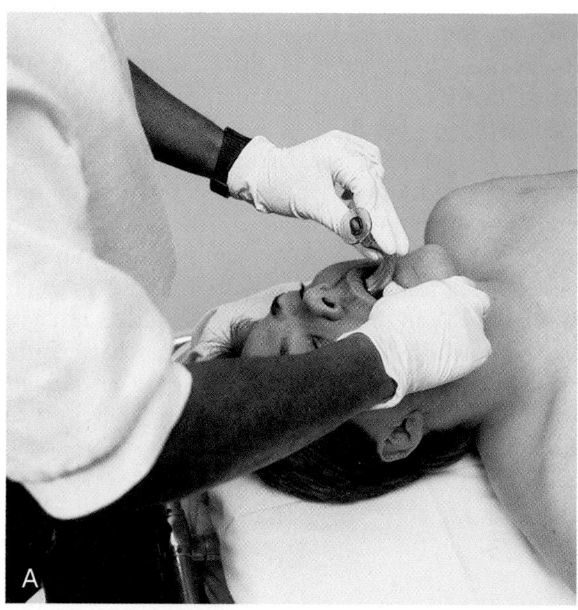

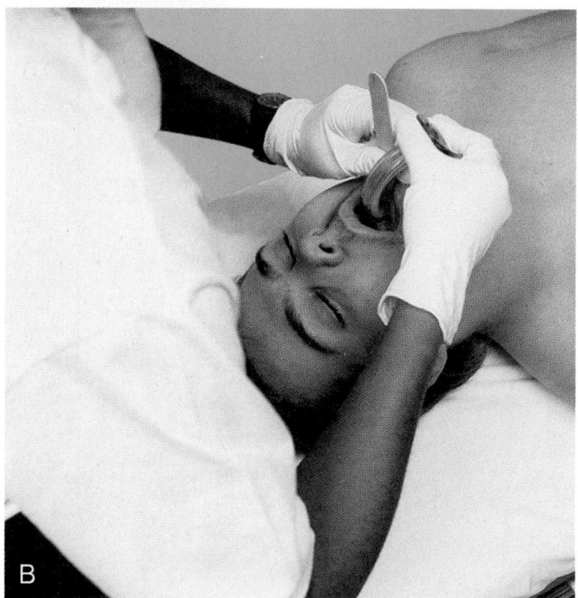

Figure 3-10

A, Insertion of an airway upside down. **B,** Alternative method of inserting an oral airway. (From Sanders M: *Mosby's paramedic textbook*, ed 3, St Louis, 2007, Mosby.)

both are designed to prevent the tongue from being pushed downward into the pharynx and creating further problems. An oral airway also may be used as protection for the tracheal tube (i.e., a bite block) as the tube is properly positioned in a biting patient's mouth.

Supraglottic (Extraglottic) Airway Devices

Airway management has come a long way since the first tracheal tube was devised in 1880. At least one or two supraglottic (now called *extraglottic*) airways are developed each year, and airway and ventilation equipment manufacturers are scrambling to decide how to classify and describe these devices (Table 3-7).

In general, extraglottic airways are inserted blindly and rest between the base of the tongue and the glottis. Because of this positioning, these devices may allow aspiration of gastric contents. Remember, this type of airway is *not* the definitive airway; rather, it has become a standard backup device for use in failed airway protocols.

The King laryngeal-tracheal airway (King LT) is an example of an extraglottic airway (Figure 3-11). The position of this airway allows for indirect ventilation. The King LT is relatively easy to insert with just the gloved hands.

A universal feature of extraglottic airways is a glottic opening, which can serve as a means of indirect intubation. This is accomplished by placing a stylet or exchange catheter through the airway and into the trachea. The extraglottic airway then is removed, and an ETT is inserted over the catheter and into position.

The Esophageal Tracheal Combitube (ETC) is included in the extraglottic airway device category. Developed many years ago as an emergency medical services (EMS) airway, the Combitube now is a dual-tube system based on the now outdated esophageal obturator airway. The large latex pharyngeal cuff creates some difficulty, especially in attempts to intubate with an ETT around the device (Figure 3-12).

Did You Know?

The term *supraglottic airway* has become confusing, because many of these devices occupy various areas in the hypopharynx. Some sit in the infraglottic area, and others are positioned in both the supraglottic and infraglottic areas. The more acceptable name for all these devices is *extraglottic airway* (i.e., located outside the glottis).

Intraglottic Airway Devices and Procedures

Inserting a soft, curved tracheal tube into a human airway with three distinct angles and sometimes a unique anatomy can be a challenge. The definitive airway is always an ETT or a tracheal tube.

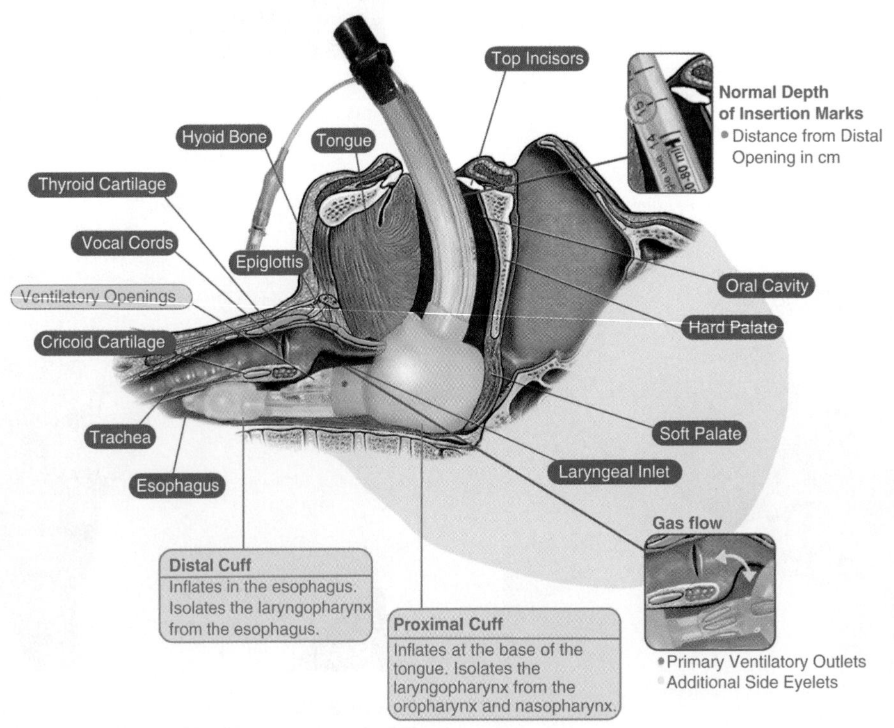

Figure 3-11

King laryngeal-tracheal airway (King LT). (Courtesy King Systems, Noblesville, Ind.)

Table 3-7 Extraglottic (Supraglottic) Airway Devices

Device and Manufacturer	Description	Special Features and Clinical Application
LMA Classic (LMA North America, San Diego, Calif.)	Oval inflatable cuff with attached tube connected to PPV; pediatric and adult sizes	Bridge or conduit to intubation for patients who are difficult to intubate and/or ventilate. Exchange catheter may be used through device to insert tracheal tube into position.
LMA Flexible	LMA cuff to smaller tube that is reinforced	Less kinking of tube and more cuff stability.
LMA Unique	Disposable LMA	Same design as the LMA Classic.
LMA ProSeal	Modified cuff and two tubes (GI, respiratory) with bite block	Second tube allows drainage of GI contents; second cuff provides a better seal; useful for bridge and route to intubation.
LMA Supreme	Same as LMA ProSeal but disposable	Same as for ProSeal.
LMA Fastrach	LMA mask attached to a stainless steel, curved tube that allows passage of a reinforced ETT	Facilitates blind or visually guided intubation with larger ETT; useful for bridge and route to intubation.
LMA CTrach	Fastrach with built-in fiberoptics; allows for simultaneous viewing and ventilation during intubation	Useful for prescreened patients found to have a "difficult" airway; reusable; useful for bridge and route to intubation.
Soft-Seal Laryngeal Mask (Smiths Medical, Kent, UK)	Similar to an LMA but is one piece and the cuff is softer and has no bars; pediatric and adult sizes	May accommodate a 7.5 mm ETT through FOB or video intubation equipment; useful for bridge and route to intubation.
Ambu AuraOnce (Ambu, Glen Burnie, Md.)	Disposable sterile LMA mask with built-in curve; one piece, molded, no bars; nondisposable	Facilitates insertion in anatomic position; may prevent mask distortion that can occur with LMA bridge and route intubation.
Ambu Aura 40	Disposable version of AuraOnce	Same as for AuraOnce.
Air-Q Laryngeal Mask (Cookgas, St. Louis, Mo.)	Disposable and nondisposable models; hypercurved with unique mask and supplied stylet	Hypercurved design resists kinking with overall larger mask with recessed anterior portion; standard ETT insertion allowed through supplied stylet; useful for bridge and route to intubation.
CobraPLA Perilaryngeal Airway (Engineered Medical Systems, Indianapolis, Ind.)	Large ID soft tube, cuffed triangular-shaped pharyngeal distal end; pediatric and adult sizes	Disposable large ID tube allows standard-sized ETTs through tube; design holds tissue away from grill that abuts the **aryepiglottic folds** and seats on the glottis; useful for bridge and route for intubation.
CobraPLUS	CobraPLA with monitoring capabilities	CobraPLA with ability to monitor core temperature in all sizes; pediatric sizes allow for monitoring of distal CO_2.
SLIPA Streamlined Liner of the Pharynx Airway (SLIPA Medical, London, UK)	Similar to LMA Unique; sized by span across thyroid cartilage; no cuff	Hollow mask allows for storage of GI regurgitation (50 mL) to prevent aspiration; available in six sizes.
Esophageal Tracheal Combitube (ETC) (Tyco Healthcare/ Mallinckrodt, Pleasanton, Calif.)	Disposable, double-lumen tube; ETT and esophageal lumens; large latex pharyngeal cuff; patient must be over 4 feet tall; two adult sizes	Blindly inserted bridge airway that combines a tracheal tube with the now outdated esophageal obturator airway. Large latex pharyngeal cuff, along with standard distal cuff; eight ventilatory holes rest against the glottis. Provides some protection against GI aspiration.
Elisha Airway Device (EAD) (Elisha Medical Technologies, Katzrin, Israel)	Molded device with three channels that allows ETT as large as 8 mm; two cuffs	Allows for ventilation, intubation, and gastric tube insertion through three separate channels; allows ventilation during intubation.
Chou Airway (Achi, San Jose, Calif.)	Two-piece, adjustable oral airway; adult sizes	Outer tube protects the inner one; the inner tube is flexible and creates an open air passage to the glottis; nondisposable.

Continued

Table 3-7 Extraglottic (Supraglottic) Airway Devices—cont'd

Device and Manufacturer	Description	Special Features and Clinical Application
Intersurgical i-gel	Nondisposable, noninflatable, cuffed extraglottic tube designed to match perilaryngeal anatomy; adult sizes	Similar to other devices with a gastric channel; minimizes epiglottic folding that sometimes occurs with an LMA; useful for bridge or route intubation with ETTs as large as 8 mm.
King Laryngeal-Tracheal Airway LT (King Systems, Noblesville, Ind.)	Latex-free, single-lumen, double-cuff design; pediatric and adult sizes	Nondisposable device that is blindly inserted as a bridge or route to intubation. Has a mask-free design but is similar to the LMA ProSeal. Smallest size (size 2) is suitable for patients <26 lb (12 kg); other sizes are 2.5, 3, 4, and 5. Both cuffs inflate with supplied syringe, which is color coded to the tube size. Considered an oropharyngeal device by the FDA.
King LT-D	Disposable King LT	Same as for King LT.
King LT-S	Double-lumen King LT	Second lumen is posterior to the ventilation port and allows gastric access for suction. Similar to LMA ProSEAL. Distal tip is narrower to allow for easier insertion.
King LTS-D	Disposable King LT-S; adult sizes only	Same as for King LT-S.

CO_2, Carbon dioxide; *ETT,* Endotracheal tube; *FDA,* U.S. Food and Drug Administration; *FOB,* fiberoptic bronchoscopy; *GI,* gastrointestinal; *ID,* inner diameter; *LMA,* laryngeal mask airway; *PPV,* positive pressure ventilation.

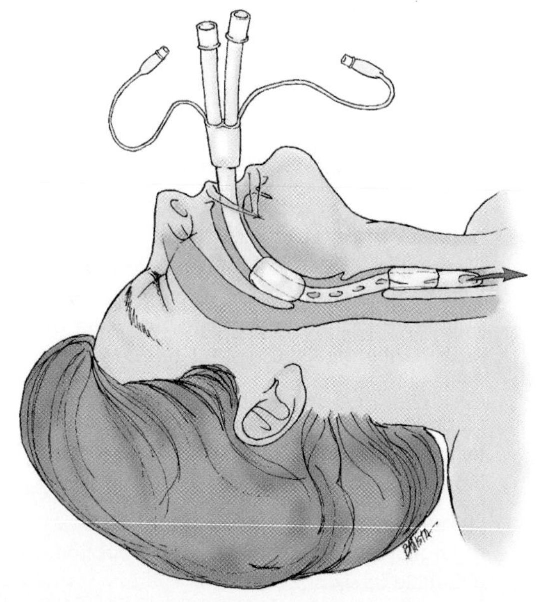

Figure 3-12

Placement of the Esophageal Tracheal Combitube (ETC) airway. (From Sanders M: *Mosby's paramedic textbook,* ed 3, St Louis, 2007, Mosby.)

The four primary indications for endotracheal intubation are:

- To protect the airway
- To clear pulmonary secretions
- To provide positive pressure ventilation
- To maintain oxygenation

Endotracheal and tracheal tubes must be designed according to certain standards. They must have a clearly marked inside diameter (ID) and outside diameter (OD), distance markers (from the tip), a Murphy eye, and **radiopaque** marker.

ETTs may be cuffed or uncuffed. The purpose of the cuff is to facilitate a seal between the tube and the tracheal wall; this prevents aspiration of liquids inferiorly and air leakage in either direction, because an air leak severely reduces or eliminates the delivery of positive pressure (e.g., PEEP). The cuff also positions the tube in the center of the trachea and prevents irritation of the mucosal lining. Uncuffed tubes are designed for emergency use in pediatric patients; cuffed tubes are the best choice for children who are mechanically ventilated. These cuffs may include special monitoring equipment to measure the cuff pressure. However, even with such equipment, cuffs may injure the tracheal wall; therefore, the cuff pressure should be monitored routinely.

Endotracheal Tube Maintenance

A cuffed ETT has distinct advantages and disadvantages for the patient. The cuff helps secure the position of the tube, but it also may lead to erosion of the mucosal membrane and disruption of mucociliary transport. A slight air leak is tolerated to maintain the health of the tracheal lining. Choosing the correct airway size in relation to the ID of the trachea further simplifies this process. With the proper-sized tube, rarely is more than 4 to 5 mL of air required to seal an airway for mechanical ventilation. This is particularly important after extubation of the patient, because a healthy tracheal mucosa is required to ensure a cough that is adequate to protect the airway in the future.

For this reason, the pressure in the inflated cuff should be kept below 25 cm H_2O, a level that allows minimal air to escape, yet prevents aspiration from above. Manometers are available that specifically measure the cuff pressure, but it can be adequately maintained by other means. Two methods are the minimum occlusion volume technique and the **minimum leak technique.** Both techniques are simple, quick, and surprisingly accurate.

Minimum Occlusion Volume Technique

Minimum occlusion volume technique: Beginning with a deflated cuff, the cuff is slowly inflated with air just to the point where no leak is heard by auscultation.

Minimum Leak Technique

Minimum leak technique: Beginning with an inflated cuff, air is withdrawn from the cuff to the point where a minimal leak is heard by auscultation.

Did You Know?

Injecting 10 to 12 mL of air into the cuff of an endotracheal tube can generate pressures higher than 90 cm H_2O on the surrounding tissue.

The cuff pressure also must be sufficient to protect the airway from aspiration. The body perceives the tube as a foreign body, which results in constant production of oral secretions. These secretions normally are swallowed and managed by the gastrointestinal (GI) tract. In a mechanically ventilated patient, these secretions may pool in the vallecular space or enter the trachea and pool above the vocal cords or the cuff. Pooled secretions carry bacteria from the oral cavity that pose a threat to the lower airway and lungs. Passive aspiration of these secretions across the cuff of the ETT has been linked to **ventilator-associated pneumonia (VAP),** a deadly **nosocomial** infection commonly acquired in the ICU. About 12% of patients who need mechanical ventilation develop VAP, most often in the first few days of ventilation. For this reason, mechanically ventilated patients require vigorous oral care and frequent removal of oral secretions, not only from the mouth and oropharynx, but also from the vallecula and subglottic region. *Before transporting any patient with an advanced airway, it is a good idea to suction the oral cavity and posterior pharynx.*

Tracheostomy Tube Maintenance

The same precautions used for an ETT cuff should be taken with a tracheostomy tube cuff. The cuff should never be deflated while the patient is on mechanical ventilation unless a clinician is present. Some patients may be using a cuffed tube with the cuff deflated to allow communication (deflating the cuff on smaller diameter tubes allows air to move through the vocal cords). Other patients may be using an expiratory occlusive valve on the tracheostomy tube, which requires a deflated cuff. This is essentially a one-way valve; it allows air to enter the trachea through the tracheostomy tube and then closes to force air up through the vocal cords and out through the upper airway. The pilot balloon should be in plain view on all patients with cuffed tubes, whether inflated or deflated.

Tracheostomy tubes have several features that pose added challenges to patient care. The most common of these features is the inner cannula (or, simply, the cannula), the "tube within a tube." The outer cannula is the tracheostomy tube itself; the inner cannula is a thin-walled tube that fits inside the tracheostomy tube and locks into place, either by a screw-type mechanism or a snap lock. The inner cannula is designed so that it can be removed for cleaning without requiring removal of the airway.

Another feature of the tracheostomy tube is the *fenestration,* an opening on the posterior wall of the tube that allows airflow from the lungs to the upper airway. Fenestrated tubes usually are packaged with one fenestrated cannula, one unfenestrated cannula, and an obturator. The obturator is a blind plug that is used to insert the tracheostomy tube into the stoma. Fenestrated tubes pose a risk to the tracheal mucosa if left in place for long periods, because granulation tissue grows into the fenestration; this can cause bleeding, irritation, and stridor. Obstruction of the fenestration by secretions should also be prevented.

If a tracheostomy tube is displaced (i.e., comes out), careful thought must be given to the replacement process. If the stoma is old (generally, more than 7 days old), it may be possible to replace the tracheostomy tube using the obturator. If the old tracheostomy tube is unavailable (e.g., too soiled to use) and a new one is not available, an ETT can be placed through the stoma (remember, it will require a very shallow insertion). If the stoma is new (generally, less than 7 days old), the chances of losing the tract between the skin and the trachea are high. In general, if the stoma is new and the tracheostomy tube comes out, the patient should be orally reintubated with an ETT until the tracheostomy site can be carefully evaluated. Attempting to replace a tracheostomy tube through a fresh stoma carries a high risk of creating a false airway passage and ventilation of the mediastinum rather than the trachea; the results can be disastrous.

Regardless of the type of tube used, tube vigilance during transport cannot be overemphasized (Table 3-8). Tubes move; they shift with movement of the patient's head. Think of all the position changes a patient undergoes during a simple transport. Check the stability and security of the tube as follows:

- Before the initial move
- After entering the ambulance
- Before leaving the ambulance
- Before moving the patient to a bed or stretcher
- Before beginning cardiopulmonary resuscitation (CPR)
- After defibrillation or a seizure
- Anytime the patient becomes agitated

The best airway protection device is the healthcare provider; no mechanical device can ever work as well.

Skill 3-3 presents instructions for suctioning an ETT or tracheostomy tube, and Skill 3-4 lists the steps in the care of a tracheostomy tube.

Table 3-8 Checklist for Transporting Intubated Critical Care Patients

Item	Yes	No
1. Endotracheal or tracheostomy tube in?	☐	☐
2. Tube secure and midline?	☐	☐
3. Oropharynx and distal upper airway clear of secretions?	☐	☐
4. Cuff pressure acceptable?	☐	☐
5. Audible leak around cuff?	☐	☐
6. Breath sounds in all four zones?	☐	☐
7. Patient awake or sedated?	☐	☐
For tracheostomy patients:		
8. Tracheostomy tube adapter free of obstruction?	☐	☐
9. Speaking valve in place?	☐	☐
10. If yes to no. 8, is cuff *deflated?*	☐	☐
11. Obturator available?	☐	☐

Skill 3-3

SUCTIONING OF AN ENDOTRACHEAL TUBE OR A TRACHEOSTOMY TUBE

An artificial airway hinders the patient's ability to cough and clear secretions. Endotracheal tubes (ETTs) and tracheostomy tubes may even become completely occluded with thick secretions, creating an obstructed airway. However, the benefits of suctioning may be outweighed by the potential side effects, which include the introduction of pathogens into the respiratory system and the anoxic/apneic period required for the suctioning procedure.

Two techniques can be used to suction these airway devices: an open technique and a closed technique. Open suctioning has many disadvantages; closed (in-line) suctioning is preferred.

INDICATIONS

Clear secretions in the artificial airway

Aspiration of suspected gastric or upper airway secretions

Facilitate auscultation of adventitious lung sounds over the trachea and bronchi

Evaluate an increase in peak airway pressures during positive pressure ventilation

Address an increase in coughing or the respiratory rate (or both)

Address a decrease in oxygenation levels: arterial oxygen pressure ($Pa{O_2}$), saturation of oxygen via arterial blood ($Sa{O_2}$), or pulse oximetry ($Sp{O_2}$)

Address a sudden onset of respiratory distress

Obtain samples from the respiratory tree

CONTRAINDICATIONS

There are no absolute contraindications to suctioning of artificial airways. In patients with a high risk for intolerance of suctioning, the clinical benefit must be weighed against the risk

COMPLICATIONS ASSOCIATED WITH SUCTIONING

Respiratory or cardiac arrest (or both)

Cardiac dysrhythmias

Hypertension or hypotension

Hypoxia

Increased intracranial pressure

Bronchospasm

Pulmonary hemorrhage or bleeding **(epithelial denudement)**

Procedure for Open Technique

1. Gather the appropriate-sized sterile suction catheter, sterile water-soluble lubricant or sterile saline, sterile gloves, and a sterile solution container or basin. Wash hands and follow standard precautions.
2. Assemble the connecting tubing and turn on and test the suction unit (100 to 120 mm Hg of pressure). Organize the connecting tubing near your work surface and keep the suction on.
3. Gather the bag-mask system with oxygen reservoir, positive end-expiratory pressure (PEEP) valve, and connecting tubing.
4. Put on facial protection (open suctioning aerosolizes the patient's respiratory secretions).

5. Open the sterile catheter onto a clean work surface near the patient's head. Use the wrapper as your sterile field.
6. Open the sterile container and partly fill it with sterile saline or water using sterile technique.
7. Put on sterile gloves. Ask for assistance in hyperoxygenating the patient.
8. Using sterile technique, attach the catheter to the connecting tubing. Suction a small amount of saline from the basin as a test.

Hyperoxygenation Therapy Before and After Suctioning

For at least 30 seconds before and after suctioning, hyperoxygenate the patient by one of the following methods:

- Hold the suction hyperoxygenation button on the ventilator.
- Increase the fraction of inspired oxygen (FIO_2) on the ventilator to 100%.
- Disconnect the patient from the ventilator and have an assistant deliver 5 or 6 slow, even breaths through a bag-valve system (15 L of oxygen, PEEP).

9. Insert the appropriate-sized sterile catheter into the artificial airway until resistance is met; *then pull back slightly.*

NOTE: Premeasuring the depth of insertion of the catheter according to the artificial airway eliminates trauma to the mucous membranes but results in suctioning only of the airway and not of the respiratory tree.

NOTE: Special catheters are available that can directly suction either the left or right mainstem bronchus. Because of the airway anatomy, customary catheters usually enter the right mainstem bronchus.

10. With your nondominant hand, occlude the suction port while withdrawing and rotating the catheter with the thumb and forefinger of your dominant hand. Apply suction only on the removal phase of this process and only for 10 seconds.
11. Hyperoxygenate the patient again and monitor the person carefully.
12. If secretions remain, you may suction again as indicated in steps 9 through 11. Limit suctioning to two or three attempts and then allow the patient to rest. Rinse the suction catheter between attempts by inserting it into sterile saline or water and applying suction.
13. After the lower airways have been suctioned and ventilations to the patient have been resumed, the same catheter may be used to suction the upper airways (nose and mouth). Once the upper airways have been suctioned, the catheter is considered nonsterile and must be discarded.
14. Reposition the patient and reestablish all ventilation parameters. Wash your hands and document the procedure, including how well the patient tolerated it.

NOTE: Sterile saline or sterile water should not be instilled into the tracheobronchial tree before suctioning as a routine practice. Instillation of 5 to 10 mL of sterile saline does not thin secretions, and it may cause hypoxia and increase the risk of lower airway infection.

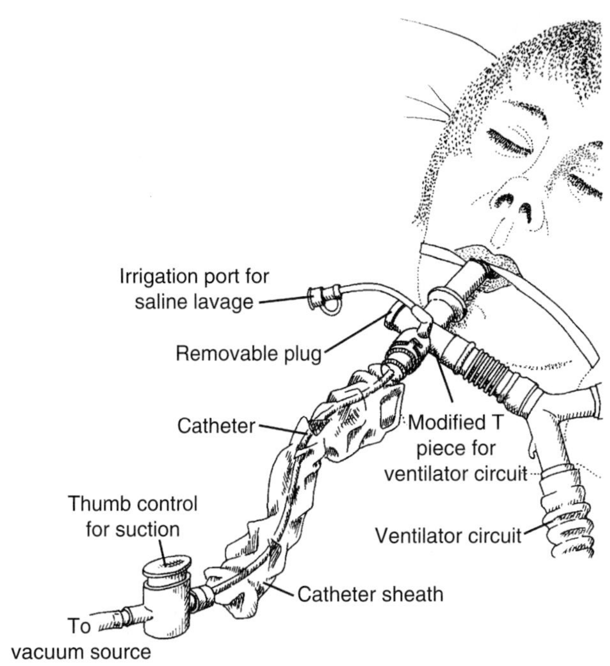

Closed suction technique. (From Sills JR: *Respiratory certification guide*, St Louis, 1991, Mosby.)

Procedure for Closed Technique

1. Wash your hands and follow standard precautions.
2. Set the suction level to that recommended by the manufacturer of the closed suction system; do not turn on the suction.
3. Attach the suction connecting tubing to the closed system port.
4. Hyperoxygenate the patient.
5. With the suction still off, gently and quickly insert the catheter into the artificial airway until resistance is met; *then pull back slightly.*
6. Use your nondominant hand to engage the suction while withdrawing (into the sleeve) and rotating the catheter between the thumb and forefinger of your dominant hand. Suction for no longer than 10 seconds.
7. Hyperoxygenate the patient and monitor the person carefully.
8. Steps 5 through 7 may be repeated, for a total of two or three suction passes at one time.
9. A separate catheter may be opened to suction the upper airways. Attach this catheter to the connecting tubing and complete the procedure.

10. Discard the disposable equipment appropriately and wash your hands. Document the procedure, including how well the patient tolerated it.

NOTE: Some patients do not tolerate suctioning, even with hyperoxygenation therapy. If complications arise:

a. Make sure 100% oxygen is being delivered.
b. If you are using the open technique, switch to the closed technique to avoid removing the patient from the ventilator.
c. Allow the patient to rest for a longer period between suctioning passes.
d. If the patient is receiving ventilator PEEP, maintain PEEP during suctioning. This is best done using a closed device, because open suctioning leads to loss of PEEP.
e. If you disconnect the patient from the ventilator for suctioning, maintain PEEP on a bag-mask device.

Skill 3-4

TRACHEOSTOMY TUBE CARE

Tracheostomy tubes have a variety of parts with distinct functions that help keep the patient's artificial airways open. A tracheostomy tube generally is smaller in diameter and shorter than an endotracheal tube (ETT). Some have a distal cuff to protect against aspiration or air leakage during mechanical ventilation.

INDICATIONS

Serve as an elective surgical airway when the primary airway is obstructed by a lesion or inflammation

Serve as an emergency surgical airway when acute airway obstruction has occurred

Allow long-term ventilation therapy (replaces the ETT, usually after 1 to 2 weeks)

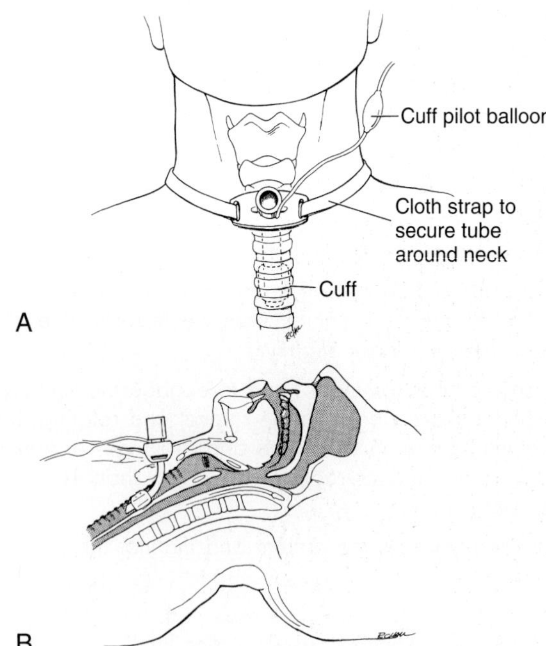

A, Anterior view of the tracheostomy tube after insertion. **B,** Lateral view of the tracheostomy tube after insertion. (From Eubanks DH, Bone RC: *Comprehensive respiratory care,* ed 2, St Louis, 1990, Mosby.)

PARTS OF THE TRACHEOSTOMY TUBE

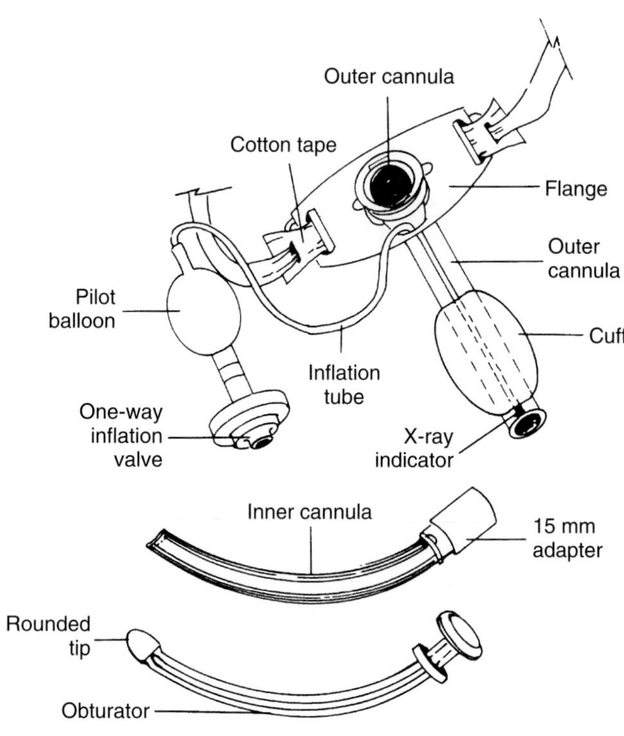

Parts of a tracheostomy tube. (From Eubanks DH, Bone RC: *Comprehensive respiratory care,* ed 2, St Louis, 1990, Mosby.)

1. *Outer cannula:* This is the body of the tube; it sometimes has a cuff (cuffs are not used in children or in adults with laryngectomies).
2. *Neck flange:* This is connected to the outer cannula. It provides stabilization against the skin of the anterior neck and allows cloth ties to be attached for further securement.
3. *Inner cannula* (optional): This is a clear tube that is inserted into the outer cannula. It has the standard 15 mm adapter for ventilation attachment.
4. *Obturator:* This is a blunt-ended, solid stylet used during insertion of the device. It should be kept near the patient in case the tracheostomy tube needs to be reinserted.
5. *Pilot balloon* (optional): If the device is cuffed, the function of the pilot balloon is similar to that of the cuff on an ETT.

PROCEDURE

1. Wash your hands and follow standard precautions. Use facial protection if you will be suctioning, if copious secretions are present, and/or if the patient is unable to cover the stoma while coughing.
2. *To cut new ties:* Cut the twill tape to a length that would circle the patient's neck twice.
3. Hyperoxygenate and suction patient as needed.
4. Remove the soiled dressing and discard it appropriately.
5. Discard your nonsterile gloves and wash your hands.
6. Prepare the sterile field and assemble the supplies: sterile saline, hydrogen peroxide, and a sterile container. Combine the sterile saline and hydrogen peroxide in the container in a 50:50 mix.
7. Put on sterile gloves.
8. Remove the inner cannula and put it in the hydrogen peroxide/saline solution (clean it with a small sterile brush if necessary).
9. Rinse the inner cannula with sterile saline, reinsert it, and lock it in place.

NOTE: While the inner cannula is cleaned, oxygen and ventilation may be applied to the outer cannula or to a second inner cannula.

10. *To clean the stoma:* Cleanse the stoma site with a sterile saline–impregnated 4 × 4 gauze square and then dry it with a clean gauze square.
11. *To clean the outer cannula:* Cleanse the outer cannula with a sterile saline–impregnated 4 × 4 gauze square and cotton swabs. Pat dry with a clean 4 × 4 gauze square.
12. Have an assistant hold the neck flange in place while you release the old neck ties and discard them.

NOTE: This is especially important if the tracheostomy stoma is less than 5 to 7 days old. If the tracheostomy tube is accidentally dislodged, the fresh opening may close. In general, ties should not be replaced or the tracheostomy manipulated in the first few days after insertion.

13. Insert one end of a new tie through the neck flange and pull it until one half the length is through the slot. Slide the double tie around the back of the neck and insert it through the other slot, looping one end back to the original slot. Double square knot on that side (see the illustration).
14. Apply a fresh dressing to the site.
15. Discard the disposable supplies and your gloves appropriately and wash your hands.
16. Document the appearance of the stoma site and the amount and color of the drainage.

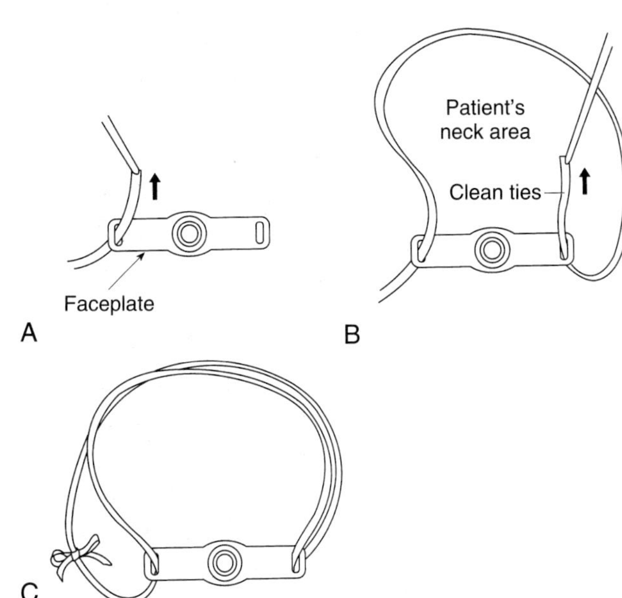

Placement of the tracheostomy twill tape. **A,** The twill tape is threaded through the faceplate (to prevent decannulation, another person must stabilize the faceplate as the tape is applied). **B,** The tape is passed around the back of the neck and looped through the other side of the faceplate. **C,** The tape is doubled and secured in a knot.

Sizes and Types of Endotracheal Tubes

According to the Magill system of measuring for ETT size, a tube with a 7 to 7.5 mm ID generally should be used for females, and one with an 8 mm ID should be used for males. Various formulas have been developed to help determine the correct size in pediatric patients (see Chapter 9).

As with extraglottic devices, many types of endotracheal tubes have been designed to meet the needs of the operating room, ICU, and special emergency situations. Single- or double-lumen tubes with flexible tips that can be used for the nasal or oral route (or both) are available. Tubes used in the operating room during laser procedures are even fire-resistant. The critical care transport team should be familiar with some of these designs.

Hi-Lo Evac Endotracheal Tube

The Hi-Lo Evac ETT with an evacuation lumen (Figure 3-13) was designed to prevent ventilator-assisted pneumonia (VAP). It allows intermittent or continuous evacuation of secretions above the cuff; this prevents aspiration of these secretions, which can lead to VAP. An adaptation of the Hi-Lo, the jet endotracheal tube (JET), was designed for pediatric **jet ventilation** through the main tube; this ETT has a side lumen for monitoring airway pressures and the $PETCO_2$ and for providing irrigation.

Double-Lumen Endotracheal Tube

The double-lumen tube (DLT) is designed to provide separate ventilation to each lung. This may be done to protect one

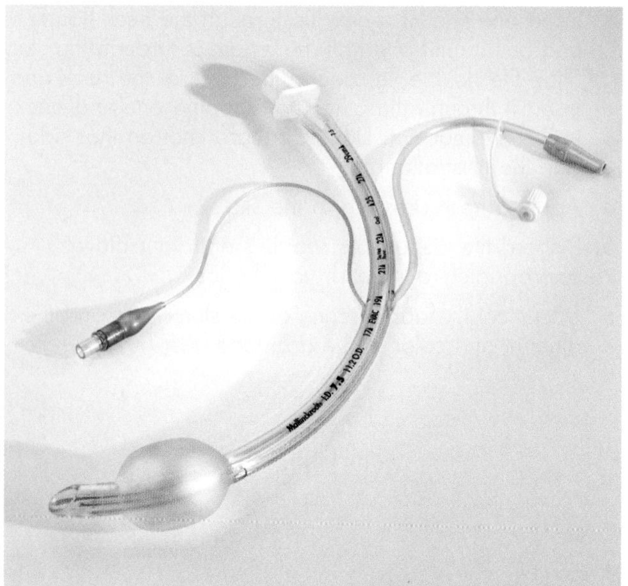

Figure 3-13

Hi-Lo Evac tube. (Nellcor Puritan Bennett [Mallinckrodt], Boulder, Colo.)

lung or to facilitate surgery. These tubes may be further categorized as DLT or tubes that allow ventilation of only one lung (while blocking the other). Endobronchial tubes (EBTs), bronchial blockers (BBs), and certain types of DLTs are specially designed for thoracic surgery, and some require bronchoscopy for correct placement.

Replacing Tracheal Tubes

In airway and breathing management, you are attempting to protect the airway and recreate the natural act of ventilation. However, the mere presence of any artificial airway creates thoracic **dead space,** airflow turbulence, and **airway resistance.** Turbulence is increased when a high inspiratory airflow is required from positive pressure ventilation (PPV) and is passed through the tracheal tube; this creates the overall effect of a small airway diameter and increases the resistance to breathing. The length and curve of the tube add to this phenomenon. Fat, short, straight tubes would be better for PPV, but they are more difficult to place properly.

After you have assessed the ABCs in a patient with a tracheal tube, you must determine whether the tube is the correct size, patent, and functioning properly. If the tube is functioning poorly (e.g., has an air leak or a cuff leak) or a patient who is difficult to ventilate has a small tube, you may need to insert a new or a larger tube. Many tools are available that can help you change the ETT without having to start from the beginning and add risk to airway management.

These tools generally are called *exchange catheters,* but even introducers and stylets may be used. For this process, the intubated patient is preoxygenated, and the proper-sized exchange catheter is inserted to the predetermined depth (to prevent tracheal damage). The preexisting ETT cuff is deflated, and the tube is gently removed. (Some exchange catheters allow for temporary ventilation through the catheter while awaiting the new ETT.) The new ETT is inserted over the exchange catheter to the proper depth, the cuff is inflated, and the tube's position confirmation is confirmed according to protocol. The exchange catheter then is gently removed, and the new ETT is secured.

Endotracheal Tube Guides and Stylets

In general, an ETT can be placed without the aid of surgery in one of three ways:

- Blindly (i.e., digitally), without the use of an intubation instrument (laryngoscope).
- Using visualization (with the aid of a laryngoscope, fiberoptics, or bronchoscope)
- Indirectly with the aid of an indicator, hearing, sensing, or lights (lighted stylet)

The correct equipment can significantly ease the process of intubation (see Tables 3-5 to 3-7).

Digital Intubation

Placing the ETT with your fingers has some benefit if you cannot see the vocal cords (because of blood or secretions) and/or the patient is unable to move the head or neck. You do not need to overcome the three angles to view the cords. Instead, palpate the epiglottis and guide the tube into position by feel. The most significant obstacles to digital intubation are the gag reflex and/or a conscious patient. Once the gag reflex has been stimulated, the patient has no choice but to bite down.

To begin this procedure, place a lighted or standard stylet inside the ETT and mold the tube into a J or hockey stick configuration. You know that the epiglottis sits behind the base of the tongue; therefore, "walk" the first and second fingers of your dominant hand to the base of the tongue. Use one finger to identify and retract the epiglottis. Angle the preconfigured ETT into the patient's mouth and toward your finger. Once in the entrance of the glottis, use the second finger to trap the tip of the ETT and "drive" it through the glottis. When it is engaged, remove your walking fingers and hold the ETT in position; alternate short withdrawals of the stylet and advancement of the ETT until the tube has been properly positioned and the stylet has been removed. Confirm placement and secure the device.

Nasotracheal Intubation

The nose is a secondary route for an ETT. Correct placement through the vocal cords can be achieved either blindly or, in adults, by direct visualization. Regardless of the technique used, the most common complication is nasal bleeding. Nasotracheal maneuvers usually are more complicated and take longer to accomplish; however, an advantage is that oxygenation can be maintained during the procedure by providing supplemental oxygen through the tube.

Because of the unique anatomy of the area, the ETT must be at least one-half size smaller than normally would be chosen for the oral route. Use a special tube with a ringlike apparatus that allows anterior deflection in the tip of the tube, if one is available. Thoroughly lubricating both the tip of the tube and the chosen nostril facilitates movement and reduces trauma. If time permits, the lubricant can be mixed with 2% lidocaine and 0.25% to 0.5% phenylephrine to provide local anesthesia and help prevent nasal bleeding.

Blind nasotracheal intubation

Blind nasotracheal intubation may be used when direct visualization of the trachea is difficult or impossible (e.g., the teeth are clenched) and when the service has no protocol for rapid sequence intubation (RSI) or there is no vascular access to administer RSI drugs.

Your patient may be either seated or supine but must be self-ventilating well enough to guide the insertion. Position the tube bevel out and at a right angle; then, insert it through the nostril and into the oropharynx. At this point, listen over the ETT for breath sounds; if they are present, slowly advance the tube while applying cricoid pressure and feeling and listening for tube position. When the tip enters the glottis, you will hear a tubular sound and the patient may cough (described as a "bovine cough"). To help yourself use "hearing" the breath sounds as your guide, you can put a special whistle (such as that used on a teakettle) over the end of the tube. As an alternative, you can remove the bell from a single tube stethoscope and insert the distal part of the tube into the ETT.

You may need to make several attempts to place a tracheal tube through the glottis via the nose successfully. To help move the distal part of the tube into position, move the patient's head into a flexed position or pull the mandible forward with the thumb and forefingers of your nondominant hand.

Nasotracheal intubation through direct visualization (adults)

A laryngoscope and Magill forceps are required for nasotracheal intubation by direct visualization. Have the Magill forceps immediately available. Lubricate the ETT and insert it appropriately; then insert the laryngoscope in a standard manner. When you can view the cords, with your dominant hand insert the forceps, grasp the tip of the ETT, and direct it anteriorly. Take care not to damage the ETT cuff with the forceps.

Fiberoptic and Video Intubation

Bronchoscopes are rigid or flexible devices that are used to aid direct visualization of the intraglottic airway for placement of an ETT or for surgical tracheostomy. The flexible type is referred to as a **fiberoptic bronchoscope (FOB)** or flexible fiberoptic bronchoscope (FFB). An FOB is used when intubation with a direct laryngoscope is impossible or is expected to be problematic or when a standard intubation attempt has failed.

Problems with intubation can be expected with abnormal anatomic features, such as congenital anomalies, cervical spine abnormalities, **temporomandibular ankylosis,** or a **Mallampati score** of class III or class IV. Video-assisted FOBs are available that can aid emergency intubation procedures. However, scope of practice regulations usually restrict the use of these devices to physicians and Certified Respiratory Nurse Anesthetists (CRNAs).

The fiberoptic laryngoscopes that have been entering the healthcare field over the past few years (and the new ones coming out) give the critical care team the advantage of a bronchoscopic view of the airway that is obtained in a manner well within the crew's scope of practice. These airway cameras allow direct laryngoscopy, provide a mechanism for confirming ETT placement, and allow direct visualization for upgrading from an extraglottic to an intraglottic airway (Figures 3-14 and 3-15; Tables 3-9 to 3-11).

Special Airway Techniques

The decision to go beyond direct or fiberoptic visualization of the airways, using extraglottic or intraglottic devices, usually is made during a highly stressful, extremely difficult airway

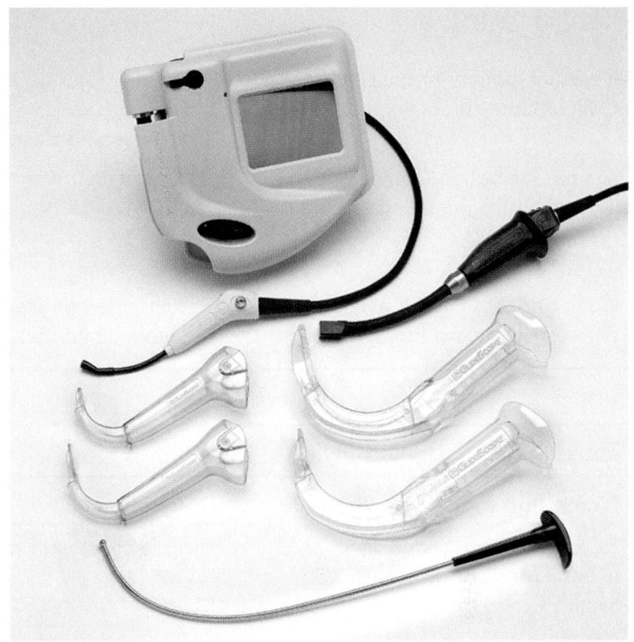

Figure 3-14

Glidescope Ranger. (Courtesy Verathon, Bothell, Wash.)

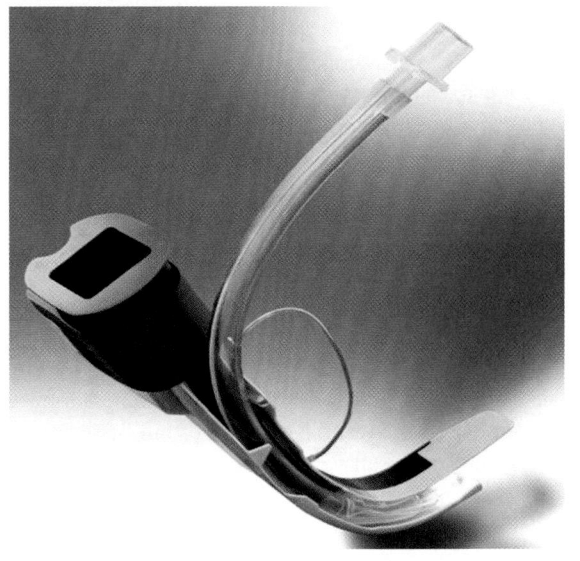

Figure 3-15

AirTraq. (Courtesy AirTraq.)

Table 3-9 Endotracheal Tube Guides

Name and Manufacturer	Description	Special Features and Clinical Application
Gum elastic bougie (also known as the Portex Venn Tracheal Tube Introducer) (Smiths Medical ASD, Keene, N.H.)	Long guide with 35-degree **Coude tip;** can also be used to guide endotracheal tube (ETT)	Introducer for anterior larynx or those with difficulty opening their mouth; used over extraglottic airways. Used either to intubate the trachea directly or as a stylet to facilitate intubation. In direct intubation of the trachea, clicks confirm placement.
Single-use bougie (Smiths Medical ASD, Keene, N.H.)	Coude tip with hollow lumen	Used as an introducer that allows for oxygenation and ventilation during placement; nondisposable.
Parker Flex-It Articulating Tracheal Tube Stylet (Parker Medical, Englewood, Colo.)	Articulating stylet for both pediatric and adult ETTs	Based on standard stylet design but has a button at viewer's end that allows a bougie-like angle at distal end of ETT; allows one-handed distal control of ETT; also facilitates video intubation.
Frova Intubation Introducer (Cook Critical Care, Bloomington, Ind.)	Angled distal tip with two side ports; allows for stiff or malleable design	Acts as an introducer, stylet, or exchanger in both pediatric and adult ETTs with adapters that allow ventilation during intubation procedure.
Aintree Intubation Catheter (Cook Critical Care, Bloomington, Ind.)	Large lumen with angled tip, two side ports, and adapters	Acts as introducer, exchanger, and stylet. Allows fiberoptic bronchoscopy (FOB) during procedure for direct visualization; also allows ventilation during procedures.
Cook and AEC (adult exchange catheter) EF (extra firm lumen)	Exchange catheter for double- lumen tubes	Extra firm catheter made for exchange of double tubes.

Table 3-10 Lighted Stylets

Name and Manufacturer	Description	Special Features and Clinical Application
Flexible Airway Scope Tool (FAST) (Clarus Medical, Minneapolis, Minn.)	Flexible stylet with rigid tip	Designed for adult exchange from intubation LMA or other extraglottic airway; confirms ETT placement.
FAST Plus	Flexible stylet with a hand adjustable atraumatic tip	Used for nasal intubation.
Shikani Optical Stylet (SOS) (Clarus Medical, Minneapolis, Minn.)	Resembles a flexible fiberoptic bronchoscope (FOB) but has a J-shaped stylet	Used to intubate or with other devices in difficult cases. Portable device with more applications in emergency setting. Allows oxygen insufflation through device; has moveable tube stop and oxygen port.
Levitan GLS (Clarus Medical, Minneapolis, Minn.)	Similar to SOS with no movable tube stop	Can be used as an adjunct to direct laryngoscopy or for similar purposes as an SOS.
Trachlight Stylet (Laerdal Light Medical AS, Stavanger, Norway)	Wand with three parts; can be used for pediatric and adult patients	Light wand for intubation but can be used instead of FOB in emergency setting; used for blind, direct, or indirect visualization when glottis is difficult to see or head movement is limited.

procedure. The critical care team must have protocols to guide these decisions. The difficult airway protocol is devised by the service's medical director, but it must be well rehearsed by every member of the team. Near the bottom of this decision tree are some special airway techniques that usually are categorized as surgical approaches (Figures 3-16 to 3-20).

Retrograde Intubation

According to difficult airway protocols, retrograde intubation is used when the patient cannot be ventilated or oxygenated. A large needle is used to gain access to the cricothyroid membrane, and a guide wire is introduced into the needle and directed through it superiorly. The guide wire is fed toward the mouth; because it will tend toward the nose, a second team member uses a Magill forceps to grab the guide wire in the pharynx and guide it out of the mouth. The guide wire is fed through an ETT, which then is passed over the guide wire into the trachea. The primary limitation of this emergency procedure is that it takes considerable time to perform.

Table 3-11 Fiberoptic and Rigid Laryngoscopes

Name and Manufacturer	Description	Special Features and Clinical Application
Glidescope Video Laryngoscopes (GVL) (Verathon, Bothell, Wash.)	Lightweight, angled blade (60 degrees) with camera; adult and pediatric sizes	Built to military and emergency medical service (EMS) specifications. Provides real-time visualization of airway; rechargeable battery. Feeds live information to a small camera.
DCI Video Laryngoscope System (Karl Storz, Tuttlingen, Germany)	Interchangeable blades (Miller or Mac) in larger sizes	Handle has snap-in, wide-angle camera with fiberscopes that allow greater visibility with less head positioning. Good for difficult airways and obese patients. Verifies endotracheal tube (ETT) placement. Intubates exchanges and introduces endoscope.
Viewmax Laryngoscope Blade (Rush, Research Triangle Park, N.C.)	Optic side port onto Mac blade; adult and pediatric sizes	Prism mounted; gives "fish eye" appearance of cords with Mac view.
McGrath Video Laryngoscope (LMA North America, San Diego, Calif.)	Portable, lightweight, wireless laryngoscope with disposable blades	Good for obese patients, those with limited mouth opening, and head movement with anterior airways. Adjustable blades allow for multiple patient sizes.
Pentax Airway Scope	Wireless video; laryngoscope with special suction blade	Similar to McGrath device but has one blade size that allows for suctioning through the blade.
AirTraq (Prodol Meditex SA, Vizcaya, Spain)	Disposable optical laryngoscope with ET guide	Self-contained unit with fiberscopic guide for routine and difficult airway management. ETT is mounted in device, and operator guides it in while watching.
Bullard Elite Laryngoscope (Gyrus ACMI, Southborough, Mass.)	Indirect fiberoptic laryngoscope; adult and pediatric sizes	Allows for oxygen insufflation and suctioning during use. Can be used with standard handle or fiberoptic source. Optical metal stylets attached.
UpsherScope Ultra (Mercury Medical, Clearwater, Fla.)	Indirect rigid fiberoptic laryngoscope; adult size	Same as Bullard Elite device but must use the Upsher handle or fiberoptic source.

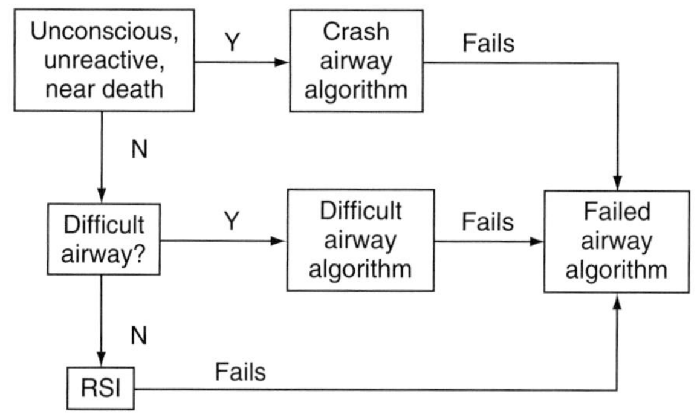

Figure 3-16

Universal emergency airway algorithm. (From Walls RM, Luten RC, Murphy MF, et al, editors: *Manual of emergency airway management: a companion manual for the National Airway Management Course*, Philadelphia, 2000, Lippincott Williams & Wilkins.)

Cricothyrotomy

Cricothyrotomy may be the final lifesaving procedure for a patient you cannot intubate, ventilate, or oxygenate. Some commercially designed devices are available to assist with this procedure.

Needle Cricothyrotomy

Needle cricothyrotomy should be performed with a large needle and catheter system. Cook's Emergency Transtracheal Airway Catheter (Cook, Bloomington, Indiana) is an example of a large, nonkinking catheter that is introduced with a needle. Another very simple system is a 14-gauge, 2-inch IV catheter that is inserted into the cricothyroid membrane with an attached syringe. Once the trachea is entered, the stylet is removed and the 15 mm adapter from a 3 mm ETT can be inserted into the top of the catheter to provide direct ventilation by means of a bag-valve system. Because the 14-gauge catheter has no fenestration, it is used only in crisis situations and for short-term therapy.

Percutaneous Cricothyrotomy

Percutaneous cricothyrotomy may involve the **Seldinger technique.** A needle is used to gain access, and the opening is subsequently dilated to allow insertion of the catheter.

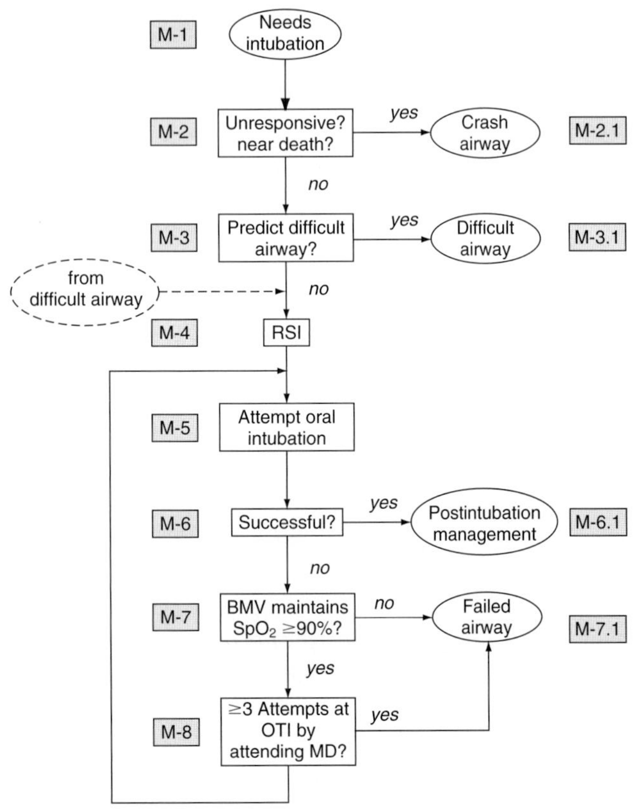

Figure 3-17

Main emergency airway algorithm. (From Walls RM, Luten RC, Murphy MF, et al, editors: *Manual of emergency airway management: a companion manual for the National Airway Management Course,* Philadelphia, 2000, Lippincott Williams & Wilkins.)

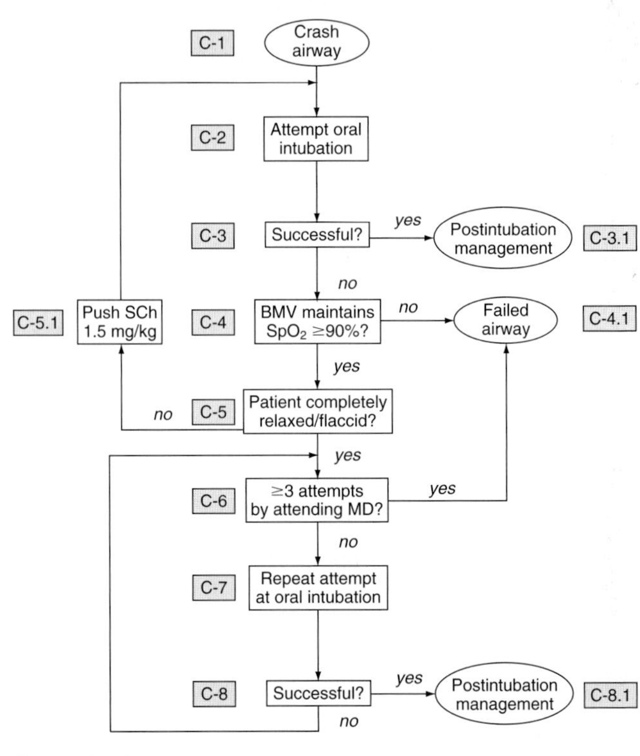

Figure 3-18

Crash airway algorithm. (From Walls RM, Luten RC, Murphy MF, et al, editors: *Manual of emergency airway management: a companion manual for the National Airway Management Course,* Philadelphia, 2000, Lippincott Williams & Wilkins.)

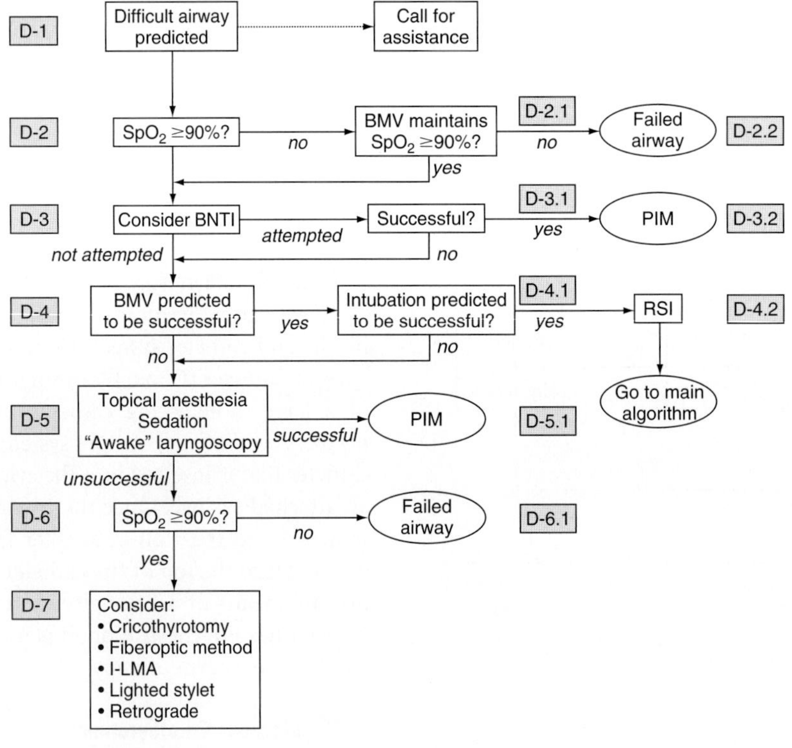

Figure 3-19

Difficult airway algorithm. (From Walls RM, Luten RC, Murphy MF, et al, editors: *Manual of emergency airway management: a companion manual for the National Airway Management Course,* Philadelphia, 2000, Lippincott Williams & Wilkins.)

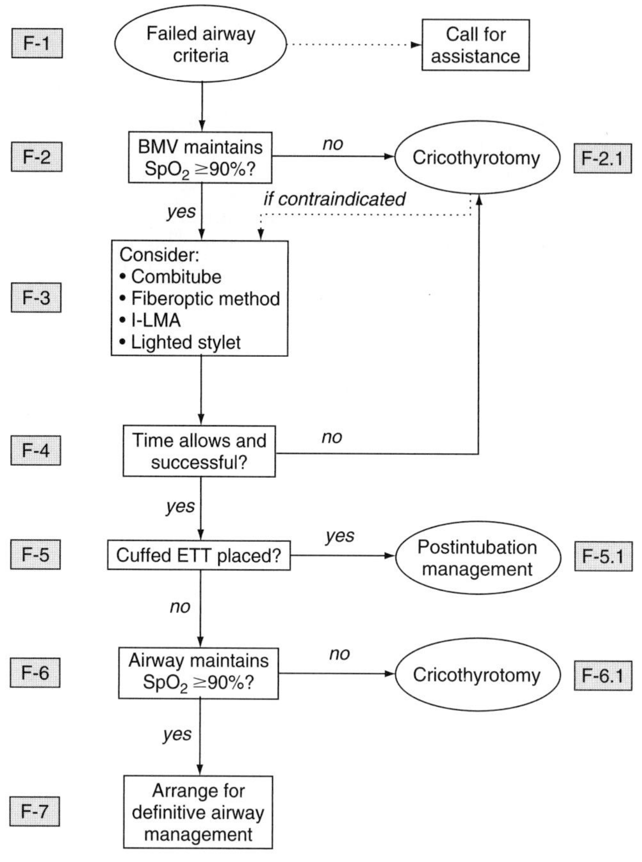

Figure 3-20

Failed airway algorithm. (From Walls RM, Luten RC, Murphy MF, et al, editors: *Manual of emergency airway management: a companion manual for the National Airway Management Course,* Philadelphia, 2000, Lippincott Williams & Wilkins.)

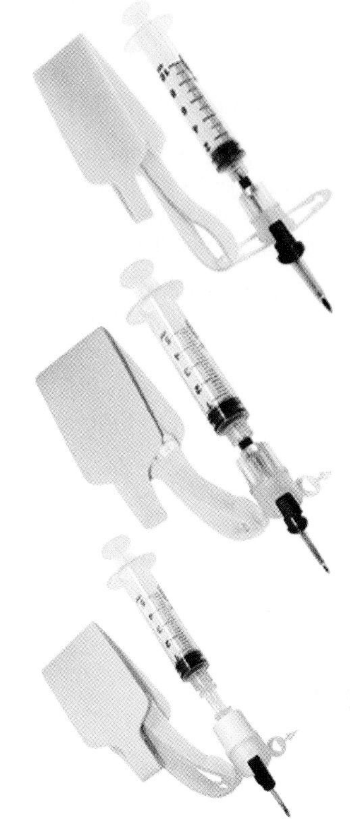

Figure 3-21

Quicktrach II with cuff. (Courtesy VBM Medizintechnik, Sulz, Germany.)

Examples of devices used for this purpose include the Melker Cuffed Emergency Cricothyrotomy Catheter Set (Cook) which houses a 5 mm cuffed airway catheter. The QuickTrach I and QuickTrach II (VBM Medizintechnik, Sulz, Germany) provide an uncuffed or cuffed tracheal tube through a large, trocarlike needle; both pediatric and adult sizes are available (Figure 3-21).

Surgical Cricothyrotomy

For a **surgical cricothyrotomy,** an incision is made first through the skin and then through the cricothyroid membrane. A tracheotomy tube or standard ETT is then inserted through the opening. This is the fastest surgical technique, especially when no other commercial products are available. Skill 3-5 presents the steps in the surgical creation of an airway.

Tracheostomy

For an emergency **tracheostomy,** incisions are made through the skin and into the trachea just beneath the cricoid cartilage. This technique is considered for children under 10 years of age and for patients with lesions or infections that have altered the airway anatomy. Note that this technique falls within the physician's scope of practice.

Skill 3-5

CREATING AN AIRWAY SURGICALLY

Surgical creation of an airway is required when "standard" mechanisms of providing an airway are unsuccessful.

INDICATION

Provide a rescue airway in cases of complete airway obstruction and failed intubation and when major facial trauma prevents intubation or ventilation through the mouth or nose

CONTRAINDICATIONS

Should not be the initial airway management procedure

Child under 12 years of age (contraindication to cricothyrotomy because of the pediatric anatomy; percutaneous transtracheal ventilation is recommended instead)

Laryngeal or tracheal pathologic condition in the cricothyroid area

PREPARING FOR A CRICOTHYROTOMY

1. Examine the cricothyroid area for any pathologic conditions. Obtain the patient's history and identify landmarks while ventilations are attempted with a bag-mask device. To identify the cricothyroid membrane:
   a. Identify the area above the thyroid cartilage (the thyrohyoid space) and palpate inferiorly to find the thyroid cartilage and then the cricoid ring; *or*
   b. Identify the tracheal rings; move superiorly to first the cricoid ring and then to the membrane (see the illustration).

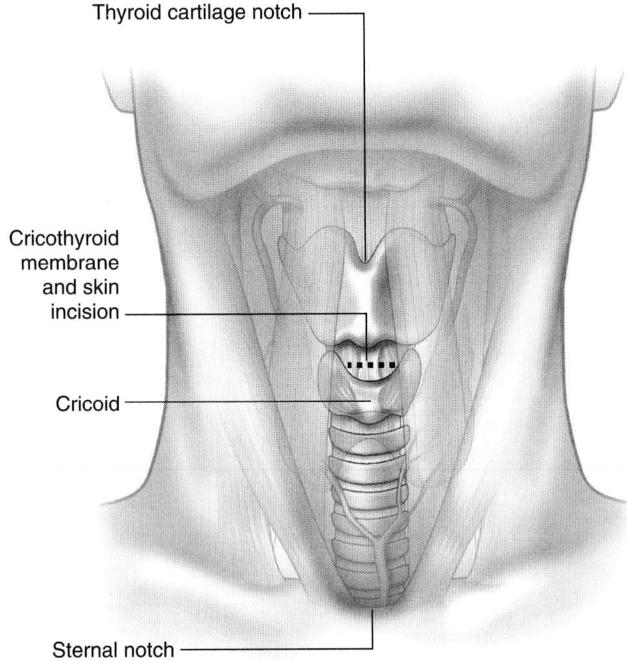

Using the thyroid notch and the cricoid cartilage as reference points, palpate the cricothyroid membrane through the skin. (From the American Association of Critical Care Nurses: *AACN procedure manual for critical care,* Philadelphia, 2011, Saunders.)

2. Gather and prepare your equipment. A "cric kit" should be preassembled and available in your airway kit. This equipment might include a commercial kit or: Betadine skin prep sticks, 4 × 4 sponges, a disposable scalpel (no. 11 blade), two Kelly clamps, a tracheal hook, a cuffed tracheotomy tube (no. 4 Shiley kit), or a 6 mm ETT and syringe. Attach one side of the tie to the flange of the device.

PROCEDURE

1. Cleanse the skin around the cricothyroid membrane with Betadine in a circular fashion; include the thyroid, cricoid, and upper tracheal rings.
2. Provide local anesthetic with 1% lidocaine injected in the skin over the cricothyroid membrane (if the patient is awake and time allows).
3. Assemble the cricothyrotomy kit on a sterile surface. Put on sterile gloves and face protection.
4. With your nondominant hand, use several digits to immobilize the thyroid cartilage. Keep one finger available to palpate the cricoid ring during procedure.
5. Incise the skin from superior to inferior with the cricothyroid membrane at the center. This is a midline incision in the superficial skin that extends from the thyroid cartilage to the upper rings of the trachea.

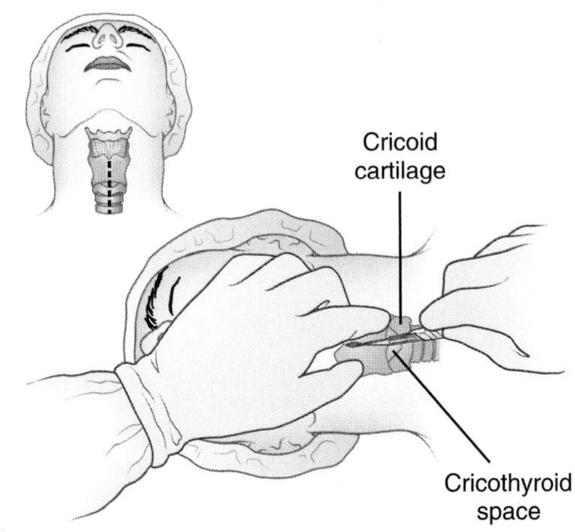

Standard surgical cricothyrotomy. (Redrawn from Walls RM: Cricothyrotomy. In Rosen P, Chan TC, Vilke GM, Sternbach G, editors: *Atlas of emergency procedures,* St Louis, 2001, Mosby.)

6. The Kelly forceps can be used for blunt dissection of the overlying tissue to allow a direct view of the cricothyroid membrane.
7. After you have identified and palpated the cricothyroid membrane, use the scalpel to make a horizontal, 1 cm incision across the lower part of the membrane (see the illustrations).

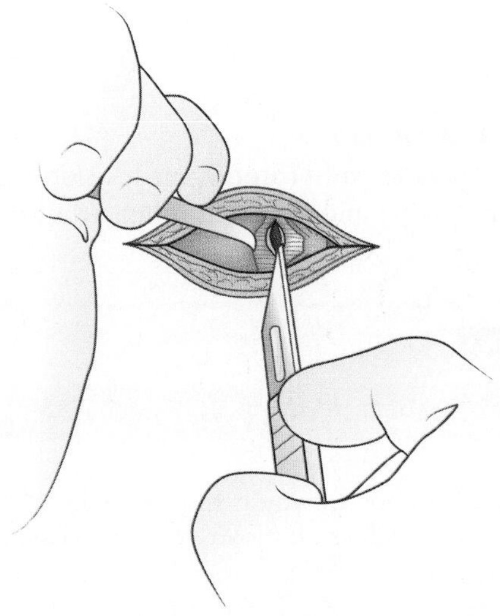

Standard surgical cricothyrotomy. (Redrawn from Walls RM: Cricothyrotomy. In Rosen P, Chan TC, Vilke GM, Sternbach G, editors: *Atlas of emergency procedures,* St Louis, 2001, Mosby.)

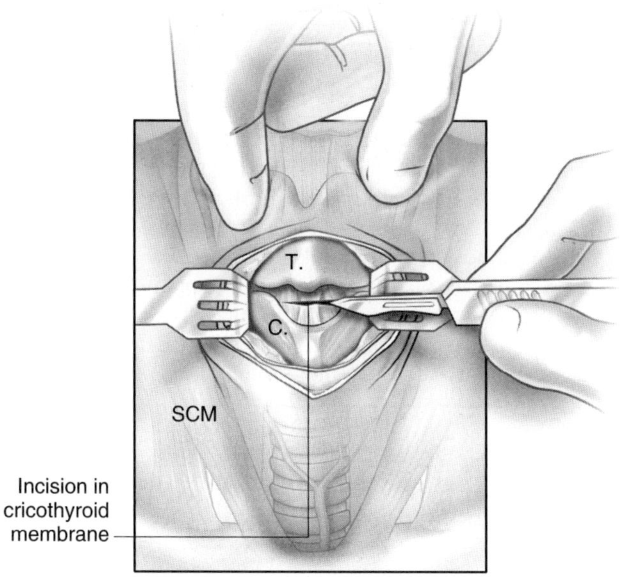

Using the thyroid notch and the cricoid cartilage as reference points, palpate the cricothyroid membrane through the skin. *T*, Thyroid cartilage; *C*, cricoid; *SCM*, sternocleidomastoid.

8. Grasp the upper margin of the cricothyroid membrane with the tracheal hook (a skin hook will do) and retract it superiorly. An assistant can retract with the hook.
9. Use the Kelly forceps (or a Trousseau dilator) to widen the opening while inserting the tracheotomy tube into the gap. Insert the tube with the obturator locked in place. Advance the tube gently and slowly, following the anatomic curve, until the flange is seated on the skin surface. (A second tracheotomy hook may be used on the inferior aspect of the opening to provide retraction from both sides.)
10. When the tracheotomy tube flange is positioned against the skin, inflate the cuff, remove the obturator, and insert the inner cannula. Attach a bag-valve device to this 15 mm adapter and gently ventilate while checking for correct positioning (the position can be confirmed by the same methods used for an ETT).
11. Position the tracheotomy tie around the patient's neck from the prepared, secured side to the other flange of the tube and tie the opposite side.
12. Continue ventilation and oxygenation.

Medication-Assisted Intubation

Many tools are available to critical care paramedics for managing the airway. Your service's choice of tools depends on a number of factors, such as cost, familiarity, and the medical director's preference. However, "hardware" is only one element of airway management; a second element is the use of medications to facilitate initial and continuing airway maneuvers.

The use of medications to facilitate passage of a tracheal tube through the upper airway is a process typically called *rapid sequence intubation (RSI)*. Although there is really nothing rapid about it, the title has stuck, and many use the term to quickly refer to the procedures used to medicate and then intubate a patient.

Dr. Ron M. Walls refers to RSI as, "the administration of a potent induction agent followed immediately by a rapidly acting **neuromuscular blocking agent (NMBA)** to induce unconsciousness and motor paralysis for tracheal intubation(1)." Several steps can help make this procedure successful. Walls RM, Ed., *Manual of Emergency Airway Management* page 8, Published in 2000, Lippincott Williams and Wilkins, Philadelphia, PA.

Crew preparation for performing RSI procedures can last months. The team must be taught and must practice the techniques and scenarios in the operating room or in simulation laboratories. Remember, intubation is not just a 30-second skill. The provider must be able to make good decisions, a skill gained through practice with simulation in multiple scenarios that rehearse the various complications that can arise in the RSI protocols.

Standard RSI Process

You have gone through the education and credentialing program to prepare yourself for RSI. Your service has a protocol in place for RSI, along with a backup plan in case of problems (i.e., a difficult or failed RSI protocol). Now, you can begin.

Step 1: Evaluation of the Patient and Preparation of the Equipment

Your patient must be intubated, and you want to avoid causing pain and complications. Assess the patient carefully for signs of a difficult airway. While evaluating the patient, administer 90% to 100% oxygen (discussed later).

Assessment of the Patient to Predict a Difficult Airway

As part of the preparation for RSI, the relevant anatomy is rapidly assessed to predict whether a patient may be difficult to ventilate, oxygenate, and intubate. This assessment is crucial to correct decision making in the RSI protocol (Figure 3-22). Figure 3-23 shows the Mallampati classification system, which is a method of assessing oral access for intubation. Access is graded as class I through class IV; classes I and II indicate no difficulty with access; class III indicates moderate difficulty, and class IV indicates severe difficulty.

Next, assess for airway obstructions and neck mobility. For example, a hematoma or epiglottitis can obstruct the glottis, preventing intubation. A neck stiff from disease causes problems in aligning the head and neck, resulting in a very difficult intubation. Fiberoptic scopes or guides can help facilitate intubation in patients with limited neck mobility. Box 3-1

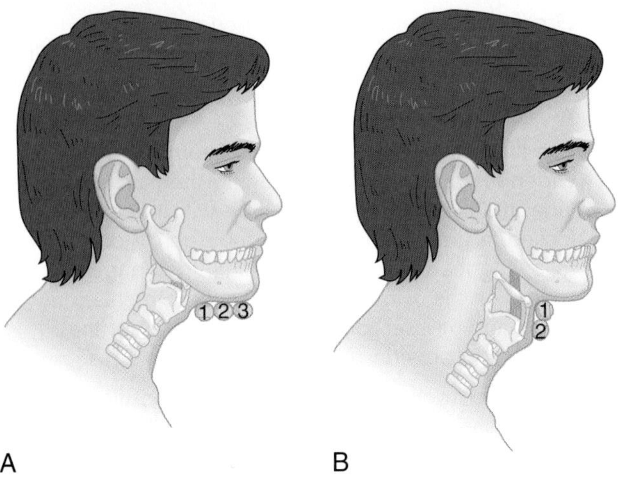

Figure 3-22

Final two steps of the 3-3-2 rule. **A,** Three fingers are placed along the floor of the mouth, beginning at the mentum. **B,** Two fingers are placed in the laryngeal prominence (Adam's apple). (Modified from Murphy MF, Walls RM: Identification of the difficult airway. In Walls RM et al, editors: *Manual of emergency airway management,* Philadelphia, 2004, Lippincott Williams & Wilkins.)

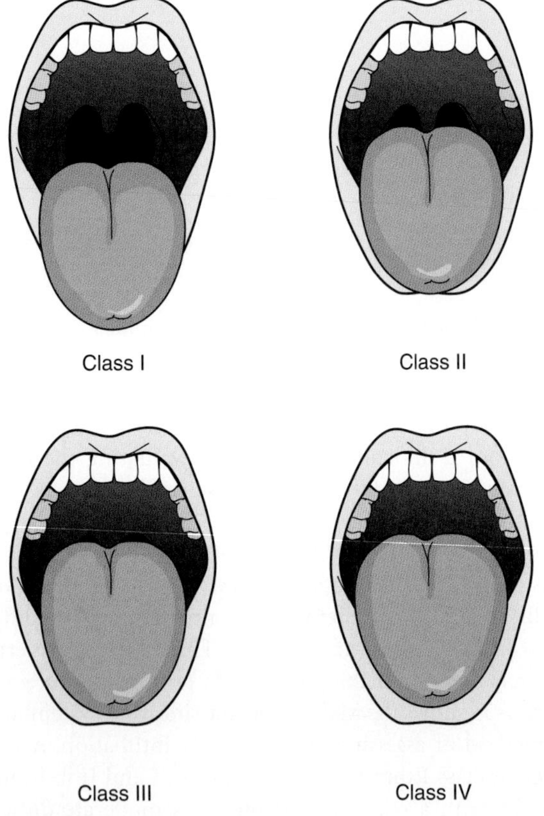

Figure 3-23

The Mallampati scale is an assessment of oral access for intubation. *Class I:* The soft palate, uvula, fauces, and pillars are visible—no difficulty. *Class II:* The soft palate, uvula, and fauces are visible—no difficulty. *Class III:* The soft palate and base of the uvula are visible—moderate difficulty. *Class IV:* Only the hard palate is visible—severe difficulty. (From Phillips N: *Berry and Kohn's operating room technique,* ed 11, St Louis, 2007, Mosby.)

Box 3-1 The LEMON Law

The acronym LEMON is a quick way to remember how to perform an emergency evaluation before rapid sequence intubation (RSI); it helps gauge the difficulty of intubation.

Look externally (e.g., facial hair, which hinders a mask seal; cachexia; edentulous mouth; buck teeth; short "bull" neck; morbid obesity)

Evaluate the 3-3-2 rule (look at the angles)

Mallampati evaluation (for space in the mouth)

Obstruction (look for tumors, edema, abscess, epiglottitis, and high cervical spine injury with hematoma)

Neck mobility (Can you move the neck? Chin to chest?)[2]

presents information on the "LEMON law," an emergency evaluation before RSI. Box 3-2 provides a recap of the RSI process.

Step 2: Preprocedural Hyperoxygenation of the Patient

As soon as the prospect of intubation arises in your management plan, make sure a high percentage of oxygen is being delivered to the patient. Think of the lungs as bags full of room air, composed mostly of nitrogen; your goal is to displace the nitrogen, making those bags a reservoir of oxygen. This reservoir usually allows for longer periods of apnea during the intubation procedure.

Did You Know?

Five minutes of 100% oxygen allows for 8 minutes of apnea in a healthy adult (4 minutes in a small child) before the hemoglobin desaturates to 90%.

Providing 100% oxygen to a patient can be a challenge. A nonrebreather mask with the flowmeter set to deliver enough oxygen to keep the mask's reservoir full actually delivers about 70% to 75% oxygen to the patient. Using a non-self-inflating bag-mask system (anesthesia bag) with the mask over the patient's mouth and nose provides a higher percentage of oxygen to the patient. If you do not have 5 minutes for this process, have the patient quickly complete eight full respiratory cycles (as deep as possible) through the anesthesia bag-mask.

Preventilating a patient in preparation for RSI provides PPV to the esophagus and stomach, which adds to the risk of regurgitation and subsequent aspiration. If at all possible, do not use positive pressure just to preoxygenate the patient. Box 3-3 provides a recap of the RSI sequence.

Certain drugs need to be given to prepare the patient for the RSI procedure. The process or the medications themselves can cause complications in certain patients. Pre-RSI therapy can help prevent these complications.

Box 3-2 Recap of the RSI Sequence: I

Now that you have assessed the patient to see whether the person fits the difficult or failed intubation protocol, you should gather your equipment in preparation for the procedure.

1. *Make sure all monitors are on the patient.* This includes sidestream end-tidal carbon dioxide ($PETCO_2$), if available; pulse oximetry; and three- or five-lead cardiac monitor.
2. *Have your service's recommended airway tools ready.* These might include an extraglottic airway and the endotracheal tube (ETT), in the appropriate sizes, and the appropriate syringes for the devices. Check all cuffs. The backup airway must be as ready as the ETT.
3. *Make sure the laryngoscope is ready and has the appropriate blade; check both.* Be sure the fiberoptics, bougie, guide, or stylet is ready. Make sure the ETT confirmation devices/diagnostics and the ETT securement device are ready.
4. *Make sure the suction device has been prepared and turned on and that a rigid tip is available to your right hand during the intubation procedure.* This generally means that the suction has been assembled and is on, and the rigid tip has been placed under the edge of the mattress near the patient's head.
5. *Have at least one (two are better) intravenous (IV) line prepared or an intraosseous (IO) line and make sure it is functioning.* Make sure all the drugs chosen have been drawn up and labeled; this includes the induction drugs (initial attempt RSI) and the drugs needed for ongoing sedation or paralysis or both.
6. *Have a bag-mask with oxygen-connecting tubing assembled and ready.* Also have the ventilator circuit assembled and the ventilation parameters dialed in.

Being prepared means that backup plans have been determined and equipment (e.g., lamps, blades, tubes) is ready to go. Thorough preparation pays great dividends in a smooth RSI procedure.

Box 3-3 Recap of the RSI Sequence: II

You have prepared yourself. You have made the decision to use RSI to intubate your patient. The equipment has been prepared, and the backup devices and plans are ready. The patient has been receiving 100% oxygen to wash out nitrogen. At least two drugs need to be calculated, drawn up, and prepared for administration: a drug for sedation and a drug for paralysis.

Step 3: Preprocedural Drug Administration

Many RSI protocols include the use of pretreatment drugs to try to blunt the effects of the paralytics that will be given and/or to increase the heart rate. Your medical director's protocol for RSI may call for the use of several different drugs for these purposes in certain patients. These drugs must be given *before* the paralytic agents are administered.

Lidocaine

A standard IV dose of lidocaine (1 to 1.5 mg/kg) may be given before sedation and paralysis are administered to blunt the effects of depolarizing paralytics. Given 3 to 5 minutes before the RSI drugs, lidocaine can reduce bronchospasm and laryngospasm in patients with reactive airway disease (asthma). In patients with increased intracranial pressure (ICP), lidocaine can blunt the rise of intracranial pressure, which can occur during the intubation procedure itself or as the expected side effect of succinylcholine administration (depolarizing drug).

Opioids

Opioids can diminish the expected sympathetic discharge associated with pain (intubation) and a rise in organ pressure (depolarizing agent) with RSI. Sublimaze (fentanyl) usually is used because of its short half-life. The standard dose is 0.5 to 50 mcg/kg IV. Watch for rare but frightening respiratory muscle paralysis with large IV doses (more common in children). If this occurs, PPV is used while the sedative and paralytic are quickly given to allow intubation of the patient.

Atropine

Succinylcholine (SCh) binds to acetylcholine receptors at the neuromuscular junction; the result is stimulation of some receptors, which can cause bradycardia, especially in children. Atropine is the standard pretreatment drug for all children under 10 years of age, because pediatric patients depend on the heart rate for cardiac output (the dosage is 0.02 mg/kg IV, given about 3 minutes before SCh). Atropine also may be used for any patient with relative or absolute bradycardia (the adult dose is 0.5 to 2 mg IV). Atropine is given before SCh because after administration of SCh, if bradycardia occurs, uptake of atropine may be blocked for a short time.

Did You Know?

If you must give a second dose of succinylcholine (SCh) during RSI, the risk of bradycardia increases dramatically. Just before giving the second dose of SCh, always administer atropine, regardless of the patient's sinus heart rate at the time.[2]

Defasciculation as Pretreatment Therapy

Depolarizing paralytics such as SCh cause fasciculations through stimulation of nicotinic acetylcholine receptors. **Fasciculation** is a phenomenon in which muscle bundles contract in brief excitatory waves; this causes a rise in pressure in many organs. In the stomach, it can cause passive vomiting (and aspiration); high intraocular pressure occurs in the eye; and the brain suffers from high ICP. Administration of 10% of the dose of a nondepolarizing paralytic just before the actual RSI sequence may blunt this effect; this is called **defasciculation.** The defasciculating dose of vecuronium is 0.01 mg/kg (with rocuronium, the dosage is 0.1 mg/kg). Administration of SCh at a dosage of 0.15 mg/kg IV can result in defasciculation, but there is less evidence of its effectiveness in preventing increases in the ICP and intraocular pressure. Box 3-4 provides a recap of the RSI sequence.

Table 3-12 Intravenously Administered General Anesthetics

Agent	Typical Adult Dose Range for Induction	Onset	Duration	Possible Adverse Effects
Barbiturate				
Thiopental sodium (Pentothal)	3-5 mg/kg	30-60 sec	5-30 min	Respiratory depression, tachycardia, ↑ ICP bradycardia, hypotension, paradoxical excitation, confusion, pain at injection site
Benzodiazepines				
Midazolam (Versed)	0.5-2 mg slow IV over 2-3 min	1-5 min	Variable; 30 min to 2+ hr	Respiratory depression, hypotension, paradoxical excitation
Diazepam (Valium)	2-10 mg slow IV over 2-3 min	1-10 min	Variable; more pronounced "hangover"	Confusion, pain at injection site
Lorazepam (Ativan)	1-4 mg slow IV over 2-5 min	1-10 min	Variable	Similar to other benzodiazepines
Opioids				
Alfentanil (Alfenta)	8-20 mcg/kg, then 5-15 mcg/kg	<2 min	10 min	Respiratory depression, bradycardia, atrial fibrillation
Fentanyl (Sublimaze)	0.5-50 mcg/kg	Almost immediate	30-60 min	Hypotension, respiratory depression
Remifentanil (Ultiva)	0.5-1 mcg/kg	1-3 min	3-10 min	Paradoxical excitation, confusion, ↑ bradycardia
Sufentanil (Sufenta)	1-30 mcg/kg	1-3 min	36 min	Nausea/vomiting
General Anesthetics				
Etomidate (Amidate)	0.2-0.3 mg/kg over 30-60 sec	1 min	4-10 min	Nausea/vomiting, pain at injection site, muscle/eye movements
Propofol (Diprivan)	0.5-1 mg/kg over 10-60 sec	10-50 sec	3-10 min	Apnea, hypotension, pain at injection site, anaphylaxis
Dissociative Anesthetic				
Ketamine (Ketalar)	1-4.5 mg/kg single dose	1-2 min	5-10 min	Hypertension, tachycardia, ↑ intracranial pressure, hallucinations, muscle movements, abuse potential

Data from Lacy, C.F., et al. (2004). *Lexi-Comp's drug information handbook* (12th ed.). Hudson, OH: Lexi-Comp, and Micromedex, accessed March 17, 2011.

Box 3-4 Recap of the RSI Sequence: III

You have administered 100% oxygen and have evaluated the patient for a difficult airway. The equipment has been set up, and backup devices are nearby. You are following your protocol for the possibility of pre-RSI therapy. (If the patient is under 10 years of age, you have administered atropine.) The patient now needs to lose consciousness promptly with sedation.

Step 4: Induction of Sedation and Paralysis

Ideally, the drugs given in the RSI sequence would have a quick onset of action, few side effects, and a short half-life. This would allow the patient to recover spontaneously if you cannot ventilate or intubate the individual. Table 3-12 presents the standard sedation (preanesthesia) drugs, and Table 3-13 presents the depolarizing and nondepolarizing paralytics.

Inducing Sedation in the RSI Sequence

As mentioned, the ideal sedative for RSI would be quick to act, quick to wear off, and have no side effects. It also would provide some analgesia, would not alter cardiac output, and would respond reliably to a reversal agent in a very short time. Unfortunately, such an agent does not exist. However, these effects can be obtained through a combination of some of the more commonly used sedatives in the RSI sequence.

Benzodiazepines

Benzodiazepines control the **neuroinhibitor transmitter** and provides **anxiolysis,** central muscle relaxation, sedation,

Table 3-13 Neuromuscular Blockers

Agent	Onset (min)	Half-Life (min)	Duration (min) of Bolus Dose
Depolarizing Drug			
Succinylcholine (Anectine)	0.5-1	<1 min	4-8
Nondepolarizing Drugs			
Mivacurium (Mivacron)	1.5-3	2	12-20
Atracurium (Tracrium)	2-3	20	20-45
Cisatracurium (Nimbex)	2-3	20-30	40-60
Rocuronium (Zemuron)	1-1.5	60-70	30-60
Vecuronium (Norcuron)	2-3	50-80	20-40
Doxacurium (Nuromax)	4-6	100-200	100-160
Pancuronium (Pavulon)	3-5	100-170	60-100
Pipecuronium (Arduan)	3-5	120-180	60-120
Tubocurarine	3-5	100-120	60-90

anticonvulsant effects, and hypnosis. Some of these drugs are more amnestic than others, because there are differences in their onset of action. Midazolam (Versed) acts the most quickly (30 to 60 seconds), but its half-life can be as long as 1 to 2 hours (see Table 3-12).

The dosing of these drugs can be challenging, because each patient can have a variable response. Generally, the induction dose of midazolam is 0.07 to 0.3 mg/kg IV push, but this also depresses the pumping action of the heart and systemic vascular resistance (resulting in hypotension). Midazolam is the most commonly used sedative in the RSI sequence, especially for continued sedation and paralysis during transport. It is given in doses of 1 to 2.5 mg IV over 2 minutes, with repeat doses titrated to the patient's needs. Dosages as high as 0.3 to 0.35 mg/kg IV are recommended. A continuous IV infusion can be established at 0.02 to 0.10 mg/kg/hour (1 to 7 mg/hour) and titrated to the patient's needs.

Etomidate (Amidate)

Etomidate, a hypnotic agent, has a quick onset of action (20 to 30 seconds) and a short duration (7 to 14 minutes) but does not create the hemodynamic instability that midazolam can. The combination of etomidate and SCh in the induction phase of the RSI sequence can blunt the rise in ICP that SCh can cause. The recommended dose for induction is 0.3 mg/kg IV.

Etomidate can cause classic **myoclonic movement (myoclonus)** as a result of stimulation of the brain stem, but this effect often is masked by the immediate injection of SCh, which causes paralysis. Hiccups and vomiting can occur after administration. If the ETT is not passed successfully on the first attempt, suction must be available for the unprotected airway.

A concern with etomidate is the possibility of a decrease in the levels of both **cortisol** and **aldosterone** with repeated administration. To prevent this side effect, inject etomidate only once. If an airway attempt fails, consider using another sedative for subsequent attempts. In patients who would benefit from a second dose of etomidate, consider using methylprednisolone to prevent this side effect. Etomidate should be avoided in those patients with sepsis, especially children.

Did You Know?

The most commonly used sedative and paralytic induction agents are etomidate (0.3 mg/kg) and succinylcholine (1.5 mg/kg), administered IV in quick succession.

Ketamine (Ketalar)

The sedative state induced by IV administration of ketamine is called *dissociative anesthesia,* because the brain's pathways are interrupted before sensory blockade. Just after injection of the drug, the heart rate and blood pressure rise; they return to normal within approximately 15 minutes. This effect may cause a rise in ICP; therefore, patients with hypotension would benefit, but not if they also have high ICP. The most valued effect of ketamine is its ability to relax bronchial smooth muscle and cause bronchodilation; it therefore is the sedative of choice for patients with asthma. Another important attribute is its ability to allow the body to maintain respiratory drive, even though it is considered a sedative. The most infamous side effect of ketamine is hallucinations. However, this is not usually a factor in the RSI sequence, because the benzodiazepines commonly injected for continued sedation blunt this effect.

The induction dose of ketamine is 1 to 2 mg/kg IV. The onset of action is 15 to 30 seconds, and the duration is 10 to 15 minutes. Keep suction available, because secretions increase after injection. Concomitant use of drying agents (e.g., atropine, glycopyrrolate (Robinul)) may blunt this "wet effect."

Propofol (Diprivan)

Propofol is a thick, white lipid solution that is often called "mother's milk." It is a hypnotic sedative that can reduce cardiac output by depressing the pumping function. It also can reduce bronchospasm. Propofol is rarely used in the induction phase of the RSI sequence; it can cause hypotension, and its use for induction purposes is restricted by scope of practice regulations to anesthesiology professionals or physicians. It is encouraged for continued sedation of an intubated patient. The dosage is 0.2 to 0.6 mcg/kg, given as an IV infusion.

Inducing Paralysis in the RSI Sequence
Neuromuscular Blocking Agents

Some of the effects and side effects of SCh have already been briefly discussed. However, critical care team members

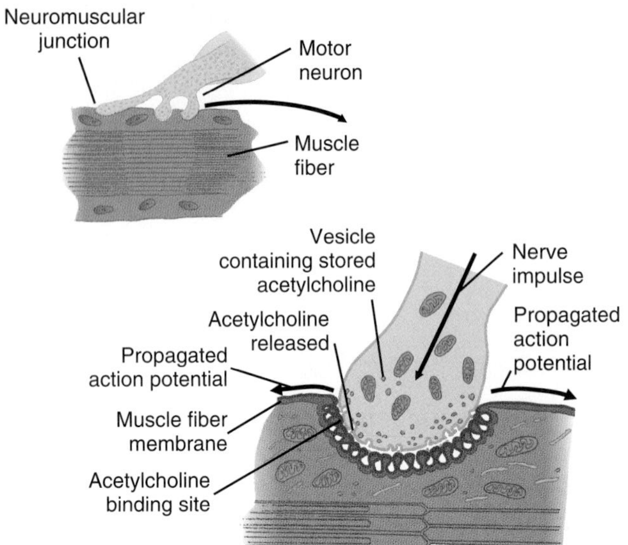

Figure 3-24

Neuromuscular junction. (From Black JM, Hawks JH: *Medical-surgical nursing: clinical management for positive outcomes*, ed 7, Philadelphia, 2005, Saunders.)

also must understand the difference between depolarizing and nondepolarizing paralytics. Generally, two classes of muscle relaxants are used for RSI: **noncompetitive (depolarizing) neuromuscular blocking agents (NMBAs)** and **competitive (nondepolarizing) neuromuscular blocking agents.**

Noncompetitive (depolarizing) neuromuscular blocking agents

The only practical drug to list in this category is succinylcholine. Designed to mimic acetylcholine, SCh blocks **nicotinic receptors** and **muscarinic receptors,** which are types of **cholinergic receptors.** As long as the patient's body has pseudocholinesterase, this drug is processed away from the neuromuscular end plates fairly quickly (Figure 3-24).

Medical directors commonly choose SCh as the initial RSI paralytic because of its short half-life. However, it has some serious side effects. The Drug Guide on the Evolve site for *Transport of the Critical Care Patient* presents a synopsis of the uses of SCh, along with its adverse effects. Because only a small proportion of the SCh actually reaches the neuromuscular junction, larger doses are recommended.

Competitive (nondepolarizing) neuromuscular blocking agents

Competitive NMBAs compete with or block acetylcholine at the neuromuscular junction. Unlike SCh, nondepolarizing agents do not stimulate this site and do not cause fasciculations. The two types of nondepolarizing drugs are aminosteroid compounds and benzylisoquinolinum compounds.

The aminosteroid compounds are the drugs most commonly used in the emergency and transport settings. In general, these drugs have a somewhat longer onset of action (1 to 2 minutes) and longer duration of action (20 to 45 minutes) than SCh, but they have fewer side effects. These agents are given when SCh is contraindicated or when a longer duration of action is needed, such as with continued ventilation during transport.

You might ask, if nondepolarizing drugs have fewer side effects, why not use them more for RSI? The answer is, quick-acting, short-duration drugs are used when possible because of the chance of failure to ventilate and intubate. Box 3-5 provides as recap of the RSI sequence.

Box 3-5 Recap of the RSI Sequence: IV

You have evaluated the patient and preoxygenated or hyperoxygenated the person. You have set up and checked all equipment, including backup devices. You have drawn up the appropriate pretreatment, sedative, and paralytic drugs and have them all clearly identified on the syringe. You now are ready for induction for intubation.

Did You Know?

With nondepolarizing drugs, increasing the dose can speed up the onset of action; however, this also lengthens the drug's duration of action.

Step 5: Administration of the Drugs, Positioning of the Patient, and Intubation

At 3 to 5 minutes before administration of the sedative/paralytic drug combination, you have already given the pretreatment drugs. Once the team is ready, the sedative and paralytic are administered, usually in rapid succession. Observe the patient for myoclonus or fasciculations. Monitor vital signs and watch for muscle relaxation and anticipated apnea. Once apnea occurs, do not provide PPV until after the standard intubation attempt, unless the patient suffered from hypoxia.

Did You Know?

Two classes of drugs are routinely administered in RSI: sedatives and paralytics. However, neither relieves pain. When you use these drugs, remember to provide analgesia to patients in pain, because they cannot complain either verbally or nonverbally.

Just after you administer the sedative, another member of the team may apply cricothyroid pressure in order to facilitate a clear view of the cords. The assistant positions the first finger and thumb on the palpated lateral edges of the cricoid ring and applies approximately 10 pounds of pressure straight downward; this ring is somewhat moveable and can be adjusted to view the cords.

Did You Know?

For most medical patients, the proper position for intubation is a sniffing position, for which a pillow is placed strategically beneath the shoulders, upper back, neck, and head. This partly helps to resolve the three airway angles that obstruct a view of the vocal cords. Also, the heavier the patient's upper torso, the higher the upper body should be. With a morbidly obese patient, you may need to put the patient in reverse Trendelenburg position and, using a foot stool, look over the patient's shoulder.[2]

As you position the laryngoscope blade or fiberoptic device, your assistant should apply *b*ackward, *u*pward, and to the patient's *r*ight *p*ressure (BURP technique) to facilitate a central view of the vocal cords. As the intubator views the cords, the assistant's thumb and forefinger guide the pressure and direction. If the patient has a small mouth cavity, the assistant can use his or her other hand to retract the right side of the mouth; this facilitates insertion of both the laryngoscope blade and the approaching ETT, which are coming from the right side. The ETT is inserted to the proper depth and manually held in position while the stylet or fiberoptic device is removed and the cuff inflated. PPV then is applied.

If the assistant notices a change in the patient's vital signs, the intubation procedure should be stopped and the patient ventilated. The next step is determined by your failed or difficult airway protocol. In most cases, this means a second attempt at endotracheal intubation.

Did You Know?

Difficult or failed intubation protocols follow a step-by-step decision tree that guides the crew through RSI if intubation fails on the first attempt. The backup plan might include an extraglottic airway device as a bridge to a second attempt or as a final destination for airway control. A crucial element in backup plans is your partner. For a safe RSI system, both crew members should have strong skills in airway and ventilation management.

Step 6: Confirmation of Tube Placement and Securement of the Device

Correct placement of an ETT can be confirmed in many ways. However, no single procedure determines absolutely that the tube is in the correct location. Therefore, most standards recommend the use of two methods of confirmation initially and after each move of the patient. However, many of these methods are not practical in the transport setting.

Considerations in ETT Placement Confirmation

1. Esophageal tube checks (bulb or syringe) may be used as the *initial* means of confirmation in patients over 4 to 5 years of age.
2. Colorimetric detectors may not change color if perfusion to the lungs and body are compromised. A false color change may occur in morbidly obese patients and those with a large amount of carbonated beverage in the stomach. The disposable devices should be used only for a short time, because the chemical paper loses its effectiveness as it is exposed to the air.
3. A chest radiograph is the gold standard for confirming the placement of an ETT. It usually is done daily for mechanically ventilated patients in the ICU. A malpositioned ETT is found in 12% to 14% of these patients. The chest radiograph can confirm the depth of placement much more reliably than for tracheal versus esophageal placement as the AP view of a chest x-ray "sees" the ETT in one dimension but the esophagus rests directly behind the trachea. If the ETT is positioned too deeply, the x-ray will "see" the tube in the right mainstem bronchus—confirmed as a tracheal tube because of depth of placement.

   However, the use of chest radiography to confirm ETT placement has many disadvantages:
   - It is expensive.
   - The patient is exposed to radiation.
   - Time is required to take and interpret the film.
   - Specialized personnel are needed to take the film.
   - An experienced physician is required to interpret the film

   Consequently, this means of confirming ETT placement is not practical for the critical care team. If the ETT cuff is inflated with saline, B-mode ultrasound can be used to confirm placement more cheaply and without patient irradiation and personnel and time costs. Direct visualization with a laryngoscope or fiberoptic device is a much more practical method for obtaining a quick answer to the confirmation question.
4. The $PETCO_2$ should be monitored in all mechanically ventilated patients throughout all transfers. Initial and ongoing monitoring of the $PETCO_2$ (capnography) also provides information on ventilation and perfusion.
5. Auscultation of at least three points initially is often the method of choice for verifying tube placement among transport personnel. Epigastric and bilateral auscultation can identify esophageal and tracheal positioning of the tube and can help determine the depth of placement in adults.

NOTE: Esophageal intubation can create enough sound throughout the chest (and stomach) to make auscultation unreliable for confirmation of placement, and a second confirmatory method is required.

6. Other methods of indirect confirmation include observation of thoracic movement (chest rise and fall) and palpation of a tracheal tube in the suprasternal notch. These are less reliable methods.

Anyone who has some experience in intubating patients has accidentally placed the tracheal tube in the esophagus. It happens. The actual negligent act, however, is failing to recognize that the ETT is not in the trachea. Be diligent in monitoring for incorrect placement and displacement of the ETT.

Placement of a commercially prepared product to secure the ETT is the next step. Some evidence indicates that the use of such a product is better than using tape. However, many ICUs do not use these devices, because the plastic piece against the patient's mouth causes irritation and open wounds. The decision whether to untape a secured ETT and apply a commercial device is up to you and your medical director. If such a device is used, take care that it does not crimp the tube in any way, thereby reducing the ID and creating higher airway pressures. Make sure that the centimeter (cm) marking at the lip is visible and documented for depth of placement. Addition of a bite block (commercial device or oropharyngeal airway [OPA]) should be considered if the patient has some control.

Begin the prescribed positive pressure on your ventilator and monitor the patient's vital signs. Box 3-6 provides a recap of the completed RSI procedure.

Step 7: Provision of Post-RSI Care

After completing the RSI sequence, evaluate the ABCs in your patient. The airway management section opened with that tip, and the medication-assisted intubation section ends with the same advice. You have applied a series of treatment modalities that can alter all three parameters. Make sure the patient has tolerated the change. Check for the following troublesome signs and their causes.

1. Bradycardia may be an ominous sign in all patients during and after RSI. Esophageal intubation is a differential that must be ruled out in this case.
2. Hypertension, especially with tachycardia, usually means that the patient is awake and is not happy with recent events. Administer the ongoing sedation and pain control drugs, and resort to paralysis only after these two drugs have been given and if the patient continues to fight your interventions. Reevaluate the vital signs once those drugs have taken effect. Review the side effects of the drugs given. Ketamine, for example, can create this situation.
3. Hypotension may be due to PPV or the drugs used. Rule out pneumothorax with obstructive shock immediately and treat it if found. In a patient with high airway pressures (asthma, COPD), the sometimes rapid ventilation associated with tube confirmation may have inadvertently created **auto-PEEP.** Once pneumothorax has been ruled out, review the patient's history and provide slow ventilations with reasonable tidal volumes at a 1 : 3 ratio; monitor the $PETCO_2$ and vital signs. A fluid bolus may help; most often fluids should be running throughout the intubation procedure. Vasopressors may be necessary, but they more often are related to the underlying condition that made mechanical ventilation necessary. Midazolam and propofol can cause hypotension.
4. If airway complications arise, follow your difficult or failed intubation protocol. Administer sedative and nondepolarizing paralytics based on your protocols. You also should provide analgesia to the patient.

Watch for a recovering patient during transport by checking the vital signs and watching for the onset of spontaneous respirations. Understanding the half-life of the drugs used can help you organize your management approach during transport. Be prepared with the next sedative and paralytic *before* the next spontaneous breath by the patient. An early sign of recovery from the drugs is a rise in heart rate and blood pressure. If you begin to see these signs, correlate with the expected recovery time from the drugs given and prepare for additional doses. The use of nerve stimulators also can help gauge patient recovery from paralytics. Noninvasive bispectral monitoring (BIS) of brain waves may be used to monitor the patient's level of sedation. The $PETCO_2$ waveform also can give clues to a waning neuromuscular blockade. A dip in the $PETCO_2$ waveform plateau, known as the "curare cleft," indicates spontaneous respirations. The deeper the cleft, the less neuromuscular blockade is still active.

Administering paralytics without sedation and analgesia is very bad practice and considered unethical. The patient should always benefit from the actions of the sedatives and analgesics while paralytics are used.

Table 3-14 presents a quick guide to the RSI sequence, and Box 3-7 lists suggested equipment for the critical care paramedic's airway toolkit.

Airway assessment and management can be quite a challenge. The team must prepare by acquiring a deep knowledge base, learning good protocols, and reinforcing its skills in

Box 3-6 Recap of the Completed RSI Sequence

1. You evaluated for a difficult airway and hyperoxygenated the patient.
2. You set up your equipment, devices, and medications.
3. You administered the pretreatment, sedative, and paralytic drugs as an assistant watched the patient's vital signs.
4. Your assistant applied cricoid pressure using the BURP technique. While the assistant maintained the pressure and retracted the right side of the patient's mouth, you used the intubator as a guide and intubated the patient.
5. You confirmed the tube's position by two methods and secured the tube.

Table 3-14 Quick Guide to Rapid Sequence Intubation (RSI)

Time	Zero −5 to −8 min	Zero −2 to −3 min	Zero −2 min	Zero	Zero +45 to +60 sec	Post Intubation
Preparation	Prepare equipment Suction 100% oxygen	Premedications Defasciculating agent	***Sedation*** Perform Sellick maneuver	***Paralyze***	***Intubate patient***	Confirm tube placement Release Sellick maneuver Secure tube
Routine RSI (head injury and patients with normal or elevated BP)	Evaluate anatomy Decide on backup plan Prepare and label medications Hyperoxygenate	***Atropine*** Pediatric: 0.02 mg/kg Adult: 1 mg ***Lidocaine:*** 1.5 mg/kg ***Norcuron:*** 0.01 mg/kg	***Versed:*** 0.05-0.1 mg/kg *or* ***Etomidate:*** 0.3 mg/kg	***Succinylcholine:*** 1.5 mg/kg	WAIT FOR PARALYSIS Intubate patient	Determine need for continued paralysis *and* sedation
Routine RSI (borderline or hypotensive patients)	Evaluate anatomy Decide on backup plan Prepare and label medications Hyperoxygenate	***Atropine*** Pediatric: 0.02 mg/kg Adult: 1 mg ***Lidocaine:*** 1.5 mg/kg ***Norcuron:*** 0.01 mg/kg	***Versed:*** 0.05-0.1 mg/kg *or* ***Etomidate:*** 0.015 mg/kg	***Succinylcholine:*** 1.5 mg/kg	WAIT FOR PARALYSIS Intubate patient	Determine need for continued paralysis *and* sedation
RSI without succinylcholine	Evaluate anatomy Decide on backup plan Prepare and label medications Hyperoxygenate	***Atropine*** Pediatric: 0.02 mg/kg Adult: 1 mg ***Lidocaine:*** 1.5 mg/kg	***Versed:*** 0.05-0.1 mg/kg *or* ***Etomidate:*** 0.3 mg/kg ***Norcuron:*** 0.1 mg/kg *or* ***Rocuronium:*** First dose: 1.2 mg/kg Then: 0.6 mg/kg for continued paralysis	***Norcuron:*** 0.1 mg/kg *or* ***Rocuronium:*** 1.2 mg/kg	WAIT FOR PARALYSIS Intubate patient	Determine need for continued paralysis *and* sedation

Courtesy Lee Ridge, Paramedic Specialist, FP-C. University of Iowa Hospitals' EMSLRC, Iowa City, IA.

practice scenarios as it sorts through the "what ifs" of airway emergencies.

DISEASE PROCESSES OF THE RESPIRATORY SYSTEM

It cannot be overstated: Emergency care assessment always includes the ABCs. The assessment and treatment of patients with airway failure have been thoroughly discussed; the focus now turns to patients in respiratory failure and the attendant complications.

Acute Respiratory Failure

When the respiratory system fails to maintain gas exchange, respiratory failure occurs; this can be a failure of oxygenation or ventilation. In the emergency assessment and resuscitation phase of patient care, this patient has an altered mental status, or the person may have a sensation of dyspnea or an obvious increase in WOB that does not improve despite treatment.

Many patients in the intensive care setting have already failed an intense resuscitation period and are attempting recovery from the primary disease. The resuscitation failure usually occurs secondary to another disease process, and these

Box 3-7 Suggested Contents of a Critical Care Paramedic's Airway Toolkit

- Nasal and oral airways
- Laryngoscope handles
- A range of blades (size 0 to 5), both straight and curved
- Extra batteries and lamps
- Lubricant
- Fiberoptic laryngoscope/viewer
- Stylet
- Bougie
- Tube exchanger or catheter
- Extraglottic airway in all sizes with appropriate syringe (if needed)
- 12 mL syringes
- All sizes of endotracheal tubes
- Rigid tonsil tip suction device and connecting tube
- Commercial endotracheal tube (ETT) holder
- 1-inch tape
- Tube confirmation devices
- Percutaneous cricothyrotomy kit or scalpel, tracheostomy tube, skin hook or trach hook, and Kelly forceps

failures can be classified according to whether the disease originates from the respiratory system itself (intrapulmonary cause) or from a cause outside the system (extrapulmonary cause). Respiratory failure from airway compromise has already been discussed. This section focuses on intrapulmonary diseases that cause acute respiratory failure (ARF) and on ventilation therapy.

Intrapulmonary Diseases

Three areas of the respiratory system are affected by diseases that can cause respiratory failure:

- Lower airways and alveoli (COPD, asthma, bronchiolitis, and pneumonia)
- Pulmonary circulation (pulmonary embolus)
- Alveolar-capillary membrane (acute lung injury [ALI]/acute respiratory distress syndrome [ARDS])

Lower Airways and Alveoli: Chronic Obstructive Pulmonary Disease

The fourth leading cause of death in the United States, the incidence of COPD continues to rise, and tobacco use is the single most common cause. The use of tobacco causes a chronic inflammation and then injury to the airways. Four major changes occur as the respiratory system attempts to remodel with this injury process:

1. *Remodeling of the airway:* The alveolar walls and connective tissues become permanently enlarged, and terminal airways collapse; both of these changes cause lung hyperinflation.
2. *Increased mucus production and destruction of the cilia:* These changes result in a chronic cough. A larger amount of sputum is produced, but the individual is unable to cough this sputum up and out.
3. *Chronic airway inflammation:* This constant irritation diminishes the ability to exhale totally.
4. *Thickening of the pulmonary vessels:* Thickening of this tissue, which is integral to gas exchange, causes hypoxia and hypercapnia. The vessels constrict, causing pulmonary hypertension, which results in damage to the right side of the heart as the hypertensive effects cause a thickening of the right ventricular wall.

These physiologic changes create an environment of gradual decline and chronic problems with very few reserves. Your focus will be on the patient experiencing an exacerbation of the disease or a complication with resulting ARF.

The goals of managing a patient with COPD in acute respiratory failure include providing support during the episode, treating the underlying cause, and returning the patient to the previous level of respiratory function. Management generally includes treatment of hypoxemia to attain an SaO_2 above 90% and/or a PaO_2 above 60 mm Hg. Because patients with COPD are unable to attain a PaO_2 much higher than 60 mm Hg, hyperoxygenation therapy usually is not helpful.

Many patients with ARF have a reactive airway component, which includes wheezing. Bronchodilator therapy with $beta_2$ agonists (both long and short acting) can help resolve that symptom; anticholinergics also may help. Some of these drugs must be given with caution in patients known to have cardiac disease. Corticosteroids may help eliminate acute inflammation, but the patient must be monitored for hyperglycemia and infection. Antibiotics are administered if the underlying trigger of the ARF event is an infectious disorder.

The mainstay of treatment in a patient with ARF is ventilatory support. In a patient with COPD, this may mean noninvasive positive pressure ventilation (NPPV) or invasive ventilatory support. A hemodynamically stable patient with COPD benefits from NPPV and usually attains the treatment goals much sooner. Patients with COPD who are hemodynamically unstable or who have mental status changes or severe hypoxemia benefit from intubation and mechanical ventilation; however, weaning the patient from this form of ventilation may be a challenge.

Asthma

Similar to COPD, asthma is a progressive, chronic disorder of the lower airways that involves injury to the tissues with resultant remodeling. The airways become very reactive to allergens, viruses, and irritants in the environment. This reactivity causes bronchospasm, edema, mucous plugging, and remodeling, which result in **air trapping,** prolonged exhalation, and a mismatch between ventilation and perfusion (V/Q mismatch). Although asthma is a chronic disorder, as is COPD, most acute asthma episodes are reversible.

Asthma exacerbations are classified as mild, moderate, severe, or imminent ARF. The focus here is on the patient with a severe or ARF-imminent exacerbation. When severe events occur, air trapping and hyperinflation increase with each breath. Because the patient cannot fully exhale, intrinsic PEEP is created (PEEPi). Eventually the symptoms lead to hypoxia and hypercapnia. An increased WOB with a diminished level of consciousness serves as a warning that ARF is imminent.

Management strategies for asthma are similar to those for COPD. You should maintain an oxygen saturation above 90%. Providing oxygen in a mixture with helium (heliox) may improve overall oxygenation, because this mix allows for improved gas exchange. Heliox reduces the work of breathing by creating a more laminar (less turbulent) airflow; it also allows for better drug distribution for inhaled medications.

Administration of $beta_2$ agonists by inhalation should be tried first, but patients with severe hyperinflation may not be able to get the drugs to the airways. Combining nebulized $beta_2$ agonists with anticholinergics may help dilate the bronchi. In patients who allow a mask over the face, you may drive the bronchodilators to the constricted lower airways with PPV; this can be a life-saving maneuver for patients in respiratory failure, before intubation. Also, consider using $beta_2$ agonists in IV form; continuous infusion of terbutaline or albuterol (Salbutamol) may be helpful.

Systemic corticosteroids should be administered as soon as possible in severe events, because they may reduce airway inflammation significantly. Corticosteroids take as long as 6 to 8 hours to reach full effect; therefore, administration early in the resuscitation is crucial.

Administration of magnesium in severe cases of status asthmaticus has shown mixed results. However, most experts agree that in severe cases in which the condition is refractory to beta agonist therapy, a bolus of 1 to 4 g of magnesium given IV over 10 to 40 minutes may improve respiratory mechanics. Because magnesium sulfate is a skeletal muscle relaxant, a tired patient must be monitored carefully for a period of worsening just before the person's condition improves.

PPV, whether noninvasive or invasive, can be a challenge in an asthmatic patient in ARF. Because of the high PEEPi, high inflation pressures must be avoided. PEEP on the ventilator can be used and may reduce the WOB; however, depending on the exact clinical scenario, it also may lead to clinical deterioration. Although PEEP is not contraindicated, its use requires very careful monitoring. Because the inability to exhale is intensely uncomfortable, most patients ventilated for status asthmaticus require very high levels of sedation and analgesia.

Bronchiolitis

Bronchiolitis is an inflammation of the bronchioles. It usually is seen in children under 2 years of age and usually is caused by a virus (often, respiratory syncytial virus [RSV]). The disease is not commonly seen in adults. It may present acutely with symptoms similar to those of COPD (e.g., air trapping, dyspnea) and may quickly lead to respiratory failure in children.

Pneumonia

Pneumonia is an inflammation of the lungs that can be categorized by the organism that causes the infection and/or where it was acquired. It may be bacterial, viral, fungal, aspiration, or chemical in nature; acquired through a ventilator (VAP); nosocomial in origin (hospital-acquired pneumonia [HAP]) or community-acquired pneumonia (CAP). Pneumonia is a relatively common reason for admission to the ICU, and it can be fatal for patients with chronic health problems.

The infectious agent affects the lung parenchyma and causes *consolidation*, a process through which areas of the lung become more solid as the air spaces fill with exudate. The infectious process causes capillary permeability and, as a result of an increase in inflammatory markers that promote blood flow, may increase perfusion to the area of the lung least able to participate in ventilation because of consolidation; this creates a severe V/Q mismatch. Pleural effusion may complicate the infection and lead to increased WOB, hypoxia, and respiratory failure.

Patients with altered mental status, feeding tubes, artificial airways, or GI disorders may develop aspiration pneumonia (pneumonitis). Pneumonitis usually is caused by chemical irritation of the lung tissue; bacterial superinfection occurs, but usually much later in the course of the illness.

Treatment of pneumonia includes antiinfective agents (antibiotics, antifungal drugs), oxygen, ventilatory support, fluids, electrolytes, and nutritional maintenance. Keep in mind that some lower respiratory infections are caused by agents that may be infectious to you and your team members. Consult your protocols or the referring hospital (including the infection control staff at the hospital) to determine whether the pathogen has been identified and the patient has been on an appropriate antibiotic for at least 24 to 48 hours. If not, your standard precautions should include at least a mask.

Pulmonary Circulation: Pulmonary Embolus

A pulmonary embolus (PE) is a vascular event in the lungs in which an embolus (e.g., clot, tumor, fat, amniotic fluid, cement from an orthopedic procedure) travels through the circulation to the pulmonary arterial system, disrupting blood flow to one or more sections of the lungs. Most clots arise in leg veins.

When a large embolus lodges in a lobar or larger artery, the result is high pulmonary pressures, an increased right ventricular workload, and subsequent obstructive shock. When a large PE is accompanied by shock, a true medical emergency exists, with a high risk of death. Alveolar dead space is created (ventilation but no circulation), with increased WOB and bronchoconstriction.

Mediators released at the injury site cause more local vasoconstriction, which adds to the pulmonary hypertension. The prognosis depends on the patient's overall health status, especially cardiovascular health, and the size of the PE. The diagnosis usually is made by CT angiography.

Treatment has three goals: manage the pulmonary hypertension, remove or dissolve the clot, and prevent additional clots and embolic events.

1. A patient with the combination of obstructive shock and pulmonary hypertension requires IV fluids to increase preload and inotropic agents to increase cardiac output. Fluid balance is very difficult with right-sided heart failure, because too much fluid may put the patient into right-sided congestive heart failure.

2. Administration of fibrinolytics (e.g., t-PA) may help dissolve the existing clot, but these drugs usually are reserved for patients with a massive PE who are in shock. Another treatment for massive PE and shock is pulmonary embolectomy, in which a catheter is radiographically directed to the vessel involved and the clot is removed.
3. Prevention of PE recurrence may include use of a continuous heparin infusion. This weight-based infusion usually is continued for several days until warfarin therapy can be maintained. Vena cava filters may be inserted surgically in high-risk patients and those who may not be able to take anticoagulants.

Alveolar-Capillary Membrane: Acute Lung Injury/Acute Respiratory Distress Syndrome

In 1967, ICU staff members noticed a trend in which acutely ill patients developed noncardiogenic pulmonary edema after an acute shock or hypoxic event. These patients' symptoms included dyspnea, tachypnea, decreased lung compliance, and diffuse alveolar infiltrates on chest radiographs. Initially, this disease was called **acute respiratory distress syndrome (ARDS).** According to most current criteria, ARDS is considered the worst form of **acute lung injury (ALI).** Whether called ARDS or ALI, noncardiogenic pulmonary edema is the pulmonary aspect of multisystem organ dysfunction syndrome (MODS) (see Chapter 8).

ALI is a systemic disease. It may begin with an acute episode of shock or hypoxia that initiates a systemic immune response (also called *systemic inflammatory response syndrome* [SIRS]). This response directly affects the alveolar-capillary membrane and subsequently results in respiratory failure.

ALI can have a direct or an indirect cause. Direct causes include aspiration, near-drowning, toxic inhalation, pulmonary contusion, pneumonia, oxygen toxicity, and transthoracic radiation. Indirect causes are sepsis, nonthoracic trauma, massive transfusion therapy, cardiopulmonary bypass, severe pancreatitis, PE, disseminated intravascular coagulation (DIC), and all shock states. Box 3-8 outlines the criteria for the diagnosis of ALI.

ALI is initiated by an immune response and subsequent release of inflammatory mediators, neutrophils, macrophages, and platelets in the pulmonary vessels. These humoral mediators damage the alveolar-capillary membrane. ALI has three phases:

1. *Exudative phase:* This is the acute phase of ALI, which begins 48 hours after the acute precipitating event. Pulmonary capillaries leak protein-rich fluid into the interstitial areas of the lungs. This influx of fluid overwhelms the lymph channels, and the fluid is pushed across the adjacent alveolar membrane. The pressure changes and fluids cause the alveoli to compress with constriction of the airways. Eventually, surfactant production decreases, and the alveoli collapse. Blood vessels do not perfuse blood to a collapsed alveoli, so shunting occurs.

   Patients in this phase appear restless, dyspneic, and tachypneic and have overbreathing and respiratory alkalosis. At first, the chest radiograph and PaO_2 are normal. If hemodynamic monitoring is used, the pulmonary artery (PA) pressure is high, and the pulmonary artery occlusion pressure (PAOP) is normal or low.
2. *Fibroproliferative phase:* The lungs quickly attempt to initiate healing, but with ALI, healing is dysfunctional. The alveolar-capillary membranes develop natural scar tissue (collagen, granulation) and become irregularly shaped. The lungs become stiff. Pulmonary hypertension and hypoxia continue because of this change in tissue and their functions.

   A patient in this phase has bilateral crackles in the lung fields, increasing hypoxia, hypercarbia, acidosis, signs of shock, and alveolar infiltrates on the chest radiograph. The PA pressure is high, and cardiac output is low. MODS may be apparent, marked by changes in many other organs.
3. *Resolution phase:* The lungs remodel themselves in an attempt to restore an intact alveolar-capillary membrane. Debris is removed, and fluid again is moved across the membrane by the lymph channels. Epithelial cells regenerate the tissues.

Management of ALI and ARDS can be quite a challenge, especially during transport of a patient who is difficult to oxygenate and difficult to ventilate with standard PPV. However, ICU staffs have become vigilant for the possibility of ALI in certain patients. It now is detected earlier, and strategies are implemented to prevent the disease and/or to manage it better.

Box 3-8 Criteria for Diagnosing Acute Lung Injury*

- The condition has an acute onset.
- The ratio of the partial pressure of oxygen (PaO_2) to the fraction of inspired oxygen (FiO_2) is less than or equal to 300 mm Hg (regardless of positive end-expiratory pressure [PEEP] settings) (<200 mm Hg for acute respiratory distress syndrome [ARDS]).
- Bilateral (four quadrant) infiltrates are seen on the chest radiograph (but not in the costophrenic angles).
- The pulmonary artery occlusion pressure (PAOP) is less than or equal to 18 mm Hg, or there is no clinical evidence of left atrial hypertension.

*Criteria established by the American-European Consensus Committee on ARDS, *Am J Respir Crit Care Med*, 149(1): 818-824, 1994.

Lung-Protective Strategies in ALI and ARDS

Low Tidal Volume Pressure Support and Permissive Hypercapnia

Once mechanical ventilation has been initiated, management of the patient focuses on *lung-protective strategies,* or practices aimed at reducing or minimizing further injury to the lungs. These practices include using lower tidal volumes, or **permissive hypercapnia** (5 to 8 mL/kg rather than the older settings of 10 to 12 mL/kg) and finding **ideal (optimal)**

PEEP (the level of PEEP at which recruitment of lung tissue is maximized and oxygenation is most adequate).

At larger tidal volumes, the lungs of a patient with ARDS can become markedly overdistended, leading to pulmonary vasoconstriction, unaerated lung tissue, and increased V/Q mismatch. Low V_T ventilation lowers the mean airway pressure and peak pressure and causes less volutrauma than do traditional tidal volumes. The goal with this strategy is to maintain the **plateau pressure** at or below 30 cm H_2O. During PPV, the plateau pressure is the pressure applied to the smaller airways and alveoli. Higher plateau pressures stretch these delicate tissues, causing trauma (ALI).

During low V_T ventilation, a higher frequency may be necessary (as high as 35/min) to meet ventilatory requirements. It most often is used with the addition of high PEEP (above 12 cm H_2O) to ensure adequate regulation of the $PaCO_2$ and oxygenation. Low tidal volumes also improve cardiac output by lowering intrathoracic pressure.

The mortality rate for ARDS is 40% to 50%. Before the implementation of permissive hypercapnia (in the early 1980s), the only advance in this disease was identification of the mechanisms of acute lung injury, and little progress had been made in effective treatments.

Although the focus in ARDS is on improving oxygenation, the acid-base balance also is monitored. The goal for the pH is 7.30 to 7.45, and this level may be difficult to maintain, especially when permissive hypercapnia (lower V_T) is used. The use of sodium bicarbonate ($NaHCO_3$) is limited to a pH refractory to changes in the ventilatory rate; the maximum ventilatory rate is 35 to 38/min. In some cases, the best thing to do with the resultant acidosis is nothing. When the pH is in the lower limits of the goal and the ventilator settings are at the maximum, the physician may elect to allow permissive hypercapnia, elevated $PaCO_2$ levels, and a low pH. Permissive hypercapnia is tolerated to allow the patient time to neutralize the pH at a spontaneous rate; to prevent complications, $NaHCO_3$ may be added to help normalize the pH.

The use of permissive hypercapnia for transport can be a concern. With the increase in the respiratory rate, the T_I requires adjustment to allow for a proper expiratory time, so as to eliminate air trapping caused by the ventilator. This can be done by monitoring the plateau pressure and peak inspiratory pressure for gradual increases over time. Oxygenation is accomplished by optimizing PEEP levels while taking into consideration its effect on air trapping. Attempting to meet all these objectives with a transport ventilator is difficult. A low V_T lung-protective strategy requires sophisticated ventilators that most often are found only at the bedside. For these strategies, the ventilator operator must be able to adjust the V_T, minute volume, and T_I; therefore, the selection of the ventilator for transport is a key issue.

Alternative Ventilation Strategies and Therapy in Acute Lung Injury

Conventional mechanical ventilation is only one limb of a very large decision tree in the treatment and management of long-term ALI and ARDS. Other methods involve not only different modes of ventilation, but also the use of medications, positioning, nutrition, and other therapies.

Nutrition Therapy

Nutrition therapy consists of calorie-dense supplements for tube feedings that contain 100% of the required minerals and vitamins. In addition, a large fat intake is used to support the energy expenditures of chronically ventilated patients. Supplements are calorie-dense, which means they provide calories with reduced free fluids to prevent fluid overload.

Nitric Oxide

Nitric oxide (NO) is a potent vasodilator. When inhaled, it preferentially selects the pulmonary vessels in ventilated areas that need to dilate. It is not the only drug known to have pulmonary vasodilation properties. Nitroglycerin and nitroprusside also have been used, but they do not selectively dilate only the vessels in ventilated areas, as does NO. Nitric oxide is not without disadvantages: It is very expensive, and its use is time-limited because it has carcinogenic properties. It also has been known to cause **methemoglobinemia** and pulmonary edema. Caution must be used when delivering NO/O_2 blends and a one-on-one caregiver to patient ratio must be strictly followed at all times. Nitric oxide will rarely be used during transport, but another important factor is that abruptly stopping NO (i.e., for transport) will lead to acutely worse (and often fatal) pulmonary hypertension. Thus, if you encounter a patient on NO for transport and you have no means of transporting with the NO, do a trial off NO while still at the hospital to determine how the patient will tolerate transport.

Pronation Therapy

Pronation therapy, or placing the patient face down until the requirement for a high oxygen concentration diminishes, is a controversial tactic. In the treatment of ARDS, pronation therapy is intended to shift blood flow to the anterior areas of the lungs, which are less severely injured and better ventilated; this is another tactic for recruiting new lung tissue to oxygenate. Depending on the type of bed used, prone positioning also may allow for better diaphragmatic excursion and improve ventilation. No conclusive data show that prone positioning improves survival outcomes in patients with ARDS, but it does improve oxygenation in some ARDS patients and is beneficial for those individuals.

Not all patients can tolerate pronation therapy, and it is not indicated for every patient with ARDS. The treatment requires a physician's consent, and rotating beds are needed to adequately provide positioning. Risks for critically ill patients include pressure ulcers, accidental extubation, asynchronous ventilation, and airway obstruction. Generally, even if your patient at the transferring facility has been placed in prone positioning, the individual can be positioned supine for transport. Skill 3-6 presents a step-by-step explanation of pronation therapy.

Skill 3-6

PRONATION THERAPY

Acute lung injury (ALI) or acute respiratory distress syndrome (ARDS) impairs the lungs' ability to exchange gases. Simple gravity and the weight of the diseased lungs influence the regional flow, pressure, and the gas exchange airways. A patient with ALI or ARDS who spends most of the time essentially supine needs a change of position to recruit new tissue to oxygenate. Other factors related to the patient's position while receiving positive pressure ventilation are the pressure of the heart and abdominal contents vs. the thoracic cavity and the increased weight of the diseased lungs in a supine position. Relieving that pressure can improve ventilation. About 70% of patients with ARDS responded to pronation therapy within 2 hours of turning with a 20% increase in the partial pressure of arterial oxygen (PaO_2).

INDICATIONS

ALI, ARDS

CONTRAINDICATIONS

Increased intracranial pressure

Patient unable to tolerate head-down position

Pregnant patient

Unstable spinal column

Severe obesity (weight >350 lb 160 kg)

Extracorporeal membrane oxygenation (ECMO) in progress

Open chest wall

Unstable pelvic fractures

RELATIVE CONTRAINDICATIONS

Hemodynamic instability

Agitated patient

PREPARATION

1. Determine whether the patient's girth can be moved 180 degrees within the confines of the bed.
2. Prepare five or six pillows, foam blocks, or a manufactured prone positioning device, along with lifting and moving sheets or satin movers. If you decide to use pillows or individual cushions (egg crate pads for pediatric patients):
   a. The chest pillow or cushion should be wide enough to support the chest.
   b. The pelvic cushion should be slightly smaller and narrower than the pelvis.
   c. The head pillow should support the head at a slightly higher angle than the chest.
   d. A small cushion should be placed under the distal femur.
   e. A narrow cushion should be used to support the toes off the bed.
3. Recruit five or six staff members with good body mechanics to help you.
4. Be prepared for accidental removal of any and all tubes in the patient. Plan for each step of the movement by positioning tubing, pumps, and poles for easy movement across the axis of the patient.
5. Tape a tracheal tube so that it is positioned superiorly (once the patient is in the prone position, it will be "up"). Have a bag-mask device ready for manual ventilations.
6. If possible, administer sedative and pain medication and/or paralytics to the patient.
7. Suction the patient's oropharynx and (as necessary) the tracheal tube if present.
8. Place monitoring electrodes on the lateral aspects of the patient's arms and left hip.
9. Cap all nonessential lines and gastric tubes. Attach extension tubing to lines that cannot be capped. If upper torso lines are present, align them at the shoulder. Align lower torso lines at the lower leg with excess over the end of the bed.
10. Heimlich valves may be placed on chest tubes before the patient is turned; the tubes are reconnected to the pleural drainage systems once the patient is in the prone position.

PROCEDURE

1. Follow standard precautions. Place the lifting sheets or devices under the patient; if you use a manufactured prone frame, position it under the patient according to the manufacturer's instructions.
2. Assign one healthcare assistant to one area of the body (and all tubes in that area).
3. Turn the patient's head away from the ventilator and position the ventilator tubing across the top of the bed. Lock the wheels of all beds and carts involved.
4. Turn the patient to a 45-degree up position and place all pillows or cushions. For a large patient: Pull the patient to the edge of the bed away from the ventilator and turn the person to 45 degrees; position the torso cushions and then move the patient into a prone position.
5. Talk to the patient through the turning process. Attempt to keep the patient on the ventilator throughout.
6. Make sure you have achieved the proper positioning:
   a. During the turn: Keep the patient's head aligned with the body, the arms close to the torso, and the legs together with the toes of the upper leg pointed into the turn.
   b. After the turn: Turn the patient's head to the side and cushion it (keep the ear pinna flat), cushion the chest and pelvis (keep the abdomen free), flex the arms up, and position the knees and feet off the bed.

7. If the patient has orthopedic skeletal traction in place, have one assistant apply manual traction to the leg until the turn is complete. If an orthopedic pin comes in contact with the bed, place an extra pillow or cushion to alleviate pressure points.

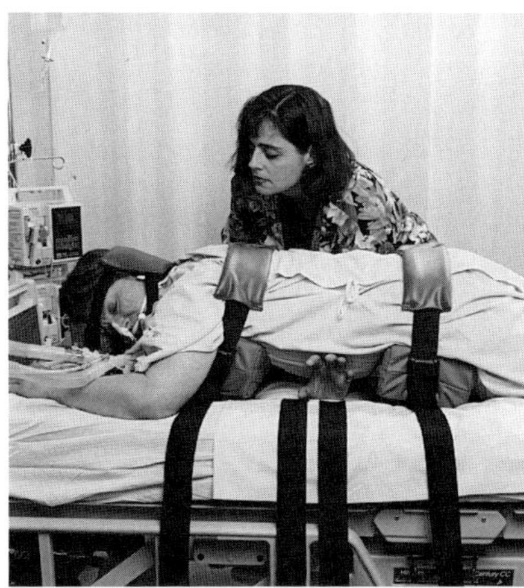

Patient lying prone on Vollman Prone Positioner. (Courtesy Hill-Rom, East Batesville, Ind.)

8. With a manufactured prone positioner, apply the device while the patient is supine and then position the straps as indicated (chest, head, and pelvis; see illustration).

NOTES

1. Patients often desaturate once in the prone position. If vital signs fail to stabilize within 10 minutes of the turn, the patient may be intolerant of the position and must be returned to supine.
2. These patients are especially prone to skin irritation and breakdown, especially on the face. Frequent movement of the head and face with padding should eliminate this risk. A special pressure-reduction bed or mattress also can lessen pressure on the skin.
3. Transport cots wide enough to perform this procedure may be difficult to acquire. The patient's girth is a primary consideration when evaluating whether a transport cot can accommodate a 180-degree turn. If your transport team has difficulty transferring a patient with ALI or ARDS from the hospital's ventilator to a transport ventilator, begin the prone positioning onto the transport cot—from bed to cot. Check for tolerance of the position before removing the patient from the hospital.

Surfactant Therapy

The extensive alveolar tissue damage in ALI allows plasma proteins to leak into the alveoli, with resulting loss of surfactant. Surfactant is an essential liquid that reduces surface tension and allows for lung compliance and gas exchange. The use of exogenous surfactant since the late 1980s has produced variable results; more recent, randomized trials have shown a reduced mortality. Some studies show that the surfactant preparation used may be an important determinant in the outcome. Surfactant is rarely used clinically for adults with ARDS; rather, it is used for neonates who may not have developed surfactant on their own.

High-Frequency Ventilation

High-frequency ventilation (HFV), or ventilation rates as high as 300/min with a small tidal volume (3 to 5 mL/kg), keeps the alveoli open and allows for the act of ventilation without the inhalation/exhalation classic to a human respiratory system. This technique has proved beneficial for neonates, but the results vary in adults with ALI.

Inverse Ratio Ventilation

Inverse ratio ventilation (IRV), mentioned earlier, is designed to prolong the inspiratory phase, which improves oxygenation in patients with ALI. However, for the patient to tolerate it, the individual must be heavily sedated and muscle paralysis must be induced.

Extracorporeal Membrane Oxygenation

Extracorporeal membrane oxygenation (ECMO) is an invasive therapy in which oxygenation is provided by bypassing the lungs. This is accomplished through a venous to arterial circuit (V-A ECMO) or a venous to venous circuit (V-V ECMO). V-A ECMO can provide oxygenation and improve cardiac output. A third method, ECMO2-R, removes CO_2 via the V-V circuit.

Liquid Mechanical Ventilation

In liquid mechanical ventilation, an experimental technique, the lungs are partly filled with perfluorocarbon liquid and ventilated mechanically. This method dissolves oxygen well and consumes less surfactant, resulting in less surface tension and inflammation.

Epoprostenol

Epoprostenol (prostacyclin; PGI2) is a powerful vasodilator. However, when given systemically, it can have hypotensive side effects through an increase in cyclic adenosine monophosphate (cAMP). When administered by nebulizer through the ventilation system, epoprostenol selects the pulmonary tissue to vasodilate more effectively and with fewer side effects than inhaled NO; it also is much less expensive. The parenteral drug is prepared in a protective bag and pumped into the nebulizer port on the ventilator; this requires frequent filter changes.

Clinical trials in regional medical centers across the United States and Europe continue to study these and other strategies for treating ALI and ARDS. The ARDSNet trials, which are supported by the National Heart Lung and Blood Institute, have published numerous studies on the effects of all these strategies. The following are some approaches undergoing evaluation.

1. Administration of granulocyte/monocyte colony-stimulating factor (GM-CSF) protein is being studied as a means to repair the alveolar layer.
2. Use of antioxidants to combat the oxidative stress on the lung and remote organs has been proposed, and N-acetylcysteine administration has been studied. Administration of albumin and of an albumin/furosemide combination to combat oxidative stress also is undergoing trials.
3. Use of the drug drotrecogin alfa (rhAPC; Xigris) is discussed with MODS in Chapter 8. This is a recombinant form of human activated protein C, similar to the natural protein in the body. It decreases inflammation and can decrease or help dissolve the formation of clots that may occur with the simultaneous inflammatory and coagulation cascade in shock.
4. The use of beta agonists in the treatment of ALI has been proposed, because these drugs stimulate reabsorption of pulmonary fluid, slow the immune response, and reduce airway resistance.
5. The use of stem cells has included applications for the alveolar epithelial cells and bronchial cells. Stem cells can repopulate the injured epithelial cells, and clinical trials are ongoing.
6. Airway pressure release ventilation (APRV), an alternative ventilation technique, is designed to increase internal PEEP by providing tidal volumes even when intrathoracic pressures are low.

The management of ALI and ARDS can be frustrating and confusing. Patients do not all respond alike to therapies, and not all strategies work for all patients. Each patient presents with a unique set of clinical problems, which makes the management of ARDS still as much an art as a science.

Complications of Respiratory Diseases

Air Leak Disorders

When a leak develops in the respiratory system, excess air must go somewhere. Most of it accumulates outside the alveoli. Two pathways are followed with air leaks:

- A pneumothorax results when air or blood accumulates in the pleural space. This may cause the lung to collapse. A pneumothorax greater than approximately 15% requires tube thoracostomy and water-seal suction systems. If air continues to leak under pressure, the accumulation of air can lead to a tension pneumothorax and subsequent obstructive shock. (Traumatic pneumothorax is described in Chapter 7.)
- **Barotrauma** or volutrauma occurs when excessive pressure (barotrauma) or excessive air (volutrauma) causes the alveolar-capillary membrane to fail. Air then enters the interstitial spaces and progresses toward the mediastinum and eventually the pleural, pericardial, and peritoneal spaces.

Box 3-9 Types of Air Leak Disease

Nontraumatic Pneumothorax (Visceral Pleura Failure; Air Enters the Pleural Space)

- *Primary:* Occurs in patients without underlying respiratory disease; known as *spontaneous pneumothorax.*
- *Secondary:* Occurs spontaneously in patients with underlying respiratory disease.

Traumatic Pneumothorax (Laceration of the Visceral or Parietal Pleura; Air Enters Pleural Space)

- *Open:* Laceration of the parietal pleura; atmospheric air enters space.
- *Closed:* Laceration of the visceral pleura; air from the lung enters space.
- *Iatrogenic:* Failure of the visceral pleura as a result of a procedure (e.g., placement of a central line catheter, thoracentesis, needle aspiration, biopsy).
- *Tension:* The pleural opening acts as a one-way valve by which air enters but cannot escape. Pressure increases, collapsing the lung, shifting the mediastinum, and squeezing the heart.

Volutrauma

- *Pulmonary interstitial emphysema:* The presence of air in the pulmonary interstitial space.
- *Subcutaneous emphysema:* The presence of air in the subcutaneous tissues.
- *Pneumomediastinum:* The presence of air in the mediastinal space.
- *Pneumopericardium:* The presence of air in the pericardial space. Air can accumulate, as in a tension pneumothorax, and pericardiocentesis is required to vent it.
- *Pneumoperitoneum:* The presence of air in the peritoneal space.
- *Pneumoretroperitoneum:* The presence of air in the retroperitoneal space.

Modified from Urden LD, Stacy KM, Lough ME: *Thelan's critical care nursing: diagnosis and management,* ed 5, St Louis, 2006, Mosby.

Box 3-9 differentiates the air leak diseases, which can be a direct result of complications of ventilator or manual resuscitation therapy.

Pleural Decompression

The presence of chest drainage systems should alert the critical care team to the potential for rapid pulmonary decompensation during transport. Water-seal drainage has been used for many years in the treatment of pulmonary air leaks. Several disposable water-seal systems are available today; we will review the principle of water-seal drainage and list the common mistakes, hazards, and complications associated with their use. Skill 3-7 presents the steps for maintaining a closed chest drainage system, and Skill 3-8 provides step-by-step instructions for performing an autotransfusion.

Skill 3-7

MAINTAINING A CLOSED CHEST DRAINAGE SYSTEM

Tubes are inserted into the mediastinum or pleural space to drain air, fluid, infectious matter, or blood in a closed setting. The tubes may be placed under emergency conditions, when pressure trauma occurs to the vacuum of the thorax, or in the operating room for certain surgical procedures. A system that allows drainage of this air or fluid from the vacuum of the thorax requires certain features to reestablish or maintain the appropriate pressure within the chest:

- Gravity, which allows negative pressure within the thorax
- A one-way valve or mechanism to prevent back flow into the chest
- A system that is maintained below the patient's chest with nonkinked tubing
- Suction connections and gauges that allow the use of portable or wall suction to improve the drainage of large amounts of air or fluid

Special features of some pleural drainage systems may include:

- Dry-dry drains (which are essentially waterless) with a one-way valve that opens on exhalation and then closes to prevent atmospheric air from entering during inhalation
- Self-sealing ports that allow the device to be accessed for samples for laboratory analysis of chest drainage or for withdrawal of excess fluid from an overfilled chamber
- Autotransfusion collection chambers
- A manometer portion that allows observation for and measurement of inspiratory and expiratory **tidaling** fluctuations

NOTES

1. The suction pressure usually is set at –20 cm H_2O; it should not be greater than –40 cm H_2O.
2. Chest tubes should not be clamped with tools or instruments.

INDICATIONS

Drain fluid, blood, and air from the pleural space or mediastinum

Restore intrathoracic negative pressure

Promote reexpansion of a collapsed lung

PROCEDURE

1. Follow the manufacturer's recommendations for setting up the pleural drainage system.
2. Follow standard precautions.
3. Depending on the setting, hang the drainage device from the lower edge of the cart or swing the unit stand into position and secure it to the floor. Keep the device lower than the patient.
4. If suction will not be used, leave the short tubing open to the air.
5. *For suction:* Fill the suction chamber with sterile water (usually provided) to the marked level on the unit. Connect the short tubing to the suction connecting tubing and suction source. (If the suction chamber becomes overfilled, insert a syringe and needle into the corresponding grommet and withdraw the excess fluid. If the chamber is underfilled, instill sterile saline through the grommet.)
6. Dial the pleural drainage system unit to the prescribed amount of suction (usually –20 cm H_2O).
7. Turn on the wall suction and check the pleural drainage unit for the indicator in the window in the suction section. Turn up the wall suction until the indicator shows the appropriate level (according to the manufacturer's recommendation).

   NOTE: You should see a constant, gentle bubbling in the chamber.
8. Uncoil the longer tubing from the drainage unit and arrange it adjacent to the sterile field established for the tube thoracostomy procedure. Keep the cap on the end of the tubing to keep the tubing sterile until it is connected to the appropriately inserted chest tube.

SECURING TUBE CONNECTIONS

All connections with tubing coming from the patient (chest tube to connector, connector to pleural drainage system tubing) are secured with tape or strapping devices.

- If tape is used, make sure it is strong and fold the ends back onto the strip for easy removal.
- If plastic straps are used, follow the manufacturer's recommendations for securing them.

PLEURAL DRAINAGE MONITORING AND MAINTENANCE

1. Follow your protocols for routine assessment of the patient's ventilation and perfusion status. However, assess it at least initially and every 2 hours or with any sudden change in the patient's condition. Include assessment of the chest tube insertion site and subcutaneous tissue for possible air leaks (sub Q air).
2. At your initial patient assessment, evaluate the pleural drainage system for proper functioning and to rule out air leaks before transport.
3. After the chest tube is inserted, the initial output should be marked with the date and time, which are written directly on the face of the pleural drainage unit. Thereafter, hourly or routine notations may be made to aid all those caring for the patient.
4. Documentation should include the initial and hourly or routine measurements (if any), the color of the drainage, and any fluctuation or tidaling.

NOTE: Surgical consultation is needed if the initial output is greater than 1200 mL and/or the hourly collection is 200 mL for more than 2 to 3 hours. Follow your service's policies for autotransfusion of blood (see Skill 3-8).

5. A syringe and 20-gauge needle can be used to aspirate a specimen from the pleural drainage system through the indicated self-sealing site.
6. To ensure the patency of the tubing:
   a. Keep the tubing free of kinks. Have it looped at the level of the patient and keep it free of thick secretions (clots) that may create an obstruction.
   b. If clots or other debris has created an obstruction, you may need to "milk" the tube: gently squeeze it between your fingers, moving the debris along toward the drainage unit. Do not strip the length of the tubing.
   c. Check for fluid fluctuations in the chamber. If no **tidaling** or fluctuations are seen, the tubing may be kinked or the patient's lung may have reexpanded.
7. To asses for air leaks:
   a. Some systems have an air leak assessment chamber.
   b. *With the suction off,* an air leak is suspected if continuous bubbling is noted in the unit.
   c. *To find the leak:* Begin at the chest wall (at the insertion site) and intermittently occlude the tubing with your fingers and hold for a few seconds; proceed toward the drainage unit. If the bubbling continues while the tubing is occluded, the air leak is between the manual occlusion and the drainage unit. Replace the tubing or drainage unit. If the bubbling stops at the insertion site, the air leak is in the patient. Make sure all chest tube eyelets are within the site and the dressing. Apply another dressing and notify the physician. Do not reposition the chest tube.
   d. If the tube is a mediastinal tube, no bubbling should ever be seen in the chamber. If an air leak is noted, this indicates false placement of the chest tube into the pleural cavity.

Skill 3-8

PERFORMING AN AUTOTRANSFUSION

Transfusing the patient's own blood (autotransfusion) back into the body eliminates the risks of a reaction and disease transmission. In a trauma patient, the pleural drainage system may accumulate pleural blood at such a rate that delivering it back to the patient with a special setup is beneficial.

INDICATION

Active bleeding from the pleural space at 1500 mL initially or greater than 200 mL/hour over 2 to 3 hours with signs of hemorrhagic shock

CONTRAINDICATIONS

Chest tube drainage from an unknown source (gastric, hepatic, splenic) because of false placement of the chest tube

Patient with known pleural malignancy

Renal or hepatic insufficiency

Known coagulopathies

Known religious prohibition of transfusion

PROCEDURE

1. Follow standard precautions. Assemble the equipment according to the recommendations of the manufacturer of the pleural drainage unit.
2. The manufacturer may provide an anticoagulating agent or may direct you to obtain one and inject it into the bag before, during, or after collecting the blood.
3. Connect and collect the pleural drainage system to the chest tube. Prepare a second drainage unit for attachment once the first bag is full.
4. Clamp the tubing, maintaining its sterility, and remove the bag of blood. Attach the second bag and open the clamps.
5. Prime the blood administration tubing and filters with normal saline solution. Attach the bag of accumulated blood to the Y port of the blood tubing and open the clamps.
6. Begin standard transfusion documentation and recording of vital signs according to your service's policy.
7. Collected blood must be transfused within 6 hours. Record the amount of blood autotransfused. Record the amounts in the pleural drainage unit routinely, according to policy.

   NOTE: The patient probably has met the criteria for surgical management and control of bleeding for the chest trauma. Moving the patient to the operating room while autotransfusion is instituted is worthwhile.

Pleural Effusion

Pleural effusion is the collection of fluid between the layers of the pleura, in the pleural space. This fluid can have multiple causes, such as infection (tuberculosis, pneumonia), cancer (lymphoma), or extrapulmonary disease (left ventricular heart failure). Fluid with a low protein level is a *transudative effusion* (most commonly caused by congestive heart failure); fluid with a large amount of protein or cellular material is an *exudative effusion* (which has multiple causes, including infection and malignancy). Regardless of the type, pleural effusions can limit ventilation and oxygenation.

When fluid or infectious debris accumulates in the pleural space, diagnostic or therapeutic thoracentesis may be done at the patient's bedside. Large volumes of fluid (as much as 1 to 2 L) can be drained from pleural effusions. If heart failure is the cause of the effusion, removal of that much fluid can cause edema to reform quickly, accompanied by cough and increasing dyspnea; this is known as *reexpansion pulmonary edema.* Be sure to monitor the patient carefully during and after the procedure.

Thoracentesis

Accumulations of fluid in the pleural space may also be removed by a procedure known as **thoracentesis.** In thoracentesis, fluid is removed from the space between the lining of the outside of the lungs (the pleura) and the wall of the chest. Normally, very little fluid is present in this space. For the procedure, the patient is positioned correctly (either sitting up or lying supine, depending on the clinical situation and the patient's comfort), and the skin is anesthetized. A licensed practitioner inserts a catheter-over-needle system through the skin of the chest wall into the pleural space. Fluid is withdrawn and collected. For a diagnostic thoracentesis, the fluid may be sent to the laboratory for analysis. A therapeutic thoracentesis is performed to alleviate shortness of breath. Indications for thoracentesis include cancer, pulmonary embolus, pancreatitis, cirrhosis, infection, and kidney disease. The risk of complications is relatively low, but pneumothorax, respiratory distress, fluid reaccumulation, infection, and bleeding at the site can develop. For this reason, a chest radiograph is done after the procedure.

Treatment of Respiratory Failure

Initiation of Ventilation

Lung Mechanics

All members of the critical care team should understand the mechanics of the lungs and how they correlate with the use of a ventilation system. When you provide ventilation to a patient, you need to recreate what is natural to the lungs.

Resistance is opposition to airflow; this may be caused by friction, increased turbulence, or a reduction in the diameter of the conducting tube (i.e., the airways). As the diameter of the airways decreases, resistance to airflow increases. Airflow follows the path of least resistance; therefore, increased resistance often leads to areas of decreased ventilation. Increased resistance often is seen with obstructive defects, such as asthma, emphysema, and laryngeal edema.

The gas laws (discussed elsewhere in the text) deserve a brief review. When a person is at rest, breathing in the normal lung stimulates the muscles of respiration to contract, causing the pressure in the alveolus to drop below atmospheric pressure. This is a reflection of Boyle's law: As pressure decreases, volume increases. This pressure gradient is what causes air to flow into the lungs. Dalton's law explains how gases behave in a mixture. When a gas is made up of several different constituents, each constituent demonstrates its individual behavior as though the other gases did not exist. If a gas mixture is made up of 80% nitrogen (N_2) and 20% oxygen (O_2), it stands to reason that 80% of the pressure is exerted by the nitrogen and 20% by the oxygen. This becomes important when you consider the fractional content of air and that multiple gases share the alveolar space. The larger the percentage of gas in the alveolar space, the more likely the gas is to diffuse into the blood cells.

With multiple gases in the alveolus, the intent is to have one (O_2) move freely into the capillary system and another (CO_2) move in the reverse direction. This is accomplished by diffusion, the result of a pressure gradient. Gases in motion can move across a permeable membrane, such as a cell wall. The pressure of oxygen in the alveolus is higher than the pressure of oxygen in the pulmonary capillary. Therefore, oxygen in the alveolus moves across the alveolar-capillary membrane into the blood until the pressure of oxygen nears equilibrium. The pressure of carbon dioxide is higher in the blood than in the alveolus. This causes the carbon dioxide molecules to move from the blood into the alveolus until a nearly equal pressure gradient is reached. This is the basis for all gas exchange: gases at a higher partial pressure move into a space with a lower partial pressure until the gas is close to equilibrium in the two places.

Lung Volumes and Ventilation

Now that you know how gases behave and that gases in mixture maintain their respective volumes and amounts, let's review lung volumes. There are four lung volumes and four lung capacities. All the capacities are made up of two or more volumes. (See Figure 3-25 for a graphic representation of lung volumes.) Remember that the basic function of any mechanical ventilator is to mimic the body's ability to ventilate the lung. Knowing how the lung volumes relate to one another is the key to using mechanical ventilation to your advantage.

Most clinicians recognize the term **tidal volume (V_T)**, which describes the volume of air that moves into and out of the lung with calm respirations. We use the tidal volume as the basis for a description of the other lung volumes and capacities. A normal tidal volume ranges from 250 to 500 mL, based on a person's height, gender, and ideal body weight. *The tidal volume generally is smaller than we think, and it varies from breath to breath.* This principle is important in mechanical ventilation, for which ventilator parameters must be set. It is especially important for patients with ALI caused by blunt trauma, barotrauma, or ARDS. The use of smaller tidal volumes protects the lungs from barotrauma during mechanical ventilation.

Did You Know?

Most lung volumes (and medication doses) are based on a patient's ideal body weight (IBW). The following formulas can be used to find the ideal body weight:

***Men:* Ideal body weight (kg) = 50 + 2.3(Height [in] – 60)**

***Women:* Ideal body weight (kg) = 45.5 + 2.3(Height [in] – 60)**

The Hamwi formulas are another means of calculating the IBW.

Hamwi Formula for Men[3]

106 lb for first 5 feet + 6 lb for each inch over 5 feet (medium frame)
Small frame (–10%)
Large frame (+ 10%)

Hamwi Formula for Women

100 lb for first 5 feet + 5 lb for each inch over 5 feet (medium frame)
Small frame (–10%)
Large frame (+10%)

The **inspiratory reserve volume (IRV)** is the maximum volume of air that can be inhaled from the peak of tidal breath; this is the volume we inhale during a sigh. It averages about 2 to 3 L. The IRV is the amount of space available to be recruited if a greater tidal volume is needed (e.g., during exercise).

The **expiratory reserve volume (ERV)** is the maximum volume of air that can be exhaled at the end of a tidal breath. It averages about 1 to 1.25 L. This volume is the amount of air usually expelled during a cough, and it is considered the first volume of gas exhausted during respiratory failure. Because the ERV is easily depleted, loss of ERV often prevents weaning from mechanical ventilation.

The residual volume (RV) is the amount of air left in the lungs at the end of a forceful expiration. The RV maintains inflation of the alveoli so that the intrapulmonary pressure is not a significant obstacle to the next tidal breath. It also contributes to compliance. If not for the RV, we would have to generate huge pressures to breathe at rest.

The lung capacities are sums of various combinations of lung volumes. The **vital capacity (VC)** is the sum of the IRV, V_T, and RV. This is the maximum amount of air that can be moved in a single deep breath. The VC is an indicator of the ability to cough and of expiratory muscle strength, and it is routinely measured when patients are weaned from mechanical ventilation.

The inspiratory capacity (IC) is the maximum amount of air that can be inhaled after a normal expiration. It is the sum of the IRV and V_T. A reduced IC is a manifestation of restrictive disease.

The **functional residual capacity (FRC)** is the amount of air remaining in the lungs after a normal expiration (ERV + RV). The FRC is an indicator of air trapping, commonly seen in obstructive disease. As terminal airways are constricted and collapse on expiration, air is trapped behind the obstruction and remains in the alveolus; this contained air increases the FRC, and the increased lung volume decreases compliance, which makes the lung more difficult to inflate. It may also lead to increased WOB and respiratory inefficiency. However, in some disorders (e.g., pneumonia, ARDS, and trauma to the chest or abdomen), the FRC may be decreased as a result of atelectasis or consolidation. The primary problem in such patients is maintaining oxygenation.

The total lung capacity (TLC) is the sum of all four lung volumes. It averages 4 to 6 L, and it is calculated by two different (yet mathematically identical) methods: VC + RV = TLC or IC + FRC = TLC. The ratio of the RV to the TLC is a measurement of the volume of air that cannot be expired. As the RV increases, ventilation must be increased to maintain adequate gas exchange. The patient may increase tidal breathing, the respiratory rate, or both to meet the need. Chronic increases in the RV often result in decreased O_2 or elevated CO_2 levels (Figure 3-25).

Patient-Ventilator Interface

Emergency medical personnel are quite familiar with endotracheal tubes and their insertion. However, critical care team members must remember that the ultimate outcome of every intubation should be successful *extubation*. Likewise, the ultimate outcome of every case in which a patient is placed on a ventilator is a patient who has been weaned from the ventilator.

Ventilation

Noninvasive Ventilation

Noninvasive positive pressure ventilation (NPPV) can be provided in several forms; it often is referred to as **continuous positive airway pressure (CPAP)** or **bilevel positive airway pressure (BiPAP).** This form of ventilation is considered noninvasive because a tracheal tube usually is not required; instead, the patient may use a special nose or face device or a standard mask. CPAP uses a single pressure, generated by constant flow, and it allows the patient to breathe spontaneously. Envision yourself sticking your head out the car window while the vehicle is traveling 50 to 60 mph. CPAP blows the airways open.

BiPAP uses two pressures, one on inspiration to deliver volume and one on expiration to increase the FRC to improve oxygenation. On a standard ventilator, this is a combination of pressure support ventilation (PSV) and PEEP; on a standalone BiPAP machine, it is a combination of inspiratory positive airway pressure (IPAP) and expiratory positive airway pressure (EPAP). EPAP with PEEP is equivalent to CPAP. In a spontaneously breathing patient, the result is PSV or IPAP to increase the tidal volume (and overall minute ventilation),

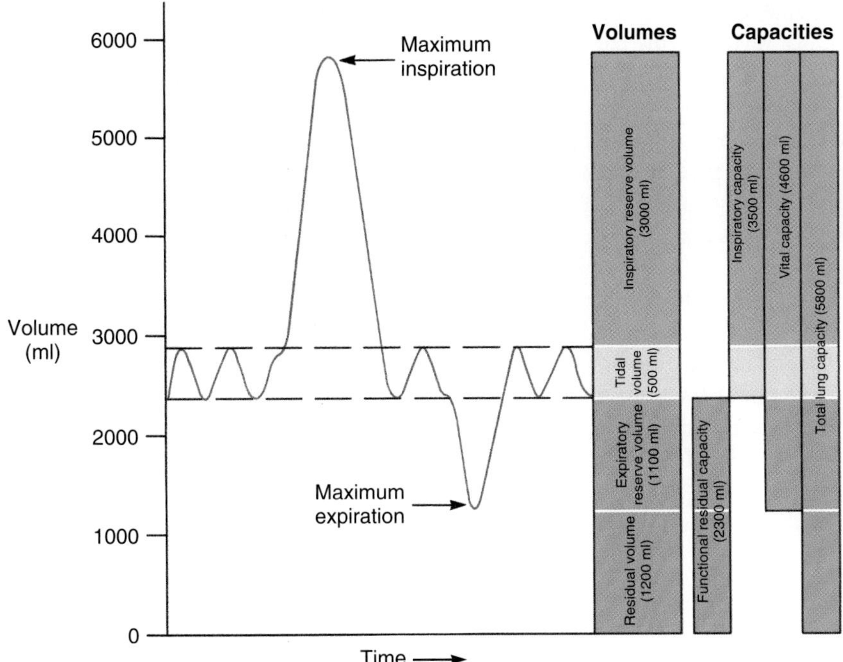

Figure 3-25

Lung volumes and capacities. Tidal volume during resting conditions. (From Seely R: *Anatomy and physiology,* ed 2, St Louis, 1992, Mosby.)

thereby increasing alveolar ventilation and decreasing the $PaCO_2$. In a patient with respiratory distress, BiPAP lessens the use of accessory muscles and relieves dyspnea. With the PEEP or EPAP on the exhalation side of the bilevel support, the PaO_2 increases.

Traditionally, noninvasive ventilation has been used to treat sleep-disordered breathing, such as sleep apnea. It is growing in popularity in the critical care field as a means of correcting ventilatory defects and hypoxemia. It is particularly helpful for patients with heart failure who have acute pulmonary edema.

The ventilator settings include inspiratory pressure, expiratory pressure, and oxygen concentration (FiO_2); these should be adjusted to provide the lowest inspiratory pressure possible, to make it as comfortable as possible for the patient while maintaining adequate oxygenation. Several protocols for the management of NPPV are available. Initially, inspiratory pressures generally are 12 to 15 cm H_2O, and expiratory pressures range from 5 to 8 cm H_2O. Titration of the inspiratory pressure may be necessary to achieve patient comfort.

A proper mask fit is important. The mask should fit tightly enough to form a gentle seal when pressure is applied, but not so tightly that it irritates the skin. Some transport ventilators with CPAP and BiPAP have special masks that have an exhalation port through the ventilation circuit. Masks are made so that the pressure from the flow of air helps create a good seal; therefore, excessive tightening of the straps is not necessary. Bronchodilators can be delivered by placing the nebulizer in the patient line at the mask. The use of positive pressure to deliver medications may enhance particle deposition and distribution of medication.

Complications of NPPV include ulceration of the nasal bridge, nasal congestion, eye irritation, gastric distention, and aspiration. A nasogastric tube can be used to alleviate gastric distention, but the tube makes maintaining a seal with the mask difficult. Aspiration can be prevented by using NPPV only in patients who are awake and alert. Contraindications to NPPV include hemodynamic instability, dysrhythmias, apnea, uncooperativeness, intolerance of the mask, and inability to maintain a patent airway, clear secretions, or properly seal the mask.

Improvement in the patient's dyspnea, respiratory rate, and breath sounds should be evident within 1 to 2 hours of therapy. The acid base balance and $PaCO_2$ should be monitored by ABG analysis at 1 hour and as needed for the first 24 hours.

Invasive Positive Pressure Ventilation

A patient may need to be placed on a ventilator for a number of physiologic and clinical reasons. For the critical care team, such patients include those who have been found to be in respiratory failure, those already on a ventilator in a critical care setting, and those in acute care settings whose condition warrants airway management (and thus PPV).

You have been taught that providing PPV to a patient by mechanical means is superior to providing it manually, except when chest compressions are being performed. All hospitals and ambulance companies *should* use ventilators rather than manual resuscitators whenever a patient requires artificial respiration; in critical care transport, ventilators are a must.

This section reviews ventilator terms and parameters and their definitions; the use of ABG results to guide the choice of ventilator settings; and the characteristics of a good transport ventilator. First, however, is a review of the bag-valve system of ventilation.

Manual Positive Pressure Ventilation

Regardless of the type of manual resuscitator system you use, some key points apply. You must have and use the correct-sized bags and masks for all patients transported by your service. For example, if your patient is a 7-year-old who weighs 40 kg, a "preemie" 250 mL bag will not provide the necessary tidal volumes. At minimum, your service should have a 450 to 500 mL bag and a 1 L bag, Many misinterpret the generic "pediatric" and "adult" designations for bags; there are many sizes of pediatric bags and at least two sizes of adult bags. Your service should research its needs based on the patients it will be transporting.

A manual resuscitator should have PEEP valve capability. If you need to temporarily ventilate a patient manually and the patient just came off the ICU's bedside ventilator with PEEP, that parameter needs to be maintained. Oxygenation is improved when a reservoir bag or tube is added *and* the person using the device ventilates the patient slowly and with just enough tidal volume to raise the chest.

Another misconception about manual (self-inflating) bag-valve systems is that they all deliver 100% oxygen if you add 12 to 15 L of oxygen with the reservoir. If you ventilate slowly with a moderate tidal volume, you can approach 100% oxygen with these devices, but it is difficult. For most of these systems, the oxygenation range is 65% to 80%. As previously mentioned, non-self-inflating devices (anesthesia bags) deliver 100% oxygen to the patient. Although these bags are not "user friendly," many critical care professionals prefer them, because they allow the user more of a sense of the compliance of the patient's lungs during ventilation. Anesthesia bags provide built-in PEEP capability with the flow-control valve.

Mechanical Ventilators

Mechanical ventilators are categorized as positive pressure ventilators or negative pressure ventilators. Currently, all emergency and critical care ventilators are positive pressure ventilators; the classic example of negative pressure ventilation is the iron lung.

The ventilator must complete four phases of ventilation to mimic a standard respiratory cycle for your patient: (1) pause and change from allowing exhalation to triggering positive pressure; (2) inspiration; (3) change from blowing positive pressure into the patient to stopping; and (4) exhalation. This process is accomplished by means of volume, pressure, flow, and time.

Trigger

The trigger for a spontaneous inspiratory effort is the pressure gradient between the intrathoracic pressure and the atmospheric pressure, along with chemoreceptors in the body. In a ventilator, this trigger can be created by time, pressure, or flow changes.

Sensitivity

The sensitivity must be set on the ventilator to tell the machine when to initiate a breath. This setting tells the machine when the patient has taken a breath (patient triggered) so that another breath is not stacked on top of it, causing lung trauma. The machine-triggered breath may be based on time or on flow. The trigger for a time-based breath requires a sensitivity setting adjusted by the rate you dial into the ventilator. For instance, a rate of 12/minute means that one breath will be delivered every 5 seconds. Flow- or pressure-triggered breaths are patient-assisted ventilations. When the sensitivity is set (the standard setting is −2 cm H_2O), the machine is triggered by a negative or decreasing flow within the circuit if the patient makes enough inspiratory effort in the A/C mode of ventilation.

Limit

The setting that maintains the inspiration is called the *limit;* this setting also may be based on pressure, flow, or volume. In a pressure-limited breath, a preset pressure is maintained during inspiration. In a flow-limited breath, a preset flow is reached before the end of inspiration. In a volume-limited breath, a preset volume of air is delivered on inspiration.

Cycle

Cycle is the variable that ends the inspiration. Four general types of ventilators are available, and the name of each of the four types is derived from the cycle it uses to stop the inspiration: volume cycled, pressure cycled, flow cycled, and time cycled.

Baseline

The baseline is the exhalation phase of mechanical ventilation. In this phase, the pressure setting indicates to the machine where exhalation should occur. This pressure setting is almost always zero unless you want to allow for PEEP.

Ventilator Modes

A ventilator's *modes* describe how the ventilator will deliver a breath to the patient. A number of choices are available, because different patients have different ventilatory needs. For example, two terms may be used as a prefix to the ventilator mode: *pressure control* and *volume control.* In pressure control ventilation, the inspiratory pressure is maintained at a constant level and the tidal volume varies. In volume control ventilation, the V_T is constant but the inspiratory pressure varies (Tables 3-15 and 3-16).

The most common modes available on transport ventilators are A/C, PSV, continuous mandatory ventilation (CMV), mandatory minute ventilation (MMV), and synchronized intermittent mandatory ventilation (SIMV). Some references further categorize these as assist or control modes, and new devices come on the market yearly. Many variations of these ventilatory modes are becoming available.

Other parameters besides the mode may need to be selected on the ventilator. These may include the rate, I:E ratio, V_T, %

Table 3-15 Comparison of Volume Control and Pressure Control

Variable	Volume Control	Pressure Control
Tidal volume	Set by clinician; constant	Variable; based on patient effort and compliance
Peak inspiratory pressure	Variable; based on patient effort and compliance	Set by clinician; constant
Inspiratory time	Set; function of respiratory frequency and inspiratory flow	Set by clinician; constant
Inspiratory flow	Set; function of respiratory frequency and inspiratory flow	Variable; based on patient effort and impedence

Modified from 2nd Ed. Critical Care Skills by Mims; Taken from Branson, Campbell's Mode of ventilator operation from *Mechanical Ventilation*, WB Saunders.

oxygen delivery, and PEEP. A transport ventilator should monitor the mean airway pressure and should have alarms for high and low pressure and disconnection.

Ventilator Settings

As mentioned, the ventilator's rate determines how often the ventilator will deliver breaths. For this reason, it is referred to as the **frequency** (f). The frequency can be controlled to some degree by the mode of ventilation. It also must be designated as either a *mandatory rate* (the number of times per minute the ventilator will deliver the tidal volume) or a *spontaneous rate* (the number of times the patient initiates breathing without control from the ventilator). A mandatory rate often affects other parameters, such as the minute volume, peak inspiratory pressure (PIP), and I:E ratio. A spontaneous rate affects the minute volume and mean airway pressure.

The **inspiratory to expiratory (I:E) ratio** (the relation of T_I to T_E) usually is derived from flow and frequency (force and speed). The standard or normal I:E ratio is 1:2; that means that if you set a timed rate on the ventilator of 12/min, one breath is given every 5 seconds. Each of the 5-second intervals

Table 3-16 Modes of Ventilation

Mode	Special Features	Goal of Ventilation	Concerns
Assist-control (A/C)	Allows spontaneous breathing but delivers controlled breaths at a minimum rate; all volumes are preset.	Alveolar recruitment and limiting of barotrauma.	Development of auto-PEEP Prevention of atelectasis
Synchronized intermittent mandatory ventilation (SIMV)	Allows spontaneous breathing with a lower mandatory rate. Spontaneous breaths generate spontaneous volumes.	Allows patient to bear some of the burden of respiration.	Minute ventilation may not be adequate; sedation must be managed to prevent hypoventilation.
Pressure-regulated volume control (PRVC)	Much like A/C, but each breath is adjusted according to compliance, and volume varies breath to breath.	In patients with high airway resistance or low lung compliance, PRVC manages minute volume delivery.	Use of higher ventilatory rates and lower tidal volumes requires additional monitoring.
Pressure support ventilation (PSV)	Set inspiratory pressure is delivered when patient initiates a breath or with a set rate over a baseline of PEEP.	Spontaneous ventilation; goal is to allow patient to bear more of burden of breathing; typically used in weaning from ventilation.	Not to be used for sedated patients with little or no spontaneous effort. Constant monitoring is advised.
Pressure control ventilation (PCV)	Volume delivered is determined by a preset inspiratory pressure.	Limits volume, maintains mean airway pressure.	Limited volume may lead to atelectasis; inspiratory pressure must be adjusted for changes in mean airway pressure.
Airway pressure release ventilation (APRV)	High PEEP level released by time control valve and reestablished when valve closes again; implies an inverse I:E ratio	Reduction of lung volume and preservation of spontaneous breathing.	Not suitable for patients with high airway resistance or extended expiratory times.

I:E, Inspiratory to expiratory; *PEEP*, positive end-expiratory pressure.

is divided between the T_I and T_E. If the V_T is delivered over 1.7 seconds and the exhalation phase lasts 3.3 seconds, the I:E ratio is essentially 1:2. A 1:3 ratio is recommended for patients with diseases such as emphysema, who require a longer time to get the air out.

An abnormal I:E ratio can develop if the minute volume is set too high (rate and V_T) and the time needed to deliver a large breath is inadequate, causing air trapping and possibly auto-PEEP. An example would be a rate set at 20/min (one breath every 3 seconds) and a V_T set at 1000 mL; delivering 1 L of gas to a patient in less than 1 second and then allowing less than 2 seconds for exhalation back to zero would be extremely difficult. Occasionally, the I:E ratio can be altered as a therapeutic tactic in patients who are difficult to ventilate.

Inverse ratio ventilation (IRV) uses an inspiratory to expiratory ratio that is greater than the standard 1:2 or 1:3 (i.e., 1:1 or 2:1). The goal of IRV is to improve oxygenation by providing a longer inspiratory time. As mentioned previously, the high flow rate and high frequency associated with IRV mean that most patients require heavy sedation and often muscle paralysis to tolerate this mode.

As you know, the V_T is the amount of air delivered in a single breath. The tidal volume is a mandatory setting in volume control modes; it is not affected by the rate or I:E ratio, but it is limited by the peak airway pressure in pressure-regulated modes (e.g., pressure control, APRV, pressure-regulated volume control [PRVC], and BiPAP). The spontaneous volume may or may not be equal to the mandatory tidal volume. It is a component of the minute volume (V_E), which is the product of *f* and V_T. The V_T is affected by the rate and flow in ventilator modes that are based on the minute volume.

The **mean airway pressure** reflects the alveolar pressure and alveolar compliance. It is measured by breath-hold maneuvers. In ventilation for patients with ARDS, mean airway pressure is closely controlled by reducing the V_T and increasing the frequency to prevent barotrauma or, more aptly, volutrauma.

Positive end-expiratory pressure (PEEP) is the resting level of volume maintained in the lung at the end of expiration. **Intrinsic PEEP** is created from airflow through the nasal passages; in normal, spontaneously breathing patients, PEEPi is 2 to 3 cm H_2O. Here, we consider PEEP as a function of mechanical ventilation. PEEP that is set on a ventilator is called **extrinsic PEEP.** PEEP increases the functional residual capacity, aids in the recruitment of alveolar volume, reduces alveolar fluid, and improves oxygenation. PEEP affects the MAP, PIP, and in some respects, compliance. Most patients require low levels of PEEP to achieve a sufficient increase in the FRC, but patients with ARDS may require higher levels because of their decreased diffusion capability. The bottom line is, PEEP means oxygen to the patient.

Most in-hospital ventilation is begun with 60% to 70% oxygen (FiO_2 of 0.6 to 0.7). If oxygenating the patient becomes difficult, the oxygen percentage usually is increased first. Otherwise, the standard admission PEEP setting is 3 to 5 cm H_2O.

High levels of PEEP (above 12 cm H_2O) are initiated when oxygenation is difficult. As mentioned earlier, optimal PEEP is the level at which gas exchange is maximized and the possibility of overdistention is minimized. Once established, PEEP should not be interrupted by breaks in the circuit. As FRC is recruited and oxygenation improves, PEEP may be reduced incrementally. An FiO_2 below 0.5 is preferable before reductions in PEEP are started. In manual ventilation, PEEP is accomplished with the addition of a tension valve on the expiratory port of a manual resuscitator.

Did You Know?

You are assessing and treating a critical care patient who is difficult to ventilate. The patient is receiving >70% oxygen with a high PEEP (>10 cm H_2O). A break in the ventilator circuit (tubing) would release all the PEEP in the patient, creating a very unstable condition. What do you do?

Gently pinching the tracheal tube to trap the PEEP while quickly attaching the transport ventilator circuit may help prevent this complication.[4]

Auto-PEEP is the development of end-expiratory pressure caused by airflow limitation. It is seen in patients with airway disease (emphysema or asthma) and when the expiratory time allowed is inadequate. Auto-PEEP increases the WOB and contributes to barotrauma, hypotension, and decreased cardiac output by squeezing the heart and reducing preload back to the heart. Auto-PEEP usually can be corrected by increasing the expiratory time and reducing the frequency.

Setting and Understanding Common Ventilator Alarms

Alarms in the ventilator should be set to at least two pressure limits: low pressure and high pressure. The low pressure alarm usually is set at 20 cm H_2O. Most low pressure alarms are triggered because the patient has become disconnected from the circuit (or the circuit from the ventilator). This alarm also may sound if the circuit is torn or has a hole.

The high pressure alarm should be set at 40 to 60 cm H_2O. Triggers for the high pressure alarm include obstructed (kinked) circuits; a patient who is "bucking" the ventilator (dyssynchrony); coughing; and mucous plugs or other heavy secretions that block the path for a breath. High pressure can cause pneumothorax or barotrauma and must be investigated quickly and efficiently.

Box 3-10 discusses several elements that should be considered in the purchase of a transport ventilator.

Box 3-10 Important Factors in the Purchase of a Transport Ventilator

1. *Physical features:* Dimensions, weight, configuration, fittings, portability, and durability. Does the ventilator have an internal barometer for high altitude or variable altitude use? Is it capable of the same modes as ventilators used at transferring or receiving hospitals? Does the device contain ferromagnetic components (cannot be used for a patient undergoing MRI)?
2. *Settings:* Does the unit have a variable tidal volume (V_T), from 100 to 1500 mL? Rate settings of 2/min to 30/min? Minute ventilation from 4 to 20 L/min? Intermittent mandatory ventilation (IMV) and controlled mechanical ventilation? Demand or sigh settings?
3. *Mechanical load:* Is the unit powered by gas or electricity? How much gas (L/min) does it use? Will the batteries be sufficient? Does the mode of ventilation affect these two variables? (Some electric ventilators have more precise controls and less fluctuation in pressure than gas models.)
4. *Patient-ventilator interface:* Are pressures, volumes, sensitivities, and triggers external or internal? Is a PEEP leak compensation available (trigger sensitivity accounts for PEEP)? High- and low-pressure alarms?
5. *Monitoring and dials:* Does the unit have separate dials for rate and VT? Does it include other types of monitoring, such as the end-tidal carbon dioxide pressure ($PETCO_2$) and the oxygen saturation (SpO_2)? Are alarms visible as well as audible? Are gauges easy to read, no matter the light source?

Did You Know?

Transport ventilators may deliver breaths from a pressurized source (45 to 55 psi). According to Boyle's law, a certain mass of gas expands as it reaches higher altitudes. In fact, the expanding mass of gas is multiplied twice at an altitude of 18,000 feet. With major changes in altitude, you should move the patient from mechanical to manual ventilation as you recalibrate settings according to your protocols. Some newer transport ventilators have internal barometers that automatically recalculate this pressure change.

Hazards and Complications of Mechanical Ventilation

Sudden worsening of respiratory distress or arterial oxygen desaturation (or both) is a common clinical indicator of patient decompensation. *Your first priority in any ventilator-associated decompensation is to ensure correct patient positioning and the patency of the airway.* This development should prompt you to take the patient off the ventilator and manually ventilate the person while you troubleshoot the problem. Most resuscitation courses now teach the provider to prioritize and evaluate the decompensation using the acronym DOPE: *d*isplaced tube, *o*bstructed tube, *p*ressure or pneumothorax, and *e*quipment failure.

Note the ventilator alarms, airway pressures, and tidal volume; these should point you in the direction of the problem. Check the patient's vital signs and perform a rapid physical examination (including pain assessment), noting any dyssynchrony or diminished or absent breath sounds. You may need to suction the patient. Return the patient to the ventilator only after verifying proper function. Reassess the patient and, if necessary, increase the level of support provided by the ventilator. If dyssynchrony is noted, evaluate the patient's sedative, analgesic, and/or paralytic drug levels; bucking the ventilator triggers high pressure alarms and causes unstable vital signs.

Barotrauma or Volutrauma

Barotrauma is associated with high airway pressures, high levels of PEEP, and auto-PEEP. It may cause tension pneumothorax, pneumomediastinum, pneumopericardium, air embolism, or subcutaneous emphysema. Volutrauma may cause acute lung injury. *Free air in the thorax is a life-threatening development, and the air must be evacuated immediately.* Insertion of a chest tube will most likely be necessary.

Ventilator-Associated Pneumonia

The disease process of the lower airways has already been discussed. However, pneumonia acquired through a ventilator deserves special consideration, because this is a serious complication of mechanical ventilation. In the United States, the incidence of VAP in surgical ICUs is about 5% to 7%; for all ICUs, the incidence is 12% to 15%.

The development of pneumonia in a ventilated patient has been attributed to several factors, including prolonged ventilation, aspiration of oral or gastric contents around the ETT, frequent disconnects in the patient circuit, and poor oral care during intubation. Following recommendations made by the Centers for Disease Control and Prevention (CDC), many intensive care units are becoming more vigilant about preventing VAP through increased monitoring and changes in bedside practices. Some of the recommended preventive measures include maintaining the head of the bed at 30 degrees or higher to reduce the likelihood of aspiration of gastric contents; oral care protocols to reduce oral secretions and prevent infection; prophylaxis for venous thromboembolism to prevent the development of deep vein thrombus during prolonged bed rest (which results in increased time on the ventilator); prophylaxis for peptic ulcer by reducing acid reflux; and regular "sedation holidays," during which sedation is reduced and the patient is allowed to rouse and breathe spontaneously. Assessment of the patient's readiness to wean begins within the first 48 hours and is repeated during the sedation holiday so that weaning from mechanical ventilation can be started as early as possible.

Failure to Wean

Another complication of mechanical ventilation is a condition called "failure to wean." This and the inevitable tracheostomy are serious complications of mechanical ventilation and are noted here for the incidence of tracheostomy. Tracheostomy is one of the most frequently performed procedures in critically ill patients; approximately 24% of ventilated patients in medical ICUs will have a tracheostomy, and the likelihood that these patients will require out-of-hospital transport is very high.

Air Leaks and Mechanical Ventilation

Patients who require mechanical ventilation often have massive air leaks from chest tubes. This blow-through effect can be challenging to understand. You are providing ventilation under positive pressure, and the flow rate of the leak may exceed the capability of the drainage unit. Increasing suction from the suction source may increase the airflow *through* the system and will not affect the suction of the unit. Rapid bubbling in the water chamber with little or no bubbling in the suction chamber is an indication that airflow from the chest tube has overwhelmed the system's capacity.

Scenario Conclusion

You continue to prepare this very unstable patient for transport. You administer 5 mg of midazolam and 1.2 mg/kg of rocuronium so that you can take over complete control of ventilation. You preset your transport ventilator to PSV parameters. While transferring the ventilation tubing to the patient's ETT, you trap the PEEP by squeezing the tube for a brief time. This time, the patient tolerates the maneuver and does not decompensate. Continuous monitoring throughout transport allows a safe transfer to the medical ICU of the receiving hospital and the patient's subsequent recovery.

SUMMARY

Airway and breathing assessment and the management of the critical care patient through resuscitation and transportation are essential phases of your team's care. Ongoing education, skills, scenario practice, and strong protocols guide the provision of this care.

KEY TERMS

acute lung injury (ALI) A systemic process, considered the pulmonary phase of multiple organ dysfunction syndrome (MODS), that is characterized by noncardiogenic pulmonary edema. The most severe form of ALI is acute respiratory distress syndrome.

acute respiratory distress syndrome (ARDS) Fulminant pulmonary interstitial and alveolar edema that usually develops within a few days after the initiating trauma. It is thought to result from alveolar injury, which led to increased capillary permeability. Also called *adult respiratory distress syndrome* and *shock lung*.

adventitious Accidental or acquired; not natural or heredity. With regard to lung or breath sounds, the term refers to abnormal sounds.

air trapping A condition in which the lungs do not or are not allowed to exhale completely.

airway resistance The overall effect of a small airway diameter that increases the resistance to breathing. This effect is created by the increased turbulence that results when high inspiratory airflow is required from positive pressure ventilation and is passed through the tracheal tube.

airways The route for the passage of air into and out of the lungs.

aldosterone The major mineralocorticoid secreted by the adrenal cortex; it promotes the retention of sodium and bicarbonate, the excretion of potassium and hydrogen ions, and secondary retention of water. Large excesses can result in plasma volume expansion, edema, and hypertension. Secretion of aldosterone is stimulated by a low plasma potassium concentration and by angiotensin II.

anatomic dead space The volume of air that remains in the conducting airways and does not contribute to gas exchange.

anxiolysis The cessation of anxiety; an anxiolytic drug helps to relieve anxiety.

aryepiglottic folds Termed arytenoepiglottic; this pertains to the arytenoid cartilage and to the epiglottis, structures of the upper airway.

asynchronous ventilation A respiratory pattern demonstrated by the inability to synchronize spontaneous ventilation with mechanical ventilation. Also called *dyssynchrony*.

auto-PEEP Positive end-expiratory pressure (PEEP) that is created by the patient's respiratory system rather than set on the ventilator. PEEP keeps the distal airways open during exhalation and adds to overall oxygenation. Auto-PEEP occurs when the ventilation rate and tidal volume are set so that the patient is not allowed to exhale fully; this can create high intrathoracic pressures, barotrauma, and hypotension. Also called *intrinsic PEEP*.

barotrauma Injury caused by pressure, especially to enclosed cavities of the body such as the eustachian tubes, middle ear, paranasal sinuses, or lungs.

bilevel positive airway pressure (BiPAP) A type of noninvasive positive pressure ventilation (NPPV) that provides ventilation assistance with higher pressures on inhalation and lower pressures on exhalation. NPPV allows the patient to get more air into and out of the lungs.

bronchoscopy An invasive procedure for visualizing the upper and lower respiratory tract for diagnostic and treatment purposes.

capnograph (capnography) The measurement of carbon dioxide (CO_2) expressed as a waveform and recorded over time; this measurement is considered more valuable to the critical care provider.

capnometer (capnometry) A device that measures the amount of CO_2 and projects a number; this measurement is not placed on a graph.

cholinergic receptors Cell surface receptors that bind the neurotransmitter acetylcholine and mediate its action on postjunctional cells. Types of cholinergic receptors include parasympathetic autonomic effector cells, sympathetic and parasympathetic autonomic ganglion cells, striated muscle, and certain central neurons.

competitive (nondepolarizing) neuromuscular blocking agents Neuromuscular blocking agents that compete with and block the action of acetylcholine at the neuromuscular junction receptor site, thereby causing paralysis. Also called *nondepolarizing paralytics.*

conducting airways The lower and upper airways together, from the nares to the terminal bronchioles.

continuous positive airway pressure (CPAP) Ventilation assistance that provides a single continuous level of pressure. Also called *noninvasive positive pressure.*

CO oximetry Carbon monoxide oximetry. Oximetry is a measurement of hemoglobin and oxygen gas exchange, including oxyhemoglobin and oxygen saturation. CO oximetry measures the so-called dyshemoglobins, carboxyhemoglobin and metahemoglobin.

cortisol An important natural glucocorticoid that is synthesized in the zona fasciculata of the adrenal cortex. Cortisol affects the metabolism of glucose, protein, and fats and has appreciable mineralocorticoid activity. It also regulates the immune system and affects many other functions. When used as a pharmaceutical, it usually is referred to as *hydrocortisone.*

coudé tip A tip that is bent like an elbow; it is used on catheters and other devices to help shape or manipulate the placement of a tube or catheter.

dead space The portions of the respiratory system that are in contact with ventilating gases but not with the pulmonary blood flow; the air in these parts does not contribute to the exchange of oxygen and carbon dioxide.

dead space ventilation The areas of the lung that are underventilated.

defasciculation Administration of 10% of a nondepolarizing paralytic just before rapid induction and intubation (RSI) to prevent involuntary contractions and relaxation of small, local muscles (i.e., fasciculations).

denervation Resection or removal of the nerves to an organ or part.

distal A term that means "away from" (e.g., the airways distal to the mainstem bronchi).

epithelial denudement Pulmonary hemorrhage or bleeding.

epoprostenol A prostaglandin used to reduce pulmonary artery pressure.

excursion The movements that occur from a normal, or resting, position of a movable part in performing a function, such as the movements of the chest wall in respiration.

expiratory reserve volume (ERV) A pulmonary function parameter; it is a measure of the maximum volume of air that can be exhaled from the end of a normal breath.

expiratory time (E time, TE) The time required to exhale in one respiratory cycle.

extrinsic PEEP PEEP applied by positive pressure ventilation.

fasciculations The uncoordinated, uncontrollable twitching of a muscle group that occurs when a depolarizing neuromuscular blocking agent is administered. Fasciculations, which are visible through the skin, represent a spontaneous discharge of a number of fibers innervated by motor nerve filaments.

fiberoptic bronchoscope (FOB) A flexible bronchoscope that uses fiberoptics. Fiberoptics is the transmission of an image along flexible bundles of coated parallel glass or plastic fibers that propagate light by internal reflection.

forced vital capacity Part of a series of diagnostic tests for pulmonary function, this test evaluates the maximum amount of air forcefully exhaled from the lungs after maximum inhalation.

fremitus A palpable vibration, a thrill. Pleural fremitus is a vibration caused by a friction rub between the opposing surfaces of the pleura that can be palpated on the wall of the thorax.

frequency (f) The number of occurrences of a process per unit of time; a rate.

functional airways The airways involved in the act of respiration, or the exchange of oxygen and carbon dioxide.

functional residual capacity The volume of air in the lungs after a normal tidal volume exhalation.

ideal (optimal) PEEP The minimum amount of PEEP necessary to provide oxygenation but also prevent the complications of high intrathoracic pressures.

inspiratory reserve volume (IRV) A pulmonary function parameter; it is the measure of the maximum volume of air that can be inhaled above the standard inhalation in a normal breath

inspiratory time (I time, TI) The time it takes complete inhalation; the inspiratory portion of the inspiratory to expiratory (I:E) ratio.

inspiratory to expiratory (I:E) ratio A proportion of the time required to inhale and exhale in a given time unit. A normal human I:E ratio is 1:2 or 1:3.

intrinsic PEEP See *auto-PEEP.*

inverse ratio ventilation (IRV) A mode of ventilation in which the inspiratory time is longer than the expiratory time (i.e., the inverse of the normal I:E ratio). An inverse

I:E ratio is used for patients with ARDS to prevent barotrauma; the long, sustained inspiration reduces the mean airway pressure while increasing the partial pressure of oxygen (PaO_2). This prolonged TI would be uncomfortable for a conscious patient.

jet ventilation The high-velocity insufflation of gas (air) into the airway by means of a catheter. Jet ventilation is used during a failed airway protocol. *High-frequency jet ventilation (HFV)* is the delivery of high-flow, short pulses of pressurized gas, usually to a patient with pulmonary hypertension.

Mallampati score A score that predicts the ease or difficulty of intubation based on the anatomy of the oral cavity, from the base of the uvula and the faucial pillars to the soft palate. Class I and class II scores indicate airways that likely will allow easy intubation; class III and class IV scores indicate difficult airways.

maximum occlusion technique A process in which air is injected into the tracheal tube cuff until no leak is heard; next, air is withdrawn until a small leak is heard on inspiration, and then more air is added until no leak is heard on inspiration. This technique reduces the risk of aspiration.

mean airway pressure (MAP) The average pressure over one inspiration/exhalation cycle; the value displayed on a ventilator is the average of this calculation over 1 minute.

methemoglobinemia An excess of methemoglobin in the blood, which results in cyanosis and headache, dizziness, fatigue, ataxia, dyspnea, tachycardia, nausea, vomiting, and drowsiness; it can progress to stupor, coma, and occasionally death. Methemoglobinemia may be caused by toxic exposure to a chemical or drug, including nitrates, sulfonamides, and aniline dyes.

minimum leak technique A process in which the tracheal tube cuff is slowly inflated until all leaks stop; then, a small amount of air is removed slowly until a small leak may be heard on inspiration. This technique reduces mucosal injury.

minute volume The volume of gas exhaled from the lungs in 1 minute; the tidal volume multiplied by the respiratory rate.

muscarinic receptors Cholinergic receptors that are stimulated by the alkaloid muscarine and blocked by atropine. Muscarinic receptors are found on autonomic effector cells and on central neurons in the thalamus and cerebral cortex. Three types may be distinguished on the basis of pharmacologic specificity and five types on the basis of molecular structure.

myoclonic movement (myoclonus) Shocklike contractions of part of a muscle, an entire muscle, or a group of muscles; the contractions may be restricted to one area or may appear synchronously or asynchronously in several areas. Myoclonus may be part of a disease process (e.g., epileptic or postanoxic myoclonus) or a normal physiologic response (e.g., nocturnal myoclonus).

nasal turbinates Any of the nasal conchae (concha nasalis or turbinal concha), the shell-shaped, bony plates that project from the nasal walls.

neuroinhibitor transmitter Any of a group of substances that are released on excitation from the axon terminal of a presynaptic neuron of the central or peripheral nervous system and travel across the synaptic cleft to inhibit the target cells.

neuromuscular blocking agent (NMBA) A drug that interferes locally with the transmission or reception of impulses from motor nerves to skeletal muscles.

nicotinic receptors Cholinergic receptors that initially are stimulated (and at high doses are blocked) by the alkaloid nicotine and blocked by tubocurarine. These receptors are acetylcholine-gated ion channels and are found on autonomic ganglion cells, striated muscle, and spinal central neurons.

nitric oxide (NO) A gas that in combination with oxygen reduces pulmonary hypertension.

noncompetitive (depolarizing) neuromuscular blocking agents Neuromuscular blocking agents that compete at the motor end plate by simulating acetylcholine and creating an impulse (depolarization) but then blocking the nerve's ability to be reset for subsequent stimulation; this results first in fasciculations and then in paralysis. Also called *depolarizing paralytics*.

noninvasive positive pressure ventilation (NPPV) Ventilatory support that does not require an advanced airway (e.g., BiPAP and continuous positive airway pressure [CPAP]).

nosocomial Pertaining to or originating in the hospital; the term usually refers to a disease or other pathologic condition (e.g., a nosocomial infection is one acquired in the hospital).

occlusion technique A technique for determining the minimal cuff pressure for a tracheal tube.

parenchyma The functional part of an organ in the body (e.g., the lung parenchyma).

percutaneous cricothyrotomy Percutaneous means that it is performed through the skin with a needle. In this case, it is the introduction of a needle through the cricothyroid membrane in order to create an airway in an emergency.

permissive hypercapnia A deliberate decrease in alveolar ventilation that allows the arterial carbon dioxide pressure ($Paco_2$) to rise.

$PETco_2$ The pressure of CO_2 near the end of exhalation. Also called the *end-tidal* CO_2.

physiologic dead space The portions of the airway, from the nose and mouth to the terminal bronchioles, in which exchange of oxygen and carbon dioxide does not occur.

plateau pressure A pressure value that is maintained constant during a portion of the inspiratory phase of the breath. It represents the pressure at the alveolus and therefore is the best predictor of barotrauma.

pleural effusion The presence of fluid in the pleural space. Types of pleural effusion include chylothorax, hemothorax, hydrothorax, and pyothorax (empyema).

positive end-expiratory pressure (PEEP) Pressure maintained above the level of atmospheric pressure at the end of exhalation. This is achieved by preventing the complete release of gas during exhalation, usually by means of a valve in the circuit. The purpose of PEEP is to increase the volume of gas remaining in the lungs at the end of exhalation, thereby reducing the shunting of blood through the lungs and improving gas exchange.

radiopaque Referring to the quality of being impenetrable by x-rays or other forms of radiant energy; radiopaque areas appear light or white on exposed film.

resistance With regard to respiration, the opposition of the tracheobronchial tree to airflow; the mouth-to-alveoli pressure difference divided by the airflow.

respiration The cellular metabolic process by which oxygen is taken in, substances are oxidized, energy is released, and carbon dioxide and oxidized products are given off.

Seldinger technique A method of introducing a catheter into a lumen or body cavity: a narrow needle is used to enter the lumen or body cavity, a guide wire is passed through the needle, the needle is removed, and the catheter is advanced over the wire.

spirometry The measurement of the breathing capacity of the lungs, such as in pulmonary function tests.

surgical cricothyrotomy A tracheotomy created by an incision through the skin and cricothyroid membrane to secure a patent airway; it is performed for emergency relief of an upper airway obstruction.

temporomandibular ankylosis Immobility and consolidation of the temporomandibular joint as a result of disease, injury, or a surgical procedure.

thoracentesis A procedure in which the thoracic cavity is entered with a needle or a catheter over a needle to aspirate fluids. Also called *pleurocentesis.*

tidaling The rise and fall of fluid in a chest tube; it is synchronized with the respiratory cycle.

tracheostomy The creation of an opening in the anterior trachea to allow insertion of a tube to relieve upper airway obstruction and facilitate ventilation. In this context, the terms *tracheotomy* and *tracheostomy* are used interchangeably.

V/Q The ratio of ventilation to perfusion.

V/Q mismatch An anatomic or a physiologic shunt that indicates impaired gas exchange.

ventilation A passive activity in which air is moved into or out of the lungs for the purpose of exchanging oxygen for carbon dioxide.

ventilator-associated pneumonia (VAP) A nosocomial pneumonia acquired during mechanical ventilation. Also known as *ventilator-assisted pneumonia.*

vital capacity A measurement of pulmonary volume, VC is the sum of the inspiratory reserve volume, the tidal volume, and the expiratory reserve volume.

work of breathing (WOB) The use of accessory muscles of respiration; WOB is an indicator of respiratory muscle fatigue and impending ventilatory failure.

REFERENCES

1. St John R: End-tidal carbon dioxide monitoring, *Crit Care Nurse* 23:83-88, 2003.
2. Walls R, editor: Manual of emergency airway management, Philadelphia, 2000, Lippincott Williams & Wilkins.
3. Hamwi GJ: Therapy: changing dietary concepts. In Danowski TS, editor: *Diabetes mellitus: diagnosis and treatment,* vol 1, New York, 1965, American Diabetes Association, pp 73-78.
4. EMS Learning Resources Center: Critical care paramedic curriculum, 1996, University of Iowa Hospitals & Clinics.

Bibliography

AARC clinical practice guideline: in-hospital transport of the mechanically ventilated patient—2002 revision and update, *Respir Care* 47:721-723, 2002.

Arroliga A: Noninvasive ventilation in respiratory failure: Does it improve outcomes? *Cleve Clin J Med* 68:677-680, 2001.

Bautin A, Khubulava G, Kozlov I, et al: Surfactant therapy for patients with ARDS after cardiac surgery, *J Liposome Res* 16:265-272, 2006.

Blonshine S: New applications of capnography, *AARC Times* 4:36-39, 1999.

Clinical practice guideline: bronchoscopy assisting—2007 revision and update, *Respir Care* 52:74-80, 2007.

Des Jardins T, Burton G: *Clinical manifestations and assessment of respiratory disease,* ed 5, St Louis, 2005, Mosby.

Dorland MW: *Dorland's medical dictionary,* ed 31, Philadelphia, 2007, Saunders.

Edwards JR, Peterson KD, Andrus ML et al: NHSN [National Healthcare Safety Network] report: data summary for 2006, *Am J Infect Control* 35:290-310, 2007.

Ellison RT: Intrahospital transport triples the risk for ventilator-associated pneumonia in critically ill, mechanically ventilated patients, *Journal Watch: Infectious Diseases (online),* January 13, 2006. www.jwatch.org. Accessed April 30, 2010.

Greenberg RS, Kay NH: Cuffed oropharyngeal airway (COPA) as an adjunct to fibreoptic tracheal intubation, *Br J Anaesth* 82:395-398, 1999.

Hache M et al: Inhaled prostacyclin (PGI2) is an effective addition to the treatment of pulmonary hypertension and hypoxia in the operating room and intensive care unit, *Can J Anaesth* 48:924-929, 2001.

Hagberg C: *Current concepts in the management of the difficult airway.* Fifty-second annual refresher course lectures from the Clinical Updates and Basic Science Reviews; annual meeting of the American Society of Anesthesiologists, Los Angeles, October, 2001.

Hatlestad D: Transport ventilation. *RT Magazine (online)*, October/November 2002. www.rtmagazine.com/issues/articles/2002-10_01.asp. Accessed May 5, 2010.

Heinonen E, MerilaÈinen P, HoÈgman M: Administration of nitric oxide into open lung regions: delivery and monitoring, *Br J Anaesth* 90:338-342, 2003.

Helm M, Schuster R, Hauke J et al: Tight control of prehospital ventilation by capnography in major trauma victims, *Br J Anaesth* 90:327-332, 2003.

Hsu C, Chang CH, Jerng JS et al: Timing of tracheostomy as a determinant of weaning success in critically ill patients: a retrospective study, *Crit Care* 9:R46-R52, 2005.

Ingham J, Macnaughton PD: Measurement of pO_2, pCO_2, pH, pulse oximetry and capnography, *Anesth Crit Care Med* 6:12, 2005.

Levitsky M: *Pulmonary physiology,* ed 6, New York, 2003, McGraw-Hill.

MacIntyre NR: Evidence-based guidelines for weaning and discontinuing ventilatory support: a collective task force facilitated by the American College of Chest Physicians, the American Association for Respiratory Care, and the American College of Critical Care Medicine, *Chest* 120:375-396, 2001.

Marrie TJ: Community-acquired pneumonia in the elderly, *Clin Infect Dis* 31:1066-1078, 2001.

Martin G: *ALI/ARDS new developments.* American Thoracic Society 2005 International Conference. www.medscape.com/viewarticle/507211. Accessed April 30, 2010.

Miller D, Camporata L: Advantages of ProSeal and SLIPA airways over tracheal tubes for gynecological laparoscopies, *Can J Anaesth* 53:188-193, 2006.

Nathens AB, Rivara FP, Mack CD et al: Variations of tracheostomy in the critically ill trauma patient, *Crit Care Med* 34:2919-2924, 2006.

Payen JF, Chanques G, Mantz J et al: Current practices in sedation and analgesia for mechanically ventilated critically ill patients, *Anesthesiology* 106:687-695, 2007.

Rossaint R, Falke KJ, Lopez F et al: Inhaled nitric oxide for the adult respiratory distress syndrome, *N Engl J Med* 328:399-405, 1993.

Ruppel G: *Pulmonary function testing,* ed 8, St Louis, 2003, Mosby.

Sherman SC, Schindlbeck M: When is venous blood gas analysis enough? *Emerg Med* 38:44-48, 2006.

Shi-ping L, Chi-huei C: Acute lung injury/acute respiratory distress syndrome (ALI/ARDS): the mechanism, present strategies and future perspectives of therapies, *J Zhejiang Univ Sci B* 8:60-69, 2007.

Sinha PK, Misra S: Supraglottic airway devices other thank laryngeal mask airway and its prototypes, *Indian J Anaesth* 49:281-292, 2005.

Sood A: Respiratory failure presentation (website). www.siumed.edu/medicine/pulm/patinfo/facipres/RespiratoryFailurePPT.pdf. Accessed February 27, 2008.

Stoller J, Bakow E, Longworth D: Critical diagnostic thinking in respiratory care: a case-based approach, Philadelphia, 2002, Saunders.

Tobin M: *Principles and practice of mechanical ventilation*, New York, 1992, McGraw-Hill.

Vaida S, Gaitini D, Ben-David B et al: A new supraglottic airway: the Elisha airway device—a preliminary study, *Anesth Analg* 99:124-127, 2004.

Weavind L, Wenker OC: Newer modes of ventilation: an overview, Internet Journal of Anesthesiology 4:4, 2000. www.ispub.com/ostia/index.php?xmlFilePath=journals/ija/vol4n4/ventilation.xml. Accessed April 30, 2010.

Wiegand D, Carlson K, editors: *AACN procedure manual for critical care*, ed 5, St Louis, 2005, Mosby.

Woodruff DW: How to ward off complications of mechanical ventilation, *Nursing* 29:34-39, 1999.

REVIEW QUESTIONS

1. You have determined that a patient has a difficult airway. What assessment findings confirm this?
   A. The 3-3-2 rule showed that the patient's vocal cords would be difficult to view with a large tongue and a smaller mouth.
   B. The 3-3-2 rule showed that the patient's neck could not be moved.
   C. The patient was in spinal immobilization.
   D. The patient's vital signs were unstable.
2. You are in the middle of following the difficult airway protocol. You are unable to intubate on your first attempt, and 1 minute has elapsed since administration of etomidate. What is your next step, according to the crash airway and difficult airway algorithms?
   A. Quickly administer succinylcholine at a dosage of 1.5 mg/kg and attempt fiberoptic intubation.
   B. Perform a tracheotomy.
   C. Transport the patient as is.
   D. Quickly administer a second dose of etomidate at 0.3 mg/kg and a dose of rocuronium at 0.6 mg/kg and attempt orotracheal intubation.
3. What type of postintubation sedation and/or paralysis is appropriate for a stable, euvolemic, 70-kg adult patient on a 60-minute transport?
   A. Etomidate at 0.3 mg/kg with succinylcholine at 1.5 mg/kg every 5 minutes.
   B. Midazolam, 2 mg every 30 minutes, and rocuronium infusion, 1 mg/min.
   C. Propofol infusion of 30 mcg/kg/min IV.
   D. Vecuronium, 10 mg IV push every 30 minutes.
4. Extraglottic airway devices:
   A. May be used to bridge the patient to intubation.
   B. Should not be used in an obese patient.
   C. May not be used in children at all.
   D. Protect the patient from aspiration of gastric contents as well as an ETT.

5. A local physician placed a 6 mm ETT in a female patient with asthma who is 18 years old, weighs 80 kg, and is 68 inches tall. Ventilating the patient has been difficult; she has had intermittent bradycardia and hypotension with continued hypercapnia and hypoxia. Your partner thinks you should reintubate the patient with a larger-sized tube. What do you think?
   A. Your partner is wrong; the patient has a secure airway.
   B. You should remove the tube, hyperoxygenate the patient, and perform RSI to place a 7.5-mm ETT.
   C. You should increase the minute volume and PEEP, switch to pressure support on the ventilator, turn off the alarms, and transport the patient.
   D. You should use your tube exchanger and upgrade to a 7.5- or 8-mm ETT.
6. In the chapter scenario, what disease process has complicated the pneumonia patient's ability to be ventilated?
   A. Aspiration
   B. Shock
   C. Acute respiratory distress syndrome
   D. Renal failure
7. What alternative ventilation techniques might you use to recruit new alveoli and maximize oxygenation of a patient with ALI?
   A. Inverse ratio ventilation
   B. SIMV
   C. BiPAP
   D. CPAP
8. A patient has been ventilated with a bag-valve system for approximately 1 hour. As you observe the manual ventilations, you note that the healthcare provider is ventilating 30 times a minute with fairly high tidal volumes. The capnometer shows 20 mm Hg, and the patient's BP has been steadily dropping. What phenomenon may be present?
   A. Pneumothorax
   B. Oxygen toxicity
   C. VAP
   D. Auto-PEEP
9. In the chapter scenario, the ventilator was set at a rate of 18/min with a V_T of 900 mL and PEEP of 12 cm H_2O. What is the I:E ratio?
   A. T_I of approximately 1.5 seconds and T_E of 1.8
   B. 1:2
   C. Unable to calculate
   D. 1:4
10. A patient receiving 100% oxygen is on A/C ventilation with 12 cm H_2O of PEEP. To prevent desaturation and bradycardia, what must you avoid?
   A. Administering paralytics
   B. Administering sedatives with paralytics
   C. Allowing a break in the ventilator circuit
   D. Allowing the patient to awaken or have a spontaneous respiratory effort
11. You are given the following information about your patient. Select the most appropriate treatment.
   Patient's weight and height: 100 kg, 72 inches tall
   Ventilator settings: O_2, 50%; V_T, 600 mL/kg; rate, 10/min; PEEP, 5 cm H_2O
   ABG results: pH, 7.36; PaO_2, 130 mm Hg; $PaCO_2$, 38 mm Hg; HCO_3, 15 mEq/L; BE, −8 mEq/L
   Monitoring: Sinus tachycardia; SpO_2, 100%; $PETCO_2$, 33 mm Hg
   Vital signs: Pulse, 140 beats/min; BP, 72/40 mm Hg; temperature, 100.6° F (38.1° C)
   A. Administer IV fluids and vasoactive agents for septic shock.
   B. Reduce the oxygen level to 40%, reduce PEEP to 2 cm H_2O, increase the V_T to 700 mL/kg, and increase the rate to 11/min. Administer a Tylenol suppository.
   C. Keep the oxygen level as is; increase both the V_T and rate to compensate for the metabolic acidosis.
   D. Increase the V_T to 1000 mL/kg, increase the rate to 15/min, and keep the oxygen level as is to compensate for the respiratory acidosis.
12. You are given the following information about your patient. Select the most appropriate treatment.
   Patient's weight and height: 80 kg, 60 inches tall
   Ventilator settings: O_2, 100%; V_T, 800 mL/kg; rate, 15/min; PEEP, 10 cm H_2O
   ABG results: pH, 7.48; PaO_2, 100 mm Hg; $PaCO_2$, 30 mm Hg; HCO_3, 24 mEq/L; BE, 0
   Monitoring: Sinus tachycardia; SpO_2, 100%; $PETCO_2$, 28 mm Hg
   Vital signs: Pulse, 100 beats/min; BP, 100/70 mm Hg; temperature, normal
   A. Give IV fluids to reduce the heart rate.
   B. Maintain the current ventilator settings.
   C. Reduce the rate and V_T on the ventilator.
   D. Reduce the O_2 setting.

13. You are given the following information about your patient. Select the most appropriate treatment.
Patient's weight and height: 70 kg, 70 inches tall
Ventilator settings: O_2, 80%; V_T, 600 mL/kg; rate, 11/min; PEEP, 6 cm H_2O
VBG results: pH, 7.40; PaO_2, 40 mm Hg; $PaCO_2$, 40 mm Hg; HCO_3, 24 mEq/L; BE, +2 mEq/L
Monitoring: Sinus rhythm; SpO_2, 96%; $PETCO_2$, 45 mm Hg
Vital signs: Pulse, 72 beats/min; BP, 140/90 mm Hg; temperature, normal
   A. Maintain all treatment as is.
   B. Increase the rate and V_T.
   C. Reduce the rate and V_T.
   D. Increase the O_2 to 100% and the PEEP by 2 cm H_2O.

14. Patients with COPD may need a longer T_E in the I:E ratio.
   A. True
   B. False

15. A multisystem trauma patient needs to be transported to a Level 1 trauma care facility. The patient has been intubated because her Glasgow Coma Score is dropping, and she has a chest tube on the left for a hemopneumothorax. On arrival, and after you assess the patient, you move the tracheal tube onto your transport ventilator with $PETCO_2$ monitoring. The pleural drainage unit has continuous bubbling in the second chamber; the suction is off and there is no bubbling in the first chamber. The collection chamber has 300 mL of blood. Choose the most correct statement about these findings.
   A. High PPV may push pressure through the system, creating an air leak.
   B. The physician should insert a second chest tube to fix the air leak.
   C. You should assess for a system leak by clamping the drainage tube with your fingers, working your way toward the pleural drainage system.
   D. All of the above

16. You are preparing to perform RSI and want to pretreat the patient with fentanyl because he is in pain. You have just administered 100 mcg of the drug; the patient suddenly stops breathing, and ventilating him with bag and mask is nearly impossible, even though his airway is patent. What is the appropriate treatment?
   A. Begin CPR and give diphenhydramine; this is an allergic reaction.
   B. This may be chest wall paralysis; speed up the RSI sequence, give sedative and paralytic drugs, and intubate the patient.
   C. This may be chest wall paralysis; administer a narcotic antagonist.
   D. This is a side effect of narcotic overdose; stop ventilating and give a narcotic antagonist.

17. Which of the following are effective techniques for preventing VAP?
   A. Continuous antibiotics
   B. Prone positioning
   C. Supraglottic suctioning
   D. All of the above

18. You are transporting an intubated, ventilated patient who suddenly coughs and is "bucking" the ventilator (dyssynchrony). You can hear the patient moaning, and he is restless. Select the most appropriate treatment in this situation.
   A. Adjust the unit's settings until the patient tolerates the ventilator.
   B. Check the $PETCO_2$ and determine the location of the tube.
   C. Immediately give sedatives and analgesics and, if absolutely necessary, paralyze the patient.
   D. Stop the ventilations and allow for spontaneous respirations.

19. You are beginning transport of an intubated, ventilated patient with respiratory failure secondary to CAP. You have started propofol according to your service's protocols. The patient's wheezing has subsided, but her BP is falling. Choose the correct statement about this situation.
   A. These are expected effects or side effects of propofol; reduce the dose and begin a fluid challenge.
   B. This may be an allergic reaction; stop the drug and give epinephrine.
   C. Administration of a paralytic drug is required with propofol.
   D. Propofol is contraindicated in a patient with CAP.

20. You have just moved your critical care patient onto your cot. She has been intubated and is connected to your ventilator circuit and $PETCO_2$. Your ventilator sounds the high airway pressure alarm, but the patient's heart rate has risen by 30 beats/minute. The $PETCO_2$ shows dyssynchrony with a high plateau pressure (CO_2, 50 mm Hg). Select the most appropriate therapy.
   A. Disconnect the patient from the ventilator and begin bag-valve ventilation while you continue your assessment.
   B. Assess for bilateral breath sounds.
   C. Check for obstructions in the tube and suction as needed.
   D. All of the above

CHAPTER 4

Cardiovascular System

OBJECTIVES

1. Explain the concepts of cardiovascular anatomy, physiology, and pathophysiology as they relate to the assessment and management of an adult critical care patient.
2. Describe a treatment plan that includes pharmacologic, electrical, and mechanical interventions for a patient with cardiovascular compromise.
3. Discuss the indications, contraindications, equipment, techniques, and maintenance of various methods of hemodynamic monitoring, including the use of direct arterial blood pressure, central venous pressure, and flow-directed, balloon-tipped thermodilution systems.

Scenario

You and your partner are dispatched to a local intensive care unit (ICU) for transport of a 68-year-old man. He must be transferred to a downtown hospital so that the cause of his continued pericardial tamponade can be determined. This patient was brought into the transferring hospital for chest pain and was immediately taken to the cardiac catheterization laboratory for placement of a stent. Today, day 3 of his CCU stay, he began to have chest discomfort with tachycardia and dyspnea on exertion, which progressed to air hunger at rest. He became very weak, and the heart sounds were distant. The ICU physician performed pericardiocentesis, and you were dispatched shortly thereafter, because the patient now requires a cardiac surgeon.

On arrival, you find your patient lying in bed; he is pale and weak and appears ill. You introduce yourself, and when you shake his hand, you note cool skin. On reviewing his chart, you find a normally healthy man who came in 3 days ago with a massive inferior lateral myocardial infarction (MI). He was taken straight to the cardiac catheterization laboratory, where stents were put into the left anterior descending (LAD) and left circumflex (LCX) arteries.

The patient has two peripheral intravenous (IV) lines in place. He is receiving dopamine at 10 mcg/kg/min, milrinone at 0.5 mcg/kg/min, and potassium at 20 mEq/L/hour. He has a cardiac monitor, and a non-rebreathing mask (NRB) set to deliver oxygen at 15 LPM. The patient has no allergies to medications and was taking no medications before coming to the hospital. The patient smoked and has high cholesterol.

The physician has just placed a balloon pump, and the timing is referenced to the R waves. The patient's last set of vital signs was: pulse, 110 beats/min; respirations, 24/min; BP, 88/60 mm Hg; pulse oximetry (SaO_2), 92% on O_2. Blood gas results 20 minutes ago were: pH, 7.32; arterial carbon dioxide pressure ($PaCO_2$), 36 mm Hg; bicarbonate (HCO_3), 15 mEq/L; base excess (BE), −10 mEq/L. You carefully transfer this patient to your stretcher and transition him to your ambulance.

The case study just posed may challenge you on your first day as a Critical Care Paramedic (CCP). However, this is a common call, and it requires your full attention, knowledge, and patient management skills. This chapter presents a brief review of the basics and then moves into a more advanced discussion of the anatomy and physiology of the cardiovascular system. Pathologic conditions and management strategies also are presented.

ANATOMY AND PHYSIOLOGY

The size of the heart is equal to its owner's clenched fist. The heart weighs, on average, about 311 g, and it lies in the mediastinum, left of midline, resting on the diaphragm. The long axis is oriented from the right shoulder blade to the upper left quadrant of the abdomen. During inspiration and exhalation, the heart moves with each breath. When a person takes a deep breath, the diaphragm falls, causing the heart to move vertically. If we were to look at the heart on a chest radiograph during inspiration, it would look thinner. Conversely, during exhalation, the diaphragm rises superiorly, causing the heart to lie more horizontally in the thorax.

Atria

Atrial contractions contribute approximately 20% of the blood flow to ventricular filling; the other 80% occurs passively during diastole. The left atrium, although smaller than the right atrium, has thicker walls (approximately 3 to 5 mm thick). The cavity and walls of the left atrium are formed largely by the proximal parts of the pulmonary veins. The walls of the right atrium are approximately 2 mm thick and the chamber receives systemic venous blood from the superior and inferior vena cava and the coronary sinus. The atrial septum is at an angle (which makes the right atrium both anterior and to the right of the left atrium), and it also extends slightly inferior and to the left.

Ventricles

A wall of muscle, called the *interventricular septum,* separates the left ventricle from the right ventricle. The interventricular septum is functionally more a part of the left ventricle than the right ventricle, because it forms the anterior wall of the left ventricle.

Did You Know?

Up to 30% of the U.S. population has a patent foramen ovale (PFO) in the atria. A PFO can create a turbulent effect in the blood flow, leading to embolic events. About 46% of stroke patients under 55 years of age have been found to have an atrial PFO. In most cases, when a PFO is found, antiplatelet therapy is initiated until the defect can be closed, usually in the cardiac catheterization laboratory.[1]

The ventricles are the primary pumping force of the heart. A normal, healthy right ventricle is approximately 3 to 5 mm thick, and a normal left ventricle is approximately 13 to 15 mm thick. The right ventricle extends from the base of the heart toward the apex, roughly in the area of the left nipple. The right ventricle ascends to the left, reaching the pulmonary opening and supporting the cusps of the pulmonary valve. The left ventricle is a powerful pump that must generate amazing force to eject blood through the aorta. Longer and narrower than the right ventricle, it extends from the arterioventricular groove at the cardiac apex to the base (Figure 4-1).

Atrioventricular Valves

Between the atria and the ventricles are the two atrioventricular (AV) valves: the tricuspid valve on the right and the mitral valve on the left. The tricuspid valve has three leaflets, a large anterior leaf and two smaller posterior and septal leaflets. The mitral valve is made up of a long, narrow posterior leaflet (mural) and an oval anterior leaflet (aortic). The mitral valve (also called the *bicuspid valve*) has two cusps. The AV valves open during ventricular diastole (filling) and close during ventricular systole (contractions) to prevent blood flow back into the atria. A fibrous, collagenous structure, the chordae tendineae, supports the cusps of the AV valves, which attach to the tricuspid and mitral valves. This structure stabilizes the AV valves and prevents the leaflets from turning inside out during systole. The chordae tendineae is attached to papillary muscles or sometimes directly to the ventricular walls or septum (Figure 4-2).

In the right ventricle, two major papillary muscles are located anteriorly and posteriorly. A third, smaller muscle is in a more medial position, and several smaller muscles are attached to the ventricular septum. On the left side are two papillary muscles that support the mitral valve cusps. These two muscles vary in length and width, and they may be divided into two parts, or branches. The anterolateral muscle originates from the sternocostal mural myocardium, and the posteromedial muscle originates from the diaphragmatic region. During diastole, the papillary muscles relax, allowing the valves to open. The increase in ventricular pressure during systole closes the valves completely.

Semilunar Valves

The aortic and pulmonic valves, also called the *semilunar valves,* are located in the ventricles. The aortic valve, which is situated between the left ventricle and the aorta, is made up of three somewhat thicker cusps (Figure 4-3). The pulmonic valve, which is situated between the right ventricle and the pulmonary artery, is made up of three cusps.

The semilunar valves permit unidirectional blood flow from the outflow tract during ventricular systole and prevent retrograde blood flow during ventricular diastole (Table 4-1 and Figure 4-4).

Coronary Arteries

The coronary arteries comprise the network of blood vessels that carry oxygenated and nutrient-rich blood to the cardiac muscle. Three arteries run on the surface of the heart and branch several times. These arteries, when healthy, maintain coronary blood flow to the heart and the electrical conduction system. Understanding the branching of the coronary vessels can help you better understand the reasoning and methods behind patient treatment.

In most people, the coronary arteries arise from the left and right sinuses of Valsalva, one of the three dilations above the

Table 4-1 Cardiac Valves and Their Locations

Valve	Type	Location
Tricuspid	AV	Between the right atrium and the right ventricle
Pulmonic	SL	Between the right ventricle and the pulmonary artery
Mitral	AV	Between the left atrium and the left ventricle
Aortic	SL	Between the left ventricle and the aorta

From Urden LD, Stacy KM, Lough ME: *Thelan's critical care nursing: diagnosis and management,* ed 5, 2006, Mosby.
AV, Atrioventricular, *SL,* semilunar.

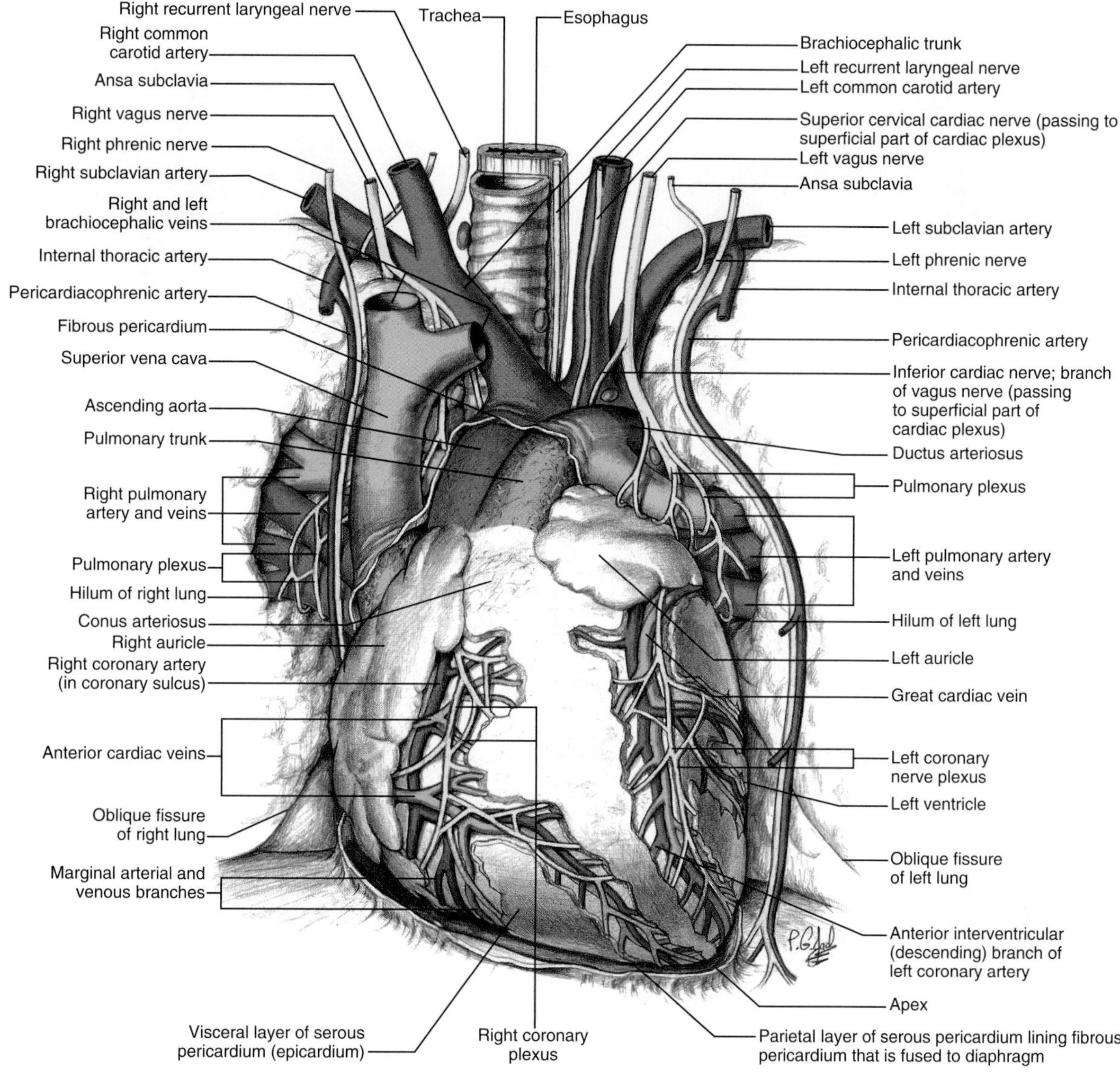

Figure 4-1

Anterior view of the heart and great vessels. (From Standring S: *Gray's anatomy: the anatomical basis of clinical practice*, ed 39, London, 2004,Churchill Livingstone.)

aortic valve. The two main coronary arteries are the left coronary artery (LCA) and the right coronary artery (RCA). The term *dominant* is used to describe the coronary artery responsible for supplying the posterior part of the heart. Depending on which artery supplies the greater portion of the myocardium, a person's coronary circulation can be classified as *right dominant* or *left dominant.*

The LCA arises from the aorta behind the left cusp of the aortic valve as the left main (LM) artery and eventually divides into two major arteries: the LAD artery (also known as the *anterior interventricular artery*), where the diagonal (D) and septal (S) branches arise, and the LCX artery, from which the obtuse marginal (OM) branch originates. The LAD artery supplies the anterior two thirds of the interventricular septum, the anterior wall of the left ventricle, the right bundle branch (RBB), and an anterior division of the left bundle branch (LBB). The LAD artery also gives off two to six diagonal branches that route at an angle away from the septum, supplying blood to the anterior surface of both ventricles.

The LCX artery travels in a groove called the *coronary sulcus,* which separates the left atrium from the left ventricle and is embedded in the epicardium on the back of the heart. The LCX artery supplies the left atrium and the lateral wall of the left ventricle. The SA node is supplied by the LCX in about one half to one third of our patients.

The RCA arises from an opening behind the right anterior aortic cusp; it travels behind the pulmonary artery and extends behind the right heart to the heart's posterior surface, where it branches to the atrium and ventricle. The RCA divides into the posterior descending (PD) artery, and several smaller

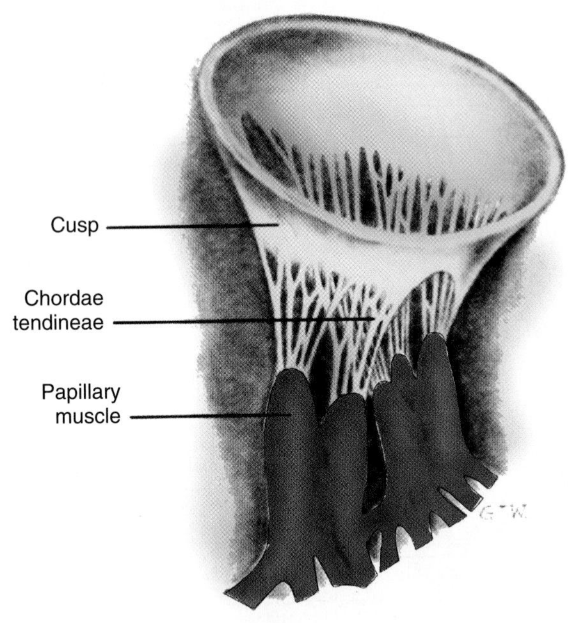

Figure 4-2

The mitral valve and the relationship of the cusps, chordae tendineae, and papillary muscles. (From Urden LD, Stacy KM, Lough ME: *Thelan's critical care nursing: diagnosis and management*, ed 5, St. Louis, 2006, Mosby.)

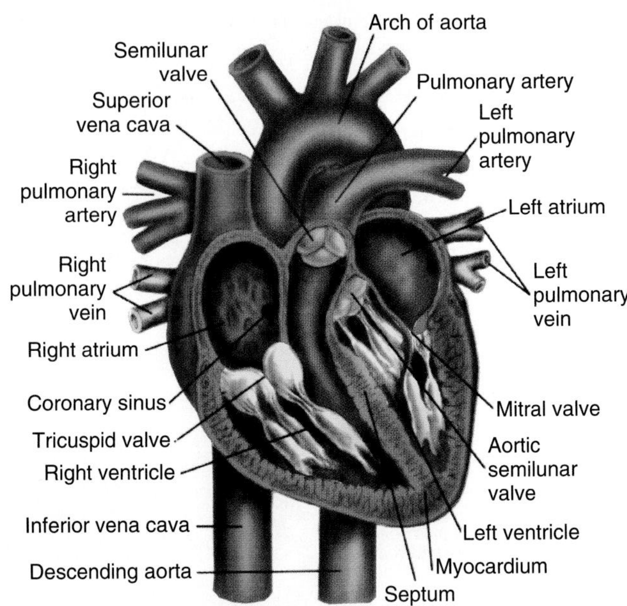

Figure 4-4

Cross-sectional view of the heart. Note the position of the four cardiac valves. (From Thompson JM, McFarland GK, Hirsch JE, Tucker SM: *Mosby's clinical nursing*, ed 5, St Louis, 2002, Mosby.)

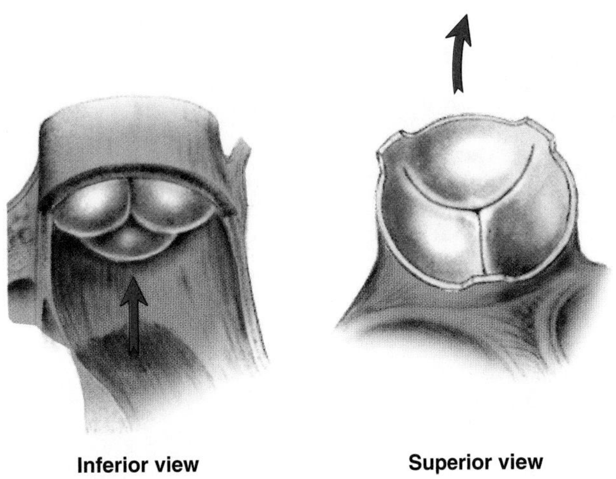

Figure 4-3

The aortic valve and its cuplike leaflets. (From Urden LD, Stacy KM, Lough ME: *Thelan's critical care nursing: diagnosis and management*, ed 5, St. Louis, 2006, Mosby.)

branches, including the conus branch (CB), the sinus node branch (SN), the acute marginal (AcM) artery, and the posterolateral left ventricular (PLV) artery.

The coronary arteries are the only blood supply to the myocardium; because there is no backup blood supply, blockage of these vessels is a life-threatening development (Figure 4-5).

Major Cardiac Vessels

The major cardiac vessels are the pulmonary trunk, the thoracic aorta, the inferior vena cava, and the superior vena cava.

Aorta

The aorta is the largest artery in the body. It has three sections: the ascending aorta, the aortic arch, and the descending aorta. The descending aorta has two distinct areas, the thoracic aorta and the abdominal aorta. The ascending aorta originates at the base of the left ventricle, level with the lower border of the third left costal cartilage. It ascends obliquely, curving forward and behind the left half of the sternum, to the upper border of the second left costal cartilage.

Three major arteries originate from the aortic arch: the brachiocephalic artery, the left common carotid artery, and the left subclavian artery. These arteries carry oxygenated blood to the head and upper limbs.

The descending aorta is the longest part of the aorta. The portion that runs down through the chest to the abdomen is called the *thoracic aorta.* Its continuation, the *abdominal aorta,* extends from the diaphragm and terminates near L4 in the umbilical region. It eventually divides into the two common iliac arteries. The abdominal aorta supplies oxygenated blood to all the abdominal and pelvic organs and the legs.

Pulmonary Artery

The pulmonary artery is the only artery in the body that carries deoxygenated blood. It carries blood from the right ventricle to the lungs. Below the aortic arch, the pulmonary artery divides into the left and right pulmonary arteries, which are almost equal in size; this bifurcation allows blood to enter the left and right lungs, respectively.

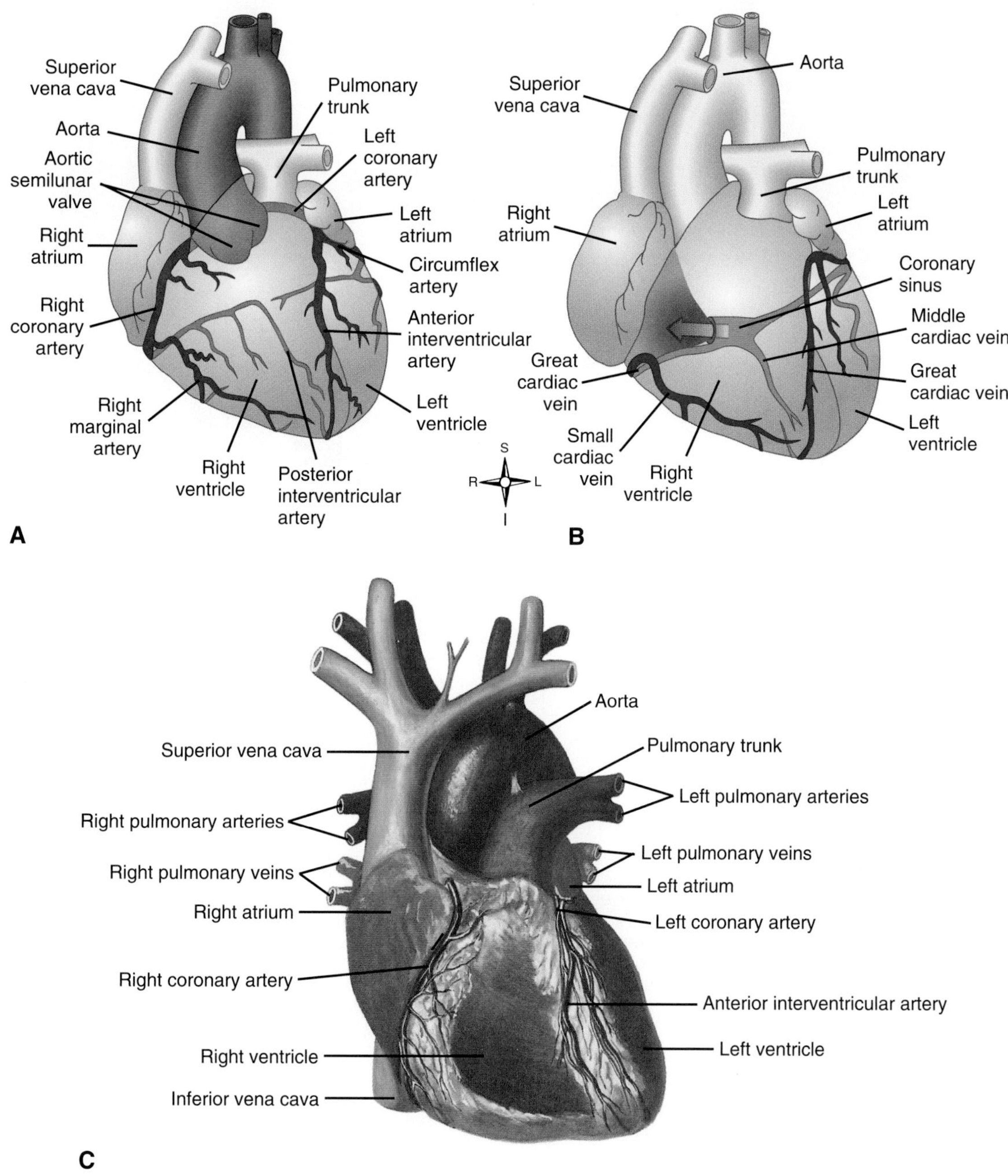

Figure 4-5

Coronary circulation. Anterior view of the heart: arteries **(A)** and veins **(B).** Vessels near the anterior surface are more darkly colored than vessels of the posterior surface seen through the heart. **C,** View of the anterior (sternocostal) surface. (From McCance K, Huether SE: *Pathophysiology: the biological basis for disease in adults and children*, ed 5, St Louis, 2005, Mosby.)

Pulmonary Veins

The four pulmonary veins return oxygenated blood from the lungs to the left atrium. These veins have no valves before entering the left atrium; therefore, filling of the left side of the heart occurs basically by means of simple hydrostatic pressure gradients. The pressure in the left atrium must be lower than that in the pulmonary circulation for flow to continue in a forward direction (Figures 4-6 and 4-7).

Cardiac Cycle

The first phase of systole is called the **isovolumetric period**. In the cardiac cycle, this is the interval during which the cardiac muscle fibers contract, or relax, but the valves remain closed, anchored by the chordae tendineae. The ventricular pressure changes rapidly while the volume remains constant. As pressure in the ventricles increases, the AV valves close, producing the first heart sound (S_1).

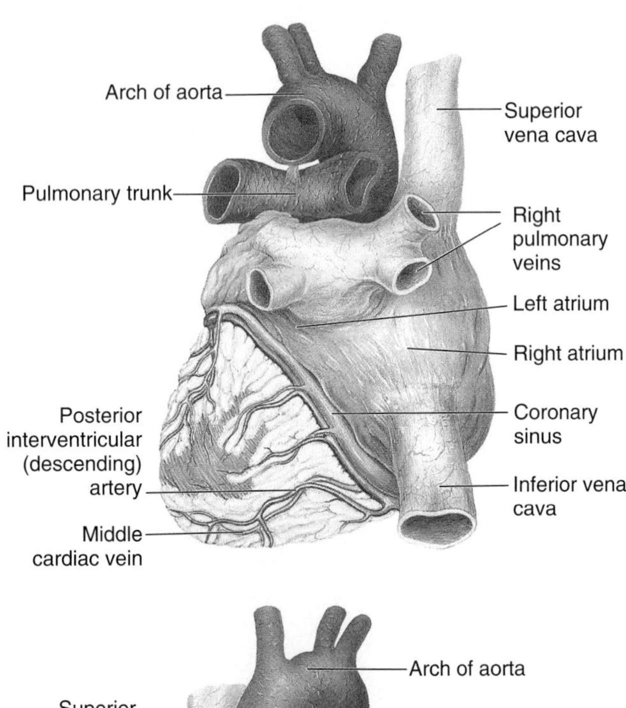

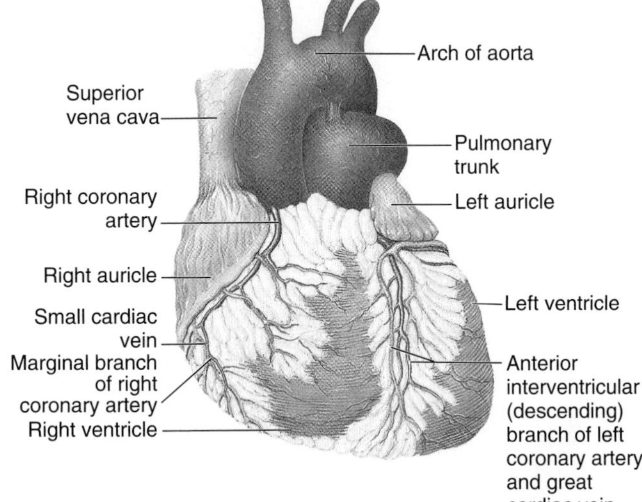

Figure 4-6

The heart and great vessels. The pulmonary veins carry oxygenated blood, and the pulmonary trunk carries deoxygenated blood. (From Standring S: *Gray's anatomy: the anatomical basis of clinical practice,* ed 39, London, 2004, Churchill Livingstone.)

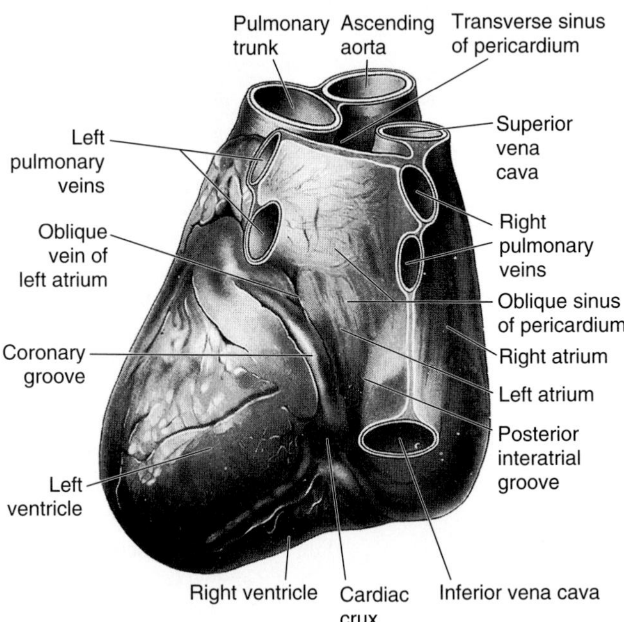

Figure 4-7

Base and diaphragmatic surface of the heart. The serosal pericardium is in situ, and its cut edge is seen around the great vessels; its disposition is highly schematic (recesses omitted). The cardiac crux results from the confluence of the posterior interatrial groove, the posterior atrioventricular groove, and the posterior interventricular groove. (From Standring S: *Gray's anatomy: the anatomical basis of clinical practice,* ed 39, London, 2004, Churchill Livingstone.)

As ventricular pressure builds, the AV valves are pushed toward the atria. The left ventricular pressure exceeds the pressure in the aorta, and the aortic valve opens. The same mechanism occurs with the pulmonic valve as systolic ejection occurs. At this point, the intraventricular pressure and ventricular volume decrease immediately.

As the ventricular pressure falls below that of the aorta, ventricular ejection stops. Because the pressure in the aorta is greater than that in the ventricles, the aortic and pulmonic valves close. Isovolemic relaxation occurs, producing the second heart sound (S_2). The aortic valve closes, pressure in the left ventricle falls quickly, and no blood enters the ventricles.

With the AV valves closed, blood now flows into the atrium from the systemic and pulmonary system. When the pressure in the ventricles is lower than that in the atria, the AV valves open to initiate the rapid filling of the ventricles in diastole. Most ventricular filling occurs through this pressure gradient change. When the atria contract, a smaller percentage of blood is propelled into the ventricle, a phenomenon called the *atrial kick*; only about 20% of ventricular filling is accomplished during atrial contraction.

Adequate time for ventricular filling during diastole is a crucial factor. Rapid heart rates with a short diastole can cause a drop in cardiac output, because the filling time is insufficient.

Factors That Affect Cardiac Performance

Four factors directly affect cardiac performance: preload, afterload, heart rate, and myocardial contractility (Figure 4-8).

Preload

Preload is the amount of blood filling the ventricle at the end of diastole; it is determined by the stretch or pull on the myocardial muscle fibers at that time. The more volume in the ventricle, the more stretch on the muscle, and the greater the next contraction (with limits) and stroke volume. This part of the stroke volume cannot be measured directly; rather, it is derived from the filling pressure of the ventricles (i.e., the right ventricular end-diastolic pressure [RVEDP]). Two primary factors determine preload: the amount of venous return to the atria and the blood left in the left ventricle after systole.

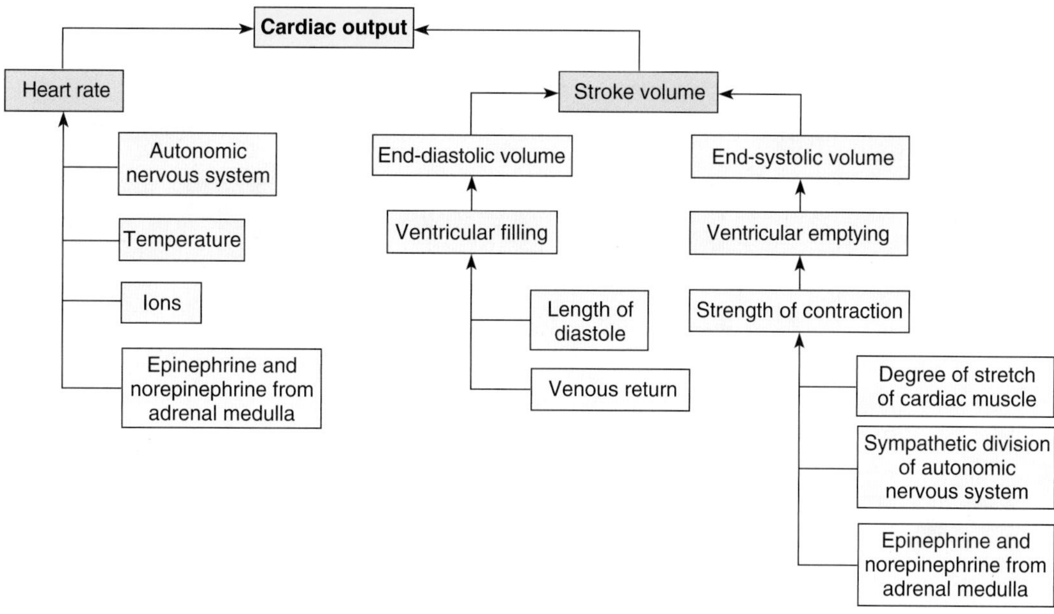

Figure 4-8

Factors that affect cardiac performance. Cardiac output, or the amount of blood (in liters) ejected by the heart per minute, is determined by the heart rate (beats/minute) and stroke volume (milliliters of blood ejected during ventricular systole). (From McCance K, Huether SE: *Pathophysiology: the biological basis for disease in adults and children*, ed 5, St Louis, 2005, Mosby.)

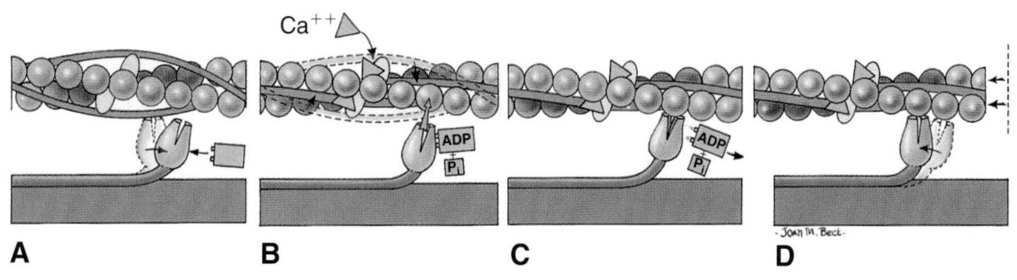

Figure 4-9

Cross-bridge theory of muscle contraction. **A,** Each myosin cross-bridge in the thick filament moves into a resting position after an adenosine triphosphate (ATP) molecule binds and transfers its energy. **B,** Calcium ions released from the sarcoplasmic reticulum bind to troponin in the thin filament, allowing tropomyosin to shift from its position blocking the active sites of actin molecules. **C,** Each myosin cross-bridge then binds to an active site on a thin filament, displacing the remnants of ATP hydrolysis, adenosine diphosphate (ADP) and inorganic phosphate (P_i). **D,** The release of stored energy from step *A* provides the force needed for each cross-bridge to move back to its original position, pulling actin along with it. Each cross-bridge remains bound to actin until another ATP molecule binds to it and pulls it back into its resting position (step *A*). (From Thibodeau GA, Patton KT: *Anatomy and physiology*, ed 4, St Louis, 1999, Mosby.)

As the ***Frank-Starling law*** of the heart explains, the myocardial fibers contract more forcefully when stretched. This ability of stretched muscles to contract with increased force is a characteristic of all striated muscles, not just cardiac muscle. Starling found that as the volume of blood entering the heart increased, cardiac output increased. According to the Frank-Starling law, the longer the initial resting length of the cardiac muscle, the greater the strength of the contraction.

However, if the cardiac muscle fibers are overstretched, cardiac output falls (Figure 4-9). Overstretching of these muscle fibers reduces the force of contraction, because actin and myosin become partly disengaged, disturbing the cross-bridges; this is the basis for the Starling curve (Figure 4-10).

If actin and myosin become completely disengaged, the force of contraction drops to zero (this is somewhat like a rubber band that is stretched over and over until it loses its elasticity). Overstretching of the cardiac muscle fibers can result in a disease process, such as heart failure.

Afterload

When the ventricles sense resistance in the arterial system (vascular resistance), the ventricular fibers shorten to correctly force blood out into the lungs and body; this is called **afterload.** Afterload can be affected by various factors, including the pressure in the arteries, the amount and viscosity of the blood, and the compliance of the arterial walls.

Afterload, stroke volume, and the workload of the heart have a proportional relationship: If the afterload increases, the stroke volume decreases (as the myocardial oxygen demand rises); if the afterload decreases, the stroke volume increases (as the myocardial oxygen demand declines).

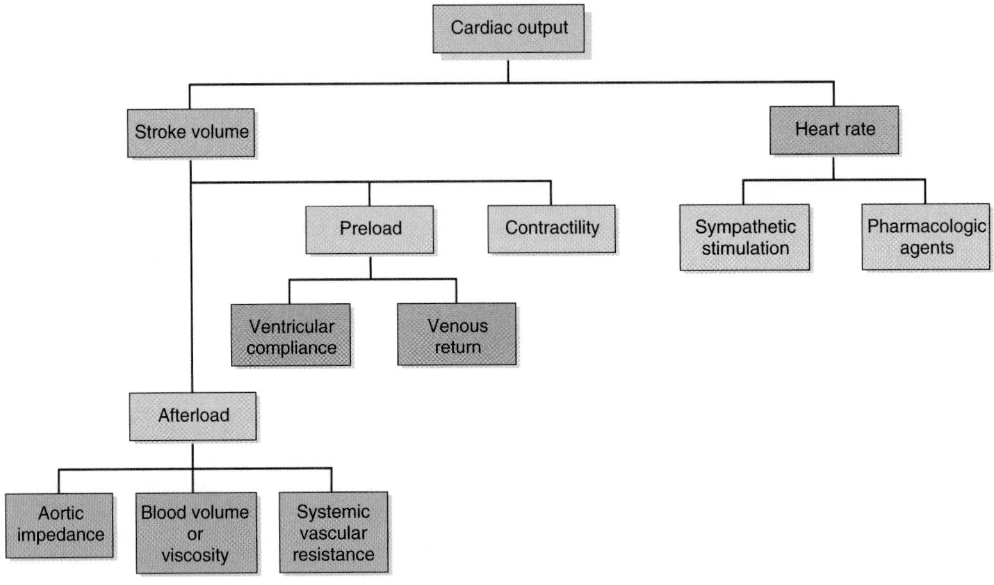

Figure 4-10

Starling curve. As the left ventricular end-diastolic pressure (LVEDP) increases, so does ventricular stroke work, or contractility. When the left ventricular filling pressure exceeds a maximum level, contractility and cardiac output diminish. (From Urden LD, Stacy KM, Lough ME: *Thelan's critical care nursing: diagnosis and management*, ed 5, St. Louis, 2006, Mosby.)

As with preload, afterload cannot be measured directly; this resistance pressure is derived from the pulmonary vascular resistance (PVR) and the systemic vascular resistance (SVR). The formula for measuring the SVR is:

$$SVR = \frac{MAP - CVP\ (\text{or RAP})}{CO} \times 80$$

where *MAP* is the mean arterial pressure; *CVP* is the central venous pressure (reflected as the right atrial pressure [RAP]), and *CO* is the cardiac output.

For example, a patient with a blood pressure of 120/80 mm Hg has an MAP of 93 mm Hg. If the RAP (which reflects the CVP) is 5 mm Hg , and the CO is 5 LPM, the SVR is calculated as follows:

$$\frac{93-5}{5} \times 80$$

$$SVR = 1408\ \text{dynes/sec/cm}^{-5}$$

A normal SVR is 770 to 1500 dynes/sec/cm^{-5}.

Clinically, a decrease in the SVR and left ventricular afterload can occur with vasodilator therapy (nitrates), distributive shock, cirrhosis, and anemia. If the SVR is decreased, the CO should increase. An elevated SVR (high afterload) creates a low cardiac output state. High afterload states can occur clinically with hypovolemia, hypothermia, and peripheral edema.

If vascular resistance is measured in the pulmonary system (PVR), the CVP is measured through a pulmonary artery catheter "wedged" into the distal vessel; this value is reflected as the pulmonary wedge or occlusion pressure (pulmonary capillary wedge pressure [PCWP], pulmonary artery occlusion pressure [PAOP]). For example, using the previous formula, if a patient's wedge pressure is 8 mm Hg, the MAP is 15 mm Hg, and the CO is 5 LPM:

$$\frac{15-8}{5} \times 80$$

$$PVR = 112\ \text{dynes/sec/cm}^{-5}$$

A normal PVR is 30 to 120 dynes/sec/cm^{-5}, because the pulmonary system is a lower pressure, lower resistance system.

An elevated afterload in the pulmonary system (i.e., an elevated PVR) can be caused by large pulmonary emboli, pulmonary edema, sepsis, hypoxia, and some valvular heart diseases. Pulmonary vasodilator therapy (e.g., epoprostenol, discussed in Chapter 3,) reduces the PVR.

Heart Rate

The heart rate, which determines the pace of the cardiac cycle, is calculated by the number of contractions per minute. The average adult heart rate is 60 to 100 beats/min. The heart rate is controlled by different activities arising from different systems and hormones, including the central and autonomic nervous systems, atrial receptors, and neural reflexes. This is important, because ventricular filling occurs during diastole, and an excessively fast heart rate (supraventricular tachycardia [SVT], rapid atrial fibrillation, or ventricular tachycardia [VT]) lessens the time between contractions for filling of the ventricles, leading to reduced cardiac output.

Myocardial Contractility

Contractility is defined as the inotropic state of the heart; it has a considerable influence both on the stroke volume and

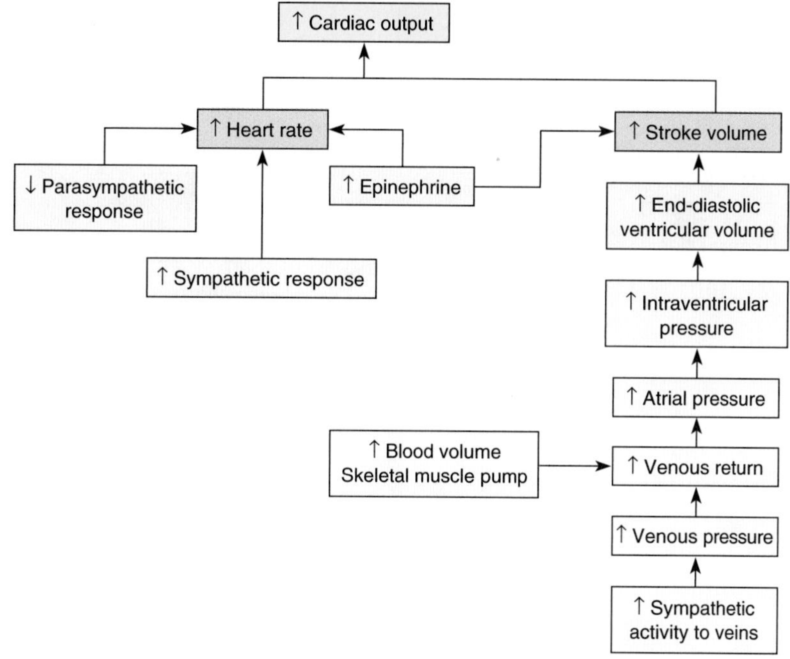

Figure 4-11

Major factors that determine an increase in cardiac output. (From McCance K, Huether SE: *Pathophysiology: the biological basis for disease in adults and children*, ed 5, St Louis, 2005, Mosby.)

on overall cardiac output. A strong contraction of the heart has positive inotropy, whereas a weaker contraction has negative inotropy. As was discussed with the Frank-Starling law, the strength of contractions is influenced by preload. Disease processes of the cardiac muscle (cardiomyopathy) and the sympathetic nervous system, in addition to drugs that stimulate the sympathetic nervous system, all can positively and negatively affect the contractile forces of the heart (Figure 4-11).

Stroke Volume

The stroke volume (SV) is the amount of blood pumped by the ventricles in one heart contraction. During ventricular contraction, only about two thirds of the blood is ejected from the ventricles; this is the stroke volume. The stroke volume depends on several factors: preload, afterload, contractility, the duration of contraction, and the size of the heart. Cardiac output is the product of the stroke volume multiplied by the heart rate (CO = SV × HR). The SV is expressed as milliliters per beat (mL/beat), and the HR is expressed as beats per minute (beats/min); the CO, therefore, is expressed as milliliters per minute (mL/min) or liters per minute (LPM).

Cardiac Output

Cardiac output can be measured by several direct or indirect methods. Hemodynamic monitoring is a method familiar to the CCP. The thermodilution technique for measuring the CO may be performed through a pulmonary artery catheter. The radionuclide and echocardiograph (ECG) techniques display real-time changes in the size of the ventricles, which helps determine the SV; that value, multiplied by the HR, gives the cardiac output.

Blood Flow

Autoregulation of blood flow is based on two mechanisms, the myogenic theory and the metabolic theory. According to the myogenic theory, as the pressure in an artery rises, the vessels stretch, stimulating vascular smooth muscle constriction; this, in turn, reduces blood flow to normal, and as the pressure decreases, the vascular smooth muscles relax. The metabolic theory states that as the pressure in an artery rises, the increased blood flow brings needed nutrients to the tissues and removes waste products that cause the vessel to constrict, such as adenosine phosphates, lactic acid, potassium, prostaglandins, and carbon dioxide (Figure 4-12).

Blood Volume

Blood volume is determined by the amounts of water and sodium that are ingested, excreted by the kidneys into the urine, and lost through the gastrointestinal (GI) tract, lungs, and skin. The amounts of water and sodium ingested and lost are highly variable. To maintain blood volume within a normal range, the kidneys regulate the amount of water and sodium lost into the urine. For example, if excessive water and sodium are ingested, the kidneys normally respond by excreting more water and sodium into the urine.

Blood Viscosity

The viscosity of whole blood is strongly influenced by three factors: the hematocrit, the temperature, and the flow rate.

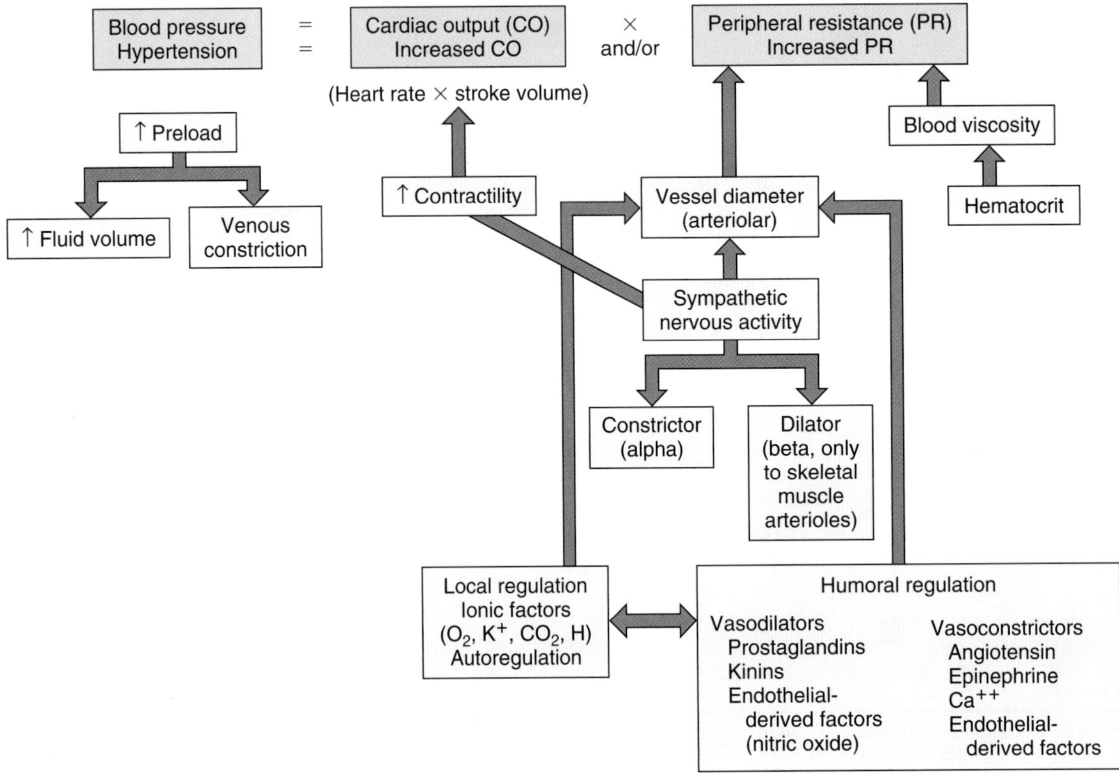

Figure 4-12

Factors that regulate blood flow. (From McCance K, Huether SE: *Pathophysiology: the biological basis for disease in adults and children*, ed 5, St Louis, 2005, Mosby.)

- The *hematocrit* is a laboratory test that measures the proportion of red blood cells to plasma. This value is important for determining the viscosity of blood. As the hematocrit increases, a disproportionate increase in the blood viscosity occurs. For example, at a hematocrit of 40%, the relative viscosity is 4; however, at a hematocrit of 60%, the relative viscosity is about 8. Therefore, a 50% increase in hematocrit from a normal value increases blood viscosity by about 100%. Such changes in hematocrit and blood viscosity occur in patients with polycythemia, or in those with plasma loss due to burns. Higher blood viscosity affects afterload.
- Temperature also has a significant effect on viscosity. As the temperature decreases, viscosity increases. For each 1° C decrease in temperature, viscosity increases approximately 2%. This effect has several implications. For example, when a person's hand is cooled by exposure to a cold environment, the increase in blood viscosity contributes to the decrease in blood flow (along with neurally mediated thermoregulatory mechanisms that constrict the vessels). The use of whole body hypothermia during certain surgical procedures also increases blood viscosity and therefore increases resistance to blood flow.
- The flow rate of blood also affects viscosity. At very low flow states in the microcirculation, as occurs during circulatory shock, the blood viscosity can increase significantly. This occurs because at low flow states, cell-to-cell and protein-to-cell adhesive interactions increase, which can cause erythrocytes to adhere to one another and increase the blood viscosity.

Shunting

Shunting is defined as a diverting or bypassing, and in the cardiovascular system, shunting occurs continuously through vessel dilation and constriction. There are more blood vessels than there is blood volume to fill them; therefore, blood is continuously pushed around through this vasoactive process to ensure adequate perfusion. In a shock or low flow state anywhere in the body, shunting to primary organs is compensatory and critical. In compensatory hypovolemic shock, shunting of available blood away from the skin, bones, muscles, GI tract, and kidneys maintains core organ perfusion to most of the brain, heart, and lungs.

Neuroregulation of the Heartbeat

The sympathetic and parasympathetic nervous systems create a sense of balance between relaxation and a "fight or flight" response. The nervous system is assisted in this by the intrinsic reflexes, which act as a feedback system for the brain. These reflexes include baroreceptors and chemoreceptors, which are located in the aortic and carotid areas. **Baroreceptors** are pressure sensors that are sensitive to vessel wall changes; they send signals to the autonomic nervous system either to raise or to lower the heart rate. For instance, when the size of a vessel increases, baroreceptors sense the change and signal the medulla to produce tachycardia and increase the cardiac output. During distributive shock states, such as anaphylaxis, baroreceptors note the change in vessel size and evoke tachycardia very early. **Chemoreceptors** maintain homeostasis by sensing the capillary bed oxygen tension, carbon dioxide (CO_2) levels, and pH; stimulation of the chemoreceptors causes an increase in the respiratory rate and depth.

Neuroregulation also affects the electrophysiology of the heart. For example, thinking about the "fight or flight" reaction has a direct effect on the heartbeat.

Electrophysiology of the Heart

Initiation of the cardiac cycle is very characteristic and specific, and it depends on the anatomy and physiology of functioning, healthy cardiac muscle and the conduction system. The cardiac action potential relies on transmission of electrical impulses that make nonstop duplication of the cardiac cycle possible. The cells in the heart are joined in a way that allows quick, efficient transmission of these electrical impulses. When the impulses are passed in a cascading fashion, the fibers of the myocardium shorten. This shortening, in turn, causes muscle contraction. After the contraction, the fibers relax and return to their resting state.

The heart cells are unique in that they have their own conduction system, which allows the heart to generate its own action potential. These cells, called *nodes,* are located throughout the heart (Figure 4-13).

Sinoatrial Node

The SA node is found at the intersection of the superior vena cava and the upper posterior of the right atrium. The SA node, which receives its blood supply from the SA node artery, has an intrinsic rate of 60 to 100 beats/min. Atrial initiation begins with the generation of an impulse in the SA node. The rate of discharge (and therefore the heart rate) depends on parasympathetic tone (via the vagus nerve) and sympathetic tone. The impulse spreads in radial mode to depolarize the right atrium, the intraatrial septum, and then the left atrium. The last part of the left atrium to be activated is the tip of the posterior-inferior left atrium underneath the left inferior pulmonary vein.

Three specialized pathways with Purkinje fibers have been identified that connect the SA node to the AV node. The internodal pathways are designated as (1) the anterior internodal tract (Bachmann's bundle), which leaves the SA node leftward and divides into branches of the left atrium and interatrial septum, ultimately connecting to the AV node; (2) the middle internodal tract (Wenckebach's bundle), which crosses the septum to connect to the AV node; and (3) the posterior internodal tract (Thorel's pathway), which crosses the crista terminalis portion of the right atrium to connect to the right superior margin of the AV node.

Typically on an ECG, the initial part of the P wave represents depolarization of the right atrium, and the later part represents depolarization of the left atrium and the right atrial wall. Because both deflections are aimed down and to the left, they tend to come together and form a single wave or deflection.

Atrioventricular Node

The AV node is situated in the right atrial wall above the tricuspid valve, on the floor of the right atrium. The AV node delays the electrical impulse and allows the atria to eject (kick) blood into the ventricles before the next ventricular contraction. The AV node has an intrinsic pacemaker rate of 40 to 60 beats/min. The delay from the end of the P wave to the

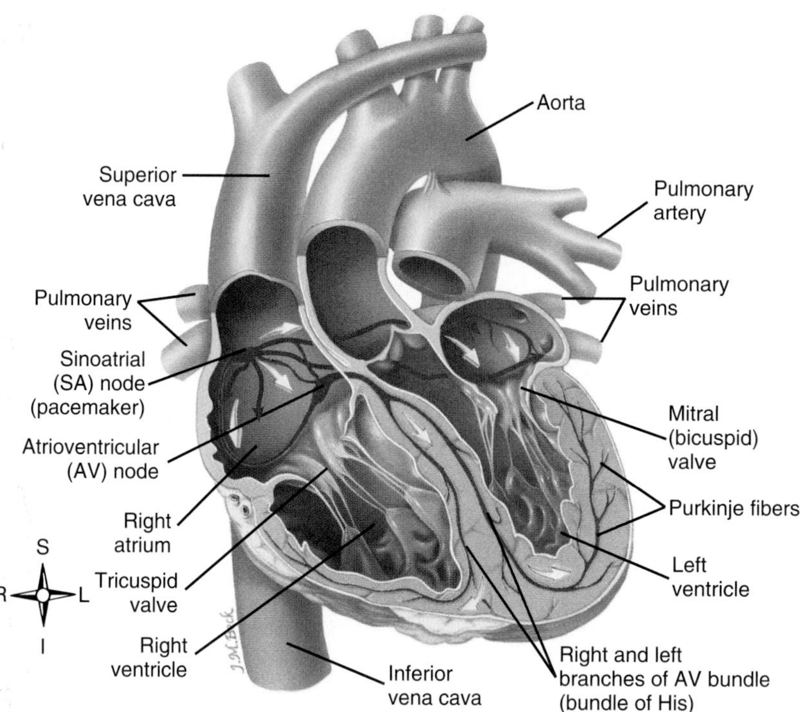

Figure 4-13

Conduction system of the heart. Specialized cardiac muscle cells in the wall of the heart rapidly conduct an electrical impulse throughout the myocardium. The signal is initiated by the sinoatrial (SA) node, the pacemaker of the heart, and spreads to the rest of the atrial myocardium and to the atrioventricular (AV) node. The AV node then initiates a signal that is conducted through the ventricular myocardium by way of the atrioventricular bundle (bundle of His) and the Purkinje fibers. (From McCance K, Huether SE: *Pathophysiology: the biological basis for disease in adults and children,* ed 5, St Louis, 2005, Mosby.)

beginning of the QRS complex creates the PR interval. This is the connection on the ECG between atrial activation and ventricular depolarization. During this period, the AV node, the bundle of His, the bundle branches, and the interventricular conduction system are activated.

Bundle of His, Right and Left Bundle Branches, and Purkinje Fibers

The bundle of His is a triangular structure that lies within the posterior border of the intraventricular septum. The left and right bundle branches originate in the lower portions of the triangle. Once the AV node has been activated, the impulse slants to the bundle of His, which conducts the impulse to the left and right bundle branches.

The right bundle branch is thin and extends to the right ventricular apex without much branching. The left bundle branch divides into two branches, or fascicles: the left anterior branch (left anterior papillary muscle to the left ventricle), and the left posterior branch (posteriorly crosses the left ventricular inflow tract to the base of the left posterior papillary muscle). The anterior fascicle activates the anterior and lateral wall of the left ventricle, and the posterior fascicle activates the inferior and posterior walls of the ventricle.

At the end of the left and right bundle branches are the Purkinje fibers, a network of small conduction fibers that penetrate the ventricular muscle mass and carry electrical impulses directly into the ventricular muscle cells. The Purkinje fibers have an intrinsic pacer rate of 24 to 40 beats/min (Figure 4-14).

ASSESSMENT

All findings from a patient encounter can be divided into four broad categories: global findings, regional findings, local findings, and cellular findings. Together, they provide an in-depth picture of the patient's state of health.

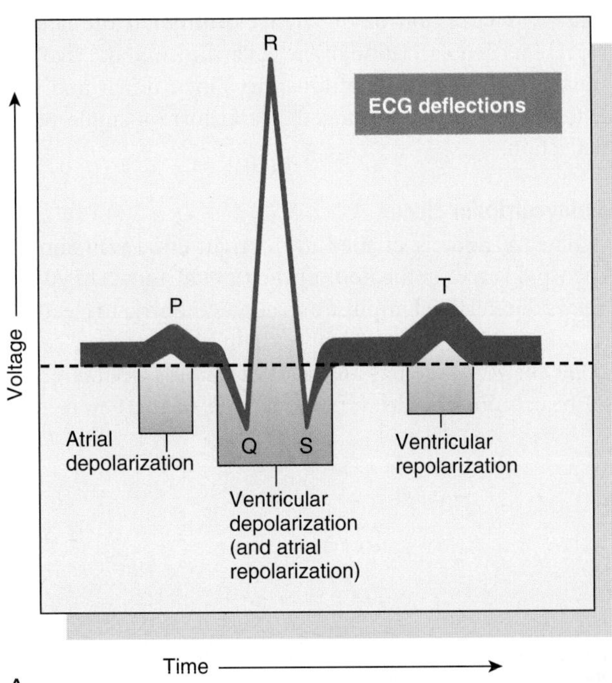

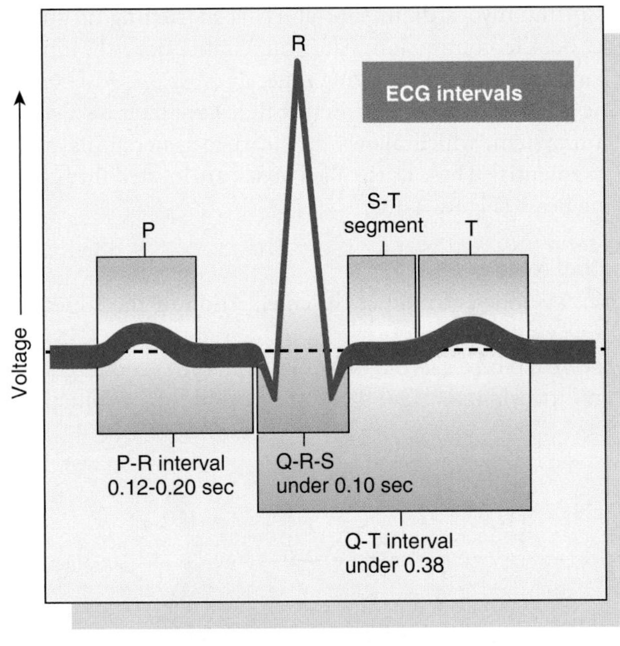

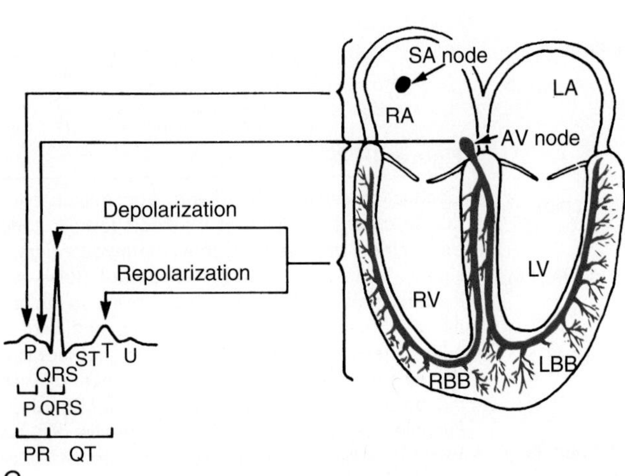

Figure 4-14

Electrocardiogram (ECG) and cardiac electrical activity. **A,** Normal ECG showing depolarization and repolarization. **B,** ECG intervals among P, QRS, and T waves. **C,** Schematic representation of an ECG and its relationship to cardiac electrical activity. *RA,* Right atrium; *LA,* left atrium; *AV,* atrioventricular; *RV,* right ventricle; *LBB,* left bundle branch; *RBB,* right bundle branch. (From McCance K, Huether SE: *Pathophysiology: the biological basis for disease in adults and children,* ed 5, St Louis, 2005, Mosby.)

Global Findings

How does the patient look? Is the person in distress? What is the respiratory effort? Is the person in pain? Has the level of consciousness changed? This is your true first impression of the patient, and it provides immediate clues to the severity of the person's condition. Assessment and clinical care are ongoing processes throughout the patient encounter. How and what you determine about your patient should be objective in nature.

When you first encounter your patient, think objectively. Your "gut instinct" may be correct, but if you cannot quantify the information, it is only subjective. Always consider your differential diagnosis and ask yourself what else this could be. Ask yourself these questions even if you are picking up a patient at a top-ranked hospital. Allow your knowledge and experience, not your surroundings, to guide you. Critically ill patients are attached to so much technologically complex equipment that you can easily be distracted. The global survey is even more important in this setting.

Regional Findings

Consider all the systems of a body and how they function separately and together. As individual components, changes may not appear significant. For instance, if pulmonary function decreases, cardiac output can decrease. This, in turn, can lead to an altered level of consciousness. Chronic changes in perfusion can lead to poor renal function.

Local Findings

Consider localized areas of the body. What do the physical signs mean? More importantly, what could have caused a change? Pedal edema and jugular venous distention (JVD) can be signs of congestive heart failure (CHF). The question you should try to answer is, "Why?" JVD and pedal edema are signs of a problem with both preload and afterload. Essentially, the right side of the heart is not able to pump out blood efficiently. The cardiovascular system is a closed high-pressure system; if JVD is present and blood is backing up, basically the pump is not doing what it needs to do.

CHF is only one cause of JVD. It also can be caused by a tension pneumothorax, pulmonary embolus, MI, cardiac tamponade, and pericarditis. Again, do not allow yourself to get tunnel vision. Localized changes also can be signs of potential global problems. Let's consider the 68-year-old male patient from the chapter scenario. During your localized assessment, you note that his right lower leg is swollen. It may seem insignificant for a patient with chest pain, but consider some causes of isolated extremity swelling. Does the patient have an underlying condition that may cause the swelling? Deep vein thrombosis (DVT), venous thromboembolism (VTE), or peripheral vascular disease (PVD) can cause isolated swelling. What if the swelling were caused by one or several clots? These clots can become dislodged from the peripheral site and end up in a pulmonary artery.

Everything about the patient is significant, but it is relevant to your patient care only if you look.

Cellular Findings

Cellular perfusion (or its absence) is an important indicator of the patient's condition. Although the global cellular perfusion status may be difficult to determine, consider what it means: Shock can be defined as inadequate perfusion to support cellular needs; that is, cells are not getting proper perfusion. A **myocardial infarction** is just that; cardiac cells have lost perfusion to the point of cell death. From a vascular standpoint, if peripheral cells have decreased perfusion, they shift into anaerobic metabolism, which increases the production of toxins and decreases the pH. With our 68-year-old patient, ask yourself how well his cells are being perfused. If the answer is they are not, you direct your care toward meeting cellular needs (Table 4-2).

Physical Assessment

All critical care transport vehicles and hospital units have a wealth of diagnostic tools available. The most important, however, is *you*. There are five senses, three of which we discuss here: sight, hearing, and touch. These are the best diagnostic tools you have. No amount of electronic gadgetry can compensate for good observation and quality clinical knowledge.

Sight

From your first impression to transfer of patient care, you see everything about your patient. Look for what is right and for what is wrong. From the global perspective, use your vision to obtain information about the patient's work of breathing

Table 4-2 Clarifying Chest Pain Symptoms by Asking Specific Questions

To Determine...	Ask...
Location, radiation	Where is it? Does it move around or stay in one place?
Quality	What is it like?
Quantity	How severe is it? How frequent? How long does it last?
Chronology	When did it begin? How has it progressed? What are you doing when it occurs? What do you do to relieve it?
Associated findings	Do you feel any other symptoms at the same time?
Treatment sought and effect	Have you seen a physician in the past for this same problem? What was the treatment?
Personal perception	What do you think causes this? Why do you think it happened now?

From Urden LD, Stacy KM, Lough ME: *Thelan's critical care nursing: diagnosis and management*, ed 5, St. Louis, 2006, Mosby.

(or ease of ventilation), general skin color for perfusion status, and level of consciousness.

Distress

Acute distress results from conditions in which a patient is on the verge of decompensation or has started to decompensate. Patient care can be easily directed to address these conditions. For patients with chronic conditions, consider whether they are in distress or whether their physiology has adapted over time. Essentially, do they look physiologically "normal"? If not, is what you see now "normal" for that particular patient?

Skin

What does the skin look like? The nail beds, lips, and mucosa are relatively consistent in all patients. The skin also reflects changes if you have an established baseline:

- Normal: The skin tone, nail beds, and mucosa are normal.
- Pale: Pallor is the result of decreased overall circulation at that locale; this can be the result of shunting, compensation, or shock.
- Ashen: The skin appears gray; the peripheral circulation is decreased, and what remains becomes deoxygenated.
- Cyanosis: A bluish hue is the classic sign of cyanosis, which results from a decrease in oxygenation and the retention of carbon dioxide. Differentiate between peripheral and central cyanosis.
- Yellowish: A yellowish tint indicates jaundice secondary to liver disease or hemolysis.

In addition to assessing the skin, you should:

1. Inspect the nail beds for **clubbing**, which can indicate intrathoracic or pulmonary disease.
2. Look at the extremities for signs of peripheral vascular disease (Table 4-3) and dependent edema. Pitting edema can be documented according to a scale*:

0	No edema present
1+	Trace (¼-inch depression with rapid return to baseline)
2+	Mild (¼- to ½-inch depression with return to baseline in 10 to 15 seconds)
3+	Moderate (½- to 1-inch depression with return to baseline in 1 to 2 minutes)
4+	Severe (greater than 1-inch depression with return to baseline in 2 to 5 minutes)

3. Position the patient appropriately (if allowed) and evaluate for increased right-sided heart pressure to determine whether JVD is present. As described earlier, JVD is an indication of elevated right-sided heart pressure. To evaluate for JVD:

- Position the patient at a 30- to 45-degree angle, head-up.
- Turn the head slightly to the left.
- Assess the internal jugular vein just above the sternal angle at the end of the exhalation phase.
- JVD is present if you can see the internal jugular vein above the sternal border for about 3 cm (Figure 4-15).

*Modified from Urden LD, Stacy KM, Lough ME: *Thelan's critical care nursing: diagnosis and management,* ed 5, St. Louis, 2006, Mosby.

Did You Know?

During neck vein evaluation, a cannon wave can be seen when the atria contract against closed AV valves. This can occur when atrial contraction is initiated while the ventricle contracts, as in complete heart block or premature ventricular contraction (PVC). To examine for a venous cannon wave, have the patient turn his or her head to the left as you evaluate the right jugular vein. If this phenomenon is present, you will note a "wave" of pressure up the vasculature. However, this evaluation is very challenging to make in the EMS environment.[2]

Hearing

Listen to your patient. When you ask questions, the way the person responds is as important as the answers given. Level of consciousness, dyspnea, distress, and pain are easily determined by the patient's responses. Audible wheezes or rhonchi are objective, but the more subtle sounds can be detected only by using a stethoscope. Listening to the heart sounds is a skill that requires practice, but when properly done, it can reveal considerable information about heart and valve function. Also listen for bruits, the sound made when the blood flow in the artery is turbulent rather than laminar. Carotid and brachial bruits often are overlooked, but they indicate plaque in the artery and, by default, an obstruction.

Touch

Do not be afraid to touch your patient. For now, take a minute and imagine yourself as a patient. A caregiver addresses you with a clipboard in hand and begins the interview. Sound normal? Now, imagine the caregiver you would want to take care of your 68-year-old family member; a caregiver who takes the time to shake your hand and introduce himself or herself. To which caregiver are you more likely to respond? Those who gain the experience to move into critical care transport have elevated themselves to the top of the game in this career field. Your assessment and professional approach to your patient are the primary tools of your critical care toolbox. If you shake hands with a patient, what have you done? Social decorum aside, you have created an environment in which your patient is likely to feel less stress about your interview. You can assess skin temperature and diaphoresis. Moving to both hands, you can check grip strength, equality, and distal neurologic response.

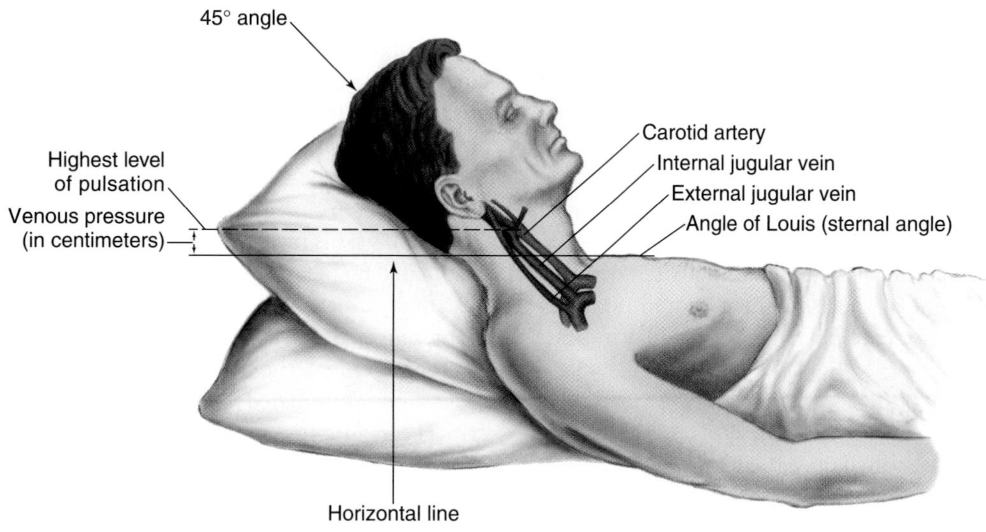

Figure 4-15

Positions of the internal and external jugular veins. Pulsation in the internal jugular vein can be used to estimate the central venous pressure. (From Thompson JM, McFarland GK, Hirsch JE, Tucker SM: *Mosby's clinical nursing,* ed 5, St Louis, 2002, Mosby.)

Table 4-3 Arterial and Venous Disease Findings on Inspection and Palpation of the Extremities

Characteristics	Arterial Disease	Venous Disease
Hair loss	Present	Absent
Skin texture	Thin, shiny, dry	Flaking, stasis, dermatitis, mottled
Ulceration	Found at pressure points; painful, pale, dry with little drainage; well-demarcated with eschar or dried tissue; surrounded by fibrous tissue; granulation tissue scant and pale	Usually found on the ankle; painless, pink, moist with large amount of drainage; irregular, dry, and scaly; surrounded by dermatitis; granulation tissue healthy
Skin color	Elevational pallor, redness in dependent extremities	Brown patches, redness, mottled cyanotic color in dependent extremities
Nails	Thick, brittle	Normal
Varicose veins	Absent	Present
Temperature	Cool	Warm
Capillary refill	>3 sec	<3 sec
Edema	None or mild, usually unilateral	Usually present foot to calf, unilateral or bilateral
Pulses	Weak or absent (0 to 1+)	Normal, strong, and symmetric

Modified from Krenzer ME: Peripheral vascular assessment: finding your way through arteries and veins, *AACN Clin Issues* 6:631, 1995.

Palpation of pulses includes all seven pairs of bilateral arterial pulsation points (carotid, brachial, radial, popliteal, dorsalis pedis, femoral, and posterior tibial arteries) and the abdominal aorta. Palpate these points separately and then compare the strength. Pulse volume is graded from 0 to 3+*:

0	Not palpable
1+	Faintly palpable (weak and thready)
2+	Normal
3+	Bounding (hyperdynamic)

*Modified from Urden LD, Stacy KM, Lough ME: *Thelan's critical care nursing: diagnosis and management,* ed 5, St. Louis, 2006, Mosby.

DIAGNOSTIC TOOLS

Your senses, training, and skills are the most important tools you have, but they are not the only aids to diagnosis. Do not forget the vital signs, coma scale, blood glucose level, capnography, pulse oximetry, and ECG. Whether you are in a clinical or an out-of-hospital environment, use all available tools, because they all provide objective information, and together they create a more detailed picture of your patient's condition. Patient assessment is a common practice that should be performed with consistency. As a critical care provider, your patient care is determined by your findings. Objective, thorough, and concise information establishes a baseline for your care and supports accurate diagnosis and treatment of your patient's condition. It also allows you to recognize and respond to any changes in the patient's condition. A cardiovascular patient requires particular attention to detail. Assessment of your patient always goes beyond a list of questions. It becomes an objective measure of the entire patient.

Vital Signs

Temperature

Measuring (and recording) the patient's body temperature is an important element of the assessment procedure. Fever may signal infection; unintentional hypothermia may indicate a shock state.

Respiratory Rate

You have already determined the patient's respiratory effort from your global evaluation: this is a cardinal finding in a cardiac patient. What is less obvious is the importance of the patient's respiratory rate. Many times, distress is accompanied by tachypnea. However, when the patient is breathing without extra effort, tachypnea also signals cardinal distress. Quiet tachypnea may indicate a patient who may be compensating for an acidotic state, as in sepsis or cardiogenic shock.

Blood Pressure

The blood pressure may be measured invasively or noninvasively. Correct use of the stethoscope and BP cuff is the key to accurate noninvasive measurements. The cuff normally is applied to the area above the brachial artery, but the BP can be measured on any section of an extremity (lower leg, upper leg, and lower arm). The arm or leg should be at the level of the heart, and the cuff should be large enough to incorporate two thirds of the extremity section. For a thorough cardiovascular assessment, the BP should be measured and recorded for both arms so that a pathologic condition near the subclavian artery can be detected. For example, if an aortic dissection has occurred near the subclavian artery, the BP in the two arms will be different.

A CCP's skills include the ability to take both palpated and automated BP measurements. Once transport begins, however, auscultation becomes quite a challenge. For ongoing assessment, sensed BP measurements should be done, and palpated BP measurement should be reserved for emergency assessment only. Automated BP systems should be part of your critical care monitor. Your service should conduct routine biomedical evaluation of the device for proper maintenance and to ensure accurate readings. Skill 4-1 presents a review of BP measurement.

Did You Know?

Although automated BP devices generally provide accurate systolic pressures, they derive the diastolic reading from the systolic and mean arterial pressures; the diastolic pressure, therefore, is considered an estimate.[2]

Skill 4-1

OBTAINING BLOOD PRESSURE MEASUREMENTS

In general, the blood pressure (BP) can be measured in three ways: the indirect manual method, indirect automated method, and invasive arterial method. The accuracy of indirect methods depends on blood flow in the extremity used for measurement, the equipment used, and the healthcare provider's skills. Some differences in the recorded blood pressures may be seen among the three techniques. The patient's underlying health history and vascular status, overall body size, and any systemic diseases also affect these measurements.

MEAN ARTERIAL PRESSURE

The mean arterial pressure (MAP) is the average pressure in the cardiovascular system. The following formula often is used to calculate the MAP:

$$\text{Systolic pressure} + 2(\text{Diastolic blood pressure}) \div 3$$

However, if indirect methods of measurement are used, and if the variables previously mentioned are a factor, this formula may not produce an accurate value. (A BP of 120/80 mm Hg produces an MAP of 93 mm Hg.)

Other common formulas used to calculate the MAP are:

$$\text{Diastolic BP} + \tfrac{1}{3}(\text{Systolic BP [SBP]} - \text{DBP})$$

$$\text{DBP} + \tfrac{1}{3}(\text{Pulse pressure})$$

With the indirect automated method of determining the BP, the MAP is displayed on the machine's screen with the systolic and diastolic readings.

Your protocols may use specific systolic and diastolic indirect blood pressure readings as a guide to certain types of therapy. Use of the MAP is preferable for four reasons:

1. The MAP is the same throughout the cardiovascular system.
2. Both the pulmonary and systemic vascular resistance are derived from the MAP.
3. The MAP is rarely affected by machine artifact and discrepancies.
4. The MAP reflects the pressure within the systemic and cerebral capillary beds.

When the MAP is used as a therapeutic determinant, an order for the use of a beta blocker to control a patient's blood pressure may be written such that the drug is given only if the MAP is greater than 130 mm Hg.

Direct Invasive Arterial Pressure Measurement

INDICATIONS

Continuous blood pressure monitoring

Monitor effects of therapeutics

Obtain serial blood gas readings

CONTRAINDICATION TO USE OF A SITE

Lack of collateral circulation in the extremity

Any artery may be cannulated for direct arterial blood pressure measurement, but the radial site is preferred. A **modified Allen test** is performed before the procedure to determine whether the distal extremity has collateral circulation. This test determines whether the ulnar artery is functioning adequately in the upper extremity chosen for the radial artery puncture.

MODIFIED ALLEN TEST

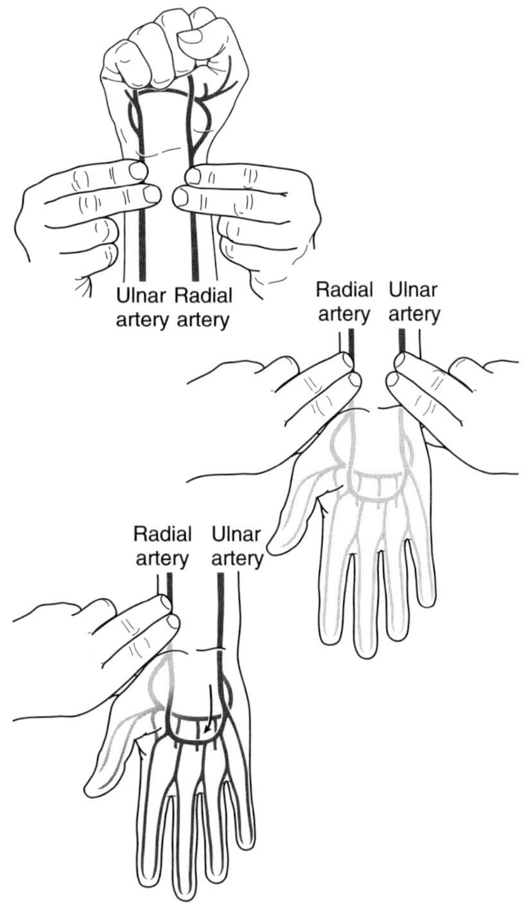

Allen test for assessing for adequate ulnar blood flow. (From Mims B, Toto KH, Luecke LE, Roberts MK, et al: *Critical care skills: a clinical handbook,* ed 2, Philadelphia, 2004, Saunders.)

1. Ask the patient to form a tight fist.
2. Apply firm pressure over both the radial and ulnar arteries.
3. While maintaining pressure over the arteries, elevate the patient's hand above the level of the heart; then have the patient open and close the fist several times. You may notice a loss of color in the hand.

NOTE: If the patient is unable to follow these commands, elevate the chosen upper extremity for several seconds while compressing both arteries.

4. Lower the patient's hand while releasing *only* the ulnar artery; maintain pressure continuously over the radial artery.
5. Observe the patient's palm for return of color. Return of color within 10 seconds indicates a patent ulnar artery (collateral circulation). If the hand remains pale for longer than 10 seconds, the radial artery should not be punctured in that extremity, because the collateral circulation is not adequate. The Allen test then may be performed on the other upper extremity; if the collateral circulation is still inadequate, an alternative site should be chosen.

ALTERNATIVE METHOD OF EVALUATING COLLATERAL CIRCULATION TO THE HAND

1. Apply a pulse oximetry probe to the forefinger of the extremity being evaluated. Compress the radial and ulnar arteries; watch for the amplitude of the oximetry pleth to disappear and then reappear as the ulnar artery pulsation is allowed to perfuse.
2. Apply a lubricated arterial Doppler head to the ulnar artery to determine whether collateral circulation to the hand is adequate.

ASSISTING WITH OR PERFORMING ARTERIAL CATHETERIZATION

Regardless of whether your critical care transport service allows insertion of arterial lines or you transport patients who already have such lines, a knowledge of the procedure is important for all who manage these devices.

1. While the practitioner prepares to insert the arterial catheter, establish a sterile field and universal precautions. Assist with skin preparation and proper positioning of the extremity.
2. Flush the **pressure transducer system**.
3. If you are inserting the catheter, wash your hands and put on sterile gloves.
4. Optional: Instill a local anesthetic intradermally and deeper around the arterial insertion site.
5. Cleanse the skin with antiseptic solution.
6. Palpate and stabilize the selected artery with your nondominant hand.
7. With the bevel up, insert the needle into the selected artery, adjusting angle as needed until blood return is noted in the hub. Slowly advance the entire

catheter about ¼ to ½ inch further to ensure full insertion.

8. Gently lower the angle of the catheter to the skin surface; then, continue to advance the cannula to its hub, with a slight rotation.
9. Pulsatile blood should be noted upon removal of the stylet.
10. Once you or the practitioner has the catheter appropriately positioned, connect it to the preflushed pressure transducer system with a Luer-Lok. Watch for a waveform. Push the button for the square wave test configuration (Box 4-1).
11. Assist with securing or suturing the catheter at the site.

Box 4-1 Dynamic Response Testing (Square Wave, Frequency Response Testing) Using the Fast-Flush System

Optimally Damped System

When the fast flush of the continuous flush system is activated and quickly released, a sharp upstroke terminates in a flat line at the proximal indicator on the monitor and hard copy. This is followed by an immediate, rapid downstroke that extends below the baseline with just one or two oscillations within 0.12 second (minimal ringing) and a quick return to the baseline. The pattern's pressure waveform also is clearly defined; all components of the waveform, such as the dicrotic notch on the arterial waveform, are clearly visible.

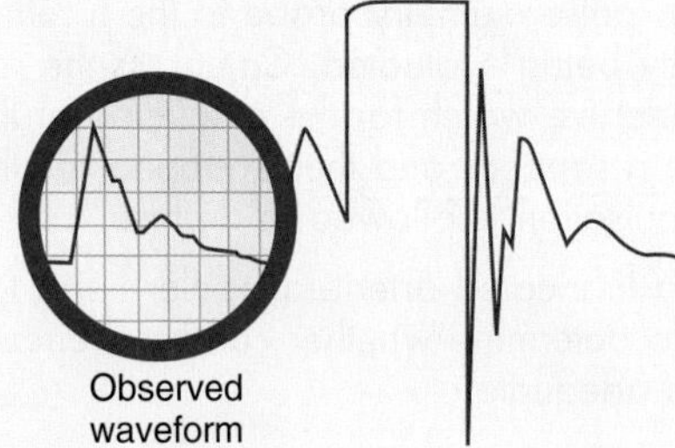

Intervention: No adjustment in the monitoring system is required.

Overdamped System

The upstroke of the square wave appears somewhat slurred, the waveform does not extend below the baseline after the fast flush, and there is no ringing after the flush. The patient's waveform displays a falsely decreased systolic pressure, a falsely high diastolic pressure, and poorly defined components of the pressure tracing, such as a diminished or an absent dicrotic notch on arterial waveforms.

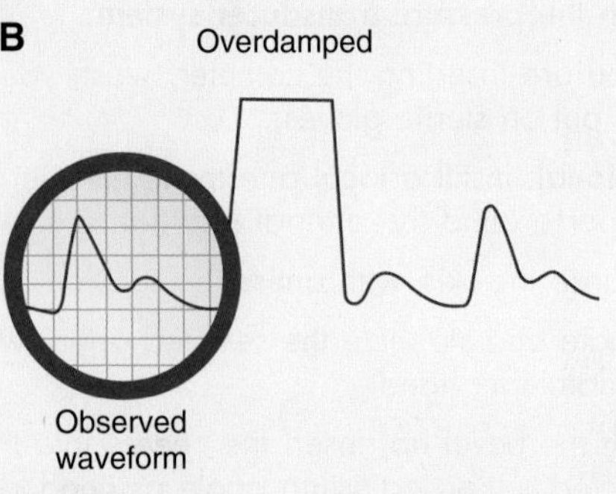

Intervention:

- Check for and clear any blood clots, blood left in the catheter after sampling, or air bubbles at any point from the catheter tip to the transducer diaphragm.
- Use low compliance (rigid) short monitoring tubing (<3 to 4 feet).
- Connect all line components securely.
- Check for kinks in the line.

Underdamped System

The waveform has numerous amplified oscillations above and below the baseline after the fast flush. The monitored pressure wave displays a falsely high systolic pressure (overshoot), possibly a falsely low diastolic pressure, and "ringing" artifacts on the waveform.

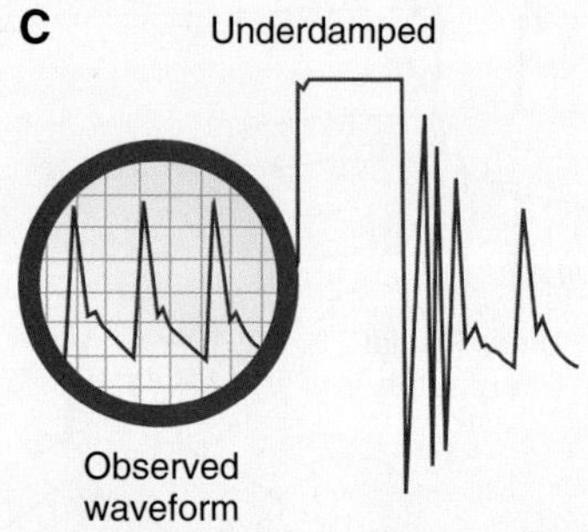

Intervention:

- Remove all air bubbles (particularly pinpoint air bubbles) in the fluid system
- Use large-bore, shorter tubing or a damping device

From Urden LD, Stacy KM, Lough ME: *Thelan's critical care nursing: diagnosis and management*, ed 5, St. Louis, 2006, Mosby.

MAINTENANCE OF AN ARTERIAL PRESSURE MONITORING SYSTEM

Did You Know?

Zeroing and leveling of the transducer are taught as two separate procedures. However, if the cables become disconnected when you reposition the patient, the two processes become one. Relevel and rezero in each instance.

1. Level the system to the phlebostatic axis.
2. Zero the system at least every 8 hours.
3. Check for an adequate amount of flush solution in the pressurized, heparinized bag.
4. Keep the pressure bag inflated to 300 mm Hg to maintain forward flow.
5. Tighten all connections and stopcock port caps. Keep the tubing and system free of bubbles.
6. If the patient has multiple "lines," label this line as "arterial."
7. Set the alarms on the monitoring system.
8. Check the distal circulation and movement in the cannulated extremity.

INTERPRETING THE ARTERIAL WAVEFORM

The arterial pressure waveform begins when the semilunar valves open and is seen as an upstroke off the baseline that should immediately ascend to the systolic (rounded) peak; this is related to the force of blood ejected from the ventricle.

Once the blood has been ejected, the pressure falls in the pulmonary and systemic arteries, and the waveform descends from the peak.

When the semilunar valves snap shut, a dicrotic notch is noted, as the wave continues descending while the pressure steadily decreases toward the end-diastolic pressure.

When this waveform is compared with your electrocardiogram (ECG) on the same screen, the QRS complex appears first, followed by the arterial pressure waveform (see illustration).

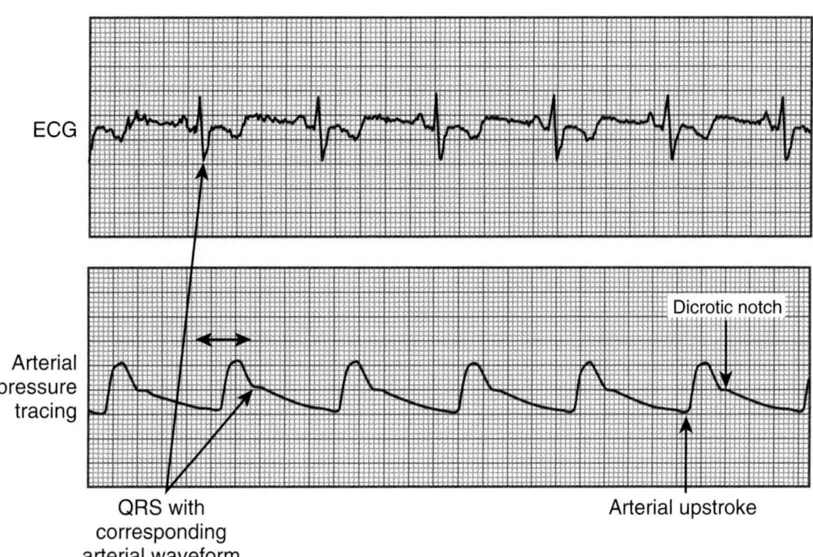

Simultaneous ECG and normal arterial pressure tracing. (From Urden LD, Stacy KM, Lough ME: *Thelan's critical care nursing: diagnosis and management*, ed 5, St. Louis, 2006, Mosby.)

Dampened Waveform

When assessing for the cause of low arterial blood pressure, always check the system for proper function, along with the patient. Monitoring systems include indirect, automated cuff measurement of the BP; therefore, correlate the arterial blood pressure with the cuff pressure.

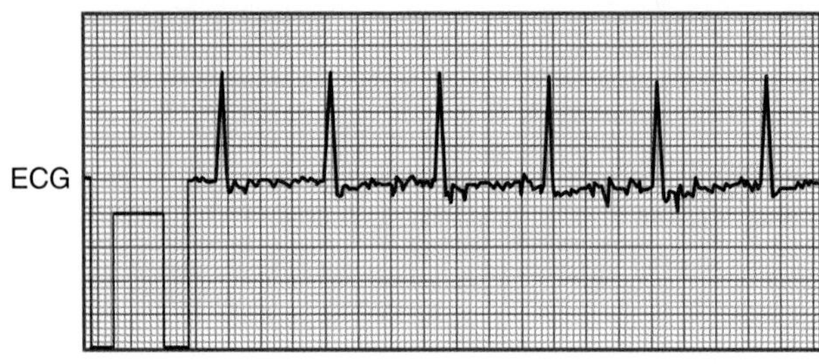

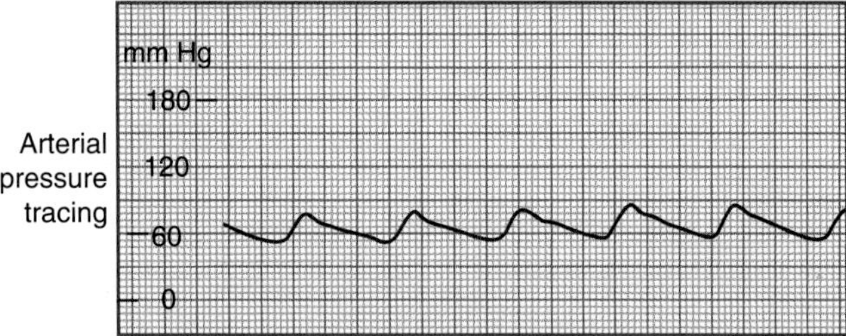

Simultaneous ECG and arterial pressure tracings show a damped arterial pressure waveform. (From Urden LD, Stacy KM, Lough ME: *Thelan's critical care nursing: diagnosis and management,* ed 5, St. Louis, 2006, Mosby.)

A dampened waveform is rounded and has no dicrotic notch. The cuff pressure is likely to be higher than the arterial pressure. A dampened waveform occurs when the communication between the transducer and the monitoring system is interrupted, resulting in false values. This type of waveform can be caused by the formation of a fibrinous piece of tissue over the tip of the catheter, a kink in the catheter, or air bubbles in the system.

Underdamped Waveform

Overshoot, fling, or an underdamped waveform is caused by distortion of the system; this creates a waveform with a sharp, narrow upswing for systole and a falsely high systolic pressure.

Loss of Waveform

Loss of the waveform usually occurs when one of the stopcocks is left open or off. Also, the tubing may be kinked, or the catheter may have moved slightly and is against the vessel wall. Make sure all stopcocks are in the correct position and the tubing is not kinked; then reposition the extremity.

PHYSIOLOGIC CHANGES THAT CAUSE DIFFERENCES BETWEEN INDIRECT AND DIRECT PRESSURE MEASUREMENTS

With a low perfusion state, cuff (indirect) BP measurement may be unreliable. Other factors that can interfere with accurate cuff measurements include edema, obesity, atherosclerotic changes, and arrhythmias. Discrepancies in arterial pressure measurements may occur with catheter migration and the location of catheter (dorsalis pedis vs. radial or distal vs. proximal readings).

MAINTAINING AN ARTERIAL CATHETER WITHOUT PRESSURE MEASUREMENT

If you determine that indirect cuff BP measurement is adequate during transport of your critically ill patient, the arterial system can be maintained without continuous measurement. Record the last arterial pressure, noting that the waveform was normal. Disconnect the transducer cable from the monitoring system. Maintain the pressure bag at 300 mm Hg and keep all stopcocks closed.

OBTAINING BLOOD SAMPLES FROM AN ARTERIAL CATHETER

The need for repeated arterial blood gas sampling may be another indication for placement of an arterial catheter.

1. Wash your hands and follow universal precautions. Explain the procedure to the patient.
2. Obtain a laboratory order and requisition. Verify the patient's identity by comparing the information on the name band and laboratory requisition and order.
3. If the sample is for arterial blood gas (ABG) measurements, open your service's blood gas sampling kit and push the plunger to rid the syringe of excess air and heparin.
4. If you are using a Vacutainer system, assemble the adapter needle in the Vacutainer and appropriate laboratory tubes. Obtain enough extra tubes to draw off a discard specimen.
5. Suspend the arterial alarms on the monitoring system.
6. Turn the stopcock off to the patient.
7. Remove the cap from the blood sampling port on the three-way stopcock closest to the patient.
8. Attach a 12 mL syringe or Vacutainer system with blood tubes for discard to this port to withdraw dead space volume from system.
9. Turn the stopcock off to the flush solution.
10. Withdraw a volume of blood to be discarded; this dead space volume is estimated as the volume from the tip of the catheter to the sampling port of the stopcock.
    - This specimen must be discarded, because it contains saline and heparin.
    - The amount withdrawn should be three times the estimated dead space (20-gauge catheter with 12.75 inches of tubing and one stopcock = 0.8 mL; the amount withdrawn for discard should be about 2.4 mL). If the laboratory samples are for the international normalized ratio (INR; also called the *prothrombin time* [PT]) or for the partial thromboplastin time (PTT), the amount discarded should be six times the dead space.
11. Turn the stopcock off to all ports; remove and discard the dead space volume into an appropriate container.
12. Attach the prepared blood gas syringe to a port or insert the appropriate tubes into the Vacutainer.

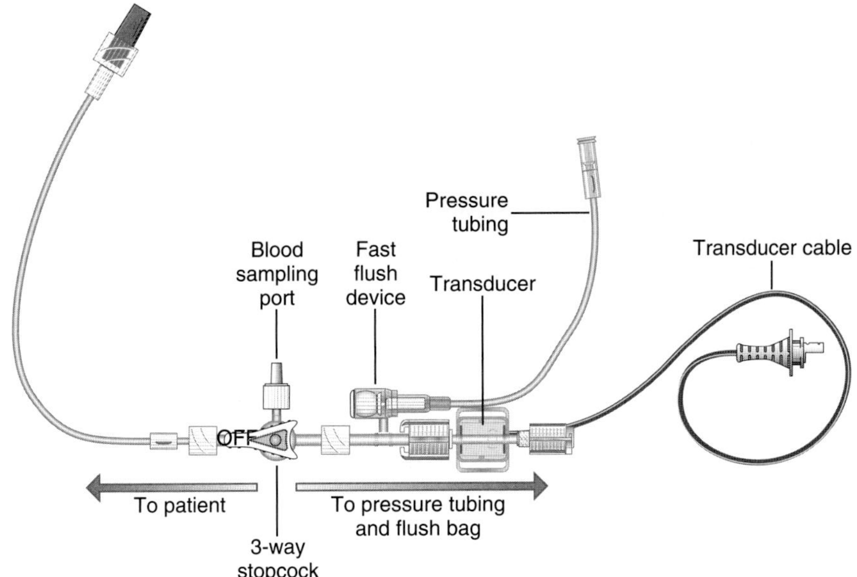

Disposable transducer with continuous flush device. The stopcock is turned "off" to the patient. (From Wiegand D, Carlson K: *AACN procedure manual for critical care,* ed 5, Philadelphia, 2005, Saunders.)

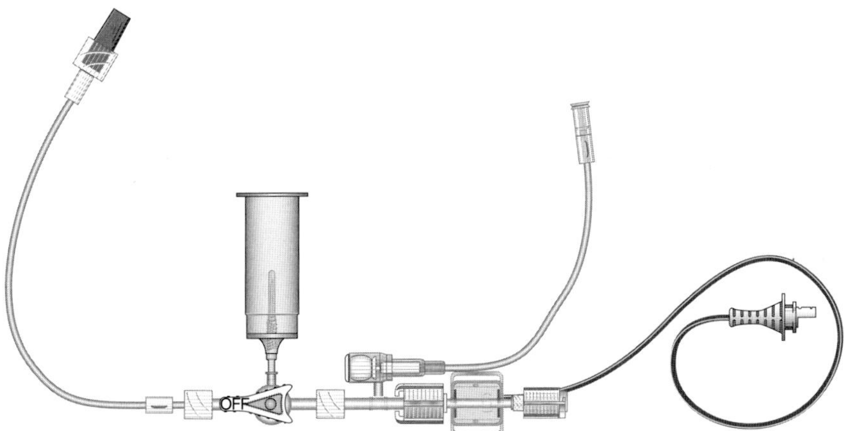

Vacutainer with "needleless" Luer-Lok needle attached to the blood sampling port of the three-way stopcock. The stopcock is "off" to the patient. (From Wiegand D, Carlson K: *AACN procedure manual for critical care,* ed 5, Philadelphia, 2005, Saunders.)

13. Turn the stopcock off to the flush solution and withdraw the required amount of blood.
14. Turn the stopcock off to all ports and remove the syringe containing the specimen.
15. Attach another 5 mL syringe to the port and turn the stopcock off to the catheter. Open the quick-flush, in-line device and flush the system to clear it of blood.
16. Turn the stopcocks off and remove the syringe. Use the in-line flushing device to intermittently push excess blood out of the system.
17. Turn on the arterial alarms and assess the quality of the waveform.
18. Label the blood specimen appropriately and transport it to the laboratory.

Pulse Pressure

As you know, the pulse pressure is the difference between the systolic and diastolic BP readings. Normal pulse pressure is 40 mm Hg (120/80 mm Hg). When compensation occurs in the low flow state, a narrow pulse pressure is noted because of arterial vasoconstriction. The purpose of this compensation is to maintain a relatively normal mean arterial pressure. Conversely, a wide pulse pressure can be seen with venodilation caused by poor vascular tone (sepsis).

Pulsus Paradoxus

The respiratory cycle, which moves the thorax with a rise and fall in pressures, affects the blood pressure in the cardiothoracic area. The systolic BP decreases slightly during inhalation and rises by the same amount during exhalation. With an elevated resting heart pressure (pericardial tamponade), this difference is much higher. With a manual system, identify the peak systolic pressure during exhalation and then reidentify it when you hear Korotkoff sounds (auscultated cuff BP sounds) during both inhalation and exhalation. If the difference is greater than 10 mm Hg, pulsus paradoxus is said to be present. A more accurate measurement for this abnormality can be obtained with pulse oximetry or an arterial waveform, which compares exhalation and inhalation.

Multilead Electrocardiogram

In recent years the electrocardiogram has advanced considerably, from the once-standard three- and 12-lead monitors to 15-lead monitors. Whether the 12-lead ECG is acquired by the referring facility or obtained during transport, advanced knowledge of the interpretation of an ECG is crucial in critical care transport.

Did You Know?

If a 12-lead electrocardiograph is not available, a standard three-lead monitor can be used to obtain a multilead (nine lead) ECG reading. (The nine-lead electrocardiogram does not include the aVR, aVL, or aVF, but it still provides valuable information about the lateral, anterior, and inferior wall.) To obtain a nine-lead reading from a standard three-lead monitor, activate the machine's diagnostic setting (if available) and follow these steps[3]:

1. **Run leads I, II, and III first. Obtain a representative sample for each lead and label it.**
2. **Leave the monitor in lead III (the negative electrode at the left shoulder) and move the left leg cable (the red lead wire) to each of the modified chest lead positions (from V1 to V6) to obtain a readout. Label each sample.**
3. **Arrange the readouts in a standard nine-lead order: I, II, and III in the first column; MCL1, MCL2, and MCL3 in the middle column; and MCL4, MCL5, and MCL6 in the last column.**

Did You Know?

All members of the cardiac care transport team are expected to know the basic interpretation of a multilead electrocardiogram.[4]

To help you master the concepts introduced in this chapter, we have included a number of 12-lead ECGs for practice on the Evolve website for *Transport of the Critical Care Patient.*

Cardiac Auscultation

As the differential diagnosis continues, many other evaluative techniques come into play. For example, the initial vital signs provide clues to possible pathologic conditions. As you move forward in the assessment, it is essential that you take note of all available data that emerge, both in the initial assessment and the ongoing assessment. Accurate assessment of heart sounds often is overlooked as part of the initial patient assessment. To develop skill in obtaining and assessing heart sounds, you must approach each patient methodically and in the same manner.

Use of the Stethoscope

Although use of the stethoscope is a noninvasive procedure, the stethoscope is a phenomenal tool for patient assessment. Many different types of stethoscopes are available, and costs range from $30 to more than $300. Depending on the examiner's preferences and needs, however, only a few features are truly significant. The earpieces of the stethoscope should be aligned with the ear canals, and they must fit snuggly and comfortably in the ears. The device that detects sound has two parts, the bell and the diaphragm. When the rim of the bell is pressed against the skin, the listener can hear low-pitched sounds. However, care must be taken to press only hard enough to eliminate air leakage; otherwise, the bell acts as a diaphragm, and the low-pitched sounds are not heard. The bell allows detection of heart sounds S_3 and S_4 and ventricular filling murmurs. The diaphragm of the stethoscope, which is flat, allows the listener to detect high-pitched sounds. The diaphragm detects heart sounds S_1 and S_2, clicks, snaps, and murmurs caused by stenotic valves.

Approach auscultation of the heart systematically, as you would any other part of the assessment. As you examine the patient, create a mental image of the location of the heart and the corresponding valves (Figure 4-16).

Begin auscultation at the point of maximal impact (PMI), which should be at the fifth intercostal space left of the sternum and close to the left nipple. This is the location for auscultation of the mitral valve. Then listen to the tricuspid valve, which is best heard in the fourth intercostal space left of the sternum, even though it is on the right side. Next, move to the aortic listening post (second intercostal space right of the sternum) and then the pulmonic listening post (second intercostal space left of the sternum). Auscultate all four areas of the heart using this same systematic approach, and use both the bell and the diaphragm to identify high- and low-pitched sounds.

Heart Sounds and Corresponding Actions

The basic heart sounds are identified as S_1, S_2, S_3, and S_4. The typical "lub-dub" sounds are identified as the heart sounds S_1 and S_2 and are considered "normal." The first heart sound, S_1, is produced by closure of the AV valve and is longer

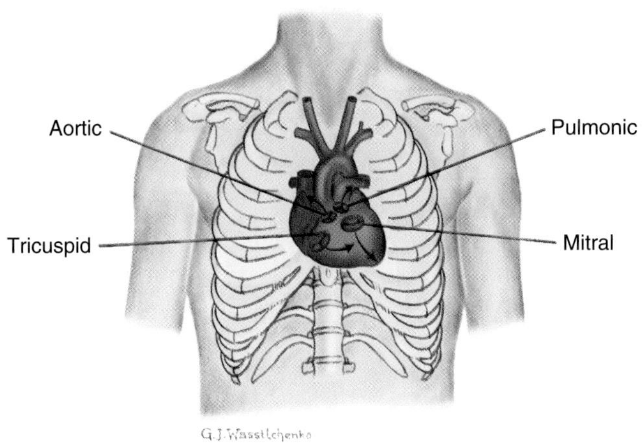

Figure 4-16

Transmission of heart sounds to the thorax and the relationship of the heart sounds to the anatomic position of the heart valves. (From Urden LD, Stacy KM, Lough ME: *Thelan's critical care nursing: diagnosis and management,* ed 5, St. Louis, 2006, Mosby.)

and lower pitched than the second heart sound. S_1 represents the onset of ventricular systole. The second heart sound, S_2, represents the end of ventricular ejection and is produced by closure of the aortic and pulmonic valves at the beginning of diastole. S_2 usually is the loudest heart sound (Figure 4-17).

Generally, each of the normal heart sounds (S_1 and S_2) is produced by the simultaneous closure of two valves. With an S_1/S_2 split, the two valves close at slightly different times. An S_1/S_2 split can be caused by pathologic or physiologic factors. In an S_1 split, the mitral valve closes before the tricuspid valve. An S_2 split is audible if the aortic valve closes early or the pulmonic valve closes late. An abnormally loud S_1 could indicate mitral valve stenosis, whereas a softer sound could signify mitral valve regurgitation. Other pathologic causes of splitting include specific cardiovascular conditions, such as pulmonary hypertension, pulmonic stenosis, and right ventricular failure with resulting right bundle branch block and premature ventricular contractions (Box 4-2).

The abnormal heart sounds, S_3 and S_4, frequently are referred to as *gallops.* Both S_3 and S_4 are low-pitched sounds that are best auscultated over the apical region. S_3 occurs in early diastole and is caused by rapid filling of the ventricles. The presence of S_3 often is considered normal in children or young adults, because their hearts are healthy and should have rapid ventricular filling. However, if the patient is older (usually over age 40) and has cardiac complaints, the presence of S_3 could signify a failing left ventricle, which may manifest in this patient as congestive heart failure. S_4, which is caused by atrial contraction, often is referred to as an *atrial gallop.* It occurs late in the diastolic phase, just before S_1. Unlike S_3, S_4 is not a normal finding and is always considered pathologic. Identification of S_4 should lead to suspicion of one or more of the following disorders: hypertension, myocardial ischemia/infarction, aortic/pulmonic stenosis, and ventricular failure (Box 4-3).

Box 4-2 Characteristics of Heart Sounds S_1 and S_2

S_1	S_2
High pitched	High pitched
Loudest in mitral area (apex)	Loudest in aortic area (base)
Split S_1	***Split S_2***
Normal split: <20 msec	Normal split: <30 msec
Split heard best in tricuspid area	Split heard best in pulmonic area
Important to differentiate between split S_1 and S_4	↑ Split with inhalation
Occurs immediately before carotid upstroke	↓ Split with exhalation

From Urden LD, Stacy KM, Lough ME: *Thelan's critical care nursing: diagnosis and management,* ed 5, St. Louis, 2006, Mosby.
↑, Increased; ↓, decreased.

Box 4-3 Characteristics of Heart Sounds S_3 and S_4

S_3	S_4
Physiologic Causes	
Related to diastolic motion and rapid filling of ventricles in early diastole	Related to diastolic motion and ventricular dilation with atrial contraction in late diastole
May be normal in children and young adults (<40 yr)	May occur with or without cardiac decompensation
Pathologic Causes	
Ventricular dysfunction with an increase in end-systolic volume (myocardial infarction [MI], heart failure, valvular disease, systemic or pulmonary hypertension)	Ventricular hypertrophy with a decrease in ventricular compliance (coronary artery disease, systemic hypertension, cardiomyopathy, aortic or pulmonary stenosis, increase in intensity with acute MI or angina)
Hyperdynamic states (anemia, thyrotoxicosis, mitral or tricuspid regurgitation)	Hyperkinetic states (anemia, thyrotoxicosis, arteriovenous fistula) Acute valvular regurgitation
Rhythmic Word Association	
Ken-tuc-ky (S_1 S_2 S_3)	Tenn-essee (S_4 S_1 S_2)
Synonyms	
Ventricular gallop	Atrial gallop
Protodiastolic gallop	Presystolic gallop

From Urden LD, Stacy KM, Lough ME: *Thelan's critical care nursing: diagnosis and management,* ed 5, St. Louis, 2006, Mosby.

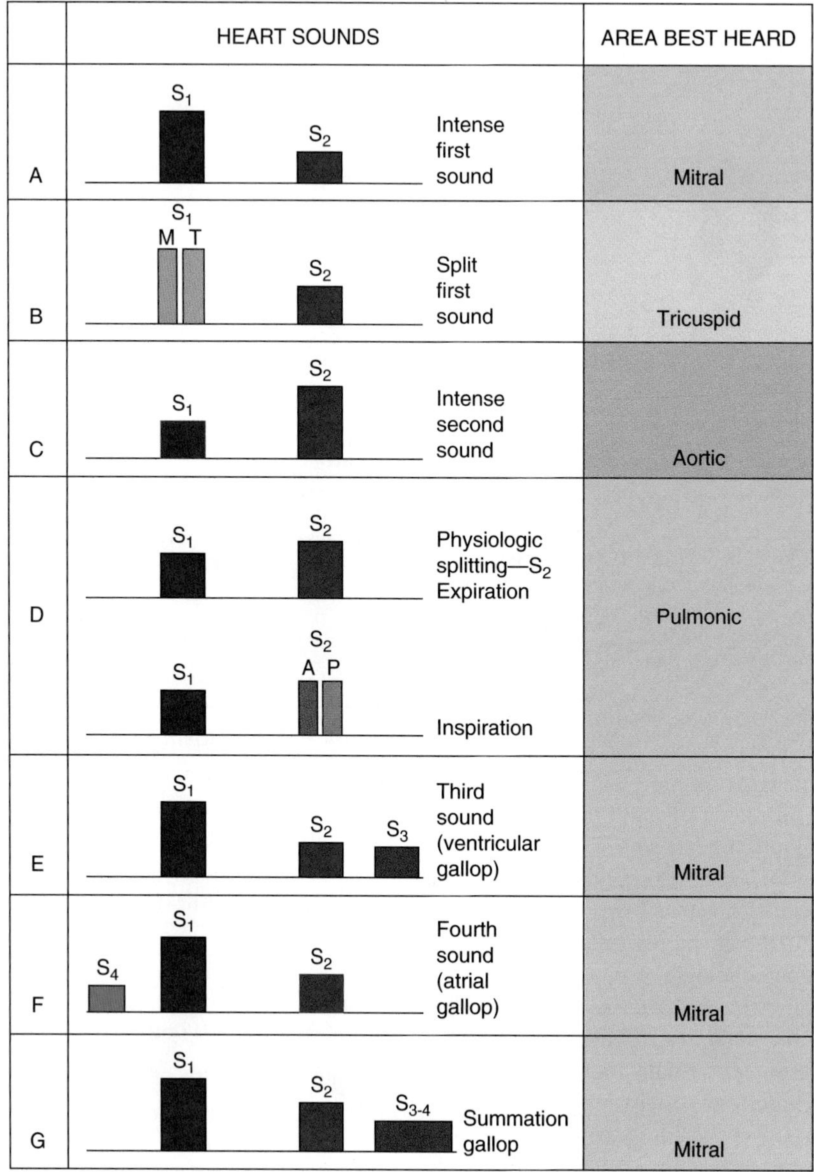

Figure 4-17

Characteristics of normal and abnormal heart sounds and the auscultatory area where each is best heard. (From Urden LD, Stacy KM, Lough ME: *Thelan's critical care nursing: diagnosis and management*, ed 5, St. Louis, 2006, Mosby.)

S_1 to S_4 are considered the most basic heart sounds that can be auscultated during a patient examination. However, other sounds also may be heard, such as clicks, snaps, friction rub, prosthetic sounds, and murmurs. *Clicks,* which are high-pitched sounds that occur after S_1, are best heard over the aortic and pulmonic areas of the heart. Clicks indicate an aortic valve that opens stiffly or mitral valve prolapse. Like clicks, *snaps* are high pitched. They are associated with opening of the mitral valve and are best heard over the left sternal border; snaps signify mitral stenosis. *Prosthetic sounds* are metallic or mechanical in nature. A prosthetic sound is heard during both opening and closing of the affected valve. A *friction rub* is generated when two layers of the pericardium rub against each other, causing a sound that has been described as two pieces of leather rubbed together, creaking, scratching, or even two balloons rubbed against each other. A friction rub is best heard with the diaphragm of the stethoscope when the patient leans forward.

Heart Murmurs

Heart murmurs (Box 4-4) are adventitious sounds created by a turbulent blood flow through the heart and its valves and associated vessels. Heart murmurs are categorized as *innocent* or *pathologic* murmurs, depending on the patient's presentation and the possible causes. Innocent murmurs are heard as faint, intermittent sounds over the affected valve. About 30% to 50% of children have an innocent murmur that resolves in adulthood. Innocent murmurs do not impair heart function and produce no outward symptoms. They typically are temporary and are caused by an increase in blood flow that can

Box 4-4 Description of Heart Murmurs

- Always systolic
- Soft, short (grade I or grade II, low pitched)
- Modified by change in position
- Normal S_2
- Most common at left sternal border

From Urden LD, Stacy KM, Lough ME: *Thelan's critical care nursing: diagnosis and management,* ed 5, St. Louis, 2006, Mosby.

be directly linked to pregnancy, fever, hyperthyroidism, or anemia.

Pathologic murmurs result from structural abnormalities of the heart and its great vessels. These abnormalities can be congenital in nature, such as a baby born with a hole in the heart or with valvular abnormalities. Structural abnormalities also may occur as a result of specific disorders that can damage the heart or valves, such as rheumatic fever, endocarditis (which causes inflammation of the inner heart lining and the related valves), and valve calcification, which occurs with aging. Patients with pathologic murmurs may have overt symptoms, such as shortness of breath, cyanosis, chest pain, dizziness, and changes in growth patterns (children with congenital defects).

Determining whether a pathologic condition exists on the basis of benign murmurs is difficult. The best practice is simply to describe what you hear in your report.

Heart murmurs are classified based on specific findings, such as when, where, what. and how.

When (Timing)

When in the cardiac cycle does the murmur occur? A systolic murmur occurs while the heart is in the contraction phase. A diastolic murmur occurs while the heart is at rest and is filling. A murmur heard throughout the entire cardiac cycle is a continuous murmur.

Where (Location)

Where on the chest is the murmur best heard? The systematic approach to auscultation ensures that you listen to the aortic, pulmonic, mitral, and tricuspid areas of the heart. The location where the murmur is heard best indicates the valve or heart chamber affected.

What (Quality/Pitch)

What does the murmur sound like? The sounds of various murmurs can be described in several ways; the most common are harsh, blowing, rumbling, and machinery-like. Describing the sounds as high, medium, or low pitched also is helpful.

How (Intensity)

How easily can the murmur be heard? Murmurs are graded by intensity on a scale of I to VI (Box 4-5) and documented accordingly (Table 4-4).

Box 4-5 Grading of Cardiac Murmurs

I/VI	Very faint; may be heard only in a quiet environment
II/VI	Quiet but clearly audible
III/VI	Moderately loud
IV/VI	Loud; may be associated with a palpable **thrill**
V/VI	Very loud; thrill easily palpable
VI/VI	Very loud; may be heard with stethoscope off the chest; thrill palpable and visible

From Urden LD, Stacy KM, Lough ME: *Thelan's critical care nursing: diagnosis and management,* ed 5, St. Louis, 2006, Mosby.

Did You Know?

In medical terms, a *thrill* is a sensation of vibration felt during the examination of a patient.[5]

The critical care paramedic should practice listening to heart sounds on all patients so as to learn to identify abnormal findings and associate them with potential causes. This is the same approach as listening to breath sounds to learn to differentiate between the normal and the abnormal. The CD with this text presents some normal and abnormal heart sounds.

Laboratory Analysis and Abnormalities in the Cardiac Patient

Electrolytes

The systemic effect of electrolytes on the body is homeostatic, and any derangement can affect many systems (see Chapter 6). Four cations affect contractility and conduction in the heart: potassium, calcium, magnesium, and sodium.

1. **Potassium (K+):** The movement of potassium across the cell membrane in the heart determines conduction. The normal serum potassium level is 3.5 to 4.5 mEq/L. Any alteration in this level can alter myocardial function.
    - *Hyperkalemia:* Hyperkalemia can be caused by many factors, such as renal failure and certain medications (e.g., angiotensin-converting enzyme [ACE] inhibitors, angiotensin receptor blockers [ARBs], and potassium-sparing diuretics). A high potassium level reduces the rate of ventricular depolarization, shortens repolarization, and depresses AV conduction. When the potassium level rises above 5.5 mEq/L, ECG changes are seen (Figure 4-18 and Box 4-6). (The treatment of this condition is described in Chapter 6.)
    - *Hypokalemia:* Usually caused by GI loss, diuretic therapy or chronic steroid therapy, a low potassium also distorts conduction by prolonging repolarization of the ventricles. A prominent U wave or PVCs of unknown etiology, along with prolonged Q-T interval might be a signal on a multi-lead ECG to warrant a lab analysis of the K+ level (Figure 4-19). (Potassium replacement therapy is described in Chapter 2.)

Table 4-4 Characteristics of Selected Heart Murmurs

Defects	Timing in the Cardiac Cycle	Pitch, Intensity, Quality	Location, Radiation
Systolic Murmurs			
Mitral regurgitation	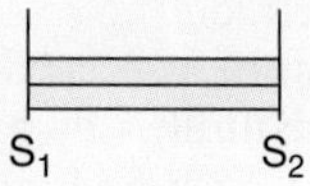 S_1 S_2	High Harsh Blowing	Mitral area May radiate to axilla
Tricuspid regurgitation	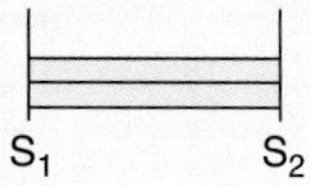 S_1 S_2	High Often faint but varies Blowing	Tricuspid RLSB, apex, LLSB, epigastric areas Little radiation
Ventricular septal defect	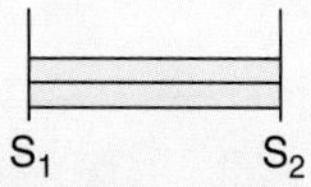 S_1 S_2	High Loud Blowing	Left sternal border
Aortic stenosis	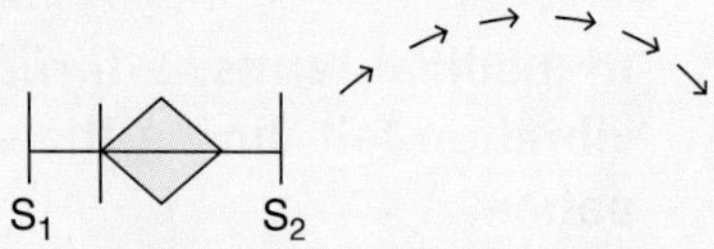 S_1 S_2	Chhhh hh Medium Rough, harsh	Aortic area to suprasternal notch, right side of neck, apex
Pulmonary stenosis	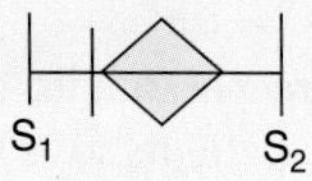 S_1 S_2	Low to medium Loud Harsh, grinding	Pulmonic area No radiation
Diastolic Murmurs*			
Mitral stenosis	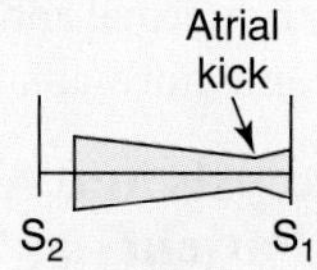 Atrial kick S_2 S_1	Low Quiet to loud with thrill Rough rumble	Mitral area Usually no radiation
Tricuspid stenosis	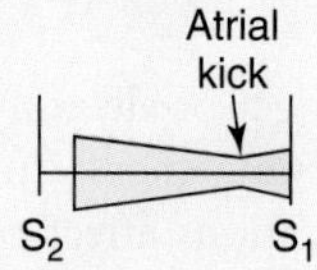 Atrial kick S_2 S_1	Medium Quiet; louder with inspiration Rumble	Tricuspid area or epigastrium Little radiation
Aortic regurgitation	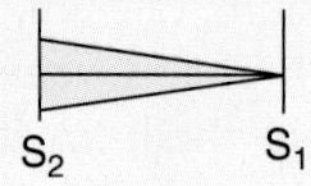 S_2 S_1	High Faint to medium Blowing	Aortic area to LLSB and aorta Erb's point (2-3 cm above clavicle at C-6, posterior border of sternocleidomastoid)
Pulmonic regurgitation	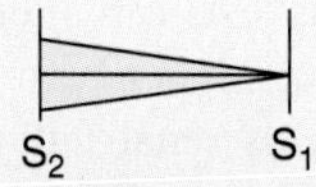 S_2 S_1	Medium Faint Blowing	Pulmonic area No radiation

From Urden LD, Stacy KM, Lough ME: *Thelan's critical care nursing: diagnosis and management,* ed 5, St. Louis, 2006, Mosby.
RLSB, Right lower sternal border; *LLSB,* left lower sternal border.
**Atrial kick* is a synonym for atrial contraction.

2. **Calcium (Ca++):** The parathyroid gland, along with the kidneys, bone, and GI tract, contribute to normal serum calcium levels. You may note two laboratory values for calcium: ionized calcium and total calcium.
   - *Ionized calcium (physiologically active calcium):* This is the preferred laboratory value, because it reflects the calcium available to the body (i.e., that is not bound to proteins). In the United States, a normal level is 4 to 5 mg/dL; in other countries, where this value is expressed in millimoles per liter (mmol/L), a normal level is 1 to 1.3 mmol/L.
   - *Total calcium:* This is a mathematically calculated value that is related to the serum albumin level. A normal level in the United States is 8.5 to 10.5 mg/dL (2 to 2.6 mmol/L elsewhere).
   - *Hypercalcemia:* An elevated calcium level can be caused by bone tumors, parathyroid disease, excessive calcium intake, and a low magnesium level. Hypercalcemia

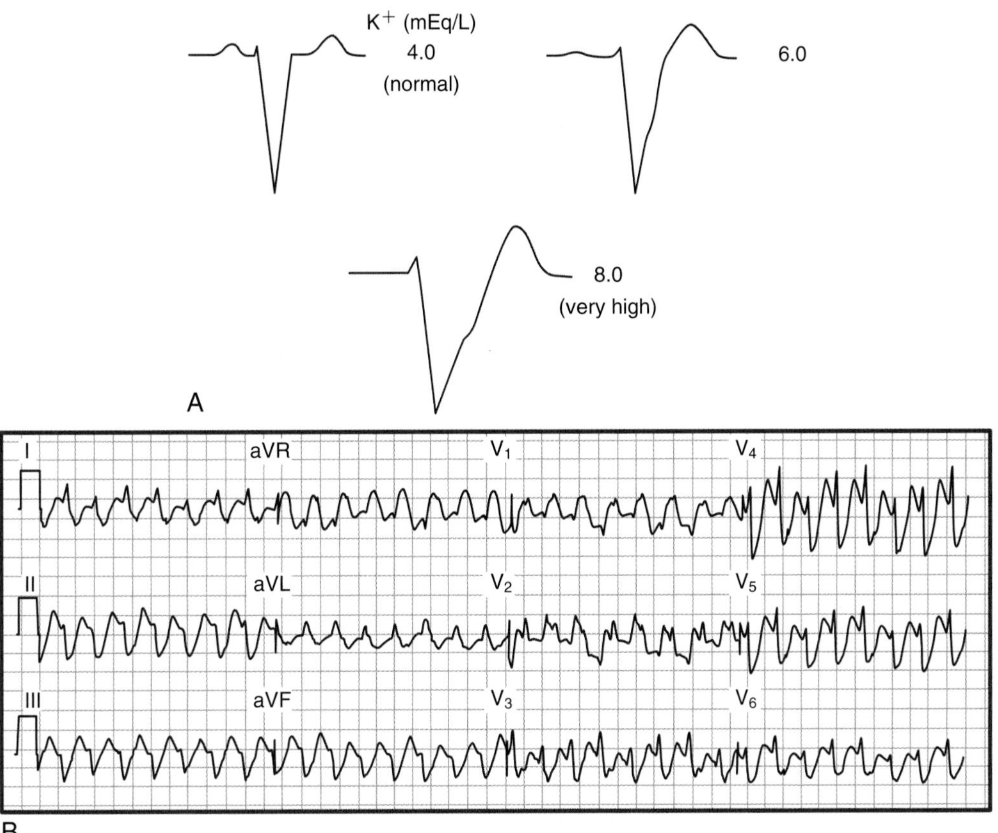

Figure 4-18

Effects of hyperkalemia. **A,** Stages of hyperkalemia, from normal potassium levels to plasma levels (measured in mEq/L). At approximately 6 mEq/L, the P wave flattens, the QRS complex broadens, and the ST segment disappears; also, the S wave flows into the tall, tented T wave. **B,** 12-Lead ECG of a patient with a serum potassium level of 9.1 mEq/L. (From Urden LD, Stacy KM, Lough ME: *Thelan's critical care nursing: diagnosis and management,* ed 5, St. Louis, 2006, Mosby.)

Box 4-6 Electrocardiographic (ECG) Changes Associated with Hyperkalemia

Serum Potassium Level	Possible ECG Changes
5.5-6.5 mEq/L	Peaked T waves, increasing PR interval
6.5-7.5 mEq/L	Flattened P waves and ST segments; wide QRS complex
7.5-8 mEq/L	Deep S wave, S-T wave merging
>8 mEq/L	Sine-wave QRS, idioventricular, ventricular tachycardia (VT)–like appearance

From Field JM: *American Heart Association ACLS resource text: professional for instructors and experienced providers,* 2008, The Association.

shortens repolarization in the ventricles and strengthens the contraction of the cardiac muscle. On an ECG, it is reflected by a shortened Q-T interval and AV or bundle branch blocks. IV fluid infusions and diuretic therapy can facilitate the excretion of calcium.

- *Hypocalcemia:* As many as 88% of patients in ICUs suffer from this common electrolyte derangement.[1] In the sickest patients, this usually can be caused by massive blood transfusions (**chelation** by citrate in blood products) or alkalosis. A low level of ionized calcium results in decreased contractility and cardiac output and can cause hypotension. Arrhythmias and ECG changes noted include bradycardia, ventricular tachycardia, and asystole. Most important, a low calcium level can prolong the Q-T interval and initiate torsades de pointes. Treatment is geared toward replacement with either calcium chloride or calcium gluconate.

3. **Magnesium (Mg++):** An integral electrolyte, magnesium plays a vital role in enzymatic reactions and energy production. It is stored in bone, muscle, and tissue. A normal level (with laboratory variances) is 1.5 to 2 mEq/L, 1.8 to 2.4 mg/dL, or 0.7 to 1.1 mmol/L.
   - *Hypermagnesemia:* This condition is rare but can occur with renal failure, overtreatment with magnesium, or tumor lysis syndrome.
   - *Hypomagnesemia:* This derangement is most commonly associated with other electrolyte imbalances, including those of potassium and calcium. Most important, hypomagnesemia causes a long Q-T interval and can

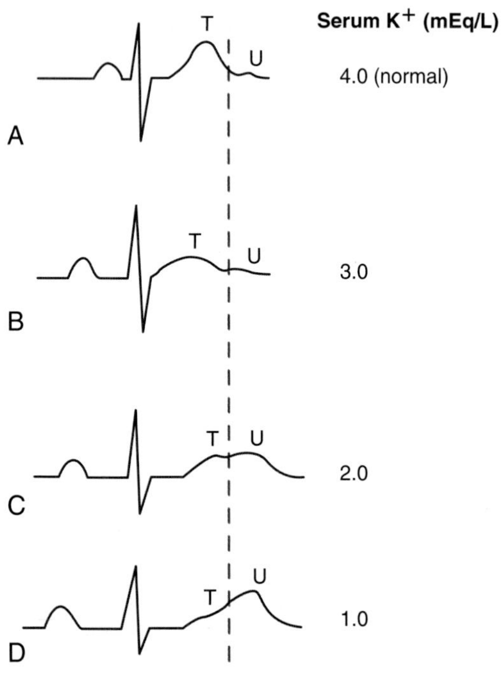

Figure 4-19

Hypokalemia. **A,** At a normal serum potassium concentration of 3.5 to 4.5 mEq/L, the amplitude of the T wave is appreciably greater than that of the U wave. **B,** By the time the serum potassium level has dropped to 3 mEq/L, the amplitudes of the T and U waves are approaching each other. **C** and **D,** With a further drop in the level of potassium, the U wave begins to tower over and fuse with the T wave. **E,** ECG tracing from a patient with a serum potassium level of 2.6 mEq/L, showing a prominent U wave. (From Urden LD, Stacy KM, Lough ME: *Thelan's critical care nursing: diagnosis and management*, ed 5, St. Louis, 2006, Mosby.)

predispose the patient to torsades de pointes. In most cases, the magnesium level must be corrected before or along with potassium or calcium replacement therapy. Hypomagnesemia can be caused by a low intake of magnesium, chronic alcohol abuse, GI loss, or use of diuretics. As with calcium, chelation by blood products can deplete magnesium. Clinically, the patient may be hypertensive and have coronary artery vasospasm, and the person is at risk of sudden death and acute myocardial infarction (AMI). The ECG changes seen with hypomagnesemia are similar to those for hypokalemia. The treatment of hypokalemia and hypocalcemia begins with magnesium replacement. IV magnesium sulfate must be given with caution to patients in renal failure.

4. **Sodium (Na+):** The chief cation and most abundant of the extracellular (ECF) body fluids, sodium is primarily responsible for shifts in body water and water levels through renal function. In the heart, sodium plays a role in the transmission of nerve impulses through the sodium pump or active transport mechanism. A normal serum value is 135 to 145 mEq/L. The large differences between the levels of sodium, potassium, and calcium, with subsequent movement, create a chemical and electrical gradient that determines the resting membrane and action potential of myocardial cells.
   - *Hyponatremia:* This condition can occur because of a net gain of water or a loss of sodium-rich fluids that are replaced by water. Typically associated with hypo-osmolality, hyponatremia is a common condition in hospitalized patients. The clinical presentation and treatment of the disorder depend on the speed of onset and the cause. The condition may be associated with a patient who has a normal, a decreased, or an increased ECF volume.
   - *Hypernatremia:* This condition may occur with water loss, water deprivation, or (in rare cases) sodium gain. In a healthy patient, thirst is the chief defense against hypernatremia; therefore, water loss or water deprivation is the primary cause of this disorder. The ability to concentrate the urine through increases in antidiuretic hormone (ADH) also helps prevent the condition. Hypernatremia causes hypertonicity and a shift of water out of the cells, which may result in central nervous system (CNS) symptoms.

Cardiac Biomarkers

Traditionally, laboratory evaluation of cardiac events has measured the "cardiac enzymes," because these tests focused on the liver enzymes released with muscle injury. More modern laboratory analysis involves cardiac-specific and non-specific laboratory values (biomarkers) that help define injury to the cardiac muscle in certain time frames. These biomarkers include creatinine kinase (and myocardial-bound creatinine kinase), troponins, lactate dehydrogenase, and myoglobin.

1. *Creatinine kinase* (CK) is a nonspecific biomarker of muscle damage in the body. It rises in response to myocardial damage a few hours after injury and returns to normal within 2 to 4 days. Normal levels are 55 to 170 units/L in males and 30 to 135 units/L in females. Three isoenzymes are specific to certain tissue: CK-M (creatinine kinase, muscle type); CK-B (creatinine kinase, brain type): and CK-MB (creatine kinase, myocardial bound), which is found in cardiac muscle.
   - *CK-MB* (CK2): Serum levels of CK-MB rise 4 to 8 hours after an MI, peak in 15 to 24 hours, and begin to fall in 2 to 3 days. A normal value for CK-MB is one that is less than 5% of total creatinine kinase (CK) activity. The normal level ranges from zero to 3.9%.
2. *Lactate dehydrogenase* (LDH): An enzyme that occurs in the cytoplasm of nearly all cells. It has muscle and heart-specific subunits; it exists as five distinct isozymes and is used for clinical diagnosis. An elevation of the LDH will be elevated days after an acute myocardial infarction. Because of this delay, troponins have essentially replaced the LDH as a cardiac enzyme. Normal serum levels are 50-150 Units/Liter.
3. *Troponins:* A troponin is a globular muscle protein. Two biomarkers are evaluated in patients with acute coronary

syndromes (ACCs): troponin I (TnI), which is found only in cardiac muscle, and troponin T (TnT), found in both cardiac and skeletal muscle. Both TnI and TnT can be used to determine myocardial muscle damage; they are the second, but most reliable and specific, biomarkers to show elevation after a cardiac event. Even then, the time to elevation ranges from 3 to 12 hours; the levels peak at 12 to 48 hours and normalize within 5 to 14 days. A normal TnI is 0.05 to 0.50 ng/mL. Elevated troponins have been seen in patients with decompensated heart failure, myocarditis, and those with rejection of transplanted hearts. Elevated levels also may be seen with renal failure and in severe sepsis. Some elevation may be detected in patients with syncopal events or prolonged tachydysrhythmias, especially with left ventricular hypertrophy (LVH).

4. *Myoglobin:* Myoglobin also is considered a nonspecific biomarker, because it is released if cardiac or skeletal muscle is damaged. This is the first biomarker to rise after an AMI (within 1 to 2 hours), and it returns to baseline in 24 hours. A normal value is 6 to 85 ng/mL. Some clinicians now consider the troponins, rather than myoglobin, to be the gold standard laboratory value.

Hematology Laboratory Studies

A number of hematology tests frequently are performed in critical care patients.

1. **Complete blood count (CBC):** This set of tests includes the hemoglobin and hematocrit values; white blood cell (WBC) and red blood cell (RBC) counts with differentials; and platelets. The CBC is used to help rule in or out differential diagnoses for ICU patients, including anemia, polycythemia, blood dyscrasias, and infection.
2. **Coagulation studies:** A generic evaluation of the effectiveness of blood clotting, this panel of tests may include the prothrombin time, the international normalized ratio, the partial thromboplastin time, and the coagulation time. A D-dimer test (fragment D-dimer or fibrin degradation fragment) also may be ordered to determine whether a clot has formed.
   - *Prothrombin time* (PT): The PT is rarely tested or reported by itself. Once the mainstay of warfarin therapy evaluation, it now is reported with the international normalized ratio (INR). The PT is a measure of the conversion of platelet factor II to its active form (thrombin) by factor X. Each laboratory has its own normal value for the PT test. The INR was developed to standardize the PT evaluation and is now used to guide warfarin therapy; a normal value is <1 (Box 4-7).
   - *Partial thromboplastin time (PTT) or activated PTT* (aPTT): The aPTT, which gauges the activity of thromboplastin (Factor III), measures the time required for blood to clot. It is used to evaluate the effectiveness of heparin (regular) therapy (however, it does not evaluate low-molecular-weight heparin therapy). A normal aPTT value is about 21 to 35 seconds. The goal with heparin therapy is an aPTT 1.5 to 2.5 times normal.

Box 4-7 Therapeutic Use of Warfarin (Coumadin)

INR	Condition Treated	Treatment
2-3	VTE, DVT, PE	None; appropriate level
2.5-3.5	Mechanical heart valve	None; appropriate level
3-5	Elevation	Hold warfarin
5-9	Elevation	Hold warfarin; give vitamin K
>9	Elevation	Give vitamin K, FFP

From Urden LD, Stacy KM, Lough ME: *Thelan's critical care nursing: diagnosis and management,* ed 5, 2006, Mosby.
DVT, Deep vein thrombosis; *FFP,* fresh frozen plasma; *INR,* international normalized ratio (prothrombin time); *PE,* pulmonary embolism; *VTE,* venous thromboembolism.

   - *Coagulation time:* Now called the *activated coagulation time* (ACT), this laboratory test is another means of evaluating heparin therapy. A normal value is 0 to 120 seconds. The goal with heparin therapy is an ACT of 150 to 300 seconds.
   - *D-dimer:* This test is also known as *fibrin degradation products* (FDP). An elevated D-dimer value indicates that fibrin degradation is occurring and that a thrombus has formed. An elevated D-dimer also is seen in the elderly, in patients who recently have had surgery, and in those with trauma, infection, liver disease, pregnancy, eclampsia, heart disease, and some cancers. However, the D-dimer should not be used as the only test to diagnose clotting disorders. A false-negative D-dimer result occurs in individuals on anticoagulant therapy.

Miscellaneous Laboratory Tests for the Cardiac Patient

Lipid studies and the glucose level, thyroid hormone level, blood urea nitrogen (BUN), creatinine, and liver enzymes also may be evaluated in critical care patients. The lipid levels help the clinician establish a treatment plan for the patient after a cardiac event to reduce cardiovascular risks. An elevated glucose level can result in numerous complications in any patient, but especially in individuals with diabetes mellitus. The most recent recommendations from the American College of Endocrinology state that the blood glucose level should be tightly maintained below 110 mg/dL. Elevated levels of the thyroid hormones triiodothyronine (T_3) and thyroxine (T_4) may aid diagnosis of hyperdynamic or hypodynamic presentations. Detection of renal dysfunction with the BUN and creatinine levels helps guide overall therapy, and liver enzyme levels may help detect liver ailments and right-sided heart failure.

Radiographic, Ultrasound, and MRI Examinations

Clinicians obtain as much information as possible to refine their list of differential diagnoses for patients with cardiovascular complaints. Often this includes a trip to the radiology department for invasive or noninvasive studies, with or without a special contrast dye or radionuclide chemicals to enhance imaging. As you depart for critical care transport of such patients, the departing hospital will provide you with various data that serve as evidence for the diagnosis. In addition, your knowledge of the results of some of these diagnostic examinations, as well as the attendant medications and their side effects, facilitates good patient care en route.

Chest Radiography

The chest radiograph is a relatively old but still reliable method of evaluating a patient with many presentations, including cardiovascular problems. The standard chest radiograph includes two views: the posterior-anterior (PA) view, in which the x-ray beam passes from posterior to anterior, and the lateral view (side to side). When a portable radiograph unit is used at the bedside, only an anterior-posterior (AP) view is obtained.

The following is a review of the standard interpretation of a chest radiograph by a nonclinician. As you know, all radiographs must be interpreted by the physician. However, members of the critical care transport team may use the chest radiograph to help determine the major pathologic condition or to verify the position of a tube or catheter.

As you know, an x-ray beam travels through the chest to the film plate (now commonly placed digitally), and different tissues absorb the beam to varying degrees. Bone appears white; dense tissue (e.g., the heart, lung tissue, and blood) appears gray; and air-filled lungs appear black. To examine a structure, look at the borders and the symmetry of the structure. Also, make sure to check the following elements.

1. The radiograph must be identified with the correct patient name and numbers.
2. The chest radiograph must correlate with the physical findings or clinical presentation.
3. *Trachea and bronchi:* Follow the borders of the upper and lower airways as they proceed inferiorly to the bronchioles. Look for signs of leakage of pleural air outside that border (black leaks into the gray or white tissues), which may indicate lacerations to the tissues.
4. *Pleural space:* Check for the following:
   a. Accumulation of fluid inferiorly
   b. Accumulation of air (black) without vascular markings (black with no gray blood vessels seen)
5. *Lung parenchyma:* May show signs of contusion (patchy, irregular air space consolidation) or laceration (hematoma consolidation).
6. *Mediastinum:* Leakage of air or blood into this space makes the outline appear out of focus or blurred. With pneumomediastinum, a **radiolucent** line outlines the structures of the area. Pneumopericardium manifests as a white line (radiopaque) surrounding the heart.
   a. Cardiac silhouette: Air or blood in the pericardium creates a blackness (lucency) around the heart, and the heart itself is enlarged.

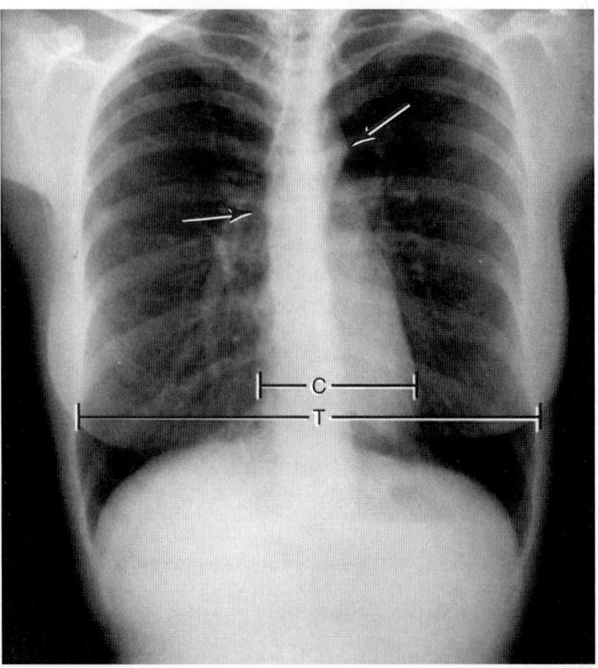

Figure 4-20

The cardiothoracic (CT) ratio is a technique for estimating heart size from a posterior-anterior (PA) chest radiograph. Normally the cardiac diameter is 50% or less of the thoracic diameter when measured during full inhalation. The width of the vascular pedicle *(arrows)* is a more accurate indicator of systemic blood volume. *C,* Maximum cardiac diameter; *T,* maximum thoracic diameter measured to the inside of the ribs. (From Urden LD, Stacy KM, Lough ME: *Thelan's critical care nursing: diagnosis and management,* ed 5, St. Louis, 2006, Mosby.)

   b. Determining normal heart size: The cardiothoracic ratio is used to determine the heart size on a chest radiograph. Normally the heart is less than one-third the diameter of the chest (Figure 4-20).
   c. Aortic disruption: In the mediastinum, injury or disease of the major vessels may distort the normal appearance. Specific criteria are used to determine whether aortic rupture has occurred; these include a widened mediastinum (greater than 8 cm at the level of the aortic arch), loss of a clear outline of the aortic knob, a depressed left mainstem bronchus, deviation of the trachea to the right, left hemothorax, fractures of the first or second rib or scapula, and deviation of a nasogastric (NG) tube to the right.
   NOTE: The chest radiograph is normal in as many as 20% of patients with an aortic dissection (Figure 4-21).
7. *Diaphragm:*
   a. Elevation of the diaphragm during full expiration (abnormal if it rises to the fourth intercostal space) may indicate a pathologic condition of the abdomen.
   b. Disruption has occurred if bowel loops or the stomach is noted (usually on the left) in the thoracic cavity.
8. *Bones of the thorax:* Look for fractures by examining the outline of each bone and compare for symmetry. Examine the scapulae, ribs, and sternum.

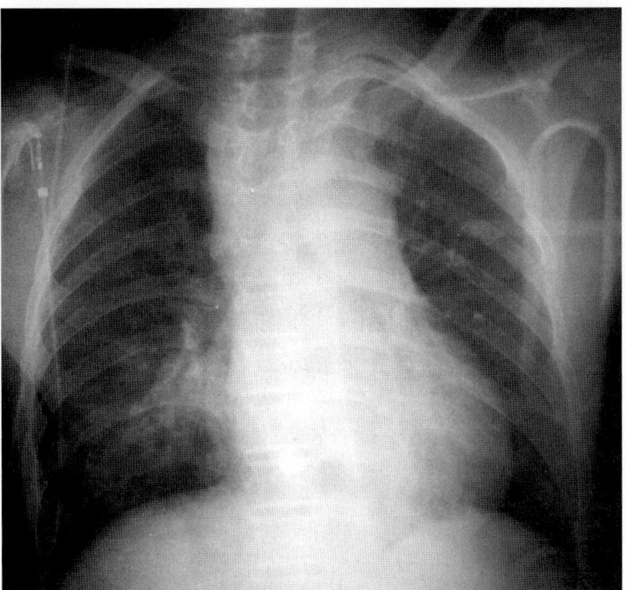

Figure 4-21

Chest radiograph from a patient with a posttraumatic aortic rupture and mediastinal hematoma. Note the widened mediastinum, the filling in of the aortopulmonary bay, and the development of a left apical pleural cap. (Courtesy Dr. L. C. Morus, Birmingham, UK.)

9. *Soft tissues:* Look for subcutaneous air
10. *Tubes and lines:* A chest radiograph should be obtained after insertion of all thoracic tubes.
    a. Central venous catheter: This appears as a radiopaque tube that extends from the insertion site to positioning of the tip at the superior vena cava (i.e., at the entrance to the right atrium but not in the right atrium).
    b. Pulmonary artery catheter (PAC): The chest radiograph verifies the location of the PAC and detects any complications (e.g., pneumothorax). The tip of the PAC must be positioned about 2 cm from the hilar point of the lung so that an accurate measurement can be obtained when the cuff is inflated and the tip is wedged.
    c. Endotracheal tube (ETT): The chest radiograph is one of eight methods of ensuring correct placement of the ETT. No one method is 100% accurate. A major advantage of the chest radiograph is that the depth of placement in relation to the glottis can be determined. Normal placement is 2 cm above the carina or between the clavicle heads.
    d. Enteric tube: The position of small-bore gastric tubes must be verified by chest radiography, particularly before any tube feeding is administered, because these tubes migrate easily toward the airways. The tube should be coiled in the stomach bubble, or at least the tip should be within the stomach itself.
    e. Chest tube: As are most tubes (e.g., ETTs, many gastric tubes, and thoracostomy tubes), chest tubes are manufactured with a radiopaque line so that locating the tube radiographically is easier. The tip of a chest tube intended for a pneumothorax or hemothorax should lie in the pleural space or cavity. After cardiac surgery, mediastinal tubes or drains typically are placed more anteriorly (i.e., the tip should rest in the mediastinum). In addition, each side port on a chest tube is radiopaque; make sure all ports are within the thorax to prevent air leakage.
    f. Intraaortic balloon pump (IABP): This device usually is inserted into the femoral artery and passed up through the descending aorta. A chest radiograph is obtained immediately after insertion and repeated if any migration may have occurred. The distal tip, which has a radiopaque marker, should be noted below the subclavian artery (just below the aortic arch).
    g. Pacemaker or implantable cardioverter defibrillator (ICD): These devices may be visualized on a chest radiograph. If the device is permanent, the entire system is seen. If it is temporary, the radiopaque wires, but not the generator, may be seen on the radiograph. Pacing wires generally are attached to the right side of the heart; however, patients with heart failure have a left ventricular wire in addition to the pacing wires.

To summarize, for a patient with a cardiovascular condition, systematically examine the chest radiograph for pathologic conditions by looking for the following:

1. *Heart size:* The normal heart is less than one third the width of the chest. The heart may be enlarged by cardiomyopathy, hypertrophy, and heart failure.
2. *Pulmonary edema:* With pulmonary edema, white, dense, cloudy areas that resemble bat wings are seen near the hilar area (pulmonary vessels). As the edema progresses, a patchy, white appearance is seen throughout the lungs. In acute respiratory distress syndrome (ARDS), the edema is distributed randomly throughout the lungs.
3. *Pneumonia:* A dense, white area (opacity) should be evaluated for pneumonia.
4. *Pneumothorax:* The two pleural layers should not demonstrate a space. The pleurae are considered part of the lungs and should not be visible. As the pleural space develops, the edge of the pleura can be seen as it traps air (black). Remember that air is also black; however, the air in the lungs should have little routes of gray vascular markings within it. The trapped air of a pneumothorax is completely black. The collapsed lung appears as a dense gray or white area below the bronchi; this is called a *pleural line.* The pleural line is created when displacement of the visceral pleura causes it to cover the lung, a development that occurs when air pushes the visceral pleura away from the parietal pleura, which covers the inside of the chest wall.

As a tension pneumothorax develops, mediastinal and airway structures are shifted away from the pressure. Remember, a chest radiograph should never be used to diagnose a tension pneumothorax; this should be diagnosed clinically because of the time required to obtain a chest radiograph.

Digital Radiographs

Nearly all radiographs are stored as images for projection onto a computer screen or printer. For patients being transferred, the radiology department usually saves radiographs on a CD or DVD that must accompany the patient to the receiving hospital.

Echocardiography

Echocardiography is a diagnostic examination of the heart's tissues and blood flow in which ultrasound waves are used to display the images. These images can be obtained by a number of methods: transthoracic, two dimensional (2D), phonocardiography, color flow Doppler, stress echo, and transesophageal, to name a few. Cardiac anomalies such as valve disease, stenosis, septal defects, an enlarged heart or hypertrophy, aortic disease, and effusions can be detected. The Doppler blood flow ultrasound study maps images of the heart and assesses for regurgitation (valve disease) and septal defects with ECG signals superimposed. The **ejection fraction** also can be determined with this diagnostic tool. Trauma assessment using ultrasound (known as *focused abdominal sonography in trauma* [FAST]) allows evaluation of the heart motion and pericardial sac.

Transthoracic Echocardiography

For transthoracic echocardiography (TTE), the lubricated transducer is placed in the third or fourth intercostal space, just to the left of the sternum, where the pericardium is in direct contact with the chest wall. If this standard location cannot achieve the desired ultrasonic picture, the clinician may change the patient's position or the position of the transducer.

Motion-Mode Transthoracic Echocardiography

Motion-mode echocardiography (M-mode TTE) maps dots as the ultrasound picks up the heart's silhouette. These dots are placed on oscilloscope paper so that they can be graphed to time. This technique is useful for looking for pericardial tamponade or effusion (Figure 4-22).

Two-Dimensional Echocardiography

Piezoelectric crystal is the active element in the ultrasound transducer that transforms the electrical energy sensed into mechanical or sound energy. In 2D echocardiography, the beam penetrates completely through the heart in a slice, demonstrating anatomic structures in relation to each other as the heart moves blood. This is particularly helpful for diagnosing wall motion abnormalities and left ventricular (LV) volume.

Phonocardiography

Phonocardiography is used to evaluate valve function. The transducer is placed on the thoracic wall to record heart sounds while the ultrasonic beam simultaneously registers heart motion. This is simply an echocardiogram with heart sounds.

Color Flow Doppler Echocardiography

Color flow Doppler echocardiography is 2D echocardiography in a color-coded format that assesses blood flow through Doppler sound waves or pulsations. This shows the speed and direction of blood flow during heart motion; one color reflects flow away from the transducer, and another color demonstrates flow toward the transducer. The brightness of the color reflects the speed of flow. This mode is particularly helpful for evaluating cardiac output and flow and for assessing for valve dysfunction.

Transesophageal Echocardiography

In transesophageal echocardiography (TEE), the transducer is mounted on a tube similar to an endoscope and inserted through the esophagus, allowing the examiner to view the heart as closely as possible. Intracardiac structures and the thoracic aorta can be seen in more detail, because the electron beam does not have to travel through skin and bone. As does any endoscopic examination, this technique requires patient preparation. Those monitoring the patient during the procedure must be vigilant about the conscious sedation practices of the hospital and must watch for vasovagal responses, which are typical for this area.

Stress Echocardiography

Viewing the heart through an echocardiogram while the patient exercises or receives a drug (usually dobutamine) to increase myocardial oxygen consumption can be helpful for diagnosing stable angina or for determining the damage caused by an MI, specifically wall motion abnormalities (which imply dead myocardium). The "stress" part of this procedure is similar to ECG stress testing.

Intravascular Ultrasound (IVUS) and Intracardiac Ultrasound

When the coronary vessels are viewed in the cardiac catheterization laboratory, a miniature ultrasound catheter can be sent to the site to view the interior of the artery or to determine whether a stent is working. Flexible ultrasound catheters also can be directed internally to the chambers of the heart.

Coronary Computed Tomography Angiography

Coronary computed tomography angiography (CTA) is a specially adapted CT imaging study that can be used to evaluate the coronary arteries for disease without requiring the use of the surgical cardiac catheterization laboratory. CTA may be used to help determine whether the patient should undergo revascularization with stents. Before the procedure, a beta blocker is given to lower the heart rate below 65 beats/min to reduce motion artifact. A contrast medium may be used to assess the amount of calcium (calcium scoring) present.

Magnetic Resonance Imaging

Magnetic resonance imaging (MRI) has been recognized as less hazardous than ionizing radiation (which is used for radiographs and CT studies), and it also provides more detailed images. MRI can be used to help diagnose many

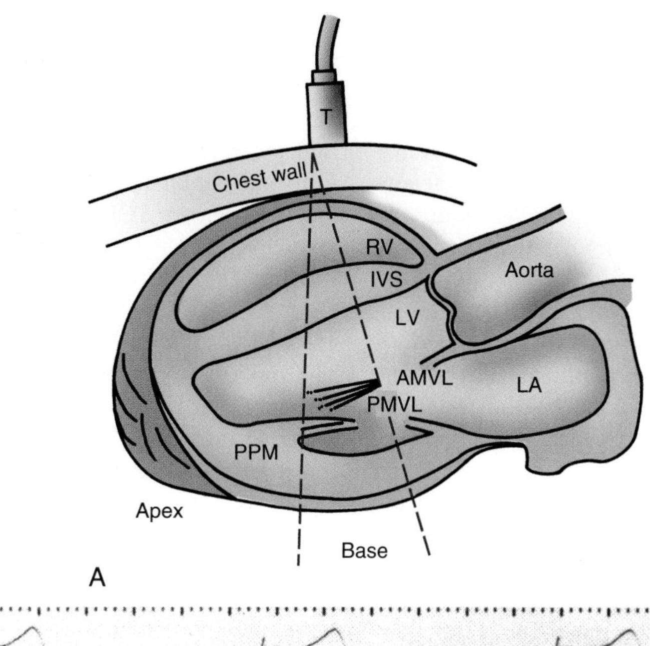

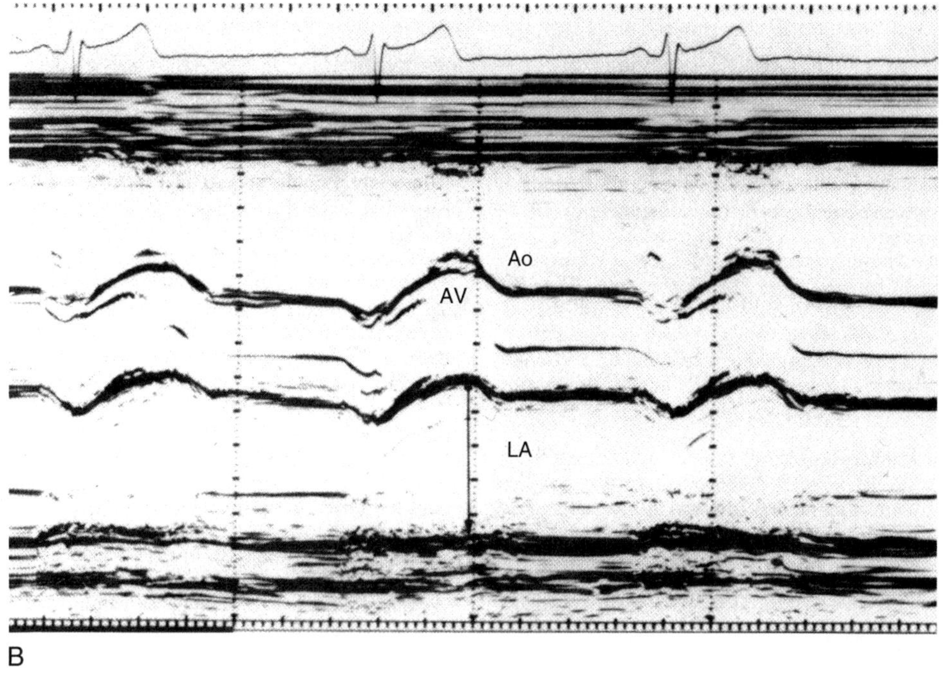

Figure 4-22

A, Schematic of cardiac structures traversed by two echo beams. **B**, Normal, M-mode echocardiogram at the level of the aorta, aortic valve leaflets, and left atrium. *T*, Transducer; *RV*, right ventricle; *IVS*, interventricular septum; *LV*, left ventricle; *AMVL*, anterior mitral valve leaflet; *LA*, left atrium; *PMVL*, posterior mitral valve leaflet; *PPM*, posterior papillary muscle; *Ao*, aorta; *AV*, aortic valve. (**A** from Urden LD, Stacy KM, Lough ME: *Thelan's critical care nursing: diagnosis and management*, ed 5, St. Louis, 2006, Mosby; **B** from Kinney MR: *Andreoli's comprehensive cardiac care*, ed 8, St Louis, 1996, Mosby.)

cardiac diseases. The disadvantages of MRI include the time required to obtain the study, the narrow confines of the tunnel in which the patient must lie (although open MRI machines sometimes can be used), and the need to use special, nonferrous healthcare devices near the magnet.

Stress Testing

Multiple diagnostic testing methods may be performed while the patient exercises both to challenge myocardial oxygen demand and to detect wall motion abnormalities.

Diagnostic Cardiac Catheterization and Percutaneous Catheter Intervention

A cardiac catheterization laboratory is a mainstay of the NSTEMI and STEMI protocols (*NSTEMI* stands for non-ST wave elevation myocardial infarction; *STEMI* stands for ST wave elevation myocardial infarction; these are discussed later in the chapter). Whether the intent is simply to diagnose a condition or to diagnose and treat it, these specialty surgical areas can provide definitive invasive management for a patient with ACS. Multifunctional catheters are inserted into the femoral artery and vein to view both the right and left sides of the heart and to detect coronary artery, valvular, and congenital heart disease. If high-risk plaque deposits are found, stents may be placed through percutaneous catheter intervention (PCI) to revascularize ischemic tissues. Special catheters may be used to repair defects found during the procedure.

The critical care transport team frequently transports patients from diagnostic-only catheterization laboratories to facilities with cardiothoracic surgeons available. These transfers usually involve very ill patients who still have femoral sheaths in place. With the personnel of the catheterization laboratory, identify which catheter is arterial and which is venous. Also, determine whether the patient has an IABP attached to reduce afterload.

If the femoral sheaths have been removed, maneuvers to control bleeding must be implemented and meticulous care to detect and prevent complications must be ongoing. This patient must remain in a flat-supine position with the affected leg extended for at least 6 hours after the procedure. A straight-leg immobilizer usually is applied to the affected leg to remind the patient not to flex it at the knee and hip. Generally, bleeding at this site is controlled by three methods: manually (sandbag), with an external mechanical compression device (C-clamp or FemStop), or by an arteriotomy closure device applied at the end of the procedure. It is important to perform routine pulse and perfusion checks on the affected leg.

Electrophysiology Studies

Often, while the patient is in the cardiac catheterization laboratory, invasive diagnostic studies are performed to detect and treat dangerous arrhythmias. Generally, for an electrophysiology (EP) study, femoral access cardiac catheterization is performed with special electrodes that allow evaluation of the heart's electrical activity. An arrhythmia may be initiated intentionally so that **ablation** procedures can be performed to eliminate aberrant pathways of conduction, such as may be seen in SVT and Wolff-Parkinson-White (WPW) syndrome.

Hemodynamic Monitoring

The application, management, and interpretation of bedside hemodynamic monitoring is routine in the critical care setting. Many of these invasive parameters can be continued while transporting the patient onto other high-level resource hospitals as long as the personnel are trained and equipped to manage these special and sometimes highly technical monitoring devices. The patients who have this special monitoring applied are usually those with poor perfusion, low cardiac output states (medical or surgical), and diseases of their pump, major vessels or volume. Interpretation of the results obtained will help you adjust therapy accurately with state-of-the-art equipment.

Skills 4-2 to 4-4 cover invasive and noninvasive hemodynamic monitoring, ranging from the simple to the complex. They also present techniques that can help the transport team (1) assist with the insertion, set-up, and management of hemodynamic lines and with interpretation of the findings; (2) discontinue monitoring before transport; (3) manage and troubleshoot monitoring equipment during transport; and (4) adjust therapy during transport.

Skill 4-2

HEMODYNAMIC MONITORING: CENTRAL VENOUS PRESSURE MONITORING

The thoracic central veins are most commonly used for measurement of the central venous pressure (CVP), either through the internal jugular or subclavian sites. Once these lines have been placed, a chest radiograph is always taken to make sure placement is correct and to rule out pneumothorax.

A pliable single-, double- or triple-lumen catheter is inserted until the tip rests in the proximal superior vena cava (SVC). During diastole, while the tricuspid valve is open, the CVP reflects the right ventricular end-diastolic pressure (RVEDP).

The standard, hard-wired bedside monitoring system measures the CVP in millimeters of mercury (mm Hg). A water manometer system measures it in centimeters of water (cm H_2O). The clinical equivalent is: 1 mm Hg = 1.36 cm H_2O. A normal CVP is 2 to 6 mm Hg (5 to 10 cm H_2O).

Generally, as venous return decreases (preload), the CVP decreases. Conversely, as venous return increases, so does the CVP. The CVP is not reliable for assessment of left ventricular dysfunction.

The CVP catheter also may be used for administration of medications and fluid and for withdrawal of blood for laboratory analysis.

INDICATIONS

Evaluate right-sided heart hemodynamics

Evaluate preload to the heart

Evaluate fluid volume status and response to therapy

RELATIVE CONTRAINDICATION

Use of this mode at the femoral line site

Procedure for Water Manometer System

1. Wash your hands and follow universal precautions.
2. Locate the phlebostatic axis (marking the skin at this site helps for subsequent readings).
3. The patient may be positioned supine in a 0 to 45-degree head-up position.
4. Attach the water manometer to the CVP tubing.
5. Turn the stopcock off to the patient.
6. Flush the tubing with saline.
7. Place the zero level of the water manometer at the phlebostatic axis.
8. Turn the manometer stopcock open to the flush solution.
9. Open the intravenous (IV) tubing clamp so that the fluid flows from the IV fluid bag into the water manometer.
10. Fill the manometer ⅔ full (above the level of the expected measurement).
11. Make sure no bubbles are present.
12. Close the IV tubing clamp.
13. Turn the water manometer stopcock open to the patient and closed to the IV solution.
14. Watch the fluid column; it should move up and down with the patient's respirations. The fluid column falls quickly and then fluctuates gently when it equalizes with the right atrial pressure (RAP).
15. Measure the CVP at the end of expiration.
16. Turn the manometer stopcock open to the flush solution and the patient. Reestablish the IV fluid infusion. Record the reading and notify the clinician if it is abnormal (see illustrations).

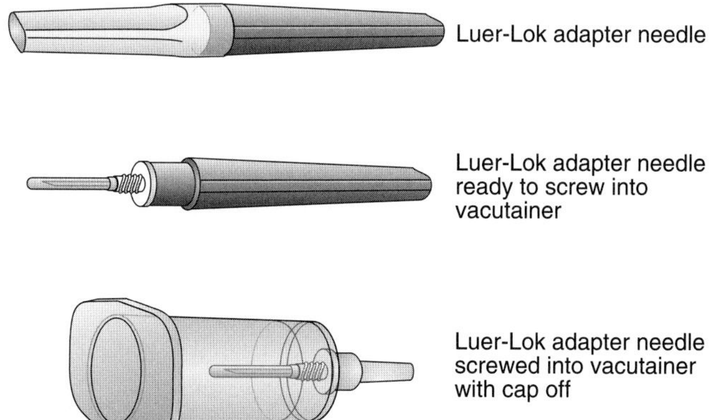

"Needleless" Vacutainer Luer-Lok adapter needle. (From Wiegand D, Carlson K: *AACN procedure manual for critical care*, ed 5, Philadelphia, 2005, Saunders.)

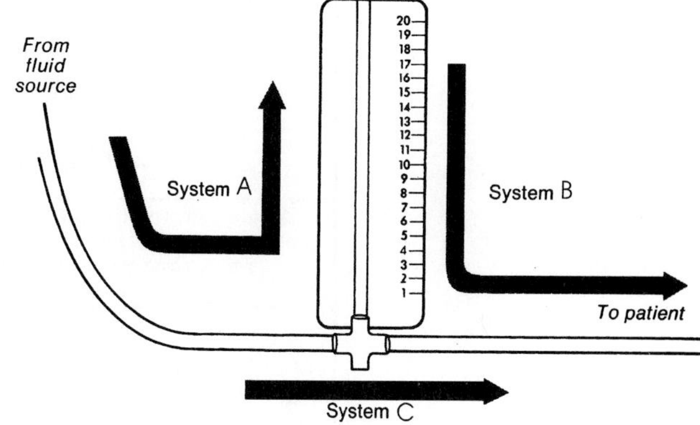

Central venous pressure measurement. **A,** The stopcock is closed to the patient for filling of the manometer. **B,** The stopcock is closed to the fluid source and open to the patient. **C,** The stopcock is closed to the manometer and the fluid system is open to the patient. (From Hucack C: *Critical care nursing: a holistic approach,* Philadelphia, 1989, JB Lippincott.)

Procedure for Hemodynamic Monitoring

1. Wash your hands and follow standard precautions.
2. Position the patient supine in a 0 to 45-degree head-up position.
3. Locate the phlebostatic axis (during transport the transducer could be taped to this site).
4. Validate the waveform on the monitor as CVP or RAP.
5. Make sure the hemodynamic monitoring system's pressure transducer has been assembled, flushed, and cable connected.
6. Level the fluid-filled interface of the monitoring system to the phlebostatic axis.
7. Run a dual-channel rhythm strip of the electrocardiograph (ECG) and right atrial waveform.
8. Measure the CVP or RAP at end-expiration.
9. Interpretation of the rhythm strip:
    - Identify the *a* wave: On the recording paper, draw a vertical line from the beginning of the P wave of one ECG complex down to the RAP waveform. Repeat on the next complex. Align the PR interval with the RAP waveform. The *a* wave occurs approximately 80 to 100 msec after the P wave and reflects atrial contraction.
    - Identify the *c* wave: The *c* wave follows the *a* wave and reflects closure of the tricuspid valve.
    - Identify the *v* wave: The *v* wave follows the *c* wave and reflects passive filling of the right atrium.
10. Measure the mean of the *a* wave against the RAP scale (usually set at 20 mm Hg).
11. Record the measurement and notify the clinician if the reading is abnormal.

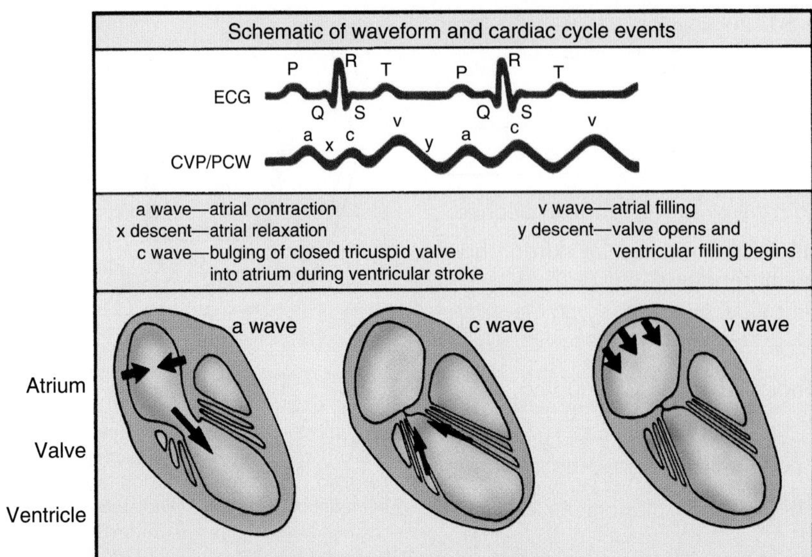

Cardiac events that produce the CVP waveform with a, c, and v waves. The a wave represents atrial contraction. The x descent represents atrial relaxation. The c wave represents the bulging of the closed tricuspid valve into the right atrium during ventricular systole. The v wave represents atrial filling. The y descent represents opening of the tricuspid valve and filling of the ventricle. (From Urden LD, Stacy KM, Lough ME: *Thelan's critical care nursing: diagnosis and management,* ed 5, St. Louis, 2006, Mosby.)

12. With hemodynamic monitoring systems, the RAP/CVP measurements can be measured and recorded continuously. Otherwise, measure the reading every 2 hours.

INTERPRETATION OF CVP MEASUREMENTS

- As mentioned, the normal range for the CVP is 2 to 6 mm Hg (5 to 10 cm H_2O).
- An elevated CVP may be caused by right heart failure (symptoms include ventricular gallops [S_3], tachycardia, narrow pulse pressure, dependent edema, liver enlargement, and possibly signs of poor distal perfusion [oliguria, weakened distal pulses, restlessness]) and by volume overload, which is marked by bounding pulses, an absence of gallop rhythm, and increased BP and urinary output (expect with renal failure).
- With a decreased CVP, hypovolemia is the common culprit. Both the CVP and MAP are used to assess the stability of a patient's condition; however, the CVP falls before the MAP in a hypovolemic patient.

Skill 4-3

HEMODYNAMIC MONITORING: PULMONARY ARTERY CATHETERS AND MONITORING

The pulmonary artery catheter (originally known as the Swan-Ganz catheter) has four lumens, which measure:

1. Right atrial pressure (RAP) or central venous pressure (CVP)
2. Pulmonary artery (PA) pressure
3. Pulmonary artery occlusion pressure (PAOP) or pulmonary capillary wedge pressure (PCWP)
4. Cardiac output (CO)

Variations on this catheter may also include continuous CO measurement, mixed venous oxygen saturation (SvO_2), and a lumen for transvenous pacing electrodes. Pulmonary artery catheters generally are size 7.5 or 8 Fr and 110 cm long. The catheter's four lumens gradually exit at different points along its structure.

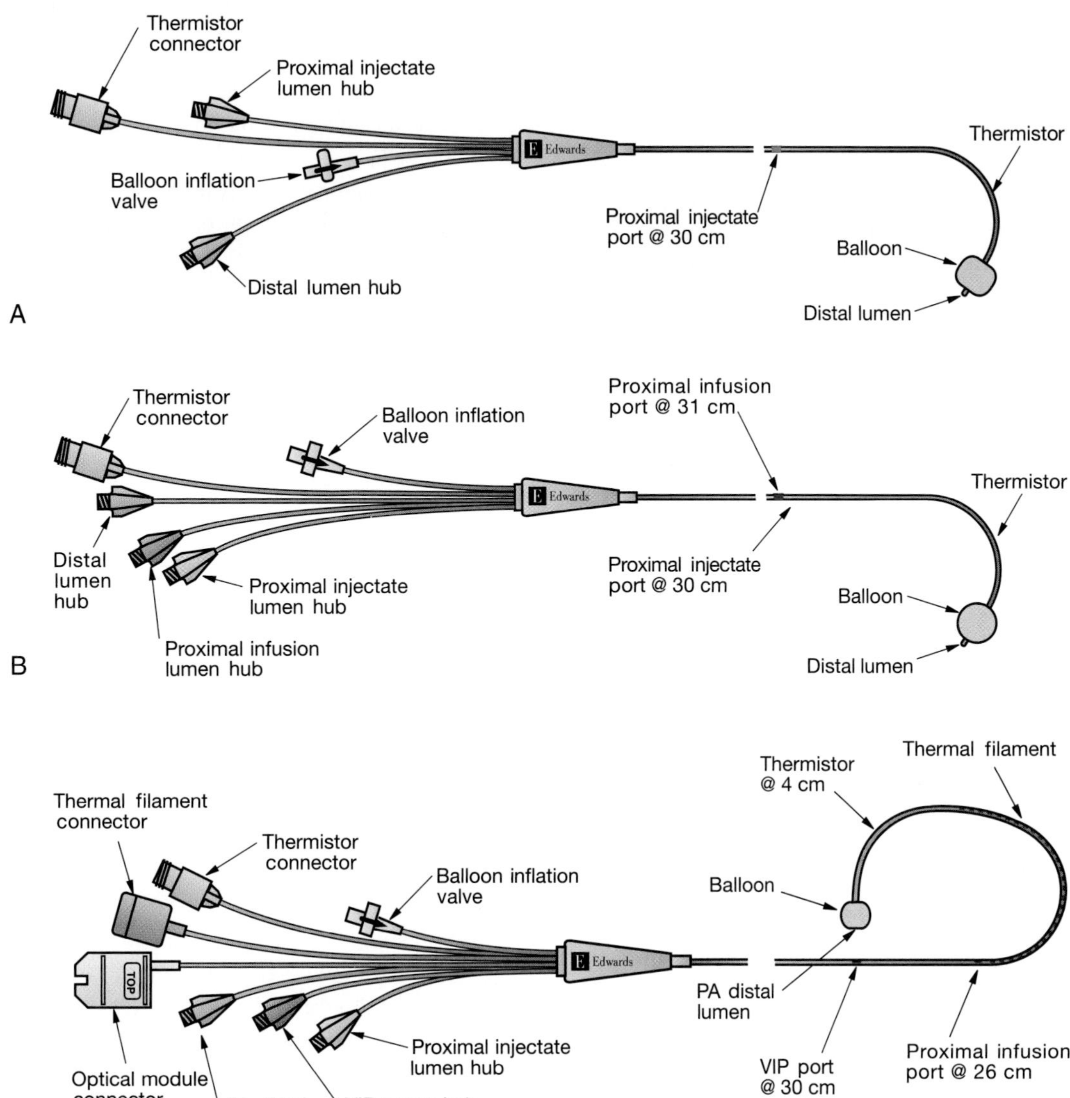

Types of pulmonary artery catheters. **A,** Four-lumen catheter. **B,** Five-lumen catheter with an additional venous infusion port (VIP) into the right atrium. **C,** Seven-lumen catheter with a VIP and two additional lumens, one for the continuous cardiac output (CCO) and thermal filament and the other for continuous monitoring of the mixed venous oxygen saturation (Svo_2) (optical module connector). The CCO filament values and the thermistor response time can be used to calculate the continuous end-diastolic volume (CEDV).

INDICATIONS

Evaluate hemodynamic status (right and left heart) in critically ill patients

Guide therapeutic intervention in the intensive care unit (ICU)

RELATIVE CONTRAINDICATIONS

Preexisting left bundle branch block

Temperature >101° F (38° C)

Mechanical tricuspid valve

Coagulopathic state

Presence of endocardial pacemaker

History of heparin-induced thrombocytopenia

PREPARATION OF HEMODYNAMIC MONITORING EQUIPMENT

Preparation is much the same as for arterial hemodynamic monitoring.

1. Use an intravenous (IV pole) with transducer holder (optional). If during transport, the pressure transducer may be placed at the level of the patient's midchest or on a rolled towel taped to the patient's arm.
2. Assemble multiple, sterile three-way stopcocks (more may be required, depending on the number of pressures monitored).
3. Obtain a bag of normal saline (NS) flush solution attached to connecting tubing with a microdrip chamber.

4. Connect the pressure transducer to the fluid-filled tubing and electronic monitoring system.
5. Prime or flush the entire system to remove all air bubbles.
6. Inflate the pressure infusor bag to 300 mm Hg and maintain it at that level.
7. Connect the pressure transducer/flush system to the distal and proximal ports of the pulmonary artery (PA) catheter and flush all lumens.
8. Connect pressure cables from the PA catheter, distal and proximal injectate transducers to the monitoring system.
9. Connect the thermistor connector of the PA catheter to the CO monitor.
10. Set all scales for pressure tracing.
11. Level the right atrial air-fluid interface (zeroing stopcock) and PA (distal) air-fluid interface (zeroing stopcock) to the phlebostatic axis.
12. Zero the system connected to the PA lumen and the RA lumen of the PA catheter by turning the stopcock off to the patient, opening it to the air, and zeroing the system.

ASSISTING WITH INSERTION OF A PA CATHETER

1. Wash your hands and follow standard precautions. During insertion of the catheter, those in direct contact with the patient during any part of the procedure should put on a gown, a mask with facial protection, a hair cover, and sterile gloves.
2. Before insertion, the catheter should be measured for the patient by comparing the packaged catheter to the distance from the insertion site to the sternal notch.
3. The practitioner inserts the catheter through a central vein introducer (see illustration). As this is introduced by the practitioner, the assistant continues to open the sterile package and allows the practitioner to withdraw the device for sterile insertion.
4. The ports of the PA catheter are handed to the critical care team member for connection to the hemodynamic monitoring system.
5. Flush all open lumens (to remove air from the catheter).
6. The practitioner inserts the manufacturer's recommended amount of air (usually 1.5 mL) into the balloon and checks for air leaks by submerging the inflated balloon in sterile water. No leaks are present if no bubbles appear and the balloon remains inflated. Withdraw the 1.5 mL of air from the balloon.
7. The PA catheter thermistor is connected to the CO monitor.
8. If the SvO_2 is being measured, calibrate all fiberoptics before insertion.
9. Zero the hemodynamic monitoring system.
10. The practitioner inserts the device through its sterile sleeve. Observe the monitor during insertion for catheter placement, along with the predetermined insertion measurements. The waveforms will change as the catheter is advanced. Insertion is performed as follows:
    a. Superior vena cava (SVC) into RA: Have the patient move the ear to the shoulder on the side of insertion; this facilitates insertion into the SVC rather than the internal jugular or subclavian vein. Watch for dysrhythmias.
    b. Inflate the balloon with 1.5 mL of air.
    c. Advance the catheter through the tricuspid valve into the right ventricle (waveform change).
    d. Continue advancing the catheter through the pulmonic valve into pulmonary artery and then into the **wedge** position.
    e. Deflate the balloon.
    f. Observe for the PA waveform (see illustration).

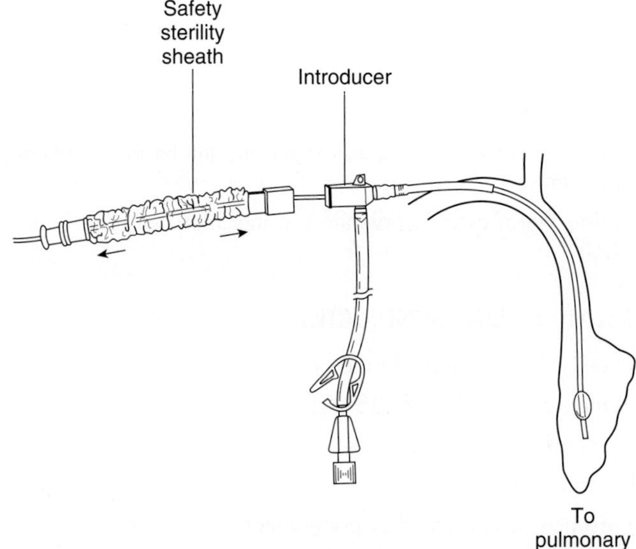

Pulmonary artery catheter inserted through a Cordis introducer catheter via a plastic sterility sheath. IV fluids may be administered through the side port connection to the introducer. (From Nakano K, Wasman K: Pulmonary artery catheterization. In Shoemaker W, Velmahos G, Demetriades D, editors: *Procedures and monitoring for the critically ill*, Philadelphia, 2002, Saunders.)

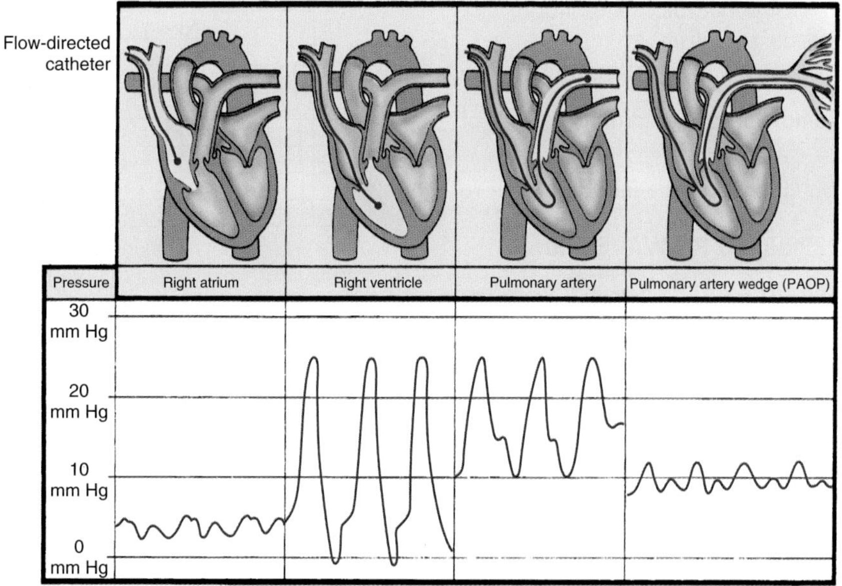

Insertion of a pulmonary artery catheter, with corresponding waveforms. (From Urden LD, Stacy KM, Lough ME: *Thelan's critical care nursing: diagnosis and management,* ed 5, 2006, Mosby.)

g. Inflate the balloon and rewedge the device to ensure proper placement.

h. Deflate the balloon.

11. Extend the sterile catheter sleeve over the device and secure both.
12. Comply with institutional policies on sterile, occlusive dressings.
13. Mark the centimeter (cm) mark on the introducer site for future reference.
14. Obtain a chest radiograph to confirm placement.

Did You Know?

The central line introducer sheath sometimes is referred to as a *sheath, Cordis introducer,* or *side port.*[2]

Did You Know?

You may infuse IV fluids through the side port of a Cordis introducer.[2]

IDENTIFICATION OF PA CATHETER PORTS

1. Right atrial (RA) lumen (also called *right atrial port, CVP port*): Proximal
   a. Used for IV infusion, CVP measurement, venous blood sampling.
   b. Used for injection of fluid for CO measurement.
2. Pulmonary artery (PA) lumen: Distal
   a. Located at distal tip of catheter in the pulmonary artery.
   b. May be used for blood sampling to measure mixed venous blood gases.
3. Balloon lumen: #3
   a. Opens into a balloon (inflated with 1.5 mL of air).
   b. Inflated only to float the catheter into position initially and then to measure the occlusion or wedge pressure intermittently.
   c. This balloon port must be locked off (manufacturer's recommendation; possibly remove syringe) to prevent inadvertent wedging.
4. Thermistor lumen: #4
   a. Temperature sensor; located 4 cm from the tip of the catheter.
   b. When CO is measured, sensing of a temperature difference determines the amount of cool fluid moving through system.
5. Additional features:
   a. If continuous SvO_2 is measured, another fiberoptic lumen is added at the tip.
   b. If a pacemaker is included, two PA catheter methods may be used (i.e., three atrial catheters and two ventricular pacing electrodes).

PATIENT MONITORING WITH A PA CATHETER

1. Routine systematic assessment should include evaluation of central and peripheral perfusion and observing and recording hemodynamic values.
   a. Level of consciousness
   b. Vital signs
   c. Heart and lung sounds

d. Monitoring for signs of pericardial tamponade, pneumothorax, and air embolism
2. Monitor the insertion site for:
a. Tissue damage (hematoma or hemorrhage, signs of induration [area of hardening tissue])
b. Migration of the cm marking on the introducer sleeve

OBTAINING AND INTERPRETING PA WAVEFORMS

1. Right atrial (RA) waveform: As described in CVP monitoring, this chamber has a distinct *a*, *c*, and *v* waveform. The RAP normal mean pressure is 2 to 5 mm Hg; *this is the proximal port of the PA catheter system.*
a. Measured at end of expiration.
b. Before entry into the tricuspid valve, the balloon is inflated to (1) cushion the distal tip against the right ventricular wall and to (2) assist insertion by allowing the device to float through from the RA to the PA.
2. Right ventricular (RV) waveform: This chamber is sensed as pulsatile and has both systolic and diastolic pressures. During blood flow through this chamber, it is not unusual for dysrhythmias to appear, even with the catheter tip cushioned. The normal RV systolic pressure is 20 to 30 mm Hg; the normal RV diastolic pressure is 0 to 5 mm Hg. Some catheters have an RA and RV infusion port for infusion of medication and IV fluids (see illustration).

Did You Know?

If the patient has no tricuspid disease, the right atrial pressure (RAP) is equal to the pressure in the right ventricle at the end of diastole (RVEDP). With the tricuspid valve open, the RAP and right ventricular pressure (RVP) equalize at the end of diastole.[6]

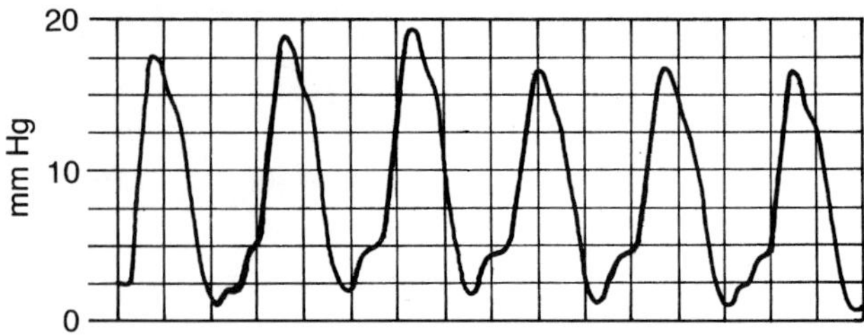

Right ventricular waveform. (From Darovic GO: *Hemodynamic monitoring: invasive and noninvasive clinical application,* ed 3, Philadelphia, 2002, Saunders.)

3. Pulmonary artery (PA) waveform: The PA waveform changes again when the catheter enters the pulmonary artery and the diastolic pressure rises. A dicrotic notch is seen on the downslope of the wave as the pulmonic valve closes (see illustration). The normal PA pressures are 20 to 30 mm Hg (systolic) and 10 mm Hg (diastolic).

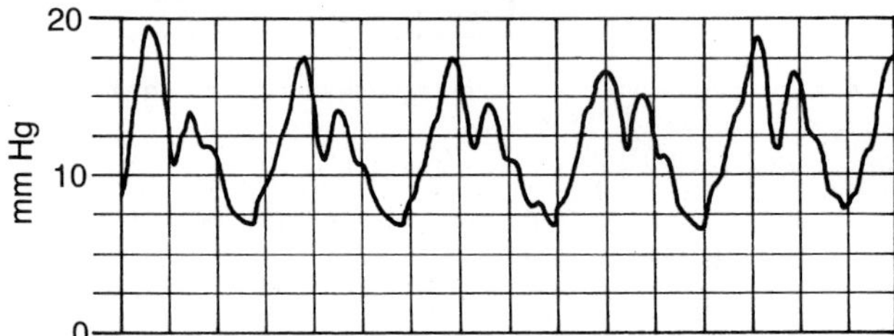

Pulmonary artery waveform. (From Darovic GO: *Hemodynamic monitoring: invasive and noninvasive clinical application,* ed 3, Philadelphia, 2002, Saunders.)

To obtain the PA pressure:
a. Position the patient supine in a 0 to 60-degree head-up position.
b. Run a dual-channel rhythm strip from the monitoring source.
c. Measure the PA pressure at the end of expiration.
d. Identify the Q-T interval on the ECG (see illustration).
e. Align the Q-T interval with the PA waveform.

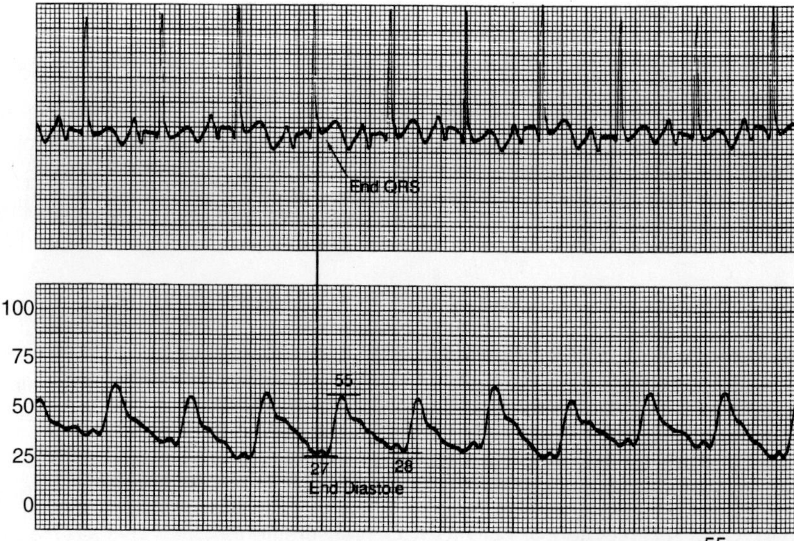

Pressure measurements in the pulmonary artery (PA). For the PA systolic pressure, align the peak of the systolic waveform with the Q-T interval on the electrocardiogram (ECG). For the PA diastolic pressure, use the end of the QRS complex as a marker and obtain the reading just before the upstroke of the systolic waveform. (From Ahrens TS, Taylor LK: *Hemodynamic waveform analysis,* Philadelphia, 1992, Saunders.)

f. Measure the systolic PA pressure at the peak of the systolic waveform.

g. Align the end of the QRS complex with the PA waveform.

h. Measure the PA diastolic pressure at the point of the intersection of this line.

4. PAWP, PAOP: The flow of blood sails or floats the inflated balloon into the pulmonary circulation out of the pulmonary artery. When the inflated balloon lodges with a segment of the artery that is slightly smaller than the inflated balloon, no blood flows into that occluded segment. The catheter tip records the pressure where vessels from the occluded and nonoccluded portions of the pulmonary circulation merge. This reflects the left ventricular end-diastolic pressure (LVEDP). The waveform changes dramatically to a low amplitude, reflecting left atrial pulsations. To obtain the PAWP/PAOP:

a. Pull up 1.5 mL of air into the PA syringe and connect to the PA inflation gate valve or stopcock.

b. Run a dual-channel strip of the ECG and PA waveform.

c. Slowly inflate the balloon until the PA waveform changes to the pulmonary artery wedge pressure (PAWP) waveform (see illustration).

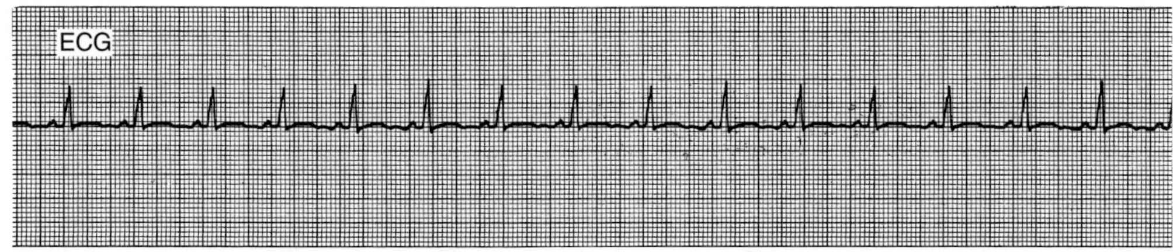

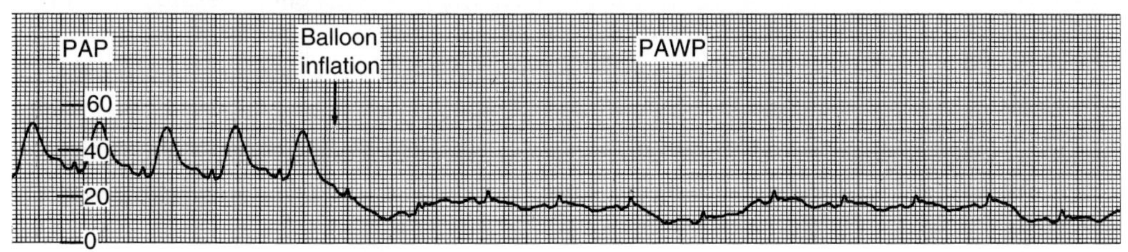

On inflation of the balloon, the pulmonary artery pressure (PAP) waveform changes into the pulmonary artery wedge pressure (PAWP) waveform. The practitioner inflates the balloon while observing the bedside monitor for the waveform change. Here, the balloon is inflated in a patient with a normal PAWP. (From Wiegand D, Carlson K: *AACN procedure manual for critical care,* ed 5, Philadelphia, 2005, Saunders.)

d. Inflate the PA balloon for no longer than 8 to 15 seconds (two to four respiratory cycles), because prolonged wedging can cause infarction of this sensitive tissue.

e. Disconnect the PA syringe from the inflation port and close the gate valve or stopcock to prevent inadvertent wedging.

f. Check that the PA waveform has reappeared on the system.

g. Expel all air from the syringe and, if allowed, reattach to the port.

h. Using the dual-channel recording strip, mark a vertical line from the beginning of the P wave of one of the ECG complexes down to the PAWP waveform. Do this for two or three complexes.

i. Align the end of the QRS complex with the PAW waveform. Identify the *a* wave. Compare the scale of the wedge tracing to the mean *a* wave tracing.

VARIABLES IN THE INTERPRETATION OF PA MEASUREMENTS

Three common variables affect PA pressure measurements and their interpretation: the position of the head of the bed, the transducer height, and respiration variants, including the use of PEEP.

- As mentioned previously, a supine position is ideal (0 to 60-degree head-up position), as long as the device is zeroed and leveled before measurement.
- Chest wall movement, with increasing and decreasing intrathoracic pressures, influences the various cardiovascular measurements through the PA catheter. Most measurements are best obtained at the end of expiration. During spontaneous breathing, negative intrathoracic pressures pull down the tracing and can produce an artificially low reading.
- If the patient is on positive pressure ventilation, during inhalation, the ventilator pushes up the tracing and can produce an artificially high value. The use of positive end-expiratory pressure (PEEP) also affects the tracings and readings of the PA catheter. PEEP pressures in acute respiratory distress syndrome (ARDS) at > 10 cm H_2O will cause the wedge and PA pressures will be artificially elevated.

CONTINUOUS VENOUS OXYGEN SATURATION MEASUREMENT

Patients with severe sepsis, shock, or ARDS or those who have had cardiac surgery may have an imbalance between oxygen supply and tissue demand. Special PA catheters may have a sensor for this at the distal tip, where it measures the SvO_2.

ADDITIONAL INFORMATION ABOUT THE PA CATHETER

Routine use of PA catheters in adult ICUs has become controversial. The complications associated with their use sometimes outweigh the benefits. Alternative means of measuring cardiovascular function and the effects of therapeutic modalities are being developed.

Skill 4-4

HEMODYNAMIC MONITORING: MEASUREMENT OF CARDIAC OUTPUT

Cardiac output (CO) is the amount of blood ejected by the left ventricle in 1 minute. It is measured in liters per minute (LPM). The CO is found by multiplying the stroke volume by the heart rate (CO = SV × HR). The normal CO is 4 to 8 LPM. The cardiac index (CI) is a more precise measurement of cardiac performance; it is the CO per square meter. The patient's body surface area (BSA) is calculated with the CO.

The pulmonary artery (PA) catheter can be used to aid calculation of both the CO and CI values. This can be done by three methods: intermittently injecting chilled fluid through the system (thermodilution CO [TDCO]); continuous CO (CCO); or noninvasive CO measurement.

INDICATIONS

Assess and monitor cardiovascular status after clinical interventions (mechanical assist devices)

Assess and monitor cardiovascular status after administration of vasoactive and inotropic medications

PROCEDURE

Thermodilution Method of CO Measurement

1. Approximately 10 mL of room temperature or chilled injectate is injected into the RA (proximal) port of the PA catheter, where it exits into the radial artery, mixes with the blood, and flows through the right ventricle (RV) and into the PA. The computer measures the temperature change and calculates the CO by measuring when most of the blood flow temperature returns to preinjectate levels.
2. This process is displayed in a curve and may be observed and printed. The computer calculates the CO in the area under the curve:
   - High CO: Small area under the curve
   - Low CO: Large area under the curve
3. The temperature difference between the injectate and the patient must be at least 10° C (50° F), and the injectate must be delivered steadily through a syringe over 4 seconds. The measurement is best taken at the end of expiration.
4. Three to five measurements are used to calculate the CO.
5. Many variables affect the calculation of the CO (see illustration).

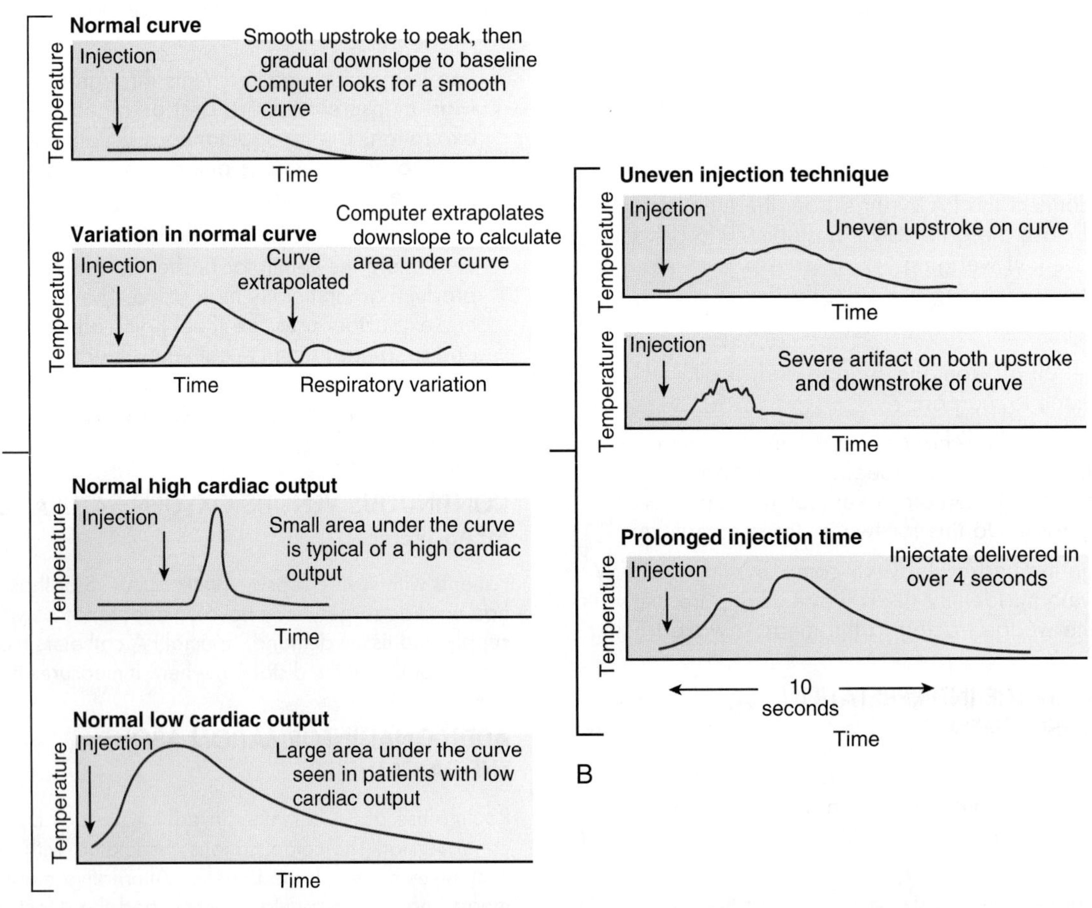

A, Variations in the normal cardiac thermodilution bolus output curve. **B**, Abnormal cardiac output curves produce an erroneous cardiac output value. (From Urden LD, Stacy KM, Lough ME: *Thelan's critical care nursing: diagnosis and management*, ed 5, St. Louis, 2006, Mosby.)

Continuous CO Measurement

1. A heat exchange catheter is used for CCO. It allows heat to mix with the blood in the RA, eliminating the need for an injectate.
2. This special PA catheter has a thermal filament close to the injection port, with the distal end near the right ventricle. Heat is generated by means of a rapid, low energy heat signal pulse.
3. Some variables affect the accuracy of CCO because of mixing of temperatures in poor blood flow areas such as intracardiac shunts or tricuspid regurgitation, or when the patient's body temperature is too high (>40-43° C) (104-109.4°).

Minimally Invasive CO Measurement

For minimally invasive CO measurement, very small (nonpharmacologic) doses of lithium chloride are injected from a central or peripheral venous line, and an arterial lithium sensor is integrated into a standard arterial pressure monitoring device.

The parameters of hemodynamic monitoring are presented in Table 4-5.

DISEASE PROCESSES AND MANAGEMENT OF THE CARDIAC PATIENT

Diagnosis of a patient with a cardiovascular condition requires more than a basic understanding of cardiac rhythms. As a critical care practitioner, you must understand the pathophysiology, clinical manifestations, and treatment of the various cardiac conditions. Although many conditions mimic each other in terms of signs and symptoms, the treatment can vary widely. This section discusses the evaluation of patients from the perspective of conductive, mechanical, and physiologic disorders.

Conductive Disorders

Bundle Branch Blocks

During normal cardiac conduction, impulses leave the bundle of His and travel into the left and right bundle branches. These branches disperse further throughout the myocardium as Purkinje fibers. When a block occurs in the bundle branches themselves, normal conduction is disrupted, either partially or fully. On an ECG, this appears as a widened QRS complex with an overt notch. However, the notch alone is insufficient indication of a bundle branch block; rather, it must be seen with the pattern of a widened QRS complex.

Mechanically, this change in conduction is manifested by an altered conductive pathway. Imagine a stream that becomes blocked by a large rock. The water continues to flow around the rock. If the rock is big enough, the water may even flow backward until it finds a way around the rock. Conduction through the myocardium also changes paths when blocked and, depending on the extent and location of the blockage, it may be diverted. This is particularly significant clinically when it results in a loss of synchronization during ventricular contraction.

Bundle branch blocks can be divided into two categories, right bundle branch block (RBBB) and left bundle branch block (LBBB) (Figures 4-23 and 4-24). Manifestations of these vary, primarily according to the location and extent of the blockage. Higher blocks cause a longer conduction delay. Any blockage is likely to be the result of an underlying cardiac problem, such as heart disease or an infarct. Among patients with coronary artery disease (CAD), an LBBB is associated

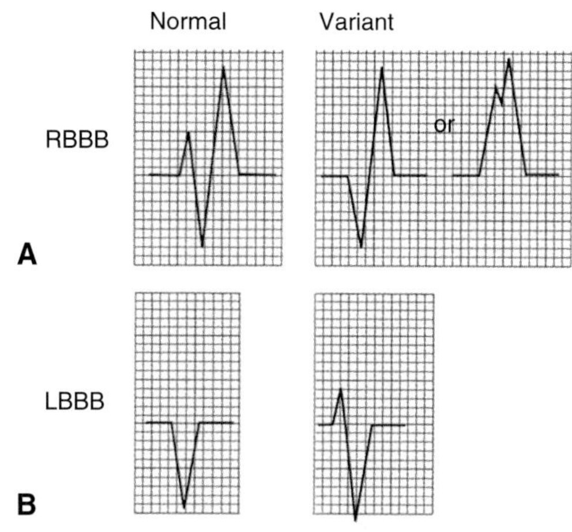

Figure 4-23

A, Right bundle branch block. **B,** Left bundle branch block. (From Phalen T, Aehlert B: *12 Lead EKG in acute coronary syndrome*, ed 3, St Louis, 2012, Mosby.)

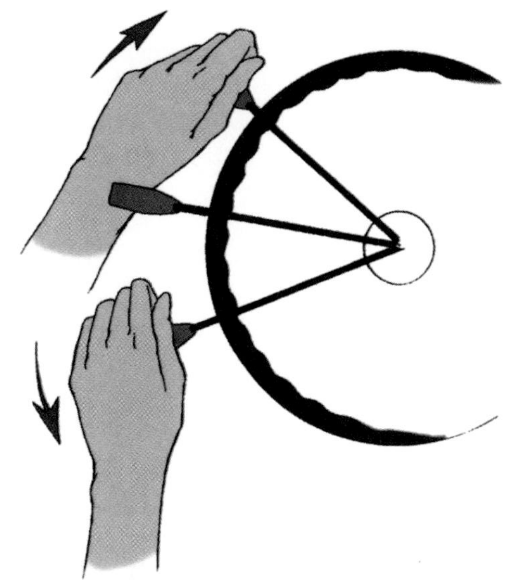

Figure 4-24

Differentiating between right and left bundle branch blocks. The "turn signal" theory is that right is up and left is down. (From Phalen T, Aehlert B: *12 Lead EKG in acute coronary syndrome*, ed 3, St Louis, 2012, Mosby.)

Table 4-5 Hemodynamic Parameters

Parameters	Formulas	Normal Value
Body surface area (BSA)	Weight (kg) × height (cm) × 0.007184	Varies with size (range, 0.58-2.9 m^2)
Cardiac output (CO)		4-8 L/min
Stroke volume (SV)	CO = HR × SV	60-100 mL/beat
Stroke volume index (SVI)	CO × 1000 ÷ HR	35-75 mL/m^2/beat
Cardiac index (CI)	SV ÷ BSA	2.8-4.2 L/min/m^2
Preload		
Central venous pressure (CVP) or right atrial pressure (RAP)		2-6 mm Hg
Left atrial pressure (LAP)		4-12 mm Hg
Pulmonary artery diastolic pressure (PADP)		5-15 mm Hg
Pulmonary artery wedge pressure (PAWP)		4-12 mm Hg
Right ventricular end-diastolic pressure (RVEDP)		0-8 mm Hg
Left ventricular end-diastolic pressure (LVEDP)		4-10 mm Hg
Afterload		
Systemic vascular resistance (SVR)	MAP – CVP/RAP × 80 ÷ CO	900-1600 dynes/sec/cm^{-5}
SVR index (SVRI)	MAP – CVP/RAP × 80 ÷ CI	1970-2390 dynes/sec/cm^{-5}/m^2
Pulmonary vascular resistance (PVR)	MPAP – PAWP × 80 ÷ CO	155-255 dynes/sec/cm^{-5}
PVR index (PVRI)	MPAP – PAWP × 80 ÷ CI	255-285 dynes/sec/cm^{-5}
Systolic blood pressure (SBP)		100-140 mm Hg
Contractility		
Ejection fraction (EF)		
Left	LVEDP × 100 ÷ SV	60% to 75%
Right	RVEDP × 100 ÷ SV	45% to 50%
Stroke work index (SWI)		
Left	SVI(MAP – PAWP) × 0.0136	45-65 gm-m/m^2/beat
Right	SVI(MAP – CVP) × 0.0136	5-10 gm-m/m^2/beat
Pressures		
Mean arterial pressure (MAP)	DBP + ⅓ (SBP – DBP)	70-105 mm Hg
Mean pulmonary artery pressure (MPAP)	PADP + ⅓ (PASP – PADP)	9-16 mm Hg

Modified from Whalen DA, Keller R: Cardiovascular patient assessment. In Kinney MR, et al, editors: AACN *clinical reference for critical care nursing*, ed 4, St Louis, 1998, Mosby; and Ahrens T: Hemodynamic monitoring, *Crit Care Nurs Clin North Am* 11:19-31. 1999.

DBP, Diastolic blood pressure; *HR*, heart rate; *MAP*, mean arterial pressure; *LVEDP*, left ventricular end-diastolic pressure; *LVEDV*, left ventricular end-diastolic volume; *MPAP*, mean pulmonary artery pressure; *PASP*, pulmonary artery systolic pressure; *RVEDP*, right ventricular end-diastolic pressure; *RVEDV*, right ventricular end-diastolic volume.

with more extensive disease, more severe left ventricular dysfunction, and reduced survival rates. Patients with associated left axis deviation have more severe clinical manifestations, and the combination of LBBB and right axis deviation has been reported as a marker of severe myocardial disease, especially dilated cardiomyopathy. RBBB is a relatively common finding, especially in older patients in general, and many have an RBBB with little clinical evidence of structural heart disease. On the other hand, new-onset RBBB is predictive of a higher rate of CAD, CHF, and cardiovascular mortality.

The treatment of bundle branch blocks involves supportive care and support of cardiac output. A high-degree LBBB (or complete blockage) can result in significant bradycardia. This not only reduces cardiac output, it also increases myocardial oxygen demand. When the blockage is caused by an ischemic event, the localized ischemia can be profound.

Multifascicular Block

The term *multifascicular block* refers to delays in conduction involving more than one component of the ventricular conduction system, which includes the right and left bundle branches and the Purkinje fibers. The left bundle branch divides into two larger branches, or fascicles, just before the Purkinje fibers begin. These generally are anterior and posterior in the myocardium and are known as the *anterior fascicle* and the *posterior fascicle.*

A conduction delay in any two fascicles is called a *bifascicular block;* if all three components (the anterior and posterior fascicles and the RBB) are blocked, it is a *trifascicular block.* A bifascicular block can present in two ways:

- As an RBBB with a left anterior fascicular block (LAFB)
- As an RBBB with a left posterior fascicular block (LPFB)

An LBBB often is considered a **unifascicular block**, because it can result from a delay in both the anterior and posterior fascicles.

Like bundle branch blocks, a fascicular block alters the conduction pathways. Unlike bundle branch blocks, the ECG change is reflected mostly by axis deviation and less by a widened QRS complex, although an intraventricular conduction delay (IVCD) may be seen.

Trifascicular blocks should be suspected when there is a permanent block in one fascicle and an intermittent block in the other two fascicles. If a patient with a chronic RBBB has a pattern of LAFB and LPFB on different occasions, the presence of disease in all three fascicles is implied. If the block in one of the three fascicles is incomplete, the ECG shows a bifascicular block with a first- or second-degree AV block. However, such an example does not always indicate whether the first- or second-degree AV block is caused by involvement of the third fascicle; the conduction delay may be at the level of the AV node or the bundle of His. A complete trifascicular block results in a complete AV block. High-degree blocks, or hemiblocks, can result in a decrease in cardiac output. Fascicular blocks largely arise from another cause, such as valvular disorders, MI, or heart disease. Fascicular blocks themselves rarely require direct intervention; instead, care should address the underlying conditions.

When signs of bundle branch and bifascicular blocks are present on the ECG, accurate evaluation of the ST segment for ischemia or injury becomes more difficult. The wide QRS complexes have oppositely conducted T waves that slur or drag the ST segment and automatically create ST segment depression or elevation. The term "MI imposter" has been coined to describe ECG conduction pathology that skews the ST segment and makes it more challenging to accurately diagnose STEMI and NSTEMI. Other imposters are described later; they include LVH, pericarditis, and early repolarization. Any ventricular rhythm or ventricularly paced rhythm also creates this illusion of ischemia or injury.

Box 4-8 Five-Step Analysis for Recognizing a Myocardial Infarction

Step 1: Rate and Rhythm

- Treat life-threatening arrhythmias

Step 2: Infarction

- Indicative changes?
- Localize
- Coronary artery involved

Step 3: Miscellaneous Conditions

- Left or right bundle branch block
- Ventricular rhythms
- Left ventricular hypertrophy
- Pericarditis
- Early repolarization

Step 4: Clinical Presentation

- Maintain a high index of suspicion, especially in the elderly and in patients with diabetics, hypertension, elevated lipids, obesity, or a history of smoking
- Remember: Infarcts also occur in women.

Step 5: Acute Infarction?

- Early notification of intervention team (PCI cath lab, fibrinolytic team)
- Anticipate complications.
- Develop a treatment plan.

Did You Know?

***Unifascicular block* is an impairment of conduction in the right bundle branch or in either the anterior or posterior limb of the left bundle branch.**

Myocardial Ischemia and Acute Coronary Syndromes

Chronic accumulation of atherosclerotic plaque eventually may result in exertional ischemia, prompting a person to see his or her healthcare provider. An acute change in the plaque stuck to the arterial walls can give rise to a number of clinical conditions, which are grouped together in a category, acute coronary syndromes. These conditions include angina, unstable angina, NSTEMI, and STEMI. The risk of sudden death is high during an acute plaque episode, which may be the first and only sign of the disease (Box 4-8).

Ischemia

Ischemia occurs when arterial blood flow is restricted to the tissue, and cellular oxygen needs are not met. *Angina* is the pain that results from restricted blood flow; *ischemia* is the physiologic effect. Although ischemia often is associated with an acute myocardial event, it frequently develops over a long period. During this time, the coronary arteries harden and plaque builds up, and eventually the cells distal to the blockage are starved of oxygen. If the condition goes untreated, cell death results.

Diagnosis of chronic ischemia in an acute setting often is difficult. Partially restricted blood flow may not produce changes on the ECG or in the laboratory results. Adequate diagnosis of silent or chronic ischemia requires further invasive testing, including cardiac catheterization, stress tests, or both.

Angina Pectoris

As previously mentioned, angina is chest pain caused by restricted blood flow to the heart. Plaque or acute coronary vasoconstriction reduces blood flow and thus the available oxygen. Whether chronic or acute, angina indicates underlying cardiac ischemia, generally caused by CAD. Angina can be categorized as stable angina, unstable angina, or Prinzmetal's angina (Figure 4-25).

Stable Angina

The chest discomfort of stable angina usually comes on during exertion and generally is relieved by rest or nitrates. ST changes may be noted, and a return to baseline may be seen after appropriate treatment. Patient care should be directed toward reducing stress on the myocardium. Although blood flow is restricted, some blood still is getting past the occlusion (Box 4-9).

Chest discomfort typically may be (1) located in the lower chest (classic presentation); (2) precipitated by exertion or strong emotion; and (3) relieved by rest and nitrates. Atypical angina may present with only two of the three typical features. (A third type of ACS chest pain is noncardiac in origin and manifests only one or none of the typical features.)

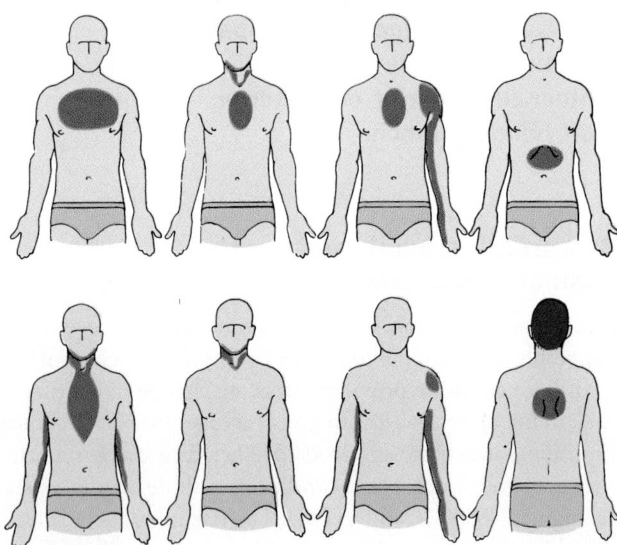

Figure 4-25

Common sites of angina. **A,** Upper chest. **B,** Beneath the sternum and radiating to the neck and jaw. **C,** Beneath the sternum and radiating down the left arm. **D,** Epigastric area. **E,** Epigastric area and radiating to the neck, jaw, and arms. **F,** Neck and jaw. **G,** Left shoulder. **H,** Intrascapular area. (From Urden LD, Stacy KM, Lough ME: *Thelan's critical care nursing: diagnosis and management,* ed 5, St. Louis, 2006, Mosby.)

Unstable Angina

When the vessel lumen begins to spasm or becomes obstructed, the patient develops angina that cannot be controlled with rest and nitrates; this is unstable angina. First-time angina also is defined as unstable angina. This condition can progress and cause major complications; therefore, it

Box 4-9 Characteristics of Angina Pectoris

Location

Beneath sternum, radiating to neck and jaw
Upper chest
Beneath sternum, radiating down left arm
Epigastric
Epigastric, radiating to neck, jaw, and arms
Neck and jaw
Left shoulder, inner aspect of both arms
Intrascapular

Duration

Less than 5 minutes
Less than 5 minutes (stable)
Longer than 5 minutes or worsening symptoms that are not relieved by rest or medication: unstable angina pectoris or preinfarction symptoms (unstable)

Quality

Sensation of pressure or heavy weight on the chest
Feeling of tightness, like a vise
Visceral quality (deep, heavy, squeezing, aching)
Burning sensation
Shortness of breath with feeling of suffocation
Worst pain ever for patient

Radiation

Medial aspect of left arm
Jaw
Left shoulder
Right arm

Precipitating Factors

Exertion or exercise
Cold weather
Exercising after a large, heavy meal
Walking against the wind
Emotional upset
Fright, anger
Coitus

Relief with Medication

Usually within 45 seconds to 5 minutes of sublingual administration of nitroglycerin

From Urden LD, Stacy KM, Lough ME: *Thelan's critical care nursing: diagnosis and management,* ed 5, St. Louis, 2006, Mosby.

should be treated as aggressively as an AMI. The presentation usually includes protracted, sustained chest pain with periods of increasing chest pain over the past 2 to 3 days and/or chest pain that awakens the patient at night. These patients may have some marginal blood flow through the diseased vessel but usually require vascular intervention. Multilead ECG changes of ischemia or injury may subside with rest, nitrates, and oxygen administration.

Prinzmetal's Angina

Prinzmetal's angina (also called *variant angina*) generally occurs at night and is due to spasm of the coronary arteries. Transient ST wave elevation may occur during these episodes of chest pain. Treatment includes rest, nitrates, and calcium channel blockers.

Acute Myocardial Infarction

Assuming an average pulse of 60 beats/min, the human heart beats 31,536,000 times a year. Basically, each beat requires a mix of oxygen, glucose, adenosine triphosphate (ATP), sodium, and potassium to be efficient. Each cell has the ability to contract and cause contraction of the adjacent cells in a three-dimensional cascade. The many conditions that comprise ACS disrupt conduction. AMI occurs when ischemia progresses and injures the myocardial cells themselves. If left untreated, this injury can lead to infarction.

When the oxygenated blood flow to the myocardium is blocked, the distal cells immediately become hypoxic. Shortly, they shift from aerobic to anaerobic metabolism. As anaerobic metabolism continues, local acidosis and waste production increase, compounding the problem. The hypoxic cells lose efficiency, and their workload must be picked up by adjacent cells. These cells, therefore, have a higher demand for oxygen. If the circulation to the disrupted area is not reestablished, these cells, too, become ischemic, and the negative effects continue. Depending on the location of the blockage, the ischemia can proceed rapidly. Imagine throwing a stone into a pond. The stone hits the water, and waves move outward in rings (Figure 4-26). In the myocardium, the blockage is analogous to that stone. The ischemia and loss of electromechanical efficiency move outward three dimensionally. If the patient survives the initial infarct, the myocardium is permanently affected by the area of necrotic cells that remains; this area becomes scar. The result is a decrease in cardiac efficiency, output, or ejection fraction and a high possibility of CHF and conductive blocks (Figure 4-27). Rapid, effective treatment, therefore, is crucial. Remember: time is myocardium (Box 4-10 and Tables 4-6 through 4-8).

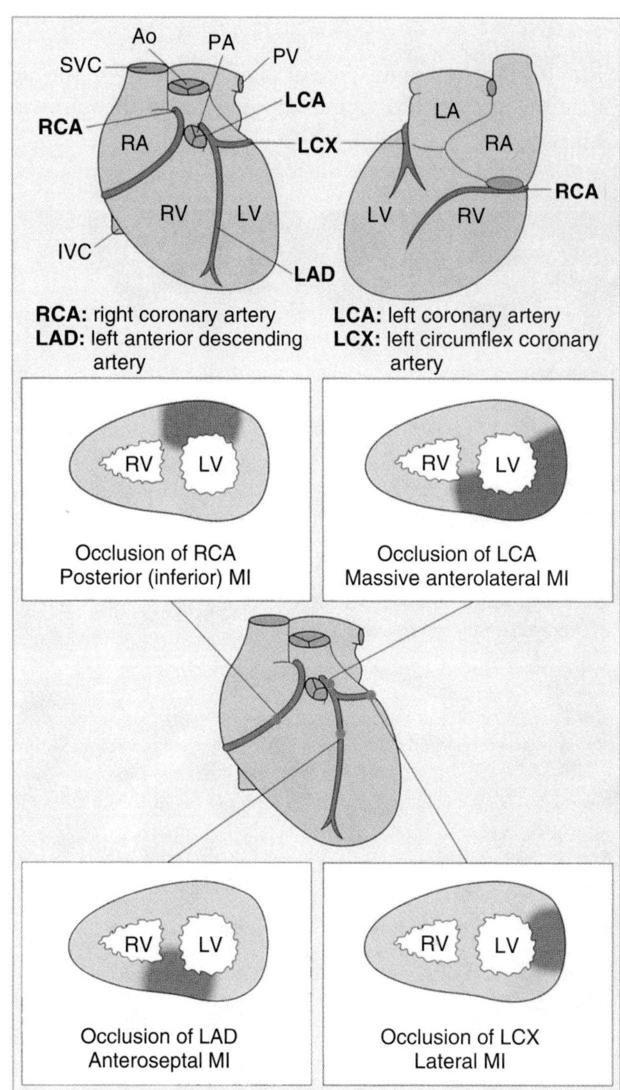

Figure 4-26

Site of a myocardial infarction (MI) and vessel involvement. *Ao,* Aorta; *PA,* pulmonary artery; *PV,* pulmonary vein; *LV,* left ventricle; *RV,* right ventricle; *IVC,* inferior vena cava; *RA,* right atrium; *SVC,* superior vena cava; *LA,* left atrium. (Modified from Stevens A, Lowe J: *Pathology,* St Louis, 1995, Mosby.)

Diagnostic ECG in Acute Coronary Syndromes: STEMI and NSTEMI

According to your protocols and the hospital's plan for management of a patient with chest pain, a multilead ECG is done and the patient is categorized into one of three groups: STEMI, NSTEMI, or unstable angina.

- **STEMI:** Two ECG presentations in a patient with chest pain indicate a high risk: STEMI and new LBBB. The ST segment becomes elevated as the myocardial cells are injured. These ECG changes may take as long as 4 to 6 hours to develop. The appearance of a new LBBB is a concern because it indicates extensive disease of the left descending and left anterior descending coronary artery, in addition to septal wall damage. Symptomatic patients also may have high-degree AV blocks (complete) and ventricular fibrillation.

However, identification of a new LBBB is problematic. To categorize the LBBB as new, you must have access to previously normal and relatively recent multilead ECGs. What you *can* say is that an LBBB is present, new or old. In such cases, the ST segment is difficult to see to identify the injury pattern; therefore, clinical judgment must be used. If the patient's symptoms are significant and new, the LBBB might also be new. The decision whether to administer fibrinolytics to the patient should be based on the fact that the person has significant ACS symptoms and an LBBB.

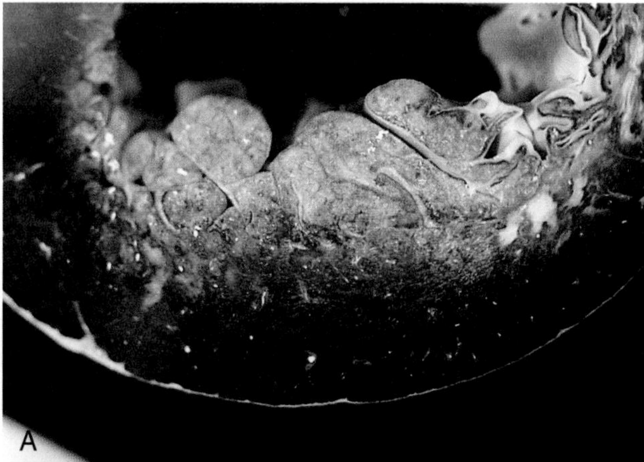

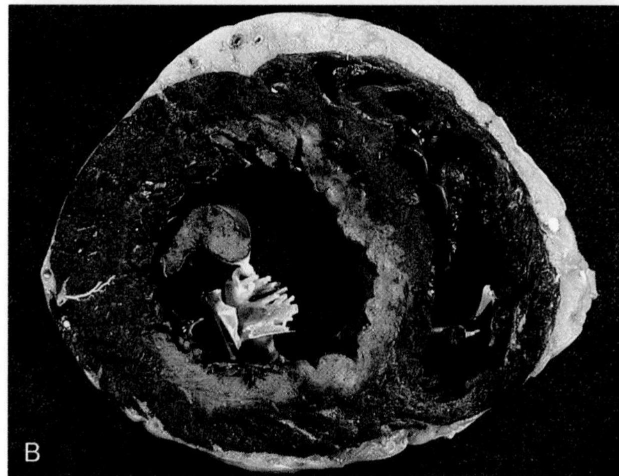

Figure 4-27

Myocardial infarction. **A,** Local infarct confined to one region. **B,** Massive large infarct caused by occlusion of three coronary arteries. (From McCance K, Huether SE: *Pathophysiology: the biological basis for disease in adults and children,* ed 5, St Louis, 2005, Mosby.)

- **Unstable angina and NSTEMI:** Signs of ischemia may be present on the ECG of a patient with chest pain, even if the pain is transient. The treatment plan may include the same diagnostics, ongoing assessment, and management as for a patient with STEMI, especially for patients with unstable angina who are clinically unstable (pump failure) or have arrhythmias and continued chest pain.

Management of STEMI and Unstable NSTEMI

Management of STEMI and unstable NSTEMI is directed at opening the partially or totally occluded vessel. This

Box 4-10 Clinical Manifestations of Acute Myocardial Infarction

- Tachycardia with or without ectopy
- Bradycardia
- Normotension or hypotension as a result of sympathetic response
- Tachypnea
- Diminished heart sounds, especially S_1
- With left ventricular dysfunction, may have S_3 or S_4 (or both)
- Systolic murmur
- Diastolic murmur
- Pulmonary crackles
- Pulmonary edema
- Air hunger
- Orthopnea
- Frothy sputum
- Decreased cardiac output
- Decreased urine output
- Decreased peripheral pulses
- Slow capillary refill
- Restlessness
- Confusion
- Anxiety
- Agitation
- Denial
- Anger

From Urden LD, Stacy KM, Lough ME: *Thelan's critical care nursing: diagnosis and management,* ed 5, St. Louis, 2006, Mosby.

Table 4-6 Electrocardiographic (ECG) Changes During Myocardial Infarction

Location of Infarction	Artery Commonly Involved	Leads Involved	ECG Changes
Anterior wall	LAD	V3, V4	Q waves, ST ↑, T ↓
Inferior wall	RCA or LCX	II, III, aVF	Q waves, ST ↑, T ↓
Ventricular septum	LAD	V1, V2	Q waves, ST ↑, T ↓
Lateral wall	LCX	V5, V6, I, aVL	Q waves, ST ↑, T ↓
Posterior wall	RCA or LCX	V1-V3 (ant); V7-V9 (post)	Tall, upright R; ST ↓, Upright T with ST ↑ (V7-V9)
Right ventricle	Proximal RCA	V4R (right)	ST ↑

From Urden LD, Stacy KM, Lough ME: *Thelan's critical care nursing: diagnosis and management,* ed 5, St. Louis, 2006, Mosby.
LAD, Left anterior descending; ↑, elevated; ↓, depressed; *RCA,* right coronary artery; *LCX,* left circumflex; *ant,* anterior; *post,* posterior; *right,* right precordium.

Table 4-7 Timing of Electrocardiographic (ECG) Changes in Myocardial Infarction

Time Frame	Change
Immediate	ST segment elevation in leads over the area of infarction or injury
Within a few hours	Giant, upright T waves; may develop Q wave
Several hours	ST segment normalizes; T waves invert symmetrically
Several hours to days	Q waves or reduced R waves; voltage may remain low permanently

From Urden LD, Stacy KM, Lough ME: *Thelan's critical care nursing: diagnosis and management,* ed 5, St. Louis,2006, Mosby.

Table 4-8 Correlations Among Ventricular Surfaces, Electrocardiographic Leads, and Coronary Arteries

Surface of Left Ventricle	ECG Leads	Coronary Artery (CA) Commonly Involved
Inferior	II, III, aVF	Right CA
Lateral	V5, V6, I, aVL	Left circumflex CA
Anterior	V2-V4	Left anterior descending CA
Anterior lateral	V1-V6, I, aVL	Left main CA
Septal	V1, V2	Left anterior descending CA
Posterior	V1, V2 V7-V9	Left circumflex or right CA (reciprocal changes)

I lateral	aVR	V_1 septal	V_4 anterior
II interior	aVR lateral	V_2 septal	V_5 lateral
III interior	aVF interior	V_3 anterior	V_6 lateral

From Urden LD, Stacy KM, Lough ME: *Thelan's critical care nursing: diagnosis and management,* ed 5, St. Louis, 2006, Mosby.

reperfusion therapy is facilitated or enhanced by the basic steps of the initial emergency medical service (EMS) or Emergency Department (ED) treatment: oxygen (target SaO2 94-99%), IV fluids, monitoring, aspirin, nitrates, heparin, pain control, and possibly beta blockers and angiotensin-converting (ACE) inhibitors. By the time a critical care team is called to transport the patient for further care, the following steps should already have been taken or should be planned for transport:

1. Administration of IV fluids and establishment of monitoring.
2. Administration of aspirin (160 to 325 mg) (or of ticlopidine [Ticlid] or Plavix (300 mg loading dose and 75 mg/day) as an alternative) for the antiplatelet effect, as early as possible.
3. Administration of nitroglycerin sublingually, followed by IV infusion of Tridal: The goal of nitrate administration in this case is to eliminate all chest pain while allowing for normal vital signs. Tridal reduces preload and afterload and may not be tolerated in patients with preload-dependent events (e.g., right-sided ACS). Strong warnings caution against allowing nitrates to reduce blood pressure and thus prevent administration of ACE inhibitors or beta blockers.
4. If the nitrates are not effective against the patient's pain, IV narcotics (e.g., morphine, fentanyl, Dilaudid) should be given. Again, do not create a hypotensive state that might preclude administration of beta blockers or ACE inhibitors.
5. Beta blockers may be given to decrease the size of the injury and to reduce mortality, especially in patients who do not receive fibrinolytics within the first 24 hours. In patients receiving fibrinolytics, beta blockers can reduce ischemia. These drugs can be administered orally or intravenously, as long as there are no contraindications, such as LV heart failure, bradycardia, hypotension, high-degree AV block, signs of poor perfusion, or a patient with respiratory disease who is also wheezing.
6. Heparin inhibits thrombin formation and when given with aspirin prevents further clotting. Two forms of heparin may be used, unfractionated heparin and low-molecular-weight heparin.
   - Unfractionated heparin (UFH) may have some disadvantages in ACS management. It has an unpredictable effect in each patient, it must be administered intravenously, and it requires subsequent monitoring of the aPTT. The increasing number of patients who develop heparin-induced thrombocytopenia (HIT) is a concern. When given to a patient with ACS, UFH usually is administered at a dosage of 60 units/kg, followed by an infusion of 12 units/kg/hour (maximum of 4000 units/bolus; 1000 units/hour IV). The aPTT goal is 60 to 70 seconds.
   - Low-molecular-weight heparin (LMWH) has become the preferred method of reducing ischemia, especially in patients with STEMI. However, it must be used with caution in patients with a creatinine above 2 to 2.5 mg/dL and also in those over age 75 because of the possibility of intracranial hemorrhage.
7. Administration of clopidogrel (Plavix): In patients with STEMI, clopidogrel (Plavix), along with aspirin, reduces platelet aggregation. Also, clopidogrel can be given both to patients who are to receive fibrinolytics and those who will not. A 300 mg oral dose of clopidogrel should be given to patients with STEMI who are under age 75

and who receive aspirin, heparin, and fibrinolytics. If the patient is to undergo PCI, consult the cardiologist in charge of the case.

8. Administration of ACE inhibitors: These drugs usually are given within 24 hours of the event, once revascularization therapy has been completed and the patient is in a monitored area of the hospital in stable condition. IV administration usually is avoided because of the risk of hypotension.
9. Administration of fibrinolytics: As part of the ischemic event in the plaque-filled coronary vessel, clot formation aggravates occlusion of the vessel. Fibrinolytics break down fibrin strands and help dissolve existing clots. The fibrinolytics comprise six drugs with a similar mechanism of action and side effects (e.g., hemorrhage). Dosing and administration vary with each drug. Commonly, alteplase (tPA) is used in an IV infusion, beginning with 15 mg, which is followed by 0.75 mg/kg (maximum, 50 mg) over 30 minutes and then 0.5 mg/kg (maximum, 35 mg) over 60 minutes. This high-risk drug administration should be started within 3 to 4 hours of the onset of ACS symptoms. TNKase sometimes is chosen as an alternative because of its ease of administration: a weight-based, 5-second bolus is given once (maximum dose, 50 mg). The healthcare provider must adjust the doses of other drugs that may be given with TNKase (e.g., heparin).

Low-Risk Unstable Angina

A normal or nondiagnostic ECG from a patient with chest pain requires further investigation. This patient should be placed in a chest pain center or a monitored area of the hospital so that serial ECGs and biomarkers can be closely watched for change, and other diagnostic tests can be performed to rule out an unstable plaque event. The old rule still applies: a normal ECG does not rule out MI.

Inflammation

Inflammation in the heart may be a condition of the heart muscle itself (myocarditis), the pericardial sac (pericarditis), or the inner lining of the heart (endocarditis). Each of these conditions is caused by an infection (viral, bacterial, parasitic, or fungal), an immune response, or a drug sensitivity. The signs and symptoms are similar. All have been associated with a fever and sharp, sometimes positional chest pain. Assuming that other causes can be ruled out, specific tests can be used as a form of differential diagnosis.

Pericarditis

The most common sign of pericarditis is sharp or stabbing, midsternal chest pain that worsens on deep inhalation. As the pericardium becomes inflamed, it increases pressure on the heart. Deep inhalation increases the intrathoracic pressure, compressing the inflamed tissue. Changing from a supine to a sitting position may relieve the pain. Pericarditis is most common in men age 20 to 50 years, and it frequently develops after a respiratory infection (Figure 4-28).

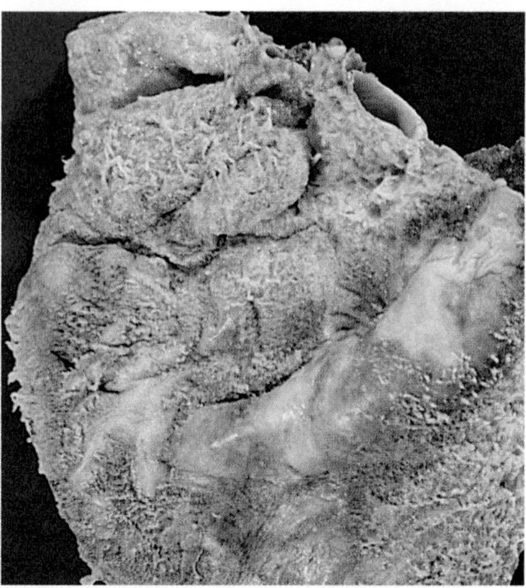

Figure 4-28

Acute pericarditis. Note the shaggy coat of fibers covering the surface of the heart. (From McCance K, Huether SE: *Pathophysiology: the biological basis for disease in adults and children,* ed 5, St Louis, 2005, Mosby.)

Pericarditis can produce a number of changes in the ECG, and diffuse ST elevation is the primary change. ST elevation is due to the inflammation of the tissues, and it can reach across any or all leads. Pericarditis is one of the STEMI imposters; therefore, diffuse ST elevations across multiple leads (not grouped according to coronary vessel), along with the history and clinical presentation, should guide you toward this differential diagnosis in a patient with chest pain. Other ECG changes may include depression of the PR segment and a notched J-point.

Myocarditis

Myocarditis is commonly caused by a viral infection. Its signs and symptoms may resemble those of ACS, but it usually is signified by sharp pain. The difference is that in myocarditis, the heart is irritated by inflammation, not direct ischemia. Because of the inflammation, cardiac output and efficiency can be decreased to the point where your patient has symptoms similar to those of CHF. The inflammation causes myocardial necrosis, which leads to myocardial dysfunction. On some ECGs, CHF can be distinguished from myocarditis by the presence of diffusely inverted T waves or saddle-shaped ST segments.

Endocarditis

A definitive diagnosis of endocarditis can be made only after extensive testing, including laboratory tests, blood cultures, radiologic studies, and echocardiograms. The signs and symptoms are directly related to the location of the infected site. Previously damaged parts of the heart are the most likely sites, and valvular dysfunction is a related indicator. Valvular disorders in themselves are not a sign of endocarditis; rather, previously damaged valves are susceptible to bacterial infections related to endocarditis.

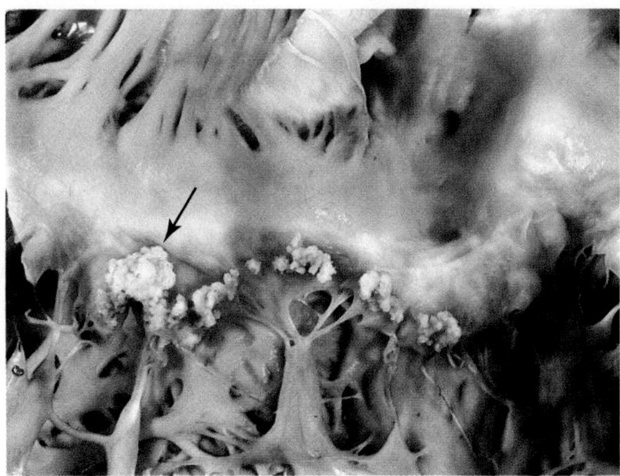

Figure 4-29

Bacterial endocarditis of the mitral valve. Lesion *(arrow)* in combination with old rheumatic valvulitis. (From McCance K, Huether SE: *Pathophysiology: the biological basis for disease in adults and children*, ed 5, St Louis, 2005, Mosby.)

Treatment of endocarditis includes antibiotic therapy and pain management. Surgical intervention sometimes is necessary to remove damaged tissue, especially any that restricts movement of the valves. In an acute setting, the focus is on treating the symptoms with supportive care. Many patients require long-term antimicrobial therapy for endocarditis (and endocarditis with valvular damage), in addition to antiplatelet and/or anticoagulation therapy to prevent an embolic event (Figures 4-29 and 4-30 and Box 4-11).

Mechanical Disorders

Congestive Heart Failure

An estimated 4.6 million people in the United States are being treated for heart failure, and approximately 550,000 new cases are diagnosed each year. This makes heart disease a fairly common disorder. A Heart Lung and Blood Institute task force on research of heart failure described this condition:

> Heart failure occurs when an abnormality of cardiac function causes the heart to fail to pump blood at a rate required by the metabolizing tissues or when the heart can do so only with an elevated filling pressure. The heart's inability to pump a sufficient amount of blood to meet the needs of the body tissues may be due to insufficient or defective cardiac filling and/or impaired contraction and emptying. Compensatory mechanisms increase blood volume and raise cardiac filling pressures, heart rate, and cardiac muscle mass to maintain the heart's pumping function and cause redistribution of blood flow. Eventually, however, despite these compensatory mechanisms, the ability of the heart to contract and relax declines progressively, and the heart failure worsens.

The right side of the heart pumps blood to the lungs, and the left side pumps it to the body. Because the vascular system is a closed circuit, failure on one side leads to a negative outcome for the other side. Heart failure occurs when a normal heart is presented with a load that exceeds capacity or when ventricular filling is impaired. Several factors can lead to heart failure, and age is one of them. Approximately 80% of patients

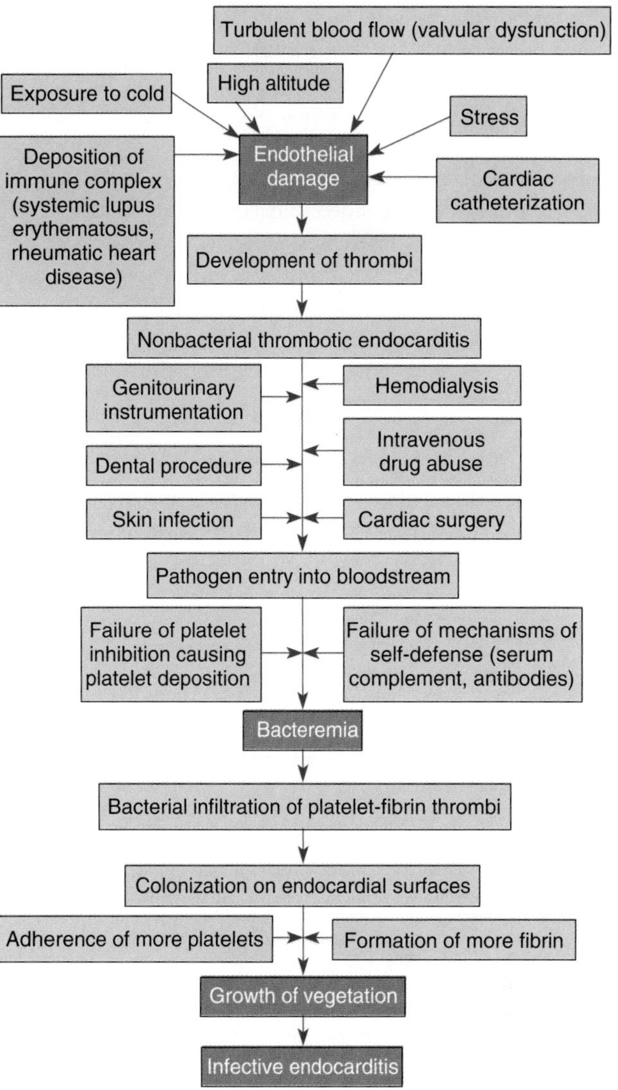

Figure 4-30

Pathogenesis of infective endocarditis. (From McCance K, Huether SE: *Pathophysiology: the biological basis for disease in adults and children*, ed 5, St Louis, 2005, Mosby.)

Box 4-11 Clinical Manifestations of Endocarditis

- Fever
- Splenomegaly
- Hematuria
- Petechiae
- Cardiac murmurs
- Easy fatigability
- Osler nodes (small, raised, tender areas most commonly found in pads of fingers and toes)
- Splinter hemorrhages in nail beds
- Roth spots (round or oval spots in the retina, consisting of coagulated fibrin, that can lead to hemorrhage)

From Urden LD, Stacy KM, Lough ME: *Thelan's critical care nursing: diagnosis and management*, ed 5, St. Louis, 2006, Mosby.

admitted to the hospital with heart failure are over age 65. Other contributory factors include the rate and degree to which the heart's performance is damaged and the ventricle that is initially involved (Table 4-9).

Left-Sided Heart Failure

The concept of left-sided and right-sided failure may be clinically useful in some cases. Otherwise, the idea that one cardiac chamber can fail without affecting the other three over time is somewhat artificial. For instance, when pulmonary hypertension leads to right-sided heart failure, the septum bulges into the left ventricular chamber. Chronic left-sided heart failure leads to pulmonary hypertension and right-sided failure.

As mentioned, differentiation of left-sided and right-sided failure can help clarify the clinical picture in a previously well patient. Fluid accumulation behind the involved ventricle is responsible for the patient's presentation. Left-sided heart failure leads to pulmonary congestion and edema, with symptoms of orthopnea and dyspnea. In addition, the left ventricle does not fill adequately, and the amount of blood ejected with each contraction is reduced. Systemically, this leads to less oxygenated blood being delivered to the body, and hypoxia ensues (Figure 4-31 and Table 4-10).

Acute pulmonary edema may be a confusing first sign in a previously well patient. Patients experiencing an anterior wall MI may present with acute pulmonary edema but will not

Table 4-9 New York Heart Association Functional Classification of Heart Failure

Class	Definition
I	Normal daily activity does not initiate symptoms.
II	Normal daily activities initiate onset of symptoms, but symptoms subside with rest.
III	Minimal activity initiates symptoms; patient usually is symptom free at rest.
IV	Any type of activity initiates symptoms, and symptoms are present at rest.

NOTE: Heart failure is typically classified using the New York Heart Association Functional Classification. Points are assigned into four groups, I-IV, depending on the degree of symptoms and the amount of patient effort to elicit symptoms.

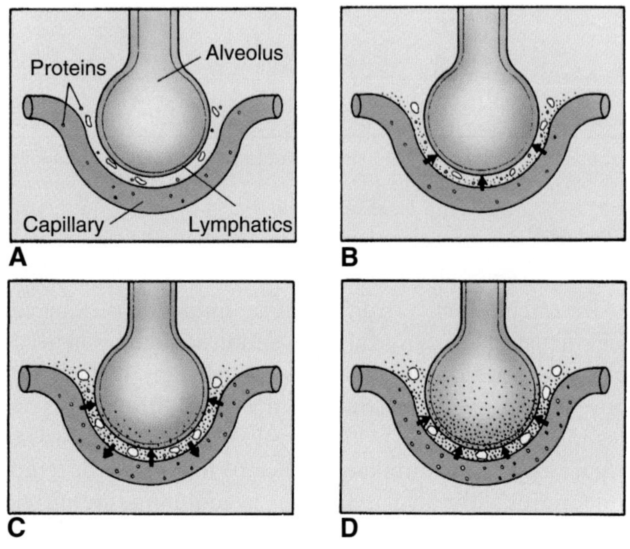

Figure 4-31

As pulmonary edema progresses, it inhibits O_2-CO_2 exchange at the alveolar capillary interface. **A,** Normal relationship. **B,** Increased pulmonary capillary hydrostatic pressure causes fluid to move from the vascular space into the pulmonary interstitial space. **C,** Lymphatic flow increases in an attempt to pull fluid back into the vascular lymphatic space. **D,** Failure of lymphatic flow and worsening of left-sided heart failure result in further movement of fluid into the interstitial space and alveoli. (From Urden LD, Stacy KM, Lough ME: *Thelan's critical care nursing: diagnosis and management,* ed 5, St. Louis, 2006, Mosby.)

Table 4-10 Clinical Manifestations of Left-Sided and Right-Sided Heart Failure

Left Ventricular Failure		Right Ventricular Failure	
Signs	Symptoms	Signs	Symptoms
Tachypnea	Fatigue	Peripheral edema	Weakness
Tachycardia	Dyspnea	Hepatomegaly	Anorexia
Cough	Orthopnea	Splenomegaly	Indigestion
Bibasilar crackles	Paroxysmal nocturnal dyspnea	Hepatojugular reflux	Weight gain
Gallop rhythms (S_3 and S_4)		Ascites	Mental changes
Increased pulmonary artery pressures	Nocturia	Jugular venous distention	
Hemoptysis		Increased central venous pressure	
Cyanosis		Pulmonary hypertension	
Pulmonary edema			

demonstrate JVD or pedal edema (which are seen with chronic CHF), because the central venous pressure remains normal.

Right-Sided Heart Failure

The atrium receives blood from the body, and the ventricle pumps it to the lungs. Patients with right-sided heart failure have systemic venous congestion, pedal edema, and hepatomegaly. With right ventricle failure, less blood is delivered to the pulmonary system. Less blood delivered to the lungs means less gas exchange, and hypoxia develops.

Signs of venous congestion can be confusing, such as JVD. Right ventricular infarction commonly presents with JVD and hypotension but no crackles. This is not a sign of failure, but of reduced ventricular preload that may be responsive to a fluid challenge (see Table 4-10).

The physical examination of the patient with signs of heart failure should focus on the person's general appearance; usually this can help you determine the severity of the condition. Patients with severe heart failure show signs of air hunger and appear very anxious. In contrast, patients with mild or moderate heart failure do not appear to be in distress after resting. Any edema should be noted and charted. The extracellular fluid volume usually must increase substantially (a minimum of 4 L in adults) before peripheral edema becomes evident. In patients confined to bed, edema most commonly is found over the sacrum. Note whether pulmonary crackles or rales are present during auscultation of the lungs. During auscultation of the heart in early diastole, immediately after the S_2 sound, listen for an S_3 gallop; it generally is heard over the left ventricle but occasionally may be heard from the right ventricle.

When the heart begins to fail, several mechanisms come into play in an attempt to compensate. These include the sympathetic nervous system (SNS), the renin-angiotensin-aldosterone (RAAS) system, and ventricular hypertrophy, which eventually causes ventricular remodeling.

- SNS effects include an increased heart rate, blood pressure elevation, peripheral vasoconstriction, and the shunting of blood from the skin to vital organs. This can lead to an increased myocardial oxygen demand.
- Overall, activation of the RAAS leads to fluid retention. Low cardiac output causes the release of renin, which converts angiotensin I to angiotensin II by means of ACE; this process leads to vasoconstriction. Aldosterone is released from the adrenal glands and stimulates sodium retention (and therefore water retention). This series of actions results not only in more vasoconstriction and fluid retention, but also in an increased myocardial oxygen demand.
- Ventricular hypertrophy, the final change to compensate for pump failure, is associated with chronic hypertension. Because of vasoconstriction and fluid retention, the afterload to the failing heart is now high. The heart muscle must change to increase the force of contraction to overcome this hurdle. This chronic change eventually dilates the heart, giving it a large (hypertrophic) appearance.

Left Ventricular Hypertrophy and Axis Deviation on the ECG

Because hypertrophy greatly increases the size of the left ventricle and eventually the entire heart, the ECG also changes. ECG clues to the presence of LVH are revealed by a step-by-step process; use these criteria once you note that the S wave or R wave is very deep or tall.

Step 1. Compare leads V_1 and V_2: Which lead shows the deepest S wave? Determine the depth of that S wave (mm).

Step 2. Compare leads V_5 and V_6: Which lead shows the tallest R wave? Determine the height of that R wave (mm).

Step 3. Add the height of the tallest R wave to the depth of the deepest S wave. If the result is 35 mm or higher, LVH may be present.

LVH, which slurs the ST segment, is one of the STEMI imposters. Indicators of LVH on the ECG may preclude recognition of any STEMI changes associated with ischemia.

Determining the heart's axis on the ECG also may yield clues to an enlarged heart. Leads I, II, III, aVL, aVR, and aVF are used for this purpose. As the electrical impulses move through the heart, these leads show which way the impulses are traveling; in a normal heart, leads I, II, and III should have an upright deflection.

Left Axis Deviation

A diseased heart may be enlarged and may skew the electrical impulses as they travel across the leads. A pathologic left axis deviation is seen with an upright complex in lead I and negative complexes in leads II and III.

Right Axis Deviation

Right axis deviation is normal in children and abnormal in most adults. It is characterized by a negative deflection in lead I; a positive deflection in lead III; and a negative, positive, or isoelectric deflection in lead II.

A 12-lead ECG can help determine axis deviation, because it calculates the positive or negative numbers as geographic axis angles, which are printed on the record.

1. An axis of −30 to −90 is left axis deviation, which may be seen with:
   - Large chest or abdomen
   - WPW syndrome
   - LBBB or left anterior hemiblock
   - Paced rhythm
2. An axis of +120 to +180 is right axis deviation, which may be seen with:
   - Right ventricular hypertrophy
   - RBBB or left posterior hemiblock
   - WPW syndrome
   - Left ventricular ectopy
3. An axis of −90 to +180 is extreme right axis deviation, which may be seen with:
   - Ventricular rhythm

Heart Failure Management

(During this discussion of heart failure and its management, refer back to the discussion of preload and contractility earlier in this chapter.) The treatment of patients with CHF depends largely on the signs and symptoms. For chronic conditions, long-term medical management should be continued. Chronic medical management includes therapy that diminishes the compensatory mechanisms described previously. Two types of drugs may be used to deter fluid retention in CHF: ACE inhibitors (the "-pril" drugs) and ARBs (the "-artan" drugs, such as irbesartan [Avapro] and losartan [Cozaar]). Spirolactone (Aldactone), a mineralocorticoid receptor antagonist, also may be used to break the RAAS mechanism.

In acute situations, use of a pulmonary artery catheter may guide management in the ICU. Care includes management of fluid overload, increasing cardiac output by increasing contractility, and reducing afterload. Skills 4-5 and 4-6 present the steps in use of an intraaortic balloon pump and ventricular assist device (VAD).

1. Diuretics reduce preload and eliminate excess fluid. These same objectives can be met without causing electrolyte disturbance by using aquapheresis.
2. Afterload is reduced with vasodilators (e.g., nitrates) or use of an IABP.
3. Contractility is increased with positive inotropic drugs (e.g., dopamine) or inodilators (e.g., dobutamine, milrinone). Nesiritide may be given to a patient with heart failure who is dyspneic at rest. Your goal should be to reduce the myocardial workload and oxygen demand while promoting cardiac efficiency.
4. Oxygenation and pulmonary edema can be improved by the use of positive end-expiratory pressure (PEEP) or noninvasive pulmonary ventilation (e.g., BiPAP or CPAP) (see Chapter 3).

Did You Know?

When dobutamine is administered to increase the heart's pumping function, arterial vasodilation occurs, sometimes causing a dramatic drop in blood pressure. Dopamine may be administered with dobutamine to counter this effect.

Aquapheresis: Emerging Technology in the ICU[7]

Aquapheresis is the removal of a predetermined amount of excess fluid from the body through peripheral or central lines. To date, two clinical trials have shown the advantages of aquapheresis over the use of diuretics in the treatment of patients with decompensated heart failure. As much as 4 L can be removed in an 8-hour period, without the electrolyte and kidney dysfunction that often accompany the typical diuretic treatment.

Aquapheresis typically is indicated for a hospitalized patient in whom the standard diuretic therapy has failed and who has:

- Fluid overload: 4 kg over dry weight, dyspnea edema
- Inadequate diuretic response: Net fluid output <125 mL/hour *or* <1500 mL in 12 hours (Net fluid output = Urine output − Fluid intake)

Aquapheresis cannot be used if venous access cannot be achieved or if requiring renal clearance (e.g., serum creatine [sCr] >3 mg/dL; Cr clearance <15 mL/minute).

The procedure requires a 6 French (Fr), dual-lumen, extended length (20 cm) peripheral catheter or a 7 Fr dual-lumen central venous catheter. Cardiologic and renal consultations are required before, during, and after the process. Other considerations include:

- Anticoagulation therapy is provided as ordered (the target partial thromboplastin time [PTT] is 80-100 seconds). Clotting of the filter may occur.
- Vital signs are monitored frequently, and treatment is adjusted if the systolic BP drops below 90 mm Hg or the heart rate exceeds 130 beats/minute.
- Postprocedural laboratory tests are obtained as ordered, and heparin therapy is discontinued as directed.
- Transport off the ICU with the aquapheresis device in place is not recommended.

Skill 4-5

INTRAAORTIC BALLOON PUMP (IABP) MANAGEMENT

INDICATION

IABP is a short-term therapy that improves myocardial oxygenation. It does this by reducing afterload through counterpulsation, thereby reducing the workload of the heart. The treatment is indicated for patients with heart failure.

CONTRAINDICATIONS

Aortic insufficiency or aneurysms

Severe blood clotting disorders

PROCEDURE

Preparation and Maintenance of the System

1. The practitioner places a sterile IABP catheter in the femoral artery and positions it in the descending thoracic aorta, just distal to the left subclavian artery. Arterial pressure hemodynamic monitoring usually

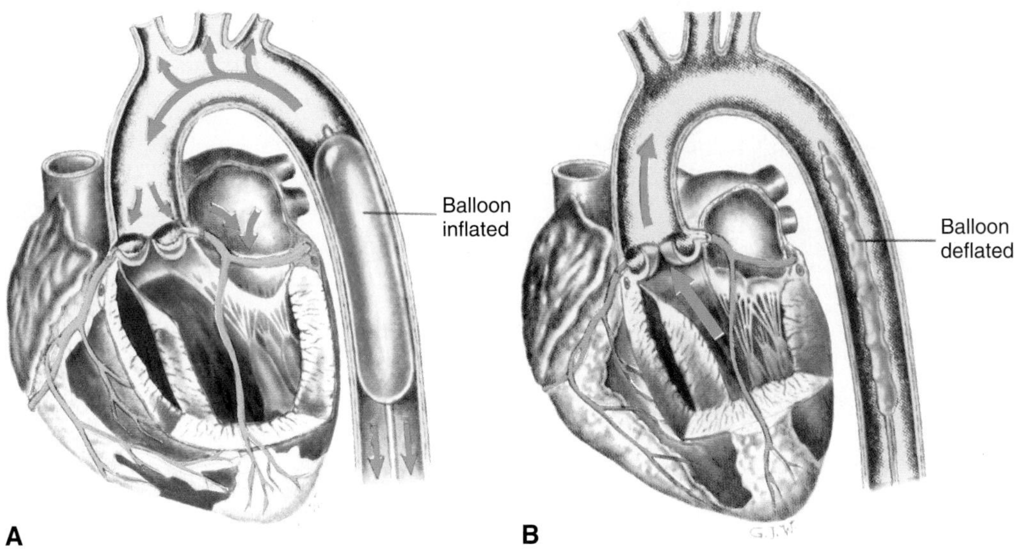

Mechanisms of action of the intraaortic balloon pump. **A,** Diastolic balloon inflation augments coronary blood flow. **B,** Systolic balloon deflation reduces afterload. (From Urden LD, Stacy KM, Lough ME: *Thelan's critical care nursing: diagnosis and management,* ed 5, St. Louis, 2006, Mosby.)

is also in place in the radial artery to assist in proper assessment and in the timing of inflation of the device.

2. The affected leg must remain extended (a full-leg knee immobilizer is effective for preventing flexion).
3. Follow the manufacturer's recommendations for the following:
   - Electrocardiogram (ECG) leads (maintain a prominent R wave for timing of the device)
   - Console maintenance (timing procedures and alarms)
   - Helium source (to inflate the IABP balloon; make sure the canister has enough gas for the duration of transport)
   - Flushing of the device to prevent thrombus formation
   - Identifying with marked tape which electrode goes to the monitor and which goes to the console
4. Follow your service's policies on the use of heparinized flush solutions.
5. Follow standard wound care, anticoagulation therapy, and dressing procedures per your policies.
6. Follow your protocols and policies for frequency of cardiovascular assessment. Assessment of the patient includes:
   - Level of consciousness (cerebral perfusion)
   - Vital signs and pulmonary artery pressure (effectiveness of IABP therapy)
   - Arterial catheter and IABP waveforms (timing effectiveness)
   - Cardiac output, cardiac index, and systemic vascular resistance (effectiveness of IABP therapy)
   - Distal perfusion (skin should be warm and dry, and urinary output should be greater than 0.5 mL/kg/hour)
   - Heart and lung sounds (to auscultate these sounds adequately, you may need to turn the IABP to standby and restart when your evaluation is completed)
7. Check all central and distal pulses to make sure the catheter has not migrated and that it is not occluding a vessel. The catheter should be measured and marked for location at the femoral site.
8. Turn and position the patient at least every 2 hours if possible.
9. Monitor the co-existing anticoagulation therapy by means of laboratory studies and clinical evidence of bleeding or clot formation. Check dressings frequently for bleeding.

Timing of the Balloon Pump

1. The ECG and arterial pressure waveform are monitored to verify proper timing of the device. Timing the inflation (during diastole) and deflation (during systole) effectively reduces the workload of the heart and improves oxygenation (see illustration).

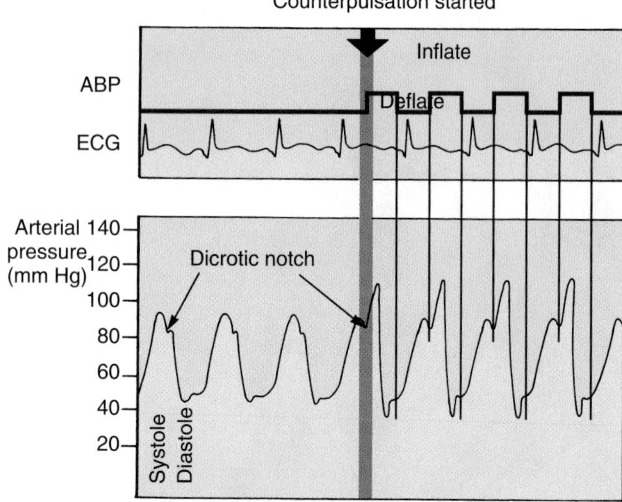

Timing and effect of balloon counterpulsations. The timing is adjusted by synchronizing balloon inflation with the dicrotic notch on the arterial waveform; this results in an elevated diastolic pressure. Inflation is maintained throughout diastole to augment coronary perfusion. Deflation occurs just before the next systole, resulting in a reduced systolic pressure and decreased afterload. (From Guzzetta CE, Dossey BM: *Cardiovascular nursing: holistic practice,* St Louis, 1992, Mosby.)

2. A prominent R wave on the ECG and a properly maintained arterial waveform signals the IABP console when to time inflation and deflation of the balloon.
3. To start, set the IABP to 1 : 2 or 50% (every other beat augmented) (see illustration).

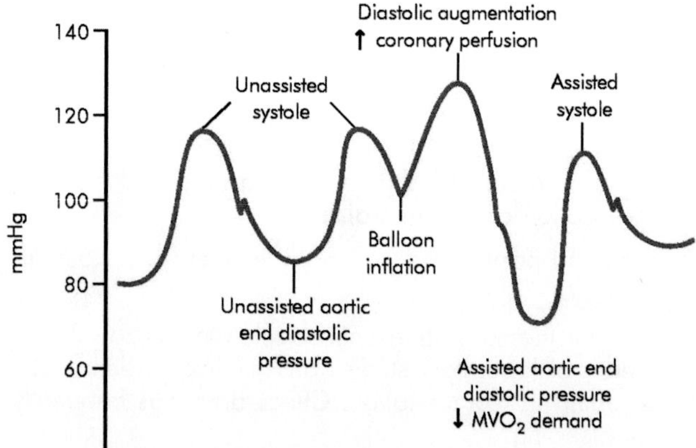

Mechanism of augmentation by intra-aortic balloon pump (IABP). (From Urden LD, Stacy KM, Lough ME: *Thelan's critical care nursing: diagnosis and management,* ed 5, St. Louis, 2006, Mosby.)

4. Inflation:
   a. Identify the dicrotic notch in the arterial waveform (aortic valve closure).
   b. Inflate the balloon after aortic valve closure; adjust inflation on the console until the dicrotic notch disappears and a sharp V wave appears (see illustration).

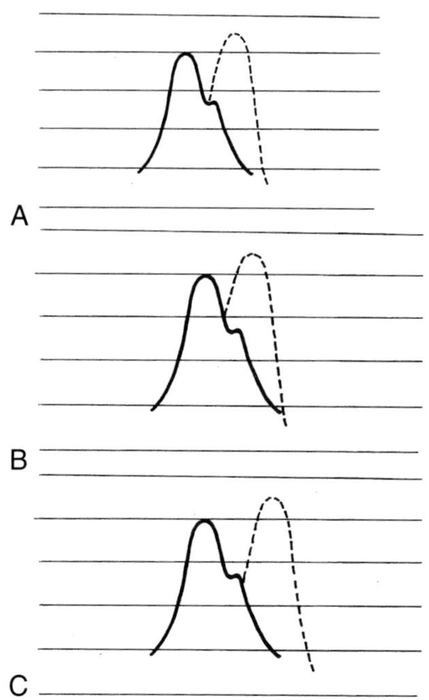

Intraaortic balloon pump inflation from 3 sites. **A,** Radial: inflate 40-50 milliseconds (ms) before the dicrotic notch. **B,** Femoral: inflate 120 msec before notch. **C,** Central aortic. (From Wiegand D, Carlson K: *AACN procedure manual for critical care,* ed 5, Philadelphia, 2005, Saunders.)

5. Compare the augmented pressure with the unassisted systolic pressure. The augmented pressure should be the same as the systolic pressure or slightly higher. If the augmented pressure is lower than the systolic pressure, the balloon is too low, the patient is hypovolemic or tachycardic, or the balloon volume is too low.
6. Adjust the console as needed to time the inflation of the balloon.
7. Accommodate the location of the arterial line as follows:
   - For a radial artery line: Time inflation to 40 to 50 msec before the dicrotic notch.
   - For a femoral artery line: Time inflation to 120 msec before the dicrotic notch.
8. Deflation:
   a. With the IABP on a 1 : 2 frequency (as above), identify the unassisted end-diastolic pressure and the assisted and unassisted systolic pressures.
   b. Deflate the balloon so that the end-diastolic pressure is as low as possible (lower than the patient's

unassisted diastolic pressure) while the optimum diastolic augmentation is maintained and *without interfering with the next systole.*

9. Now that the timing has been set, turn the console augmentation to 1 : 1 (100%).

Balloon Pressure Waveform

1. Check the IABP console for the balloon pressure waveform as helium is shuttled into and out of the catheter (see illustration).
2. Refer to the manufacturer's guidelines on inflation errors reflected in the balloon pressure waveform.

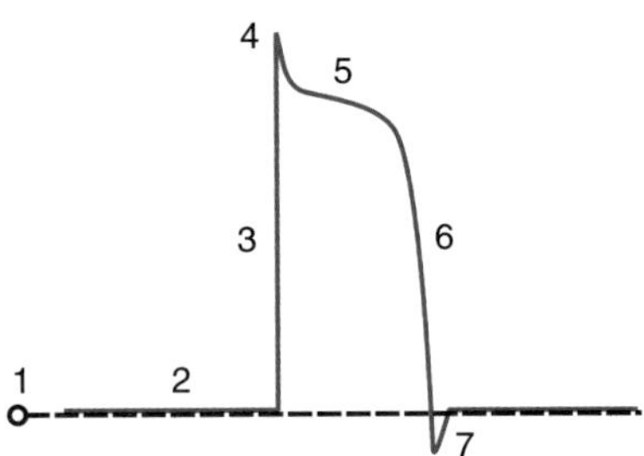

Normal balloon gas waveform. 1, Zero baseline; 2, fill pressure; 3, rapid inflation; 4, peak inflation artifact; 5, plateau pressure or inflation plateau pressure; 6, rapid deflation; 7, peak deflation pressure and return to fill pressure.

Timing the Device in a Patient with Dysrhythmias

1. Atrial fibrillation: Set the device to shuttle on most R waves or (if available) use the atrial fibrillation mode on the console.
2. Tachycardia: Set the frequency to 1 : 2 (50%).
3. Asystole: Change the trigger to the arterial pressure. If compressions do not provide an adequate trigger, set the device to internal trigger at 60 to 80/min, 1 : 2 frequency, and reduce augmentation to 50%.
4. Ventricular tachycardia or ventricular fibrillation: Cardiovert or defibrillate as necessary; the console is electrically isolated.

TROUBLESHOOTING

Timing Errors

Timing Errors
Late Inflation

Inflation of the IAB markedly after closure of the aortic valve

Waveform Characteristics:
- Inflation of the IAB after the dicrotic notch
- Absence of sharp V
- Sub-optimal diastolic augmentation

Physiologic Effects:
- Sub-optimal coronary artery perfusion

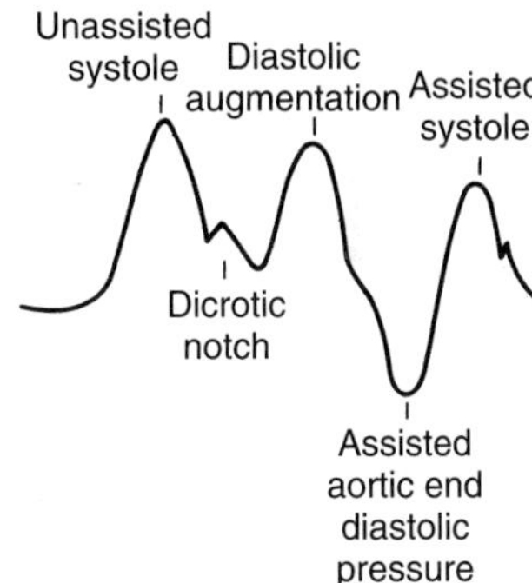

Late inflation. (Courtesy Maquet Getinge Group, Rastatt, Germany.)

Timing Errors
Early Inflation

Inflation of the IAB prior to aortic valve closure

Waveform Characteristics:
- Inflation of IAB prior to dicrotic notch
- Diastolic augmentation encroaches onto systole (may be unable to distinguish)

Unassisted systole
Diastolic augmentation
Assisted systole
Assisted aortic end diastolic pressure

Physiologic Effects:
- Potential premature closure of aortic valve
- Potential increased in LVEDV and LVEDP or PCWP
- Increased left ventricular wall stress or afterload
- Aortic regurgitation
- Increased MVO_2 demand

Early inflation. (Courtesy Maquet Getinge Group, Rastatt, Germany.)

Timing Errors
Early Deflation

Premature deflation of the IAB during the diastolic phase

Waveform Characteristics:
- Deflation of IAB is seen as a sharp drop following diastolic augmentation
- Sub-optimal diastolic augmentation
- Assisted aortic end diastolic pressure may be equal to or less than the unassisted aortic end diastolic pressure
- Assisted systolic pressure may rise

Diastolic augmentation
Assisted systole
Assisted aortic end diastolic pressure
Unassisted aortic end diastolic pressure

Physiologic Effects:
- Sub-optimal coronary perfusion
- Potential for retrograde coronary and carotid blood flow
- Angina may occur as a result of retrograde coronary blood flow
- Sub-optimal afterload reduction
- Increased MVO_2 demand

Early deflation. (Courtesy Maquet Getinge Group, Rastatt, Germany.)

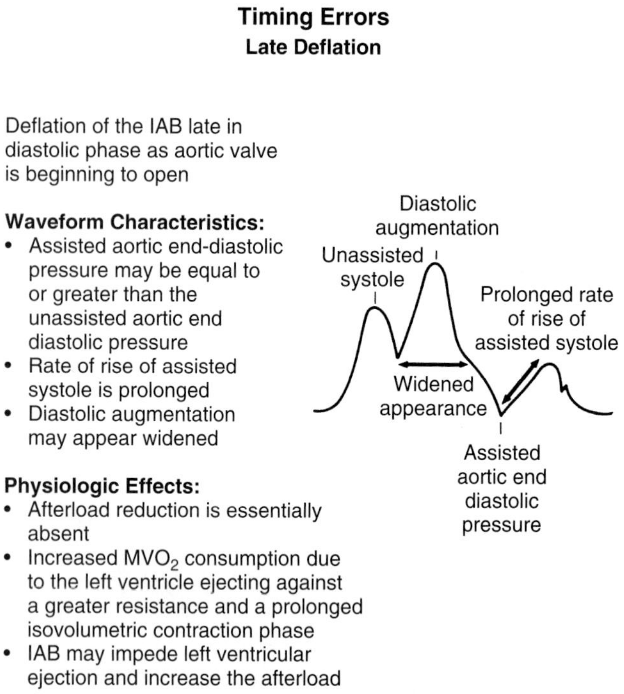

Timing Errors
Late Deflation

Deflation of the IAB late in diastolic phase as aortic valve is beginning to open

Waveform Characteristics:
- Assisted aortic end-diastolic pressure may be equal to or greater than the unassisted aortic end diastolic pressure
- Rate of rise of assisted systole is prolonged
- Diastolic augmentation may appear widened

Diastolic augmentation
Unassisted systole
Prolonged rate of rise of assisted systole
Widened appearance
Assisted aortic end diastolic pressure

Physiologic Effects:
- Afterload reduction is essentially absent
- Increased MVO_2 consumption due to the left ventricle ejecting against a greater resistance and a prolonged isovolumetric contraction phase
- IAB may impede left ventricular ejection and increase the afterload

Late deflation. (Courtesy Maquet Getinge Group, Rastatt, Germany.)

Loss of Vacuum/IABP Failure

1. Tighten all connections in the tubing
2. Check the power source on the device that drives the helium.
3. Hand inflate and deflate the balloon every 5 minutes with half of the total balloon volume to prevent clot formation.
4. Change the IABP console if possible. If the problem occurs during transport, call ahead to the receiving hospital to make sure an IABP console is available on the helipad or at the Emergency Department door when you arrive.

Suspected Balloon Perforation

1. Observe for loss of augmentation (alarms are set to sound if a diastolic drop of 10 mm Hg occurs).
2. Check the catheter; if blood is present, the balloon has been perforated.
3. Assess for a normal balloon pressure waveform on the console. The waveform will be absent if the balloon does not retain helium. The appearance of the plateau on the screen will decline if the balloon is leaking.
4. If the machine detects a leak, it will shut itself off. If it does not do so, place the console on standby and be prepared to remove the catheter within 15 to 30 minutes.
5. Clamp the IABP catheter to prevent arterial blood backup.
6. Disconnect the IABP catheter from the console (consider discontinuing anticoagulation therapy).
7. Notify the licensed practitioner and prepare for insertion of a new IABP catheter.

Skill 4-6

VENTRICULAR ASSIST DEVICES

INDICATIONS

Cardiogenic shock, severe heart failure (bridge to recovery)

Bridge to heart transplantation

Permanent placement for patient not eligible for transplantation (destination therapy)

Pneumatic device inserted for patient in cardiogenic shock secondary to IABP failure, or for high-risk percutaneous coronary intervention (PCI) or patient with end-stage heart failure

CONTRAINDICATIONS

Patient stature too small

Renal or liver failure

Comorbidity with life expectancy of less than 3 years

Psychosocial and cognitive conditions (except when used to bridge patient to recovery)

MAINTENANCE OF VENTRICULAR ASSIST DEVICE

1. See specific manufacturer's recommendations on the style and type of ventricular assist device (VAD), whether right VAD (RVAD), left VAD (LVAD), or biventricular VAD (BiVAD). All have unique ways of moving blood through a failing heart from the ventricle to the aorta.
2. A pneumatic ventricular assist device (PVAD) may be placed temporarily in the cardiac catheterization laboratory if a patient in cardiogenic shock fails to improve with balloon pump application. The clinician inserts a 21 Fr venous catheter and a 17 Fr arterial catheter in the femoral vessels, and the console suctions blood from the ventricle and then pumps the blood back to the aorta.
3. Some devices provide a nearly continuous flow, with no true pulse palpated at the arterial pulse points.
4. VADs have three main parts: a pumping chamber, cannulas, and a power source. The following illustrations show three types of VADs.

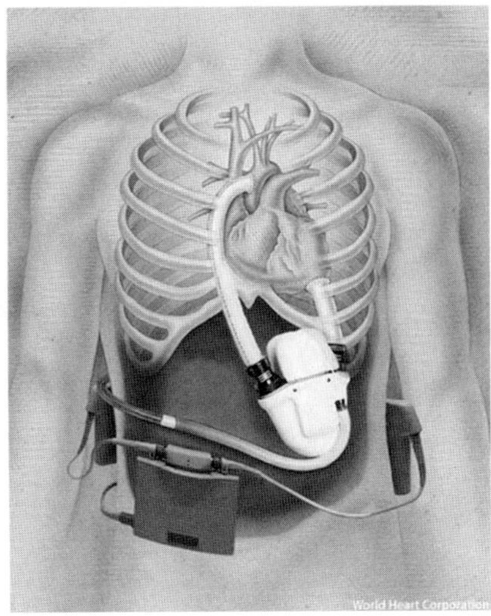

Novacor LVAS. (Courtesy World Heart, Ottawa, Canada.)

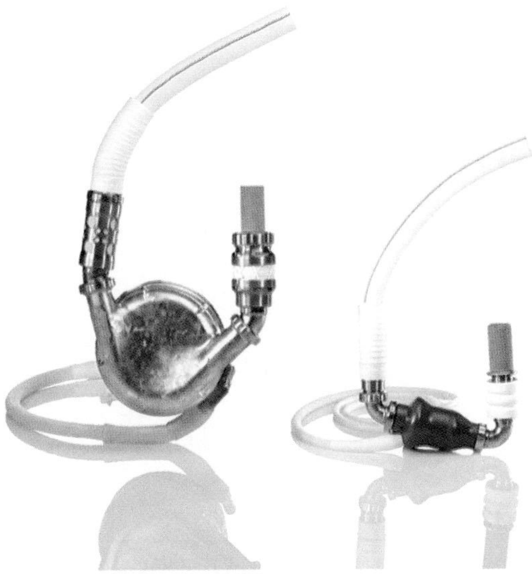

Side-by-side view of the HM-VXE (left) and the HM-II (right). (Courtesy Thoratec, Pleasanton, Calif.)

5. Early postinsertion management includes assessment for common complications: hypovolemia, right-sided heart failure, pulmonary hypertension, tamponade (mimics right-sided heart failure), bleeding and coagulopathies, arrhythmias, hypothermia, and infection.
6. Watch for clot formation and follow the manufacturer's recommendations for anticoagulation therapy (ranging from simple use of aspirin to heparin therapy).
7. Patient and family education is started early and reinforced throughout the patient's hospitalization. The patient and family are taught to plan for common troubleshooting issues: battery failure, power failure, emergency hand pumping, and so on. Keep in mind that if your critical care transport team responds to a call at a patient's private residence, the patient and family are likely to be well versed in the care of the device.

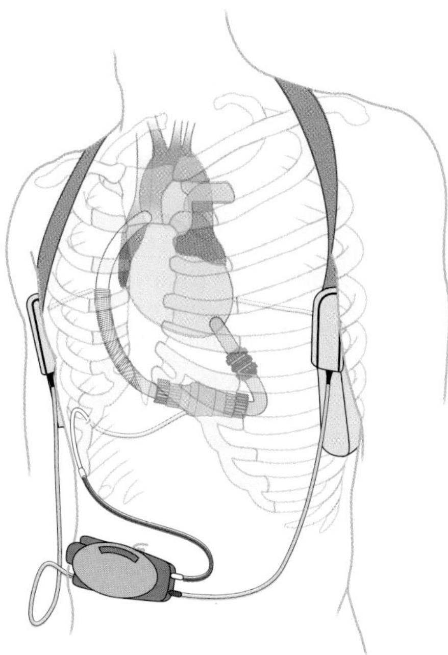

The HeartMate II continuous-flow ventricular assist device. (From Miller RD, Eriksson LI, Fleisher LA, Wiener-Kronish JP: *Miller's anesthesia*, ed 7, 2009, Churchill Livingstone.)

8. If the VAD is a continuous flow device, Doppler equipment must be used to assess the peripheral blood pressure.
9. If ventricular tachycardia or fibrillation occurs, some devices require that the power supply be disconnected from the patient before electrical therapy is applied.
10. Some transport services obtain 4 to 6 units of cross-matched blood to accompany the patient with an emergently inserted VAD in case disconnection occurs during transport.
11. Positioning a patient with an intraaortic balloon pump (IABP) or VAD console can be tricky, whether in a fixed wing or rotor wing aircraft or an ambulance. The electrodes and console catheters must not be kinked, must not become disconnected, and the console must be secured to the wall of the transport vehicle for crew and patient safety. Most ground (and some air) services load the patient into the vehicle backward to facilitate safe transport.

VAD FAILURE OR CARDIAC ARREST

1. No closed chest compressions are allowed.
2. Disconnect the controller's power source.
3. Disconnect the air filter from the percutaneous line by pressing the side release.
4. Connect the hand pump to the percutaneous line by sliding it into the coupler (air filter port).
5. Depress and hold down purge valve; then collapse the bulb with your thumb.

6. Release the purge valve and then release the bulb. Wait 10 seconds and then depress the purge valve and allow the bulb to inflate.
7. Separate the handles and swing them around so that the bulb is between the two handles. Orient the pump to the bulb so that the tubing is hanging down.
8. Squeeze the handles together to fully compress the bulb; then, release the pump at a rate of approximately 60 to 90 compressions a minute. Let the bulb fully inflate each time.
9. Every few minutes, check to see that the bulb inflates completely when released. If it does not, stop pumping and wait another 10 seconds. Press and hold the purge valve for 10 seconds more. Release the purge valve and resume pumping.
10. Contact the patient care coordinator as soon as possible and transport the patient to that location.

Emergency Hand Pumping of a First-Generation VAD

1. Remove the vent filter and connect the hand pump.
2. Push in the purge valve (which is usually white) and hold.
3. Push in the black ball (bulb) and hold.
4. Release the purge valve.
5. Release the black ball.
6. Count to 10 slowly.
7. Swing the handles around and pump 60-90 times/minute all the way to the hospital.

Valvular Dysfunction

Two mechanisms can cause dysfunction in the heart valves, stenosis and regurgitation. If a patient is brought to the ICU with valvular disease, this usually means that the patient's heart has had to compensate and heart failure remodeling has occurred.

Mitral Stenosis

Mitral stenosis (MS) is caused predominantly by aging. It is a progressive narrowing of the mitral valve, and it usually is asymptomatic. The valve leaflets fuse, preventing passive opening or closure with normal pressure changes. This dysfunction may lead to atrial fibrillation and left atrial enlargement and, frequently, CHF.

Mitral Regurgitation

Papillary muscle dysfunction, rheumatic heart disease (caused by *Streptococcus aureus* infection), age, and endocarditis may cause the mitral valve to create a backflow of blood into the left atrium; this may be a chronic or an acute condition. Chronic mitral regurgitation results in a dilated left atrium and a hypertrophied left ventricle. Acute mitral regurgitation, which is initiated when the papillary muscle ruptures as a result of MI, presents as cardiogenic shock and pump failure (Figure 4-32).

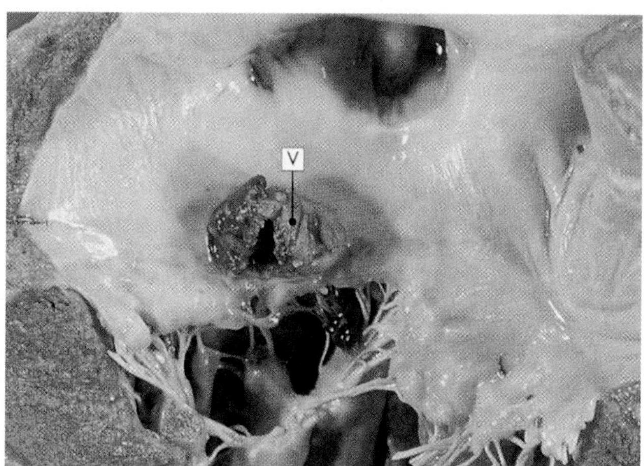

Figure 4-32

Mitral stenosis. Mitral leaflets are thickened and fused and have clumps of vegetation *(V)* containing platelets and fibrin. (From McCance K, Huether SE: *Pathophysiology: the biological basis for disease in adults and children*, ed 5, St Louis, 2005, Mosby.)

Mitral Valve Prolapse

Mitral valve prolapse (MVP) goes by many names, including systolic click–murmur syndrome, **Barlow's syndrome**, and billowing mitral cusp syndrome. In MVP, prolapse of the mitral valve, often with regurgitation, is associated with myxomatous proliferation of the leaflets of the mitral valve, a common, usually benign, and often asymptomatic condition characterized by midsystolic clicks and late systolic murmurs on auscultation. Palpitations and chest discomfort may occur, and, in some cases, progressive mitral regurgitation requires valve replacement (Figure 4-33).

Aortic Stenosis

Gradual narrowing of the aortic valve eventually slows the ejection of blood from the left ventricle into the aorta, resulting in a high LV systolic pressure, LVH, and LV dilation. Replacement of this valve is indicated when heart failure is clinically present.

Aortic Regurgitation

Backflow of blood from the aorta into the left ventricle, or aortic regurgitation (AR), is the result of insufficiency of the aortic semilunar valve; it may be chronic or acute. The condition may be caused by systemic hypertension, Marfan syndrome, or an aging valve. Usually the cusp becomes infiltrated with fibrous tissue and retracts during diastole, leading to regurgitation into the left ventricle through a defect in the center of the valve.

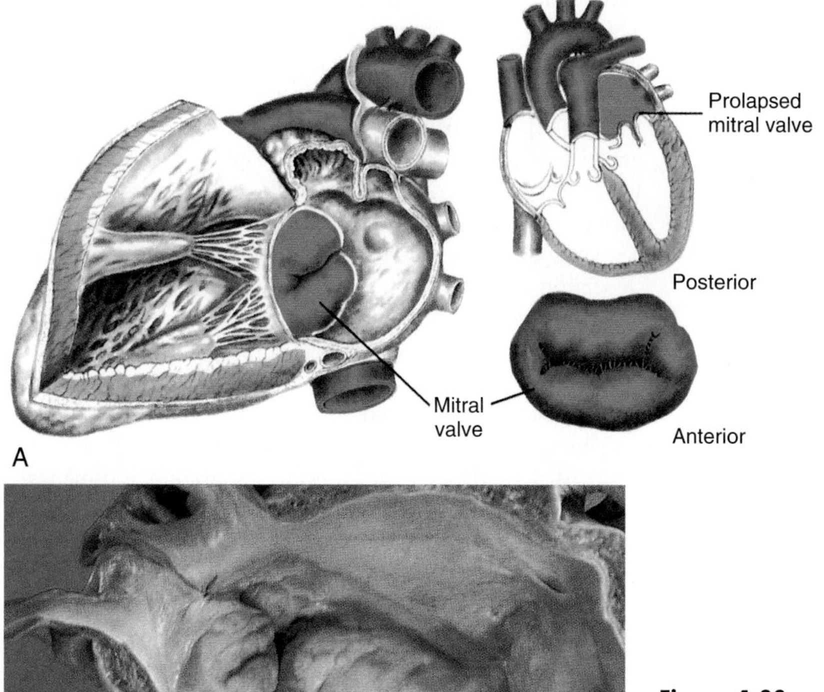

B

Figure 4-33

Mitral valve prolapse. **A,** Normal mitral valve *(lower right)* and prolapsed valve *(left)*. Prolapse allows the valve leaflets to billow back into the atrium during left ventricular systole. The billowing causes the leaflets to part slightly, permitting regurgitation into the atrium. **B,** View of the mitral valve showing ballooning of the leaflets is seen. (From McCance K, Huether SE: *Pathophysiology: the biological basis for disease in adults and children*, ed 5, St Louis, 2005, Mosby.)

Tricuspid Stenosis

Tricuspid stenosis rarely occurs by itself. It usually is paired with mitral or aortic valve disease and is caused by endocarditis or rheumatic fever. Right-sided heart failure may develop as compensation occurs.

Tricuspid Regurgitation

With advanced failure of the left side of the heart, right-sided failure eventually occurs and can cause the backflow of blood through the tricuspid valve.

Pulmonic Valve Disease

Pulmonic valve disease, most commonly associated with congenital heart disease in infants, causes right-sided heart failure. It is a rare disorder in adults.

Cardiomyopathy

In the United States, cardiomyopathy accounts for about one fourth of CHF cases. The term *cardiomyopathy* means heart muscle disease. Cardiomyopathy weakens the heart muscle, which thins and enlarges. Consequently, the entire heart muscle pumps less effectively, which eventually results in pump failure. Once failure occurs, the heart is unable to pump the appropriate amount of blood to the body. Cardiomyopathy has three basic forms: dilated cardiomyopathy (DCM, formally called congestive), restrictive cardiomyopathy (RCM), and hypertrophic cardiomyopathy (HCM). DCM accounts for about 60% of all cases of cardiomyopathy (Figure 4-34).

1. DCM results in enlarged, dysfunctional bilateral ventricles with poor myocardial muscle contraction and overall low cardiac output.
2. HCM is distinguished by an asymmetric thickening of the septal wall with left ventricular outflow obstruction (Figure 4-35). Thickening of the left ventricular wall also may be seen. This eventually results in hypertension and stenosis. Many patients with HCM develop CHF as a result of this condition. Sometimes called *hypertrophic obstructive cardiomyopathy,* HCM is genetic and has a tendency to cause arrhythmias and sudden death, frequently at a young age.
3. The least common of the myopathies, RCM causes the heart wall to stiffen, which prevents the heart from pumping effectively. RCM causes diastolic heart failure.

Management of Cardiomyopathy

The goals of treatment for cardiomyopathy include improving pump function and removing excess fluid, similar to heart failure management. Beta blockers are used to reduce the left ventricular workload; implanted defibrillators and pacers, anticoagulants, and antidysrhythmics also may be part of medical management.

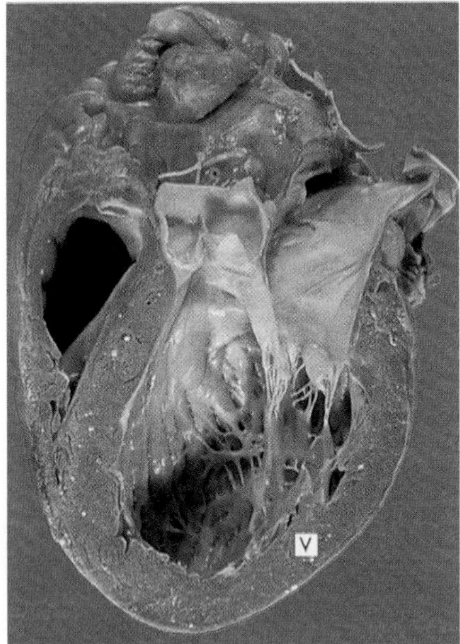

Figure 4-34

Dilated cardiomyopathy. The dilated left ventricle has a thin wall *(V)*. (From McCance K, Huether SE: *Pathophysiology: the biological basis for disease in adults and children,* ed 5, St Louis, 2005, Mosby.)

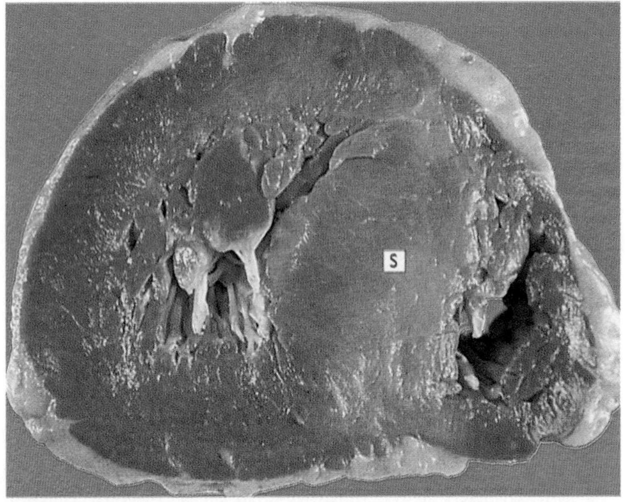

Figure 4-35

Hypertrophic cardiomyopathy. Note the marked left ventricular hypertrophy; this often affects the septum *(S)*. (From McCance K, Huether SE: *Pathophysiology: the biological basis for disease in adults and children,* ed 5, St Louis, 2005, Mosby.)

In advanced cases of cardiomyopathy, cardiac transplantation may be necessary. If the patient is unable to undergo transplantation, ventricular pumping or assist devices can be placed surgically to "bridge" the patient to transplantation or as "destination therapy" (used to assist the pump until death).

Cardiac Tamponade

Cardiac tamponade, a condition in which the pericardial sac fills with blood, pus, air, effusate, or any combination of these, results from an increase in intrapericardial pressure. Tamponade leaves the heart unable to meet its workload. Think about what happens during inspiration as the volume in the right ventricle increases: the right ventricle meets the resistance of the filled pericardium; this causes the interventricular septum to bulge to the left, which reduces the left ventricular end-diastolic volume; this reduces cardiac output, which causes a drop in the systolic blood pressure. Acute cardiac tamponade may be the result of traumatic rupture of the ventricle secondary to a procedure, blunt trauma, aortic dissection, or an MI with valve rupture. Subacute tamponade is more commonly the result of infection or uremia or develops after an MI or cardiothoracic surgery.

Management of Tamponade

The speed with which fluid (blood or effusate) enters the pericardial sac dictates the clinical presentation and management. For example, if a quick infusion of 30 mL of blood enters the pericardial sac as a result of trauma or a transmural MI, the patient rather quickly develops Beck's triad: JVD, hypotension (sometimes described with narrowing pulse pressure), and muffled heart sounds. If the effusion seeps into the sac slowly (as in third spacing from uremia), the pericardium accommodates, signs and symptoms are vague and slow in onset, and management may be more conservative.

Aortic Dissection

The aorta is made up of three layers: the tunica intima, the tunica media, and the tunica adventitia. In aortic dissection, a tear begins in the tunica intima. The higher pressure in the aortic lumen forces blood through this tear, causing the tunica intima to separate from the tunica media. As the blood volume increases between the tunica intima and tunica media, the tunica intima is pressed into the aortic lumen, restricting blood flow (Figure 4-36). The result is higher back pressure, which drives more blood and pressure into the tear. This situation rapidly worsens the patient's condition by expanding the tear farther down the aorta, possibly resulting in aortic rupture. Often the result of chronic hypertension, aortic dissection frequently is fatal despite advanced intervention. Men 50 to 70 years of age are most likely to have nontraumatic dissection, but women should not be excluded from consideration of this diagnosis, particularly with regard to pregnancy and pregnancy-induced hypertension. More than half of the cases of aortic dissection in women occur in individuals who are under age 40 and in the third trimester or postpartum.

The three major classification systems for aortic dissection are the DeBakey system, the Stanford system, and the descriptive system (Table 4-11).

Definitive diagnosis of aortic dissection requires radiologic evaluation, but some key indicators warrant a high index of suspicion. The patient usually complains of a sudden onset of sharp, severe pain, often described as "tearing." The location of the pain may be very helpful for determining where the dissection has occurred. Severe pain in the anterior chest wall may indicate a dissection only in the ascending aorta, whereas pain between the scapulas may indicate involvement only of the descending thoracic aorta. Any pain in the neck, throat,

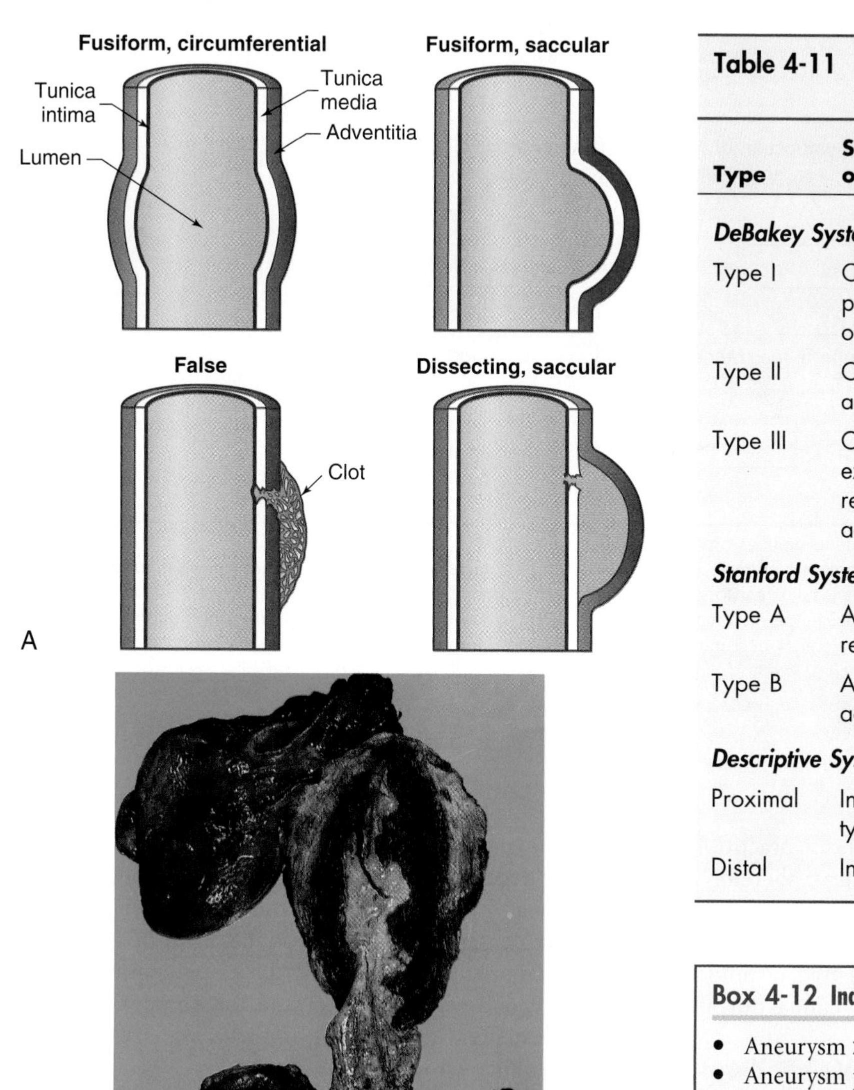

Figure 4-36

Longitudinal sections showing types of aneurysms. **A,** Fusiform circumferential and fusiform saccular aneurysms are true aneurysms, caused by weakening of the vessel wall. False and saccular aneurysms involve a break in the vessel wall, usually caused by trauma. **B,** Dissecting aneurysm of the thoracic aorta. (From McCance K, Huether SE: *Pathophysiology: the biological basis for disease in adults and children*, ed 5, St Louis, 2005, Mosby.)

jaw, or face may indicate involvement of the ascending aorta, and pain in the back, abdomen, or lower extremities predicts involvement of the descending aorta. During the physical examination, tachycardia may be noted; bilateral blood pressure measurements should be taken, and these pressures usually are high. If the patient is hypotensive, this suggests cardiac tamponade or aortic rupture. During auscultation of the heart, an aortic regurgitation murmur may be noted if the lesion is near the aortic room. The cardiac monitor usually displays sinus tachycardia, and a chest radiograph may show a widened aortic silhouette in 90% of Stanford type A dissections.

Table 4-11 Common Classification Systems for Aortic Dissection

Type	Site of Origin and Extent of Aortic Involvement
DeBakey System	
Type I	Originates in the ascending aorta and propagates at least to the aortic arch and often beyond it distally
Type II	Originates in and is confined to the ascending aorta
Type III	Originates in the descending aorta and extends distally down the aorta or, rarely, retrograde into the aortic arch and ascending aorta
Stanford System	
Type A	All dissections involving the ascending aorta, regardless of the site of origin
Type B	All dissections not involving the ascending aorta
Descriptive System	
Proximal	Includes DeBakey types I and II or Stanford type A
Distal	Includes DeBakey type III or Stanford type B

Box 4-12 Indications for Aortic Aneurysm Repair

- Aneurysm >5 cm
- Aneurysm progressively increasing in size
- Impending rupture
- Symptoms resulting from cerebral or coronary ischemia or peripheral (limb) ischemia
- Pericardial tamponade
- Uncontrollable pain
- Aortic insufficiency

Treatment of Aortic Dissection

Aortic dissection is treated either medically or surgically. The method chosen depends on the extent of the lesion and the patient's condition. If the patient is stable, you will control hypertension and anticipate an elective surgical repair (if the aneurysm is larger than 4 to 5 cm). If dissection of the aneurysm is in progress, control of blood pressure and heart rate is the goal.

Type A aortic dissection may require immediate surgical intervention that is beyond the capabilities of many hospitals. Keep this in mind when transporting these patients (Box 4-12). Extension of the dissection usually is indicated if the patient presents with new or continued pain, especially with

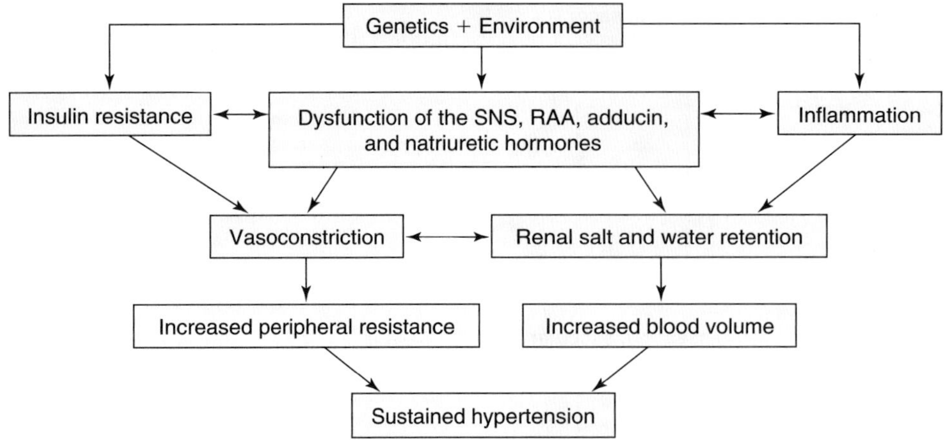

Figure 4-37

Pathophysiology of hypertension. Numerous genetic vulnerabilities have been linked to hypertension, and these, in combination with environmental risks, cause neurohumoral dysfunction (i.e., the sympathetic nervous system [SNS], renin-angiotensin-aldosterone system [RAAS], adducing, and natriuretic hormones) and promote inflammation and insulin resistance. Insulin resistance and neurohumoral dysfunction contribute to sustained systemic vasoconstriction and increased peripheral resistance. Inflammation contributes to renal dysfunction, which, in combination with the neurohumoral alteration, results in renal salt and water retention and increased blood volume. Increased peripheral resistance and increased blood volume are two primary causes of sustained hypertension. (From McCance K, Huether SE: *Pathophysiology: the biological basis for disease in adults and children*, ed 5, St Louis, 2005, Mosby.)

hypotension. The treatment goal of the critical care practitioner is to prevent further expansion of the tear; therefore, monitor cardiac rhythm, blood pressure, and end-organ perfusion. Two large-bore IV lines should be placed, and an arterial line also is usually used. If an arterial line is used, it should be placed in the right arm so that it remains functional during surgery when the aorta is cross clamped.

With the typical hypertensive presentation of aortic dissection, you must reduce the overall blood pressure and also the rise in the arterial pulse to reduce the shearing forces of the dissection. Recommendations for accomplishing this include the use of beta blockers in conjunction with a nitrate (e.g., sodium nitroprusside [Nipride]). Esmolol (Brevibloc), mixed 5 g in 500 mL of D_5W, is given as an initial bolus of 500 mcg/kg, followed by an infusion of 50 to 200 mcg/kg/min. The short half-life of this drug allows rapid, easy adjustments. The sodium nitroprusside (given to maintain the systolic BP at 100 to 120 mm Hg) is mixed 50 mg in 500 mL of D_5W and administered at a rate of 0.5 to 3 mcg/kg/min.

Patients with aortic dissection who present with hypotension should be resuscitated with IV fluids and transported as quickly as possible to a facility with a cardiothoracic surgeon. With ascending aortic dissection, pericardiocentesis may aid cardiac output and perfusion and help prepare the patient for surgical intervention.

Physiologic Disorders

Hypertensive Crisis

Hypertension is a condition the critical care team routinely encounters. It is defined as a sustained elevation of the systemic arterial BP. Hypertension can be caused by an increase in cardiac output or peripheral vascular resistance, or both. The three types of hypertension are primary hypertension, secondary hypertension, and isolated hypertension.

- Primary hypertension, also known as *essential* or *idiopathic hypertension,* usually is the result of genetics or environmental factors, and the cause cannot be pinpointed to a single or specific factor. About 90% to 95% of patients with hypertension have primary hypertension (Figure 4-37).
- Secondary hypertension usually is the result of hemodynamic changes caused by disease (Table 4-12). For example, with arteriosclerosis, reduced blood flow in areas distal to the blockage causes peripheral vascular resistance (PVR) to regulate the perfusion pressure.
- Isolated hypertension is an elevated systolic pressure with a normal diastolic pressure. This condition is due to an increase in cardiac output or rigidity in the aorta, or both.

A number of circumstances require rapid treatment of hypertension (Table 4-13). Any patient with a persistent diastolic pressure higher than 130 mm Hg and who has signs of cardiovascular, neurologic, or renal organ system dysfunction requires immediate treatment to reduce this pressure. Two such hypertensive emergencies are hypertensive encephalopathy and malignant hypertension.

Hypertensive Encephalopathy

Autoregulation of the brain (see Chapter 5) usually protects it from rises in BP. **Encephalopathy** occurs when an abrupt, sustained rise in BP exceeds the limits of autoregulation. If the mean arterial pressure (MAP) rises higher than 160 mm Hg, this rare emergency may occur, resulting in vasospasm, ischemia, small hemorrhages, and cerebral edema.

Table 4-12 Pathogenesis of Major Forms of Secondary Hypertension by Cause

Primary Disease	Pathogenesis of Hypertension
Renal Disorders	
Renal parenchymal disease	Disturbances in filtration and reabsorption of serum sodium, potassium, and calcium initiate the hemodynamics of early hypertension.
Renovascular disease	Impaired blood flow and renal ischemia evoke the compensatory renin-angiotensin-aldosterone mechanism in an effort to raise the renal perfusion pressure.
Renin-producing tumors	Elevated blood renin levels evoke elevations in angiotensin and aldosterone, which cause the blood pressure to rise.
Renal failure	Disturbances in filtration and reabsorption of serum sodium, potassium, and calcium initiate the hemodynamics of early hypertension.
Primary sodium retention	Disturbance in filtration and/or reabsorption of serum sodium initiates the hemodynamics of early hypertension.
Endocrine Disorders	
Acromegaly	Excess human growth hormone causes increased peripheral resistance.
Hypothyroidism	Mucopolysaccharide deposits in vascular tissue increase resistance.
Hypercalcemia	Calcium ion directly affects vascular tonicity; elevated serum calcium levels increase vascular tone and peripheral resistance.
Hyperthyroidism	Increased inotropic effect on the heart elevates systolic pressure; diastolic pressure decreases as a result of decreased peripheral resistance.
Adrenal disorders	Glucocorticoids facilitate sodium and water retention, initiating the hemodynamics of early hypertension.
Cortical disturbances, Cushing syndrome, primary aldosteronism	Excess aldosterone promotes sodium retention and initiation of the hemodynamics of early hypertension.
Congenital adrenal hyperplasia	Excess production of adrenocortical hormones promotes sodium and water retention.
Medullary disturbance (pheochromocytoma)	Excess catecholamines raise vascular tone and increase peripheral resistance.
Extraadrenal chromaffin tumors	Excess catecholamines raise vascular tone and increase peripheral resistance.
Vascular Disorders	
Coarctation of the aorta	Decreased blood flow in distal areas initiates maximum peripheral resistance as an autoregulatory effort to adjust perfusion pressure.
Arteriosclerosis	Loss of elasticity in vessel walls results in increased peripheral resistance.
Pregnancy-Induced Hypertension	Pathogenesis unclear.
Neurologic Disorders	
Elevated intracranial pressure (brain tumor, encephalitis, respiratory acidosis of pulmonary or central nervous system origin)	Higher systemic blood pressure is required to maintain adequate cerebral perfusion.
Quadriplegia, acute porphyria, familial dysautonomia, lead poisoning, Guillain-Barré syndrome	Interface with neural control of blood pressure initiates increased systemic blood pressure.
Acute Stress	
Surgery, psychogenic hyperventilation, hypoglycemia, burns, pancreatitis, alcohol withdrawal, sickle cell crisis, resuscitation, increased intravascular volume	Acute stress precipitates release of catecholamines and glucocorticoids.

Cotninued

Table 4-12 Pathogenesis of Major Forms of Secondary Hypertension by Cause—Cont'd

Primary Disease	Pathogenesis of Hypertension
Drugs and Other Substances	
Oral contraceptives and estrogen	Unknown; possibly caused by sodium retention, plasma retention, weight gain, changes in levels and actions of renin, angiotensin, and aldosterone.
Corticosteroids	Same as for Cushing disease.
Sympathetic stimulants, appetite suppressants, antihistamines	Raises vascular tone and increases vascular resistance.
Licorice	Contains glycyrrhizic acid, a mineralocorticoid that causes salt and water retention.
Monoamine oxidase (MAO) inhibitors	Hypertension may develop in an individual who routinely takes an MAO inhibitor and eats foods containing tyramine (e.g., aged cheese).

From McCance KL, Huether SE: *Pathophysiology: the biologic basis for disease in adults and children*, ed 5, St. Louis, 2002, Mosby.

Table 4-13 Circumstances That Require Rapid Treatment of Hypertension

Accelerated Malignant Hypertension with Papilledema

Cerebrovascular

Hypertensive encephalopathy
Atherothrombotic brain infarction with severe hypertension
Intracerebral hemorrhage
Subarachnoid hemorrhage

Cardiac

Acute aortic dissection
Acute left ventricular failure
Acute or impending myocardial infarction
After coronary bypass surgery

Renal

Acute glomerulonephritis
Renal crises from collagen-vascular diseases
Severe hypertension after kidney transplantation

Excessive Circulating Catecholamines

Pheochromocytoma crisis
Food or drug interactions with monoamine oxidase inhibitors
Sympathomimetic drug use (cocaine)
Rebound hypertension after sudden cessation of antihypertensive drugs

Eclampsia

Surgery

Severe hypertension in a patient requiring immediate surgery
Postoperative hypertension
Postoperative bleeding from vascular suture lines

Severe Body Burns

Severe Epistaxis

From Kaplan NM: Management of hypertensive emergencies, *Lancet* 344:1325, 1994.

Malignant Hypertension

Also called *accelerated hypertension,* malignant hypertension is a severe disease that damages organs. The diastolic pressure usually rises rapidly to exceed 130 mm Hg, which causes dilation of the arterioles and leakage of fluid into the tissues. These patients usually present with severe headache, blurred vision, dyspnea, and chest pain. BP readings alone should not determine this diagnosis; crackles in the bases, an enlarged left ventricle, retinal hemorrhage, and quick elevations in the BUN and creatinine with hematuria assist in the diagnosis.

Management of Hypertensive Emergencies

Invasive BP monitoring should be implemented, and reduction of the BP should be guided by judicious lowering of the MAP by 25%, with a target of 160/100 mm Hg within a few hours. Excessive and quick drops in BP can cause more end-organ damage. This management plan usually includes a constant infusion of sodium nitroprusside, because the drug has a rapid onset and a short duration of action. Infusion should begin at 0.25 to 2 mcg/kg/min; the average dose is 3 mcg/kg/min. Fenoldopam, a peripheral dopamine$_1$ receptor agonist, also may be used for this hypertensive emergency (maximum dose, 1.6 mcg/kg/min). Nitroglycerin, hydralazine, and beta blockers (e.g., labetolol) or calcium channel blockers (e.g., nicardipine) also may be used, depending on the patient's clinical status and the cause of the rise in BP.

Temporary or Permanently Implanted Electrical Devices

Pacemakers

Originally designed to stimulate faster rates in symptomatic bradycardia, the pacemaker has become another management technique for those with atrial fibrillation and patients in heart failure. For patients with paroxysmal atrial fibrillation, placing wires or sensors on the atria can stimulate a slightly faster rate in the normal rhythm, or the device can sense when arrhythmia has developed. The critical care team sometimes encounters a transvenous (endocardial) or epicardial pacing generator system and must know how to maintain the therapy.

For heart failure, cardiac resynchronization therapy is the goal of pacemaker management. As described earlier, many of these patients have ventricular conduction delays, which trigger a conduction system without synchrony, thereby making ventricular filling dysfunctional and further complicating the pump failure. Atrial and biventricular pacing (three pacing leads) resynchronizes the conduction and aids in overall pump function.

The pacing system usually is bipolar, having positive and negative leads to the heart. Stimulation is sent down the distal lead (negative) and picked up by the positive lead (sensor) on the right side of the heart. Occasionally, one lead (unipolar) can be attached directly to the myocardium through direct placement (epicardial lead) or by the IV route (transvenous or endocardial lead). Epicardial leads are sutured directly to the myocardium after heart surgery, and the wires exit the skin near the sternum. Epicardial wires are gently pulled from the site a few days after surgery.

Did You Know?

Clinicians use a special laboratory value, the brain natriuretic peptide (BNP) level, for ongoing evaluation of a patient with heart failure. The BNP level predicts congestive heart failure deterioration, sometimes before clinical signs appear. It also allows the physician to alter therapy and possibly avert admission or shorten the hospital stay. Currently, a special wireless pressure sensor is undergoing clinical trials of its ability to detect pressure changes in the heart.[8]

- **BNP levels below 100 pg/mL indicate no heart failure**
- **BNP levels of 100-300 suggest heart failure is present**
- **BNP levels above 300 pg/mL indicate mild heart failure**
- **BNP levels above 600 pg/mL indicate moderate heart failure.**
- **BNP levels above 900 pg/mL indicate severe heart failure**

Pacemaker settings include rate, output, and sensitivity (Table 4-14). The generator has a rate control setting (impulses sent to heart per minute), an output dial that regulates the milliamperes (mA) delivered to the heart, and a sensitivity control that tunes the generator's sensing abilities to the patient's inherent heartbeat, measured in millivolts (mV). Individual pacemakers may have other controls specific to the type of pacemaker and the disease process being managed.

Table 4-14 Pacemaker Terminology, Modes, and Codes

Mode	Code	Description
Asynchronous (fixed rate)	AOO	Atrial pacing, no sensing
	VOO	Ventricular pacing, no sensing
	DOO	Dual atrial and ventricular pacing, no sensing
Synchronous (demand)	AAI	Atrial pacing and sensing; inhibited response to sensed P waves
	VVI	Ventricular pacing and sensing; inhibited response to sensed QRS complex
	DVI	Atrial and ventricular pacing and sensing; both inhibited if spontaneous ventricular depolarization occurs
Universal (AV sequential; dual chamber)	DDD	Both chambers paced and sensed; inhibited response if depolarization occurs; triggered response with atrial activity to allow for natural ventricular response

From Urden LD, Stacy KM, Lough ME: *Thelan's critical care nursing: diagnosis and management,* ed 5, St. Louis, 2006, Mosby.

As with transcutaneous pacemakers, you must know whether the pacemaker stimulus beat is conducted or "captured." Loss of capture occurs when the pacing electrode becomes displaced or a high threshold develops (*threshold* is the point at which depolarization occurs with the given output). You may increase the output to regain capture or, if transvenous placement has been used, turn the patient to the left to reposition the electrodes. If battery failure or mechanical generator failure occurs, rate variances or a complete loss of pacing signal may result. Transport teams should always carry extra batteries specific to their pacemaker generator as a backup.

If the temporary pacemaker has a sensor, it may malfunction, resulting in undersensing or oversensing. *Undersensing* means that the device cannot determine the heart's inherent heartbeat and may send out paced signals in competition with normal conduction; this can cause R-on-T phenomenon and lethal dysrhythmias. This usually is caused by low R wave amplitude and can be corrected by lowering the sensitivity setting. Also check to make sure the pacemaker is in the synchronous mode. *Oversensing* is characterized by low pacing stimulus as the synchronous mode picks up errant signals and interprets them as atrial or ventricular activity. Some errant signals may come from tall T waves or electrical interference. Usually, moving the sensitivity dial toward 20 mV remedies this situation.

Implantable Cardioverter Defibrillator

An ICD is an electronic device that has sensing electrodes that recognize dysrhythmias (usually tachycardic or disorganized) and a defibrillation electrode to shock the heart. ICDs are surgically placed in patients at high risk for lethal dysrhythmias, including those with an **ejection fraction** below 30% and those who have survived a cardiac arrest. Some generators include dual, synchronous pacing and options for synchronized cardioversion. EP laboratories and the electrophysiologist are in charge of all ICD programming. Because there are many types of control generators, the sending facility may want to disconnect their device before transport. Care must be taken to have a backup generator that will receive the patient's electrodes and a backup plan, in case the wired device fails to capture. The backup plan usually includes application of transcutaneous pacemaker pads, attached to your emergency monitor/defibrillator/pacer device and ready to be used.

Scenario Conclusion

During transport, cardiac output is successfully increased through the use of dopamine, milrinone, and an IABP. However, the patient's heart rate increases to 130 beats/min, and you reduce the IABP ratio to 1:2. The distal pulses improve, along with the overall BP; the arterial reading is 98/60 mm Hg on arrival at the receiving hospital. You deliver the patient to the ICU and give a bedside report.

SUMMARY

The cardiovascular system is an incredible mechanism that allows the body to receive oxygen and nutrients and remove waste. Trillions of cells rely on a functional cardiovascular system. The critical care practitioner must have a clear understanding of the in-depth workings of the heart's anatomy and physiology as they relate to preload, contractility, and afterload for stroke volume. The stroke volume and the heart's ability to beat rhythmically at a steady rate create the necessary cardiac output that sustains life. In patients with a pathologic condition of the cardiovascular system, proper identification and management of the disease during transport are common, yet crucial challenges for the critical care practitioner.

KEY TERMS

ablation Removal or destruction of a part, especially by cutting.

afterload In cardiac physiology, the force against which cardiac muscle shortens. The force resisting shortening after the muscle is stimulated to contract in the intact heart is the pressure against which the ventricle ejects blood, as measured by the stress acting on the ventricular wall following the onset of contraction, determined largely by the peripheral vascular resistance and by the physical characteristics of and blood volume in the arterial system. It is often estimated by determining systolic arterial pressure, from which can be determined the systolic wall stress.

Barlow's syndrome Mitral valve prolapse.

baroreceptors A type of interoceptor that is stimulated by changes in pressure, particularly one located in the wall of a blood vessel; a pressure receptor.

chelation Combination with a metal in complexes in which the metal is part of a ring.

chemoreceptors A sense organ such as the carotid body, the aortic bodies, or the glomus jugulare, which is sensitive to chemical changes in the bloodstream, especially reduced oxygen content, and reflexively increases both respiration and blood pressure.

clubbing A digital deformity produced by proliferation of the soft tissues about the terminal phalanges of the fingers or toes without constant osseous changes. Clubbing is seen in various chronic diseases of the thoracic organs.

dicrotic notch A small downward deflection in the arterial pulse or pressure contour that occurs immediately after closure of the semilunar valves and before the dicrotic wave; it sometimes is used as a marker for the end of systole, or the ejection period.

ejection fraction The proportion of the volume of blood in the ventricles at the end of diastole that is ejected during systole (stroke volume divided by end-diastolic volume); it often is expressed as a percentage. The normal range for the ejection fraction is 57% to 73%; lower values indicate ventricular dysfunction.

encephalopathy Any degenerative disease of the brain.

Frank-Starling law (aka Starling's Law or Frank-Starling mechanism): The energy released with each heart contraction is a function of the length of the fibers composing its muscular walls; increased preload causes increased end-diastolic volume (or pressure) which increases the force of ventricular contraction.

isovolumetric period The interval in the cardiac cycle during which the cardiac muscle fibers are contracting or relaxing but the valves remain closed, anchored by the chordae tendineae.

myocardial infarction A cardiac event in which perfusion of the cells is inadequate.

preload The mechanical state of the heart at the end of diastole, the magnitude of the maximal (end-diastolic) ventricular volume or the end-disastolic pressure stretching the ventricles; In cardiac muscle, the force stretching the resting muscle to a given length prior to contraction; The stress on the ventricular wall at the end of diastole, determined by venous return, total blood volume and its distribution, and atrial activity.

pressure transducer system Each healthcare system creates variations but the basic system set up includes a bag of 0.9% normal saline solution (some use D_5W) as the flush. Some hospitals use 1 unit of heparin per mL of solution. Other hospitals don't use heparin. A pressure infusion cuff covers the bag of solution and is inflated to 300 mm Hg. The IV tubing includes three-way stopcocks with a manual flush device. This must be high-pressure IV tubing. The third part is the transducer that sends the pressure signal through a computer and sends the signal to the monitor.

radiolucent Permitting the passage of x-rays or other forms of radiant energy with little attention; radiolucent areas appear dark on the exposed film.

shunting To turn to one side; to divert or bypass.

thrill A sensation of vibration felt on palpation (e.g., over the heart during loud, harsh cardiac murmurs).

Wedge pressure Hemodynamic monitoring systems (pulmonary artery catheter and transducer) will measure various pressures from the left-sided and right-sided circulatory systems. Preload in the left side of the heart can be measured through this system by inflating the distal balloon on the catheter and allowing circulation to "float" the distal end into the capillary-alveolar area of the lung. The catheter tip has then been "wedged" into this area to record the pressure. Called pulmonary artery wedge pressure (PCWP). Also known as the pulmonary artery occlusion pressure (PAOP)

unifascicular block An impairment of conduction in the right bundle branch or in either the anterior or posterior limb of the left bundle branch.

REFERENCES

1. Field JM: *American Heart Association ACLS resource text: professional for instructors and experienced providers*, 2008, The Association.
2. Urden LD, Stacy KM, Lough ME: *Thelan's critical care nursing: diagnosis and management*, ed 5, St. Louis, 2006, Mosby.
3. Sanders MJ: *Mosby's paramedic textbook revised*, ed 3, St Louis, 2007, Mosby.
4. National Highway Traffic Safety Administration (NHTSA): *Paramedic curriculum, 1999 (website)*. www.nhtsa.dot.gov/people/injury/ems/EMT-P/index.html. Accessed January 8, 2010.
5. Dorland NW: *Dorland's illustrated medical dictionary*, ed 31, Philadelphia, 2007, Saunders.
6. Darovic GO: *Hemodynamic monitoring: invasive and noninvasive clinical application*, ed 3, Philadelphia, 2002, Saunders.
7. Costanzo MR, Guglin ME, Saltzberg MT, et al: *Ultrafiltration versus intravenous diuretics for patients hospitalized for acute decompensated heart failure*, *J Am Coll Cardiol* 13:49:675-683, 2007.
8. Cabuay B: *Pacemaker*. University of Iowa Heart and Vascular Center, Cardiomyopathy Treatment Program (website). www.uihealthcare.com/pacemaker. 12/15/07

Bibliography

Alspach JG: *Core curriculum for critical care nursing*, ed 5, Philadelphia, 1998, Saunders.

Braunwald E, Fauci AS, Kasper DL, et al: *Harrison's manual of medicine*, ed 5, New York, 2004, McGraw-Hill.

Braunwald E, Zipes DP, Libby P: *Heart disease: a text book of cardiovascular medicine*, ed 6, Philadelphia, 2001, Saunders.

Davis L: *Cardiovascular nursing secrets*, ed 4, Philadelphia, 2007, Saunders.

Dorland NW: *Dorland's illustrated medical dictionary*, ed 31, Philadelphia, 2007, Saunders.

Field JM: *American Heart Association ACLS resource text: professional for instructors and experienced providers*, 2008, The Association.

Gould BE: *Pathophysiology for the health care professional*, ed 3, Philadelphia, 2006, Saunders.

Grubbs N, Newby D: *Churchill's pocketbook of cardiology*, London, 2000, Mosby.

Holleron RS: *Air and surface patient transport*, ed 3, St Louis, 2003, Mosby.

Marx J, Hockberger R, Walls R: *Rosen's emergency medicine: concepts and clinical practice*, ed 6, St Louis, 2006, Mosby.

McCance K, Huether SE: *Pathophysiology: the biologic bases for disease in adults and children*, ed 5, St Louis, 2006, Mosby.

Parsons PE, Weiner-Kronesh JP: *Critical care secrets*, ed 4, St Louis, 2007, Mosby.

Phalen T, Aehlert B: *12 Lead EKG in acute coronary syndrome*, ed 2, St Louis, 2006, Mosby.

Runge MS, Ohmon ME: *Netter's cardiology*, Philadelphia, 2004, Saunders.

Standring S: *Gray's anatomy: the anatomical bases of clinical practice*, ed 39, St Louis, 2005, Mosby.

Surawiez B, Knilans T: *Chou's electrocardiology in clinical practice*, ed 5, Philadelphia, 2001, Saunders.

Young VB, Kormos WA, Goroll AH: *Blueprints: medicine*, ed 2, Malden, Mass, 2001, Blackwell.

REVIEW QUESTIONS

1. Atrial contractions contribute approximately ____% of the blood flow in ventricular filling.
2. Autoregulation of blood flow through the coronary arteries is based on two mechanisms: the metabolic theory and __________.

3. The left circumflex coronary artery (LCX) travels in a groove called the ___________.

4. The three specialized pathways that contain Purkinje fibers and connect the SA node to the AV node are the internodal pathway, the Wenckebach bundle, and the ___________.

5. Which heart tones are frequently known as gallops? ___________

6. Angina can be categorized as stable, unstable, and ___________.

7. Barlow's syndrome is also known as ___________.

8. Dilated cardiomyopathy accounts for about _______% of all cardiomyopathies.

9. What are the three major classification systems for aortic dissection? ___________

10. About 90% to 95% of patients with hypertension have what type? ___________

11. The blood gas results noted in the case study showed:
    A. Respiratory acidosis
    B. Respiratory alkalosis
    C. Metabolic acidosis
    D. Metabolic alkalosis

12. The condition noted in question 11, indicated by the blood gas results in the case study, is probably caused by:
    A. Use of the IABP
    B. Pericardiocentesis
    C. Oxygen use
    D. Shock

13. If an arrhythmia developed in the case study patient while the balloon pump was functioning, you should:
    A. Time the device by setting it to arrhythmia mode
    B. Set the ratio of shuttle to 1:2
    C. Time the device to the R waves
    D. Both A and B

14. If the IABP is timed to the arterial BP, it should be set to:
    A. Inflate just after the dicrotic notch
    B. Inflate just on the dicrotic notch
    C. Inflate just before the dicrotic notch
    D. The systolic BP of 80 mm Hg

15. The IABP is used to:
    A. Reduce afterload by inflating during systole
    B. Reduce afterload by inflating during diastole
    C. Increase contractility by deflating during diastole
    D. Increase preload by inflating during systole

16. Which of the following is/are true about a ventricular assist device?
    A. It is used for pump failure and may be a temporary management device.
    B. Newer devices power blood flow through a rotary device; therefore, the patient may not have a palpable pulse.
    C. It may be used instead of heart transplantation for cardiomyopathy.
    D. All of the above

17. The patient in the case study developed pericardial tamponade. The most common set of symptoms associated with that ailment includes:
    A. Narrowing pulse pressure, JVD, and muffled heart sounds
    B. Widening pulse pressure, JVD, and muffled heart sounds
    C. Cardiogenic shock with JVD and crackles in the lung bases
    D. Cannon waves, S_3 gallop, and ascites

18. Dopamine may be given to patients in cardiogenic shock to:
    A. Increase urinary output
    B. Increase contractility
    C. Reduce preload
    D. Increase preload

19. Milrinone is a(an):
    A. Phosphodiesterase inhibitor that aids the pumping function
    B. Vasoconstrictor
    C. Antibiotic
    D. Beta-adrenergic blocker

20. Another management technique for reducing afterload (and therefore increasing cardiac output) is:
    A. Turning the patient to the left
    B. Administering nitrates
    C. Administering alpha blocking agents
    D. Administering mineral corticosteroids

21. In the case study, the patient was noted to have an inferior-lateral MI. Which ECG findings indicate this anomaly?
    A. Q waves in all leads
    B. ST elevation of 1 to 2 mm in leads II, III, and aVF
    C. ST depression in leads I, aVL, V_5, and V_6
    D. Q waves possible in leads I, II, III, aVL, aVF, V_5, and V_6

22. The patient presents with tachycardia, and you are attempting to determine whether it is SVT or VT. Which ECG finding correctly describes a ventricular tachycardia?
    A. Extreme right axis deviation
    B. Upright R waves in V_1
    C. Downward R waves in V_1
    D. QRS width less than 1 to 2 mm

CHAPTER 5

Neurologic System

OBJECTIVES

1. Apply the principles of neuroanatomy, physiology, and pathophysiology to the assessment and management of a critically ill patient with a neurologic disorder.
2. Interpret the data collected from the neurologic assessment, diagnostic tools, and intracranial pressure monitoring to formulate an impression of the patient's clinical status.
3. List the indications, desired effects, contraindications, incompatibilities, and side effects of pharmacologic and nonpharmacologic interventions in the patient's treatment.
4. Justify a treatment plan that is within the scope of practice of the adult critical care paramedic.
5. Provide or assist in the provision of appropriate medical interventions for the patient.
6. Predict the probable physiologic consequences of the patient's condition based on serial assessment of the clinical status.

Scenario

Your critical care transport team has been contacted to transport a 22-year-old male patient from a local level III trauma care facility back to your level I facility. Within the past 30 minutes, the patient suffered high-speed, blunt force trauma in a motor vehicle collision. He has just arrived at the local hospital, and the nurse requesting the transport states, "He looks bad. We're preparing to intubate."

Sixty minutes after the initial impact, you arrive at the bedside. The patient has been intubated with an 8 mm tracheal tube (23 cm at the lip). He has bilateral breath sounds (better on the left than on the right) and a 32 Fr chest tube in the right axillary line that is connected to a closed pleural drainage system. You note 250 mL of bright red blood in the collection chamber. There are no signs of an air leak. The physician suspects intraabdominal injury, and so far 2 L of lactated Ringer's solution have been administered.

The patient's current vital signs are: heart rate, 128 beats/min; BP, 92/60 mm Hg; positive pressure ventilation, 12 breaths/min; tidal volume, 600 mL. Pulse oximetry shows 100% saturation. You apply a capnograph sensor and note normal ventilation patterns with an end-tidal carbon dioxide pressure ($PETCO_2$) of 34 mm Hg. The nurses report that the heart rate has been fluctuating between 80 and 130 beats/min in a sinus rhythm and sinus arrhythmia.

The patient's score on the Glasgow Coma Scale is 3. The pupils are 3 mm bilaterally and reactive. The patient was intubated without difficulty and with no medication assistance. No medications have been administered since his arrival. A computed tomography (CT) scan of the patient's head shows intracerebral diffuse trauma with possible diffuse axonal injury and overall edema.

Your medical control physician does not think that this patient's mean arterial pressure is high enough. He requests infusion of 2 more liters of lactated Ringer's solution. Your partner thinks you should turn down the rate on the ventilator settings. The local physician wants you to hurry up and transfer the patient to your facility.

Many assessment schemes dictate the ABCD plan (*a*irway, *b*reathing, *c*irculation, *d*isability) for evaluating and managing a patient with a critical illness or injury. This chapter focuses on the disability aspect. It reviews the normal anatomy and physiology of the nervous system and the special assessment and diagnostic tools used for neurologic conditions. It also discusses the neurologic disease processes most commonly seen in the intensive care unit (ICU) and their management.

NEUROLOGIC ANATOMY AND PHYSIOLOGY

The nervous system might be considered the computer system of the body, responsible for directing all body systems. It is the system responsible for intelligence, emotion, and thought. All sensory stimuli are evaluated by the nervous system. This complex system then generates an intellectual and/or motor response, the main goal of which is to maintain the integrity of the body. Critical care practitioners must have a sound understanding of the nervous system because of the major role it plays in normal physiologic functioning and survival.

Divisions of the Nervous System

The central nervous system (CNS) is composed of the brain and spinal cord. The peripheral nervous system (PNS) is made up of the 12 pairs of cranial nerves, 31 pairs of spinal nerves, and all other nerves throughout the body, including the autonomic nervous system.

Microstructure

Two types of cells make up the nervous system: **neurons** and the **neuroglia.** Neurons do the functional work of the nervous system, which includes receiving information, integration and sharing of data, and conduction of nerve impulses to recipient cells. Branching from these cell bodies are **neurites.** A long neurite, the *axon,* conducts information away from the cell. A shorter neurite, the *dendrite,* conducts information back to the cell.

Most of the neuronal cell bodies are located in the CNS. Neuronal cell bodies, along with dendrites and synaptic activity, are congregated in the CNS; in the brain and spinal cord, they are called *gray matter.* The axons of these cells form nerve bundles, which form into tracts in the cerebellum, cortex, and spinal cord; these specially coated axon tracts are called *white matter* because of the color of the **myelin sheath** that covers them.

The term **glia** comes from a Greek word meaning "glue" or "holding together." In the neuron, neuroglial cells provide structural support, protection, and nourishment. There are four types of neuroglial cells: astroglia (or astrocytes), oligodendroglia, ependyma, and microglia. The CNS has up to 10 times more neuroglial cells than neurons. About 40% of the brain and spinal cord is composed of neuroglial cells (Figures 5-1 and 5-2).

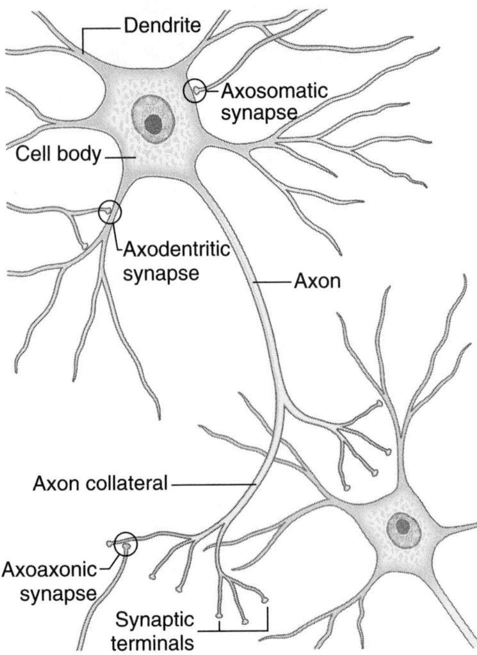

Figure 5-1

Schematic of a typical neuron. (From Standring S: *Gray's anatomy: the anatomical basis of clinical practice,* ed 40, Philadelphia, 2008, Churchill Livingstone.)

Did You Know?

Neuroglial cells are the primary source of neoplasms.[1]

This same organization of cells occurs in the spinal cord, which lies in the upper two thirds of the bony vertebral column and is continuous from the medulla of the brain. **Afferent** and **efferent** connections travel in 31 pairs of spinal nerves arranged segmentally. These attach to the cord as dorsal and ventral roots. The dorsal roots carry afferent (sensory) nerve fibers, and the ventral roots carry efferent (motor) nerve fibers back from the cord's gray matter. The spinal gray matter is configured into an H or butterfly shape in the cord.

Nerve impulses are transmitted quickly through the **nodes of Ranvier.** When a resting cell is stimulated, the membrane becomes more permeable to sodium. When sodium enters the cell, the membrane potential decreases, or moves forward from a negative value to zero; this decrease is known as *depolarization.* The cell now is more positively charged. The myelin sheath blocks the extreme sodium influx necessary for depolarization through Ranvier's nodes, which are not covered with myelin and which have ion channels built into their structure. The nodes propagate quick transmission along the course of the nerve. The depolarization-repolarization cycle is similar to cardiac physiology but can occur at 1000 times per second.

All somatic cells are polarized, with the inside more negatively charged than the outside. Sodium ions are more concentrated in the extracellular fluid, and potassium is more concentrated in the intracellular fluid. The sodium-potassium pump moves sodium and potassium across the cell membrane and changes polarity when stimulated. Electrical action potentials are created through the ion channels. At rest, the neuron is at −270 to −85 millivolts (mV). When depolarization occurs, the sodium channels open and a quick movement (from negative to zero) creates the "electricity." This movement of electricity occurs throughout the region as the sodium and potassium channels return to normal. A steady supply of adenosine triphosphate (ATP) is necessary to maintain this system.

Once an action potential reaches the end of the axon, a cascade of events, or synapse, must occur. The two forms of synapse are chemical synapse and electrical synapse. Most synapses are chemical in nature. Because no direct contact exists between the axons, neurotransmitters must be released into the void to allow for communication. Electrical synapse occurs when a small cellular bridge (e.g., metabolites or cytoplasm) is created to propagate the transmission.

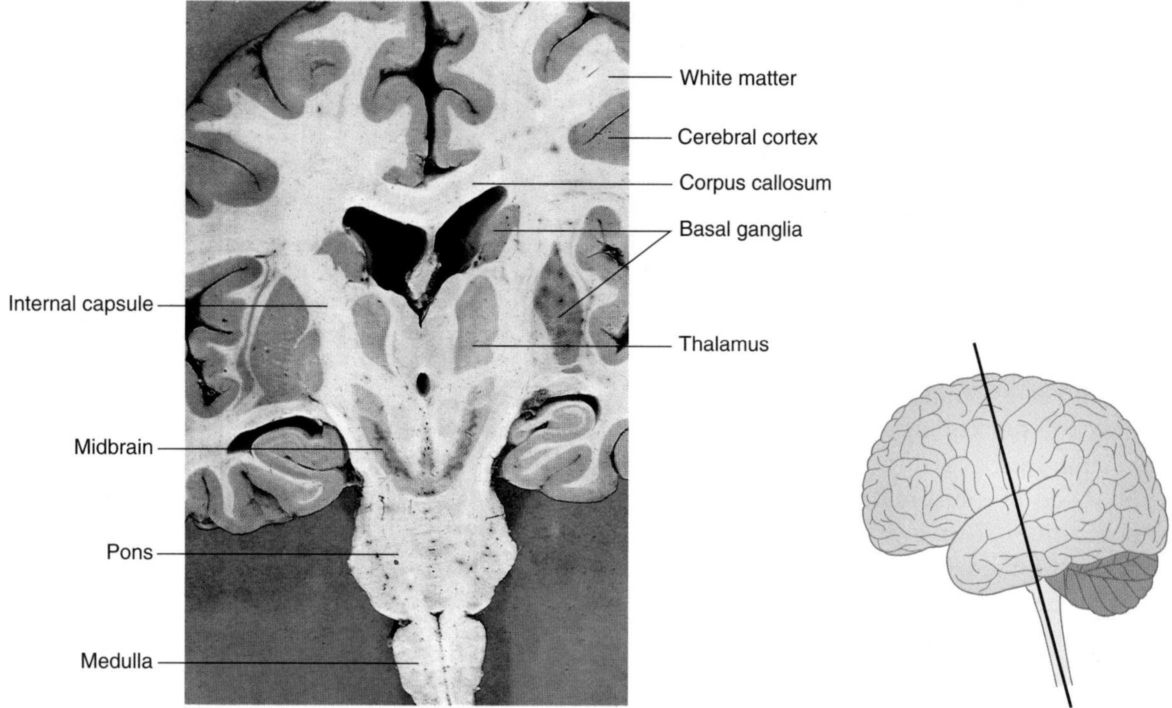

Figure 5-2

Section through the cerebral hemisphere and brain stem showing the disposition of gray and white matter, the basal ganglia, and the internal capsule. (Courtesy Kevin Fitzpatrick, GKT School of Medicine, London.)

Many disorders can develop as a result of failure of nerve impulses. For example, multiple sclerosis is a disease of the myelin sheath that results in weakness, paresthesia, and speech and visual difficulties. Infection with *Clostridium tetani* (i.e., tetanus) causes a sustained muscular contraction because of the bacterium's effect at the presynaptic level. At the postsynaptic level, chemicals such as cocaine or organophosphates can delay or stimulate pathologic processes. Local anesthesia occurs when certain drugs are injected into tissue and block the sensory nerve conductivity through sodium channels.

Central Nervous System

Extracerebral Structures

The scalp is composed of skin, a fatty layer, and a deep membranous layer that has many blood vessels. Because these blood vessels constrict poorly, the smallest laceration can bleed profusely. A freely movable, dense, fibrous tissue called the **galea (helmet) aponeurotica** covers the skull and connects the frontal and occipital bellies of the occipitofrontalis muscle.

The scalp functions as a barrier to infection and protects the integrity of the cranial bones. It helps absorb the force of external trauma, especially glancing blows to the head. Studies have shown that when the cranial vault is surrounded by an intact scalp, it can stand the application of 900 psi of force and still maintain its integrity. By comparison, if the scalp is no longer intact, the cranial vault can withstand only 40 psi of force and still maintain its integrity.

Did You Know?

A helpful mnemonic for remembering the structures of the scalp is SCALP.[2]

- **S *Skin:* The structure from which head hair grows; it is richly supplied with blood vessels.**
- **C *Connective tissue.* A thin layer of fat and fibrous tissue that lies beneath the skin.**
- **A *Aponeurosis.* The layer beneath the connective tissue (also called the *epicranial aponeurosis* or *galea aponeurotica*); a tough layer of dense fibrous tissue that runs from the frontalis muscle anteriorly to the occipitalis posteriorly.**
- **L *Loose areolar connective tissue.* This layer provides an easy plane of separation between the upper three layers and the pericranium (in scalping, the scalp is torn off through this layer); it also provides a plane of access in craniofacial surgery and neurosurgery. This layer is sometimes called the "danger zone," because infectious**

Continued

Did You Know?—Cont'd

agents can easily spread through it to emissary veins that drain into the cranium. The loose areolar tissue is made up of random collagen type I bundles and collagen type III. It contains the major blood vessels of the scalp, which bleed profusely with injuries, partly because of the absence of the venous valves found in the circulation below the neck. This layer also is rich in glycosaminoglycans (GAGs) and is composed of more matrix than fibers.

P *Pericranium.* This is the periosteum of the skull bones, which provides nutrition to the bone and the capacity for repair. It may be lifted from the bone to allow removal of bone windows (craniotomy).

The skull comprises 22 flattened, curved bones. Cranial bones are composed of two layers of hard bone that sandwich a layer of **cancellous bone**; this allows for maximum strength at a light weight. All the bones of the skull except the mandible are joined by immovable joints, called **sutures**. Eight bones make up the cranium: one frontal bone, one sphenoid bone, one ethmoid bone, two parietal bones, two temporal bones and one occipital bone. All of these bones are named for the lobes of the brain that are under them, plus the two sinus cavities (ethmoid and sphenoid). The base of the brain is very rough and is made up of three distinct compartments: the anterior **fossa**, the middle fossa, and the posterior fossa.

Once the cranial sutures have fused in childhood, the cranium is a mostly solid container. Small openings around the base of the skull allow for blood vessels and nerve fibers, but the cranium has only one large opening, the **foramen magnum**. This hole in the base of the skull allows projection of the brain stem just before it connects to the spinal cord (Figures 5-3 and 5-4).

Meninges

The meninges are nonnervous tissue that cover and completely enclose the brain and spinal cord (Figure 5-5). They separate the brain and spinal cord from the bony surface lining of the cranium and vertebral canal. Three layers provide this protection (or padding) for the brain and spinal cord. From the skull moving inward, the meningeal layers are the **dura mater, arachnoid mater**, and **pia mater**. The dura mater is a shiny, tough, inelastic membrane that is itself double layered. The outer layer serves as an internal periosteum for the cranial bones, and the inner layer forms cranial compartments by means of projections that dip toward the center of the cranial vault. There are several dural projections, but the two largest are the **falx cerebri** and the **tentorium cerebelli** (Figure 5-6). Meningeal arteries and venous sinuses lie within clefts formed by separation of the inner and outer layers.

The dura mater is separated from the bones in the vertebral canal by the **epidural space**, which contains fat, small veins, and the large meningeal arteries. A true space is found in the spinal cord but not in the cranial cavity, except when it is created artificially by bleeding between the skull and the dura mater (usually caused by tears in or injury to the middle meningeal artery). The **subdural space** is the potential space between the dura mater and the arachnoid mater. The arachnoid mater, the fine fibrous, elastic layer between the dura and pia mater, has a spider web appearance (hence the term *arachnoid*). It loosely follows the contours of the brain. The subarachnoid space (SAS) lies between the arachnoid mater and the pia mater. It contains cerebrospinal fluid (CSF). The SAS extends down the spinal cord and for some distance along the roots of nerves. In the SAS are the **arachnoid villi**, projections of the arachnoid mater that serve as channels for absorption of CSF into the venous system.

The pia mater is a delicate, soft, very vascular layer that is in direct contact with the brain. It protects and maintains the shape of the semifluid brain.

Brain

The body of the brain is a fluid-filled collection of delicate tissues and water that comprises 80% to 85% of the cranial mass. Brain tissue has the appearance of unset custard. The bulk of the brain is the cerebrum, which is divided into the right and left hemispheres. Each hemisphere is divided into four lobes: the frontal, temporal, parietal, and occipital lobes, which are named the same as their overlying skull sections (Figure 5-7).

Divisions of the Brain

Frontal Lobe

The frontal lobe is responsible for the functions of conceptualizing, thinking abstractly, and forming judgments. Functions of the frontal lobe include:

1. Prefrontal cortex
   a. Short-term memory
   b. Emotional responsiveness
   c. Abstract thinking
   d. Foresight/judgment
   e. Behavior/tactfulness
2. Primary motor cortex
3. **Broca's speech area** (dominant hemisphere)
   a. Expressive speech/vocalization
4. Intellect
5. Personality

Did You Know?

Injury to the frontal lobe may impair judgment and reasoning, and the patient may begin to shout obscene or foul language; this is known as being "frontal lobish."[3]

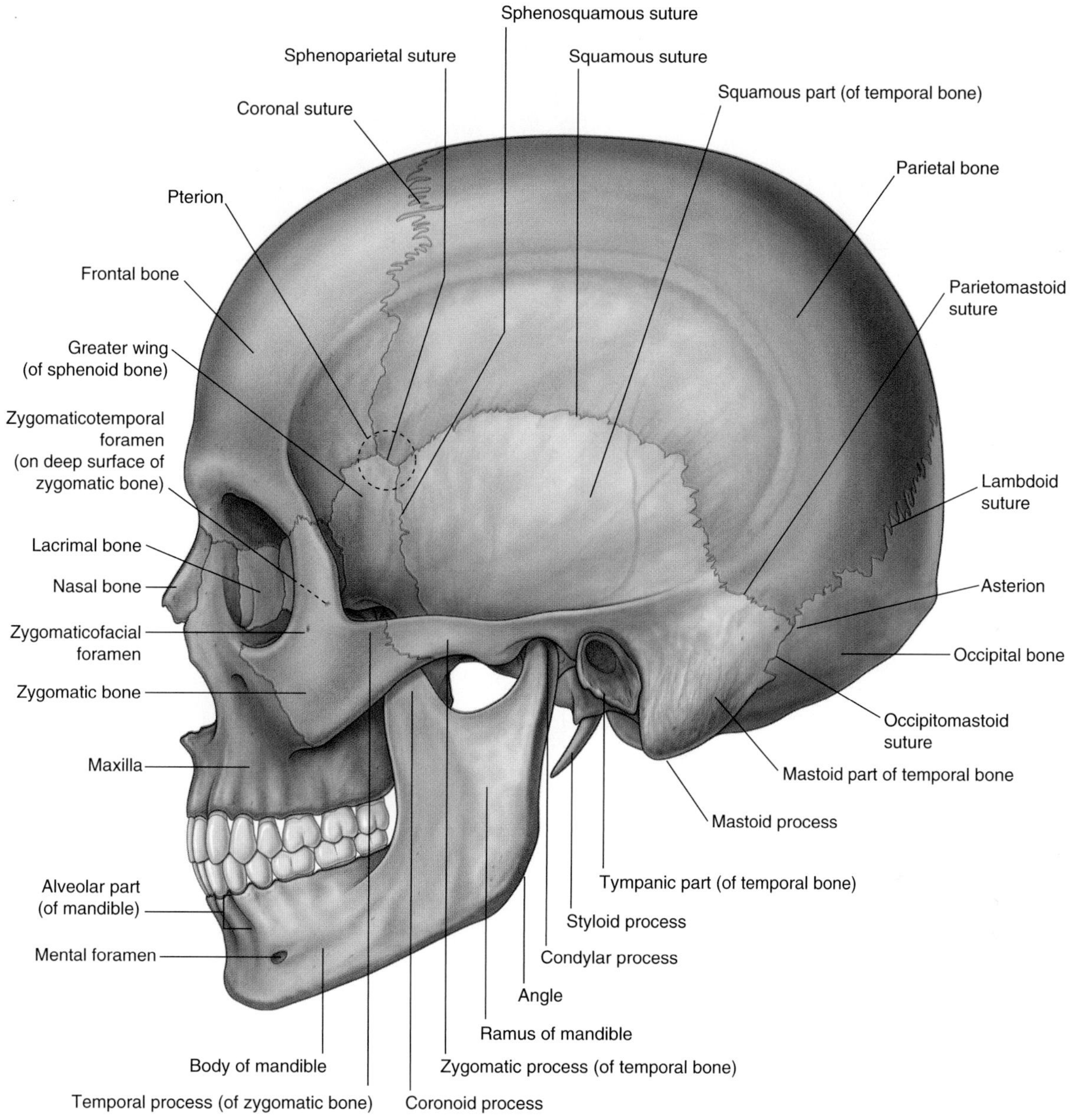

Figure 5-3

Lateral view of the skull. (From Standring S: *Gray's anatomy: the anatomical basis of clinical practice,* ed 39, Philadelphia, 2004, Churchill Livingstone.)

Temporal Lobe

The temporal lobe is actually two lobes, one on each side of the brain, that resemble the thumbs of a boxing glove. These lobes are frequently injured, because they are enclosed within relatively thin bony chambers. The bony layer is a soft **squamous bone**, which fractures easily. Functions of the temporal lobe include the following:

1. Primary auditory cortex
2. Visual task learning
3. Dominant hemisphere
   a. **Wernicke's speech area**
   b. Receptive speech/comprehension
   c. Interpretive area
   d. Intellect
4. Emotion
5. Long-term memory
   a. Dominant hemisphere: verbal
   b. Nondominant hemisphere: sensory

Did You Know?

Injury to the temporal area may cause temporary or permanent memory loss.[3]

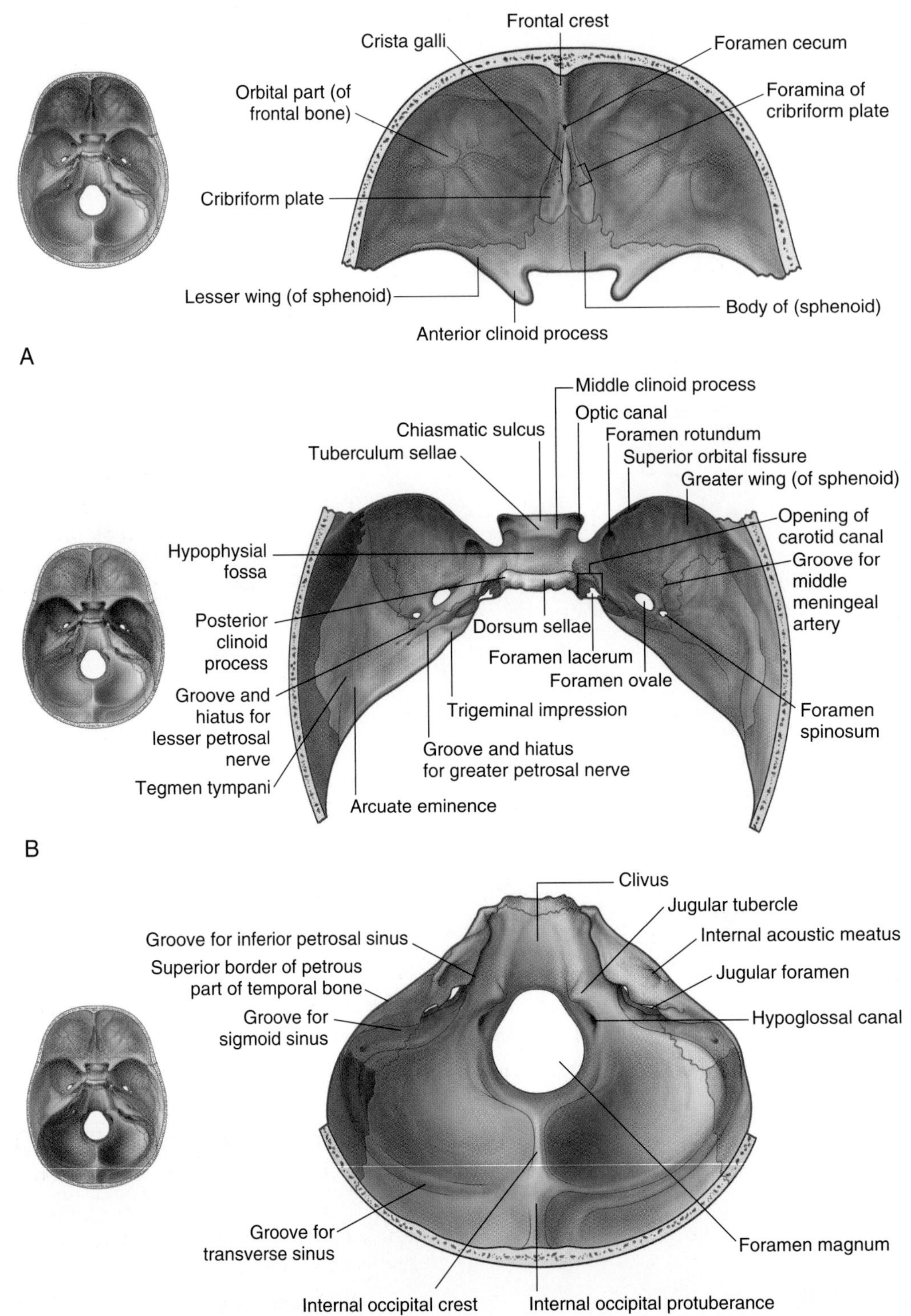

Figure 5-4

Floor of the cranial cavity, showing the cranial fossae. **A,** Anterior cranial fossa. **B,** Middle cranial fossa. **C,** Posterior cranial fossa. (From Standring S: *Gray's anatomy: the anatomical basis of clinical practice*, ed 40, Philadelphia, 2008, Churchill Livingstone.)

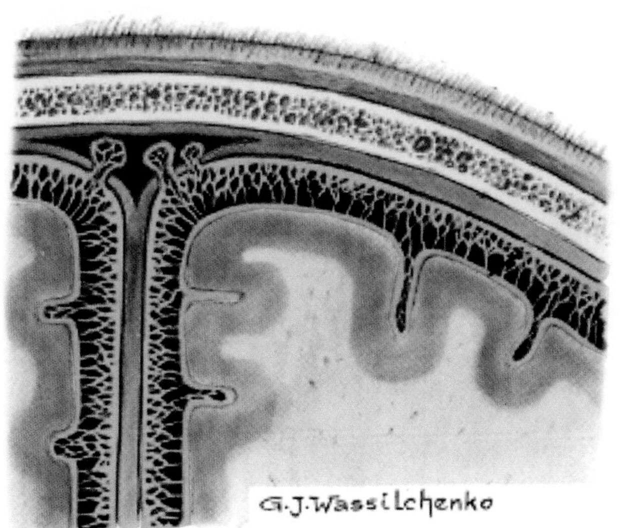

Figure 5-5

Meninges. (From Urden LD, Stacy KM, Lough ME: *Thelan's critical care nursing: diagnosis and management*, ed 5, St Louis, 2006, Mosby.)

Parietal Lobe

The parietal lobe is the area of the brain responsible for the highest integration and coordination of perceptual information and the interpretation of sensory phenomena. Its functions include:

1. Primary sensory cortex: sensory interpretation
2. **Tactile sense** and **kinesthetic sense**
3. Body awareness/body image
4. Spatial orientation/relationships

Did You Know?

Injury to the parietal lobe may cause difficulty with receptive communication.[3]

Occipital Lobe

The occipital lobe is the area of the brain responsible for vision.

1. Primary visual cortex
2. Visual association

Did You Know?

Injury to the occipital lobe may cause blurred vision, diplopia, or even blindness.[4]

Cerebellum (Hindbrain)

The cerebellum is separated from the cerebrum by the tentorium cerebelli. This area coordinates and integrates body movement. It also is responsible for maintaining equilibrium and controls posture and position sense.

Cerebral Dominance

Experts generally agree that in most people, one cerebral hemisphere is more highly developed than the other. At birth the two hemispheres have equal capacity for development. Left hemisphere dominance is found in 90% of the population; these are right-handed people. Interestingly, most left-handed people also have a dominant left hemisphere. The left hemisphere is responsible for verbal, linguistic, arithmetic, calculating, and analytic functions. The right hemisphere is responsible for geometric, spatial, visual pattern, and music functions. The right and left hemispheres are connected by a large network of white matter, the corpus callosum, which is made up of a group of commissural fibers that transfers learned discriminations, sensory experience, and memory from one cerebral hemisphere to the other.

Basal Ganglia (Basal Nuclei)

The term *basal nuclei* refers to the nuclei that lie in the inferior region of the cerebrum, just lateral to the thalamus. This area is involved in **extrapyramidal** (involuntary) motor functions and plays a major role in regulating voluntary motor function, even though they do not provide direct input to motor tracts via the spinal cord as do most voluntary control centers. Instead, they receive input from the cerebral cortex and integrate signals in order to adjust posture and allow muscle movements to be smooth. Part of this structure is the **amygdala**, which actually is associated more with the limbic system. Another section, the **striatum**, considered the principal input structure of the basal ganglia, as it receives the majority of incoming nerve signals from other parts of the central nervous system.

The functions of the basal ganglia include:

1. Fine motor movement (compensation for voluntary movement)
2. Muscle tone
3. Posture

Did You Know?

Disease or injury of the basal ganglia may result in tremor, involuntary movements, rigid or uncoordinated muscle tone, and slow movement.[1]

Diencephalon (Forebrain)

The **diencephalon** lies next to the structures that develop lateral to the third ventricle. It consists of three main parts: the thalamus, the hypothalamus, and the limbic system.

1. *Thalamus:* The thalamus, which is adjacent to the third ventricle, conducts finely organized and precisely

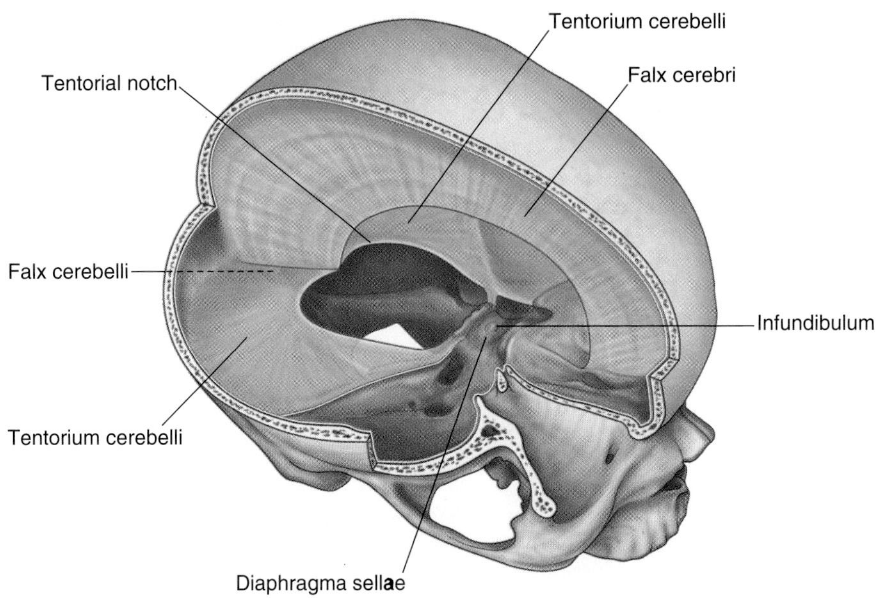

Figure 5-6

The dura mater, its reflections, and the associated major venous sinuses. (Adapted from Drake R, Vogl W, and Mitchell A: *Gray's atlas of anatomy*, St. Louis, 2010, Elsevier.)

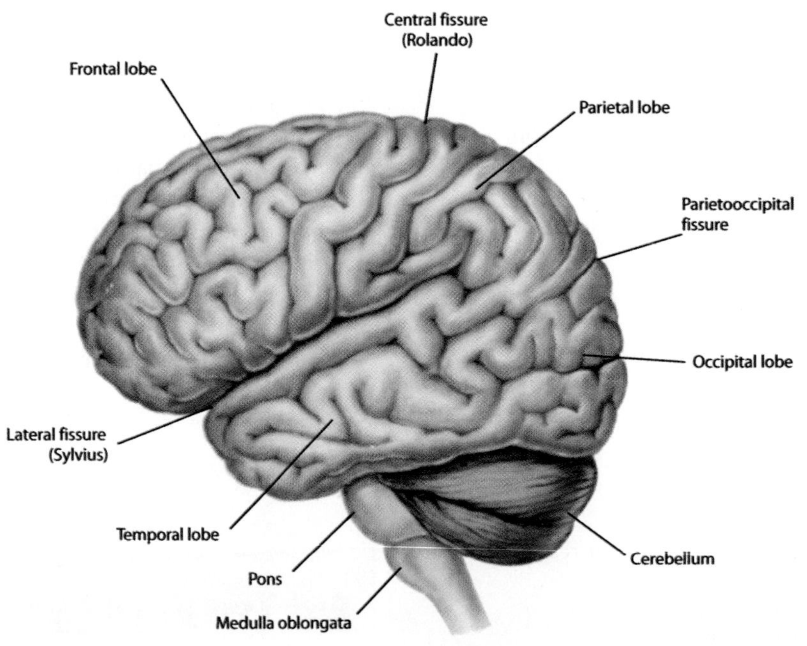

Figure 5-7

Lobes of the brain. (From Standring S: *Gray's anatomy: the anatomical basis of clinical practice*, ed 39, Philadelphia, 2004, Churchill Livingstone.)

transmitted sensory and motor information to and from the cortex. It generally is part of the arousal system and can alter its actions based on behavioral needs.

2. *Hypothalamus:* The hypothalamus, which is just beneath the thalamus, is connected to the pituitary gland and, along with the amygdala and the limbic system, provides neural control of the emotions. This area is central to homeostasis of the body, which it provides through endocrine and autonomic system control.
   a. Homeostasis
   b. Behavioral responses to emotion
   c. Temperature regulation
   d. Regulation of food and water intake
   e. Control of pituitary hormone release
   f. Augmentation of SNS and PNS

3. *Limbic system:* Sometimes referred to as a "limbic lobe," this area is near the temporal lobe. The limbic system consists of the **hippocampus** and amygdala. The frontal lobe accounts for most of the actions necessary for thinking in human beings; the limbic system is designed to keep the body safe.
   a. Recall of pleasurable, unpleasant, and dangerous events
   b. Mood modification
   c. Emotional response, interpretation of emotions
   d. Interpretation of smell
   e. Regulation of visceral processes (e.g., heart rate) associated with emotion (Figures 5-8 and 5-9)

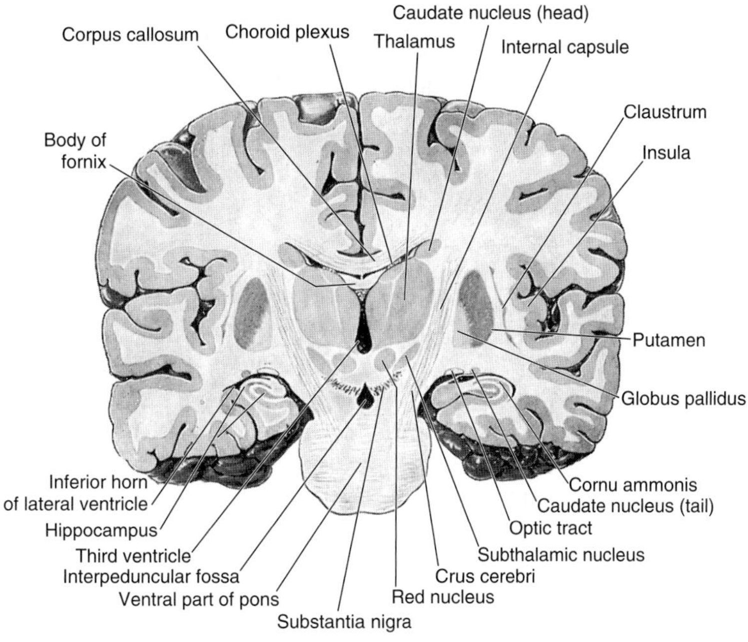

Figure 5-8

Diencephalon and basal ganglia. (From Standring S: *Gray's anatomy: the anatomical basis of clinical practice,* ed 39, Philadelphia, 2004, Churchill Livingstone.)

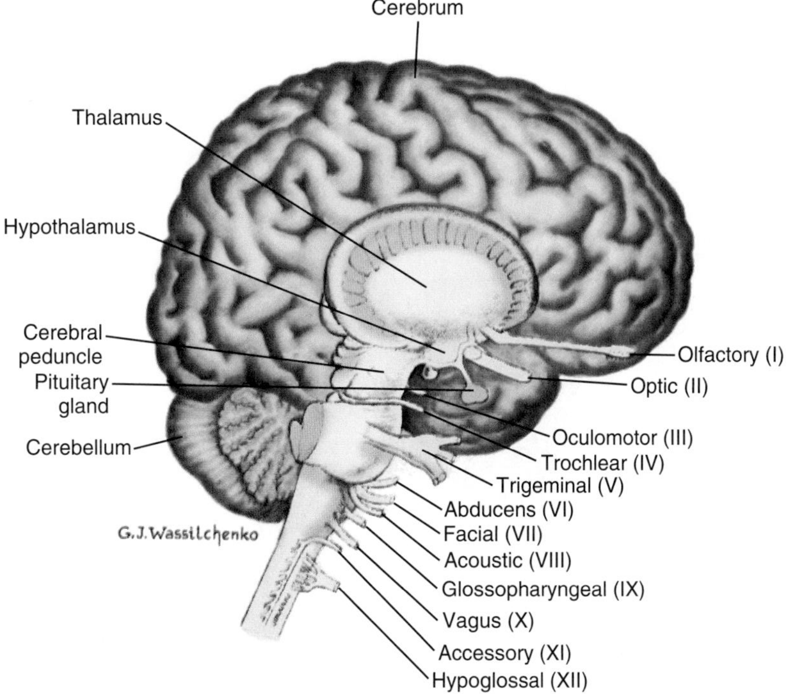

Figure 5-9

Lateral view of the brain, showing the brain stem, diencephalon, and cranial nerves. (From Urden LD, Stacy KM, Lough ME: *Thelan's critical care nursing: diagnosis and management,* ed 5, St Louis, 2006, Mosby.)

Brain Stem

The brain stem houses the axons of the original cranial nerves and provides most of the control over the head and neck sensation and movement. Autonomic fibers arise from this area. The **reticular activating system (RAS)**, a network of fibers that extends along the brain stem, is responsible for wakefulness, vigilance, and responsiveness (i.e., overall consciousness). The brain stem generally is composed of three parts: the midbrain, the pons, and the medulla oblongata.

1. *Midbrain:* The midbrain is located between the pons and the diencephalon. Cranial nerves III and IV begin here, along with the aqueduct of Sylvius. The midbrain is considered a relay station for ascending sensory and descending motor tracts.
2. *Pons:* The pons, located just above the medulla, also is a relay station. It has two special respiratory centers and the origin of cranial nerves V, VI, VII, and VIII. This area also has a special tract of fibers that connect to cranial nerves III, IV, and VI. This allows for controlled movement of the eyes in response to a sudden noise, motion, position change, or arousal.
   a. **Apneustic center**: Controls the length of inspiration/exhalation
   b. **Pneumotaxic center**: Controls the respiratory rate
3. *Medulla oblongata:* The medulla oblongata is the lower part of the brain stem and is partly situated into structural pyramids. This is the location where motor tracts cross. The bodies of cranial nerves IX, X, and XI arise here.
   a. **Medullary respiratory center**: Controls the rhythm of respiration
   b. Swallowing, coughing, vomiting, hiccoughing
   c. Heart rate, arterial vasoconstriction, respiration

Did You Know?

The term pyramidal refers to the look of part of the medulla and means voluntary motor function because of the tracts. Decussation, or crossing, of these motor fibers occurs within these tracts. The term *extrapyramidal* refers to motor functions outside this special area, which are associated with equilibrium and muscle tone. A positive Babinski's sign in a patient older than age 6 months indicates a lesion in the pyramidal tracts.[1]

Figure 5-10 shows the primary somatic sensory and motor areas of the cortex.

Ventricular System and Cerebrospinal Fluid Flow

The ventricular system, where CSF circulates, is a closed system (Figure 5-11). It is made up of four fluid-filled ventricles located in the cerebral hemispheres and the brain stem. Two lateral ventricles are connected to the third ventricle by the interventricular foramina. The third ventricle is connected to the fourth ventricle by the **aqueduct of Sylvius**. The fourth ventricle sends CSF around the brain and spinal cord through two foramina.

Expanded areas of the SAS are called **cisterns**. CSF may be aspirated from some of these cisterns for analysis. The major cisterns are the cisterna magnum and the lumbar cistern; these are located between the L2 and S2 vertebrae, the site where lumbar punctures are performed.

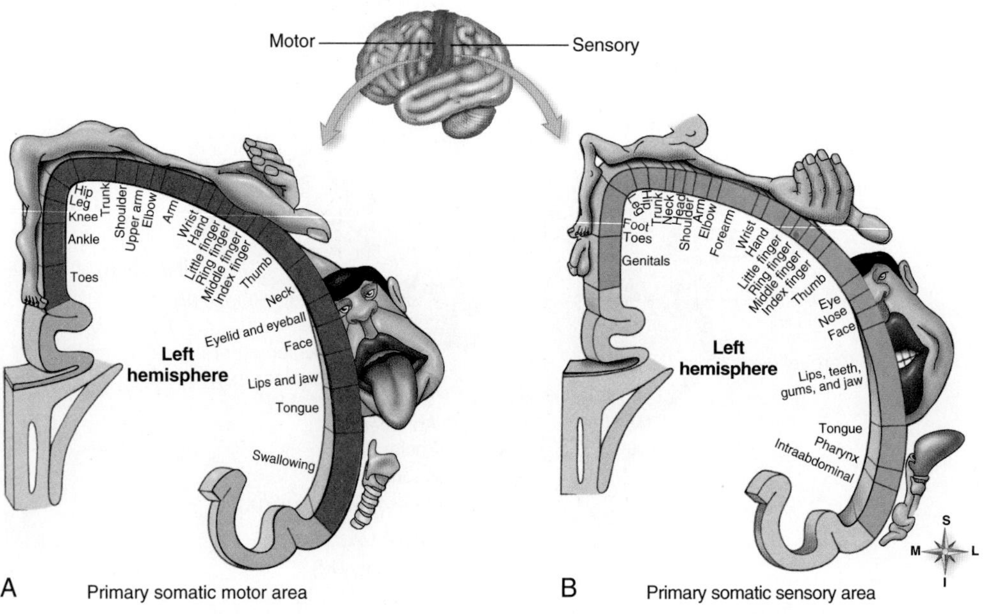

Figure 5-10

Primary somatic sensory **(A)** and motor **(B)** areas of the cortex. (From Thibodeau GA, Patton KT: *Anatomy and physiology*, ed 7, St Louis, 2010, Mosby.)

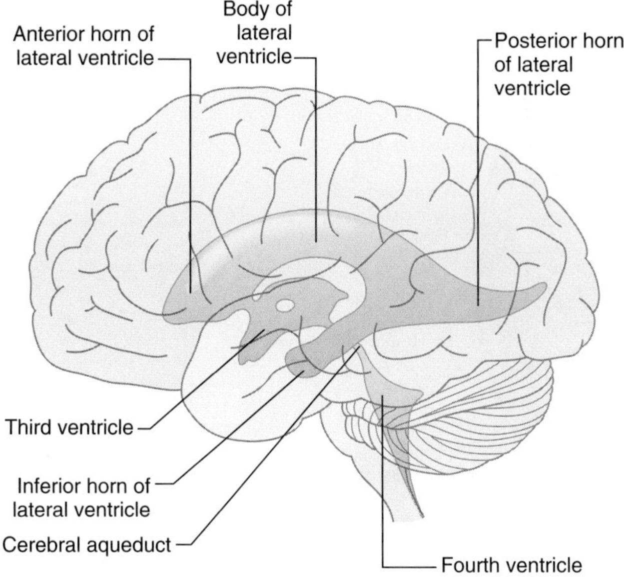

Figure 5-11

Ventricular system. (From Standring S: *Gray's anatomy: the anatomical basis of clinical practice,* ed 39, Philadelphia, 2004, Churchill Livingstone.)

The **choroid plexuses**, which are composed of tufts of capillaries covered by epithelial cells, are found in all the ventricles; these structures are the principal source of CSF. They produce approximately 20 mL/hour, although only 80 to 110 mL of CSF circulates at a given time. CSF cushions the brain and spinal cord. It also compensates for changes in the intracranial volume or pressure (or both) and plays a role in metabolism. Characteristics of CSF include the following:

- Specific gravity: 1.007
- Pressure: 76 to 200 mm H_2O (side lying); 200 to 350 mm H_2O (sitting)
- Color: Clear; xanthochromia (yellowish discoloration); cloudy (turbidity)
- Glucose level: 40 to 80 mg/dL (60% of blood value)
- Lactate level: 10 to 20 mg/dL

Most CSF is absorbed through the arachnoid villi that project from the SAS into the dural sinuses. The arachnoid villi provide the outlet through which CSF flows into the venous system. When these villi are compromised by blood or purulent matter in the CSF, blockage of CSF absorption can result. This causes the volume of CSF to increase dramatically, resulting in a communicating hydrocephalus.

The *blood-brain barrier* is the term used for a special permeability characteristic of brain capillaries and the choroid plexuses. This barrier limits the transfer of certain substances into the CSF and extracellular fluid of the brain; it also prevents some drugs from affecting the brain and spinal cord. It is very permeable to water, oxygen, carbon dioxide, glucose, and lipid-soluble compounds. Traumatic or anoxic brain injury may increase, alter, or eliminate this protective barrier.

Cerebral Circulation

The brain receives approximately 20% of the cardiac output. It receives its arterial supply from two main systems, the vertebral arteries and the internal carotid arteries.

The two vertebral arteries originate from the subclavian artery, follow the ventrolateral area of the spinal cord, and enter the skull through the foramen magnum. They unite at the level of the pons to become the basilar artery. The basilar artery divides into two posterior cerebral arteries that supply part of the cerebrum. The vertebral arteries and their branches supply the cerebellum, the brain stem, the spinal cord, the occipital lobes, the medial and inferior surfaces of the temporal lobes, and part of the diencephalon.

The internal carotid arteries originate from two different vessels: the left common carotid artery, which originates from the aorta, and the right common carotid artery, which arises from the brachiocephalic (innominate) artery off the aorta. The common carotid arteries branch out to form the external and internal carotid arteries. The external carotid artery supplies the face, scalp, and other structures outside the skull.

Did You Know?

- **The cerebral arteries have thinner walls than do arteries of comparable size in other parts of the body. The veins (other than the dural sinuses) have even thinner walls in proportion to their size and lack a muscle layer.**
- **The veins and sinuses have no valves.**
- **The venous return does not retrace the course of corresponding arteries, but rather follows its own path.**
- **The dural sinuses are unique to the cerebral circulation.**

The internal carotid artery enters the cranial vault through a foramen in the floor of the skull. The terminal branches from each carotid artery include the posterior communicating artery, the anterior cerebral artery, and the middle cerebral artery. Another important branch from this artery is the ophthalmic artery.

These two arterial systems comprise the circulation at the base of the brain known as the **circle of Willis** (some references refer to the circle of Willis as the collateral circulation of the brain). The circle of Willis permits an adequate blood supply to reach all parts of the brain, even if one or more of the four supplying vessels has been obstructed.

Venous Drainage

The venous system in the cerebrum is unlike that in other parts of the body, where the veins follow the arterial pattern closely. The venous drainage system is managed by vascular channels, called *dural sinuses.* The deep and superficial veins

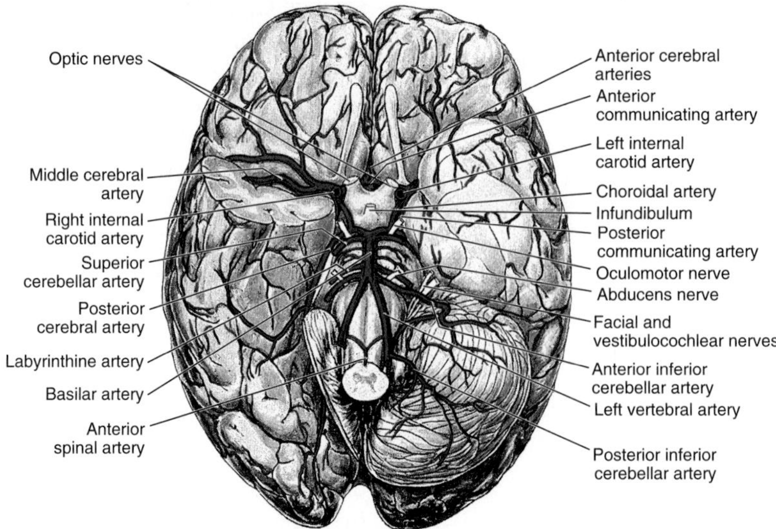

Figure 5-12

Arterial circulation of the brain. (From Standring S: *Gray's anatomy: the anatomical basis of clinical practice,* ed 39, Philadelphia, 2004, Churchill Livingstone.)

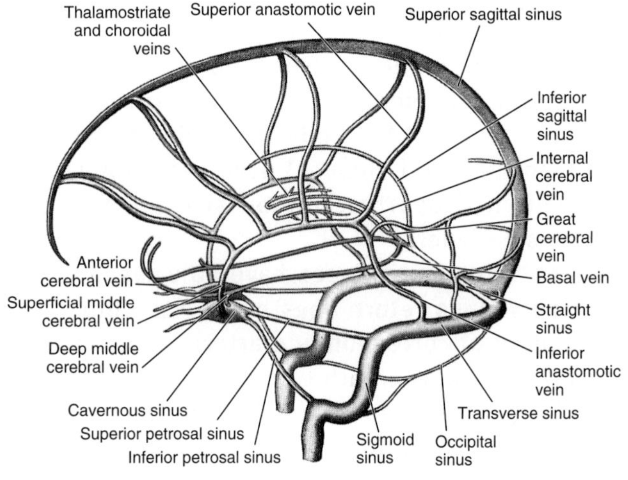

Figure 5-13

Cerebral venous system, showing the principal superficial and deep veins of the brain and their relationship to the dural venous sinuses, as viewed from the left side. (From Standring S: *Gray's anatomy: the anatomical basis of clinical practice,* ed 39, Philadelphia, 2004, Churchill Livingstone.)

in the cerebrum dump into the dural sinuses; these empty into the jugular veins, which return the blood to the heart (Figures 5-12 and 5-13).

Spinal Cord

The spinal cord is a cylindric structure about the size of your little finger that passes through the bony spinal column. It begins at the level of the foramen magnum and ends at L1 or L2. In the lower thoracic region, the cord is larger, and it reaches its maximum circumference (about 33 mm) opposite T12. It then rapidly tapers into the **conus medullaris** at L1-L2.

Spinal Column

The function of the spinal column is to protect the spinal cord and provide vertical stability for walking. The spinal column is a flexible structure made up of seven cervical vertebrae, 12 thoracic vertebrae, five lumbar vertebrae, five fused sacral vertebrae, and four fused coccygeal bones. The ends of the spinal column, where it has the most curvature, are most vulnerable when put into extreme flexion or extension. In these areas (C5 to T1 and T12 to L2), injuries are more common (Figures 5-14 to 5-17).

Although most of the vertebrae have similar structures (body, arch, pedicles, lamina, spinous process, articular process, and transverse process), the first two are unique. C1, the atlas, is a ringlike structure that supports the skull. It articulates at the occiput and helps provide for normal flexion and extension of the neck. C2, the axis, articulates with C1 at the odontoid process and provides for some of the normal rotation of the head.

The spinal column is supported by ligaments, which contribute significantly to spinal stability. The vertebrae from C2 to the sacrum are separated by intervertebral discs made of fibrocartilaginous material that is 90% water. The discs, which are highly vascular, prevent bone-to-bone contact that might jolt the cord and damage the bony vertebrae. Like the brain, the spinal cord has both white and gray matter. However, these components have nearly the opposite arrangement to that seen in the brain: the white matter is to the outside, and the gray matter is internal. Thirty-one pairs of spinal nerves exit the spinal cord (Figure 5-18).

The white matter of the spinal cord contains the myelinated ascending and descending tracts that carry information to and from the brain. Ascending columns of white matter help the body with a sense of position (**proprioception**), touch-pressure (**exteroception**), and vibration. Descending

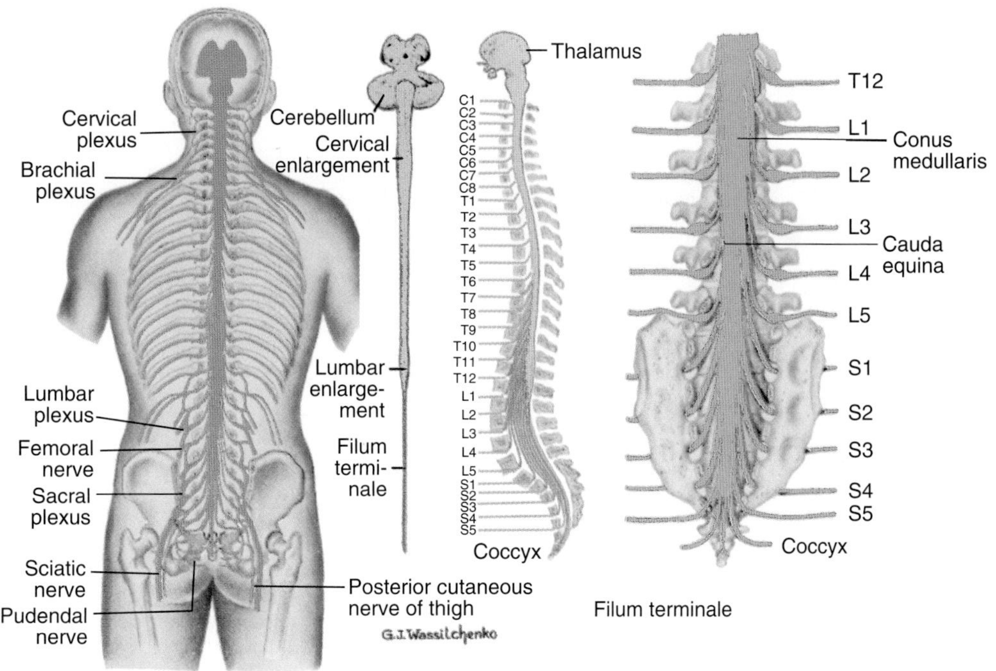

Figure 5-14

Spinal cord within the vertebral canal and exiting spinal nerves. **A,** Posterior view in situ. **B,** Anterior view. **C,** Lateral view. **D,** Cauda equina. (From Urden LD, Stacy KM, Lough ME: *Thelan's critical care nursing: diagnosis and management,* ed 5, St Louis, 2006, Mosby.)

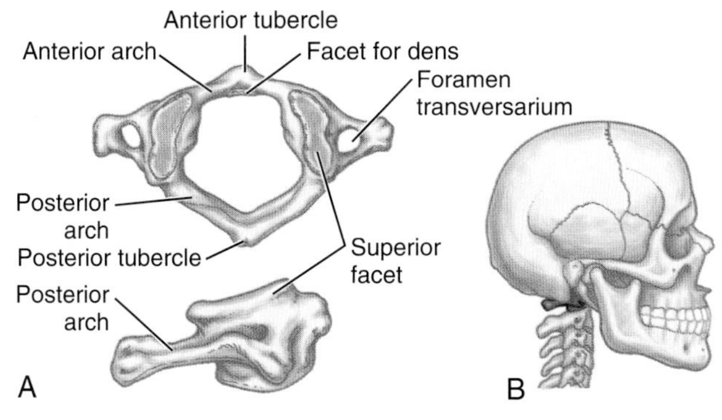

Figure 5-15

Atlas. **A,** Superior aspect *(top);* transverse aspect *(bottom).* Note the absence of the body and spinous process. **B,** Position. (From Dorland NW: *Dorland's illustrated medical dictionary,* ed 31, Philadelphia, 2007, Saunders.)

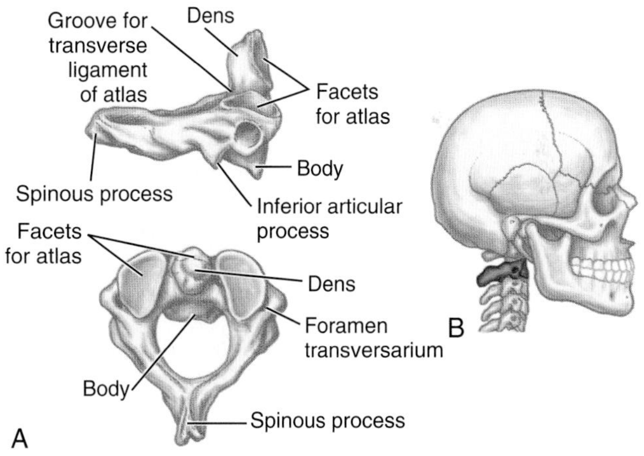

Figure 5-16

Axis. **A,** Transverse aspect *(top);* superior aspect *(bottom).* **B,** Position. (From Dorland NW: *Dorland's illustrated medical dictionary,* ed 31, Philadelphia, 2007, Saunders.)

pathways originate in the brain stem and are concerned with movement, muscle tone, and posture.

The gray matter of the spinal cord takes an H or butterfly shape within the white matter. There are two columns each of the dorsal and ventral horns. The dorsal horn contains afferent fibers and is considered a receptive zone. The ventral horn contains efferent fibers with motor function.

The lateral horn of the gray matter is seen only from T1 through L3. These fibers appear as though they are the crossbar of the H, at either side of which are the **preganglionic fibers** of the autonomic nervous system.

The 31 pairs of spinal nerves exit their corresponding vertebrae with two roots, a dorsal (afferent) root and a ventral (efferent) root. The sensory function may be evaluated through **dermatomes.** The motor functions of various spinal and cranial nerves often are grouped and can be evaluated through **myotomes** (Figure 5-19).

A unique reflex of sensation and quick action occurs through the spinal column and is considered a spinal reflex. This automatic action occurs when a sensory stretch receptor picks up a stimulus and sends the impulse to the dorsal horn via afferent nerve fibers. The afferent nerve fibers then communicate in the anterior part of the cord with the efferent

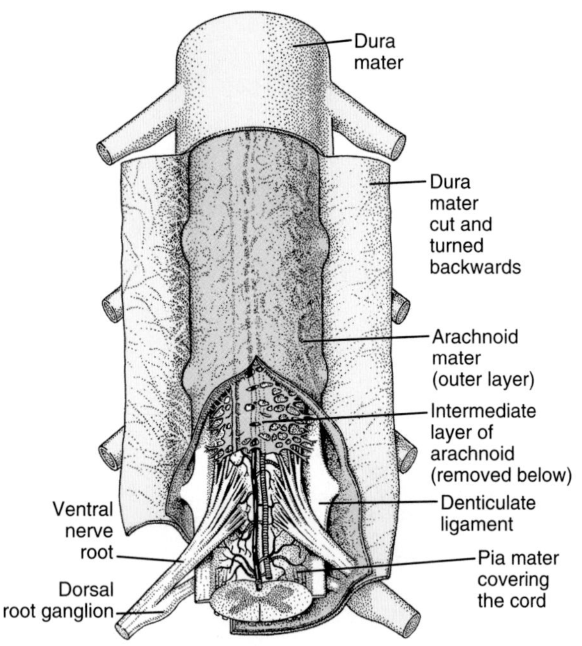

Figure 5-17

Part of the spinal cord, exposed from the anterior aspect to show the meningeal coverings. (From Standring S: *Gray's anatomy: the anatomical basis of clinical practice,* ed 40, Philadelphia, 2008, Churchill Livingstone.)

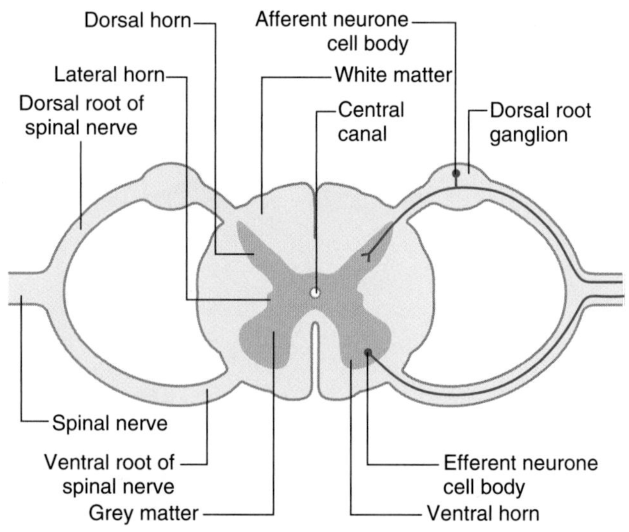

Figure 5-18

Transverse section through the spinal cord, illustrating the disposition of gray and white matter and the attachment of the dorsal and ventral spinal nerve roots. (From Standring S: *Gray's anatomy: the anatomical basis of clinical practice,* ed 40, Philadelphia, 2008, Churchill Livingstone.)

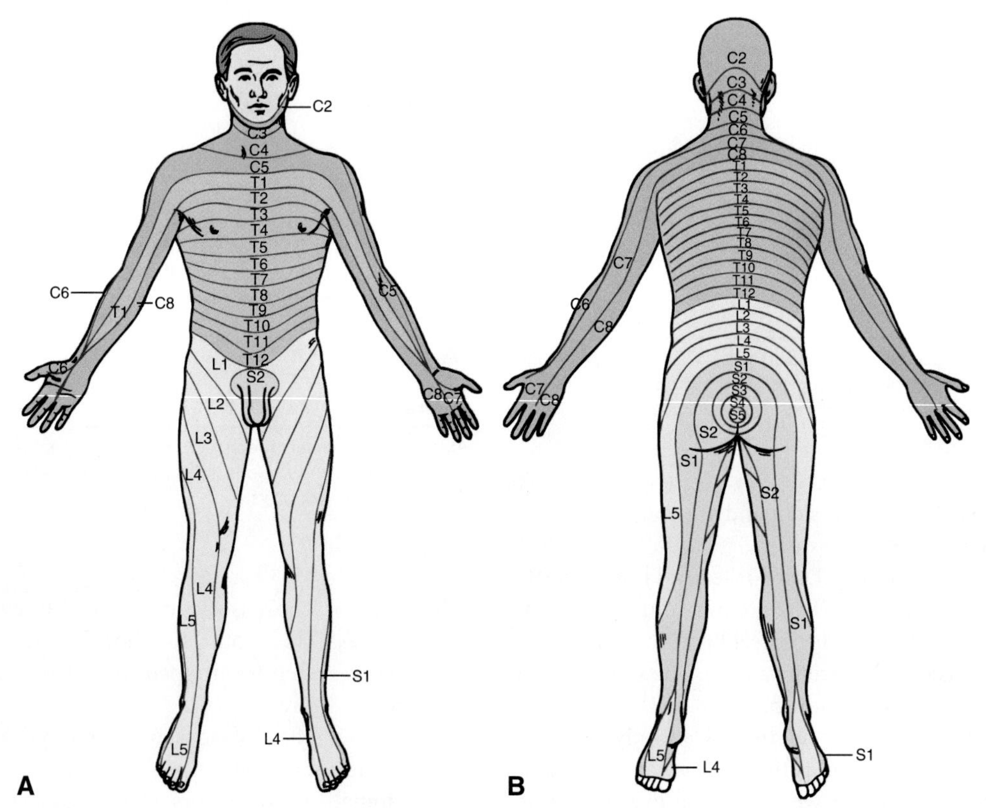

Figure 5-19

Anterior view **(A)** and posterior view **(B)** of a dermatome. (From Urden LD, Stacy KM, Lough ME: *Thelan's critical care nursing: diagnosis and management,* ed 5, St Louis, 2006, Mosby.)

nerve fibers, sending a message from the anterior horn to the muscle. There is essentially no "thought" to this action.

Autonomic Nervous System

The autonomic nervous system (ANS) arises from both the CNS and PNS through the cranial and dorsal root ganglia. The brain stem and lateral gray columns of the spinal cord have preganglionic neurons. The myelinated preganglionic axons exit certain spinal and cranial nerves and connect to their receiving ganglia. Postganglionic neurones are more numerous and can widely disperse the autonomic effects.

The three main parts of the ANS are the sympathetic nervous system, the parasympathetic nervous system, and the enteric nervous system (which is exclusive to the gastrointestinal tract). The sympathetic trunks extend from the cranial base to the coccyx and have a much wider distribution than the parasympathetic system. The preganglionic neurones release acetylcholine as the principal **neurotransmitter**. The postganglionic neurons are distributed along arteries and ducts and release norepinephrine or noradrenaline as the principal neurotransmitter.

In the parasympathetic nervous system, preganglionic neurons are located in many cranial nerves arising from the brain stem and the second through fourth sacral segments; these are considered **cholinergic**. The cell bodies are situated in the periphery, usually near the structures innervated. The oculomotor, facial, vagal, and glossopharyngeal cranial nerves are included in this system (Table 5-1 and Figure 5-20).

CSF, Intracranial, and Cerebral Perfusion Pressures and Autoregulation

Modified Monroe-Kellie Doctrine

The skull is a nondistensible, closed box filled to capacity with essentially noncompressible contents: CSF, blood (intravascular), and brain tissue. The volume of these three components remains nearly constant. If the volume of any one component increases, the volume of another component must decrease for the overall volume to remain constant; otherwise, the intracranial pressure (ICP) rises. Adequate cerebral function requires a continuous and effective blood supply, circulation, and perfusion (Figure 5-21).

Cerebral Blood Flow

The normal adult brain weighs 1350 g, and the normal cerebral blood flow (CBF) is 55 mL/100 g/min, or 750 to 800 mL/min. The brain accounts for only 2.5% of the total body weight, but it requires 15% to 25% of the cardiac output. Infants and children have a higher CBF, as high as 100 mL/100 g/min. In adults, coma results if the CBF drops below 30 mL/100 g/min.

Did You Know?

With a severe traumatic brain injury, the cerebral blood flow is lowest during the first 24 hours after injury; it can be as low as 20 to 30 mL/100 g/min.[5]

Table 5-1 Cranial Nerves and Their Functions

Nerve	Name	Function
I	Olfactory nerve	Process of smell
II	Optic nerve	Vision
III	Oculomotor nerve	Eye movement; parasympathetic innervations of the eye
IV	Trochlear nerve	Eye movement
V	Trigeminal nerve	General sensations from the head; motor to muscles of mastication
VI	Abducens	Eye movement
VII	Facial nerve	Taste; facial movement; parasympathetic innervations of the salivary and lacrimal glands
VIII	Vestibulocochlear nerve	Vestibular sense; hearing
IX	Glossopharyngeal nerve	Taste; general sensory and motor innervations of the pharynx; visceral innervations from the carotid body and sinus; parasympathetic innervations of the salivary glands
X	Vagus nerve	General sensory and motor innervations of the pharynx, larynx, and esophagus; visceral innervations from the thorax and abdomen, including the aortic body and arch; parasympathetic innervation of the thoracic and abdominal viscera
XI	Accessory nerve	Movement of the head and shoulders
XII	Hypoglossal nerve	Movement of the tongue

From Standring S: *Gray's anatomy: the anatomical basis of clinical practice,* ed 39, Philadelphia, 2004, Churchill Livingstone.

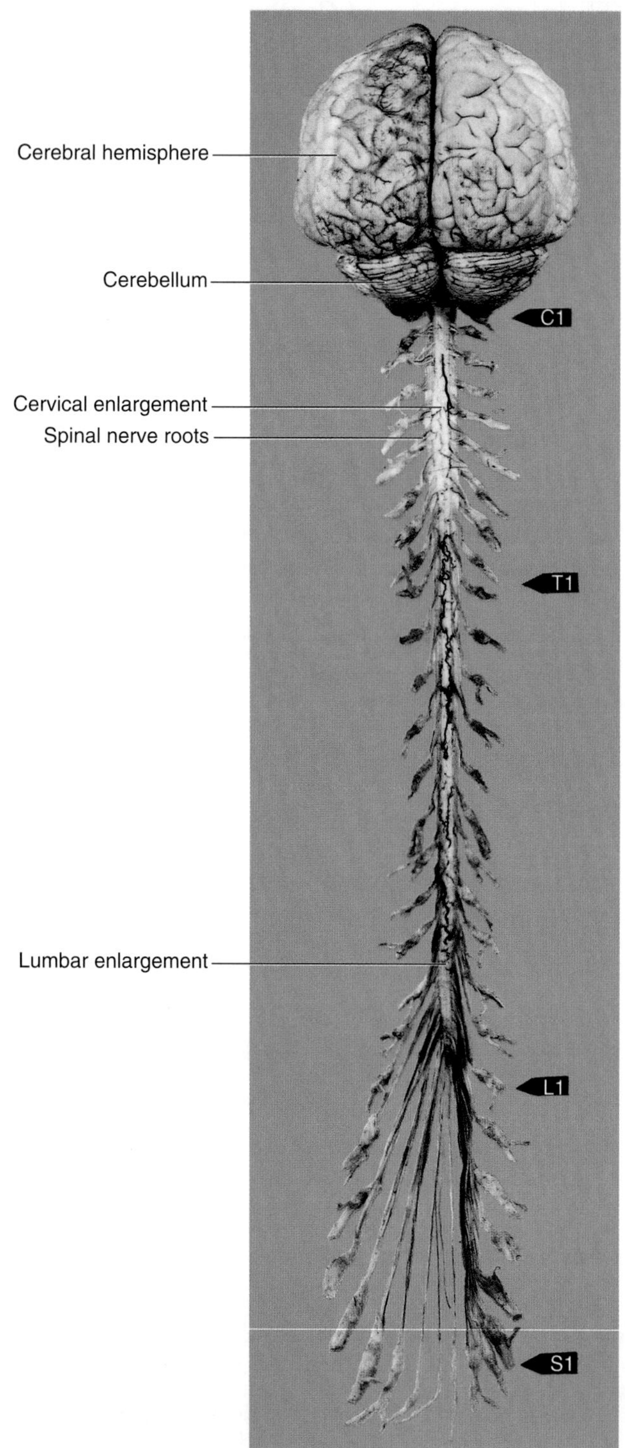

Figure 5-20

Brain and spinal cord with attached spinal nerve roots and dorsal root ganglia (from the dorsal aspect). (Courtesy Kevin Fitzpatrick, GKT School of Medicine, London.)

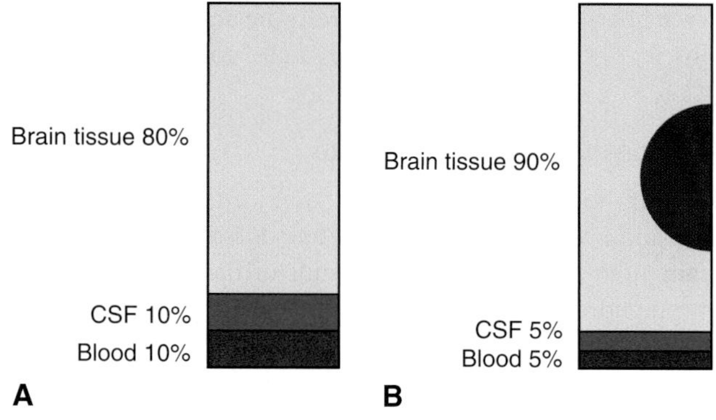

Figure 5-21

A, The cranium essentially is a box filled to capacity with noncompressible contents (i.e., cerebrospinal fluid [CSF], blood, and brain). The volume of these three components remains nearly constant. **B,** If any one component increases in volume, another component must decrease for the overall volume to remain constant; otherwise, the ICP rises.

Several factors affect cerebral blood flow.

1. *Oxygen:* The brain consumes more oxygen (O_2) per unit of weight than any other body organ (twice as much as the heart). It uses 20% of the body's total O_2 intake and has no capacity for O_2 storage. Metabolically, the brain never rests. Anaerobic metabolism causes a decrease in function. Moderate changes in the arterial oxygen level ($Pa{O_2}$) have little effect on cerebral vessels.

   If the $Pa{O_2}$ drops below 50 mm Hg, cerebral blood flow increases significantly. If it drops below 30 mm Hg, CBF doubles. Because the brain needs a high level of O_2 to function, you would think that increasing the $Pa{O_2}$ above normal would reduce cerebral blood flow; however, this results in only a slight change.
2. *Carbon dioxide:* Any variation in the arterial carbon dioxide level ($Pa{CO_2}$) causes extreme changes in cerebral blood flow. CO_2 is a potent stimulus to cerebral vasodilation. If the $Pa{CO_2}$ increases from 40 to 80 mm Hg, the CBF doubles. If the $Pa{CO_2}$ drops to 20 mm Hg, the CBF decreases by one half.
3. *pH:* Cerebral vessels are very sensitive to alterations in the pH of the extracerebral fluid of the brain. Acid solutions cause dilation, and alkaline solutions cause constriction.
4. *Glucose level:* The brain metabolizes only three carbohydrates: glucose, mannose, and fructose. It consumes 65% of the glucose used by the entire body. However, it has only very limited storage of glucose, and any sharp decrease in the blood glucose level causes drastic changes in the level of consciousness.
5. *Temperature:* Oxygen consumption rises 10% for every 1° C rise in temperature. A rise from 37° C (98.6° F) to 40.5° C (105° F) results in a 35% increase in O_2 consumption. In a patient with a brain injury, this results in cerebral hypoxia.

Cerebral Perfusion Pressure

The **cerebral perfusion pressure (CPP)** is a calculated value that represents the pressure available to perfuse the brain. It is an estimate of the adequacy of cerebral circulation. The CPP is the difference between the mean arterial pressure (MAP) and the ICP: CPP = MAP – ICP.

The formula for finding the MAP is based on the systolic blood pressure (SBP) and the diastolic blood pressure (DBP):

$$MAP = DBP + \frac{1}{3}(SBP - DBP), \text{ or}$$

$$MAP = [(2 \times DBP) + SBP] \div 3$$

For a BP of 120/80 mm Hg, the MAP would be 93 mm Hg.

Did You Know?

The mean arterial pressure (MAP) generally is displayed on the combined monitoring system. It appears next to the systolic and diastolic pressure readings, either in a small, labeled box or enclosed in parentheses.

Under normal conditions, the CPP is approximately equal to the MAP. A normal CPP in adults should be 80 to 90 mm Hg; it is always maintained at or above 70 mm Hg. In infants and young children, the CPP should be maintained at 60 to 70 mm Hg.

In all patients, if the CPP falls below 60 mm Hg, mortality from traumatic brain injury increases by 90%. If the CPP drops below 50 mm Hg, ischemia of brain tissue may occur (commonly known as *subflow*). At a CPP below 40 mm Hg, the blood supply starts to fail and the CBF is extremely compromised; below 30 mmHg, irreversible cerebral hypoxia occurs. Cerebral blood flow stops when the ICP equals the MAP.

Although the average CPP in adults is 80 to 90 mmHg, the range of normal extends from 50 to 150 mmHg. An elevated CPP (i.e., higher than 150 mm Hg) is associated with hyperemia.

Compensatory Mechanisms

A primary function of the body's systems is to maintain homeostasis. The brain has its own compensatory mechanisms for ensuring an adequate overall cerebral blood flow. It can adapt only to very small and/or transient changes in the intracranial volume and pressure (volume-pressure relationship). When the intracranial volume increases for any reason, the following normal compensatory mechanisms are triggered automatically to maintain adequate blood flow to the brain.

1. **Accommodation**: Accommodation is the primary compensatory mechanism. The spatial relationships of the skull's contents are changed or rearranged to accommodate an increase in the volume of any of the intracranial contents. This is the Monroe-Kellie doctrine put into action.
   a. CSF accommodates for increases by displacing down the spinal cord or along the roots of nerves. Also, production can be slowed or reabsorption increased. CSF accommodates best with slow-growing lesions or changes in ICP.
   b. The brain tissue accommodates by shifting.
   c. The blood volume changes by means of venous compression.
2. *Autoregulatory mechanisms:* These mechanisms regulate the diameter of blood vessels (resistance) to maintain a constant blood flow. This vital adjustment can prevent ischemia and hyperemic states. More important, it occurs totally independently of the rest of the body. The two forms of autoregulation are pressure autoregulation and metabolic autoregulation.
   a. Pressure autoregulation occurs when the cerebral vasculature compensates for changes in the CPP by altering vascular resistance. When the MAP or ICP increases, the arterioles in the cerebrum vasoconstrict to safeguard the brain from a hyperemic flow state. Just the opposite occurs with a decrease in the MAP or ICP; this results in vasodilation of the cerebral vessels, which protects the brain from subflow states and subsequent infarction.
   b. Metabolic autoregulation functions in the same manner as pressure autoregulation, but potent chemical substances trigger vasodilation of cerebral arterioles, increasing the CBF. These chemical substances (e.g., lactic acid, pyruvic acid, carbonic acid, and carbon dioxide) are metabolic byproducts of cell metabolism. They all have a dissociated hydrogen ion in common, which is a potent vasodilator.

   Autoregulation operates within a range of the MAP (50 to 150 mm Hg). Outside that range, the cerebral blood flow passively follows the perfusion pressures of the body. When autoregulation is lost, the cerebral blood vessels' ability to react and respond also is lost; the CBF then reflects changes in the MAP and CPP.

NEUROLOGIC ASSESSMENT

In emergency medicine, the neurologic examination has a high priority and is performed in the primary or initial survey. It establishes a baseline to which all subsequent examination findings are compared. With each examination, the provider must determine whether the patient is better or worse.

Obtaining the Patient History

Interviewing the patient and gathering the history directly are in themselves a neurologic examination. This is by far the best way to obtain certain information that may guide you to a field impression, nursing diagnosis, and list of pertinent differentials. If the patient cannot participate in the interview, family members or friends can be contacted. In the best case, the person who provides the patient history is someone who knows the patient well and understands the person's daily activities.

The standard SAMPLE history provides a quick overview, but a comprehensive evaluation would be helpful. A SAMPLE history includes signs and symptoms, allergies, medications, previous medical history, last intake of food and fluids, and events before the complaint. The events that occurred before the illness or injury, signs and symptoms, associated complaints, progression of disease, and family and past medical history all are information that can help you provide good patient care.

Physical Examination

The physical examination before or during critical care transport is similar to that performed in emergency medicine. Five parameters are essential in this process: respiratory assessment, vital signs, level of consciousness (LOC), pupillary response, and motor and sensory function. Some diagnostics also are important, including laboratory tests (with an emphasis on glucose levels) and imaging.

Always start with the basic assessment of the ABCDs:

A Airway patent (with cervical spine precautions in cases involving trauma)
B Breathing with supplemental oxygen
C Circulation adequate
D Disability (quick assessment of LOC and pupils)

1. **Respiratory assessment:** Airway and breathing must be evaluated for life-threatening conditions and managed immediately. Protection of the airway in a patient with an altered mental status is one of the golden rules of emergency and critical care medicine. The old standard, "If the Glasgow is less than 8, intubate (or at least insert an airway adjunct)," still plays in the medical director's protocols in transport. Assessing for cough and swallow reflexes also is important. In a patient who has had a stroke, swallowing reflexes are evaluated quite early in the process of resuscitation and care.

   Abnormal patterns of respiration can provide clues to CNS disease or trauma. The process of respiration, which moves oxygen and carbon dioxide into and out of neurologic cells, is essential to the LOC and CNS function (Table 5-2).

2. **Vital signs:** Adequate respiration, oxygenation, and perfusion are crucial to normal brain function. When you are evaluating a patient with altered mental status, the vital signs are the key to understanding whether the patient's nervous system is receiving the ingredients for basic functions and the way the body is responding to a neurologic crisis, if present.

   a. Monitor the blood pressure. As mentioned previously, cerebral blood flow is autoregulated, and the MAP is integral to determining the patient's cerebral perfusion pressure (CPP = MAP – ICP).

      Systemic hypertension, as part of an overall hyperdynamic state, is a common sign when a pathologic condition of the brain is present. When the ICP begins to increase, the pulse may fall into a range of 50 to 60 beats/min. The cardiac stroke volume increases, which causes a rise in the systolic BP to facilitate the delivery of blood to the brain despite increased resistance in cerebral vessels. The pulse pressure widens.

      A note of caution is required regarding hypertension with pathologic brain conditions. Protocols should be established that guide the provider in the management of elevated BP/MAP. When the ICP rises, the MAP must also rise to ensure an adequate cerebral perfusion pressure. Critical care standards require the provider to understand, measure, and document the patient's BP, MAP, and pulse pressure.

   b. Monitor the heart rate and rhythm. The sympathetic and parasympathetic tracts (vagus), along with the medulla, control the heart rate. When the ICP rises, a hyperdynamic state (with tachycardia) may occur, or bradycardia may present as part of Cushing's triad. Arrhythmias may be precipitated by various pathologic conditions in the brain (Box 5-1).

   c. Monitor the temperature. Hyperthermia is much more common than hypothermia. Fever is complex. It can be the result of infectious organisms or a noninfectious inflammatory response. Hypothermia can be due to spinal shock with autonomic innervation loss, metabolic or toxic coma, drug overdose (especially depressant drugs), and brain stem or hypothalamic lesions.

Table 5-2 Respiratory Patterns

	Description	Significance
Cheyne-Stokes respiration	Rhythmic crescendo and decrescendo of the rate and depth of respiration; includes brief periods of apnea	Usually seen with bilateral deep cerebral lesions or some cerebellar lesions
Central neurogenic hyperventilation	Very deep, very rapid respirations with no apneic periods	Usually seen with lesions of the midbrain and upper pons
Apneustic breathing	Prolonged inspiratory and/or expiratory pause of 2-3 sec	Usually seen with lesions of the middle to lower pons
Cluster breathing	Clusters of irregular, gasping respirations separated by long periods of apnea	Usually seen with lesions of the lower pons or upper medulla
Ataxic respirations	Irregular, random pattern of deep and shallow respirations with irregular apneic periods	Usually seen with lesions of the medulla

From Urden LD, Stacy KM, Lough ME: *Thelan's critical care nursing: diagnosis and management*, ed 5, St Louis, 2006, Mosby.

3. **Level of consciousness:** The LOC is the most important, the most sensitive, and the earliest sign of neurologic function and change. Level of consciousness has two components, arousal and cognition. The degree of alertness is assessed by applying a stimulus, usually pain or a sound, and observing the response. Generally, a minimal stimulus is used first to evoke a response, and the stimulus then is increased as necessary. Orientation is evaluated with regard to time, place, and person; it is documented as specifically as possible (do not use labels such as lethargic, obtunded, comatose, and so on).

   The Glasgow Coma Scale (GCS) relates consciousness to motor response, verbal response, and eye opening. Scores range from 3 to 15, 15 being the score for a fully awake, oriented person who has full movement in at least one extremity. Conditions marked by lower scores (less than 8) may qualify as coma. The GCS may be difficult to evaluate in patients who have used alcohol or other mind-altering drugs; who have hypoglycemia; who are in shock (systolic BP below 80 mm Hg); or who have hypothermia (temperature below 34° C [93.2° F]) (Boxes 5-2 to 5-4).

Box 5-1 Cushing's Triad

Pressure on the medulla of the brain stem produces three ominous signs, known collectively as **Cushing's triad** (or Cushing's reflex):

- Bradycardia
- Systolic hypertension
- Respiratory irregularity

Cushing's triad is seen with elevated intracranial pressure and may be an indicator of herniation syndrome.

Box 5-2 Glasgow Coma Scale*

Finding	Score
1. Eye opening response	
Spontaneously	4
To verbal command	3
To pain	2
No response	1
Untestable	E
2. Best motor response	
To verbal command	
Obeys	6
To painful stimulus	
Localizes pain	5
Flexion (withdrawal)	4
Flexion abnormal (decorticate rigidity)	3
Extension (decerebrate rigidity)	2
No response	1
Untestable	M
3. Best verbal response	
Oriented and converses	5
Disoriented and converses	4
Inappropriate words	3
Incomprehensible sounds	2
No response	1
Untestable	V
Possible total score	3-15

Modified from Jennett B, Teasdale G: Aspects of coma after head injury, *Lancet* 1:878-881, 1977.

*The Glasgow Coma Scale should be used for patients 4 years of age or older.

E, Eye opening; *M*, motor; *V*, verbal.

Box 5-3 Pediatric Coma Scale*

Finding	Score
1. Eye opening response	
Spontaneously	4
Reaction to speech/shout	3
Reaction to pain	2
No response	1
Untestable	E
2. Best motor response	
Spontaneous (or, patient > 1 yr: obeys verbal command)	6
To painful stimulus	
Localizes pain	5
Withdraws in response to pain	4
Abnormal flexion in response to pain	3
Abnormal extension in response to pain	2
No response	1
Untestable	M

Finding		Score
3. Best verbal response		
0-23 mo	2-4 yr	
Coos, babbles, smiles, follows objects, cries appropriately (consolable)	Uses appropriate words and phrases	5
Irritable crying (inconsolable)	Uses words inappropriately	4
Cries only with pain	Moans, irritable, cries/screams	3
Grunts		2
No response		1
Untestable		V
	Possible total score	3-15

Modified from Thompson SW: *Emergency care of children,* Boston, 1990, Jones & Bartlett.

*This scale is a modification of the adult Glasgow Coma Scale; it should be used for patients up to age 3 years.

E, Eye Opening ; *M*, motor; *V*, verbal.

Box 5-4 Performing the Glasgow Coma Scale Assessment

1. Record the best or highest response of which the patient is capable.
2. If you are unable to elicit a response because of causes other than depressed consciousness, do the following:
   - Eye opening response (precluded by eyes swollen shut or injured): Enter "E" on the flowsheet for the criterion Untestable in this section.
   - Best motor response (precluded by spinal cord injury or local trauma to all extremities): Enter "M" on the flowsheet for the criterion Untestable in this section.
   - Best verbal response (precluded by an endotracheal tube, trach, or dysphasia): Enter "V" on the flowsheet for the criterion Untestable in this section.

   E, M, and *V* are each scored as 1 when you total the score. Document the reason the test could not be performed in the patient care record.
3. It is better to describe a patient's level of consciousness (LOC) by recording the value of each subscale separately rather than by adding them for a total score, because the individual behaviors provide important clinical information. Two patients can have a GCS of 6 and yet have very different neurologic conditions. Suppose you have the following scores for two patients:

	Patient 1	**Patient 2**
Eye opening response	1	1
Best motor response	3	4
Best verbal response	2	V (Patient intubated)
Total GCS score	6	6

   Note that both patients have the same total GCS score, but their individual behavior scores are very different. Recording the GCS in this fashion is especially important if one or more behaviors are untestable. In the example provided, the total score for patient 2 is disproportionately low because one of the three behavior scores is missing.
4. *Stimulus.* Obtaining the best response on the GCS depends on application of the proper stimulus. Auditory and tactile stimuli are the major forms used.
   a. To elicit a reaction, always begin with the mildest stimulus, such as speaking to the patient in a normal tone of voice. If the patient does not respond at this level, increase the volume, progressing to shouting. If the patient does not respond to a verbal stimulus, apply a tactile stimulus. Gently shake the person's arm while calling the patient's name.
   b. If the patient does not respond to a tactile stimulus, apply a painful (noxious) stimulus. Painful stimuli are best applied in a standard fashion. A pain response can be elicited by many different methods. Unfortunately, many of these border on physical abuse (e.g., nipple twisting or pinching), and over the course of serial examinations, they may damage tissue and result in bruises or other trauma. To prevent these problems, nail bed pressure is the recommended method. For this method, squeeze the patient's finger or toe while holding a pen, oriented perpendicular to the nail, at the point where the nail enters the skin. Nail bed pressure usually is sufficient to elicit the best response. A painful stimulus also can be achieved by:
      - Applying pressure on the trapezius muscle on either side of the neck by squeezing or pinching it.
      - Applying pressure on the gastrocnemius muscle on the calf of the leg by squeezing or grasping it.
      - Applying supraorbital pressure by pressing on the supraorbital ridge with thumb (this form of stimulus is questionable when the patient has facial or eye trauma).
      - Pinching the axilla, nipples, or groin area; however, this method should be used only as a last resort.

      A painful stimulus must be applied to both sides of the body to allow for any difference in function. The painful stimulus should be maintained until a maximum response is obtained. For example, some patients respond when painful stimuli are applied continuously for 15 seconds, and others may respond if the stimulus is applied several times in the course of the assessment.

Eye Opening Response

5. Do not use the eyes to evaluate attentiveness or awareness. The eye opening category tests the functioning of arousal mechanisms in the brain stem.
   a. Score 4—Spontaneously: Eyes open in accordance with sleep/wake rhythms (i.e., the patient opens the eyes spontaneously and/or opens the eyes when a person enters the room without verbal stimulation).
   b. Score 3—To verbal command: Eyes open in response to speech; this is a response to any verbal approach, whether spoken or shouted, not necessarily to a command (i.e., the patient opens the eyes in response to his or her name or to a command, such as, "Open your eyes").
   c. Score 2—To pain: Eyes open only in response to pain. Pain should be tested by a stimulus to the limbs or trunk of body because a grimacing response associated with supraorbital or jaw angle pressure may cause eye closure.
   d. Score 1—No response: Eyes do not open even to painful stimuli.
   e. Score E—Untestable: If the patient cannot open the eyes for reasons other than LOC, enter "E" on the flowsheet for this category and score as described in step 2. However, a patient in a deep coma with flaccid ocular muscles may lie with the eyes open all the time; this is not a true arousal response and should be recorded as "no response."

Best Motor Response

6. Motor responses are elicited in the limbs. The arms are preferred, because they show a wider range of response. Even in patients diagnosed with brain death, the spinal reflex may cause the legs to flex briskly in response to pain. Record the best (or highest) response in any limb. A difference in responsiveness between two limbs may indicate focal damage. Note the worse response in the patient care record but record the best score on the flowsheet.
   a. To verbal command—obeys (score 6): The patient shows the proper motor response to your verbal command. Do not confuse grip with tonic grasp reflex or postural

Box 5-4 Performing the Glasgow Coma Scale Assessment—cont'd

adjustment; however, ordering the patient to "release the grip" is a valid test.

b. To painful stimulus: As mentioned, if the patient does not obey commands, a painful stimulus is applied. Initially, nail bed pressure is applied to the fingernail until a maximum response is obtained. Flexion should be observed. If it is, one of the stimuli previously described then is applied to the head, neck, or trunk of the body to test for localization.
   - Score 5—Localizes pain: A limb moves in an attempt to escape the painful stimuli when a stimulus is applied to more than one site (e.g., the patient reaches up and tries to remove your fingers as you apply pressure on the right or left side of the trapezius muscle).
   - Score 4—Flexion withdrawal: This is withdrawal from the source of pain; it is a generalized, not a localized, response (i.e., the patient withdraws or turns away from the painful stimulus but does not actively attempt to remove the source of the pain).
   - Score 3—Abnormal flexion (decorticate rigidity): This is a flexion response that is not a purposeful response. (It formerly was called "decorticate posturing," but that term is no longer used because it implies a specific physioanatomic correlation.) Abnormal flexion is characterized by flexion of the arm, wrist, and fingers with adduction in the upper extremity and by extension, internal rotation, and plantar flexion of the lower extremity. Simply stated, it is hyperflexion of the upper extremities and hyperextension of the lower extremities.
   - Score 2—Extension (decerebrate rigidity): This is the inappropriate response of extension to a painful stimulus. (It formerly was called "decerebrate posturing," but that term is no longer used because it implies a specific physioanatomic correlation.) An ominous sign, it is manifested by extension of the arms with adduction and internal rotation of the shoulder, hyperpronation of the forearms with internal rotation of the wrists, and clenching of the hands into fists. The legs are rigidly extended and show plantar extension of the feet. Stated simply, there is hyperextension of both the upper and lower extremities.
   - Score 1—No response: This is usually associated with hypotonia. It is important to exclude spinal transection and inadequate stimulus application as reasons for the lack of response.
   - Score M—Untestable: If the patient is paralyzed by injury or medication or the motor response is otherwise untestable, enter "M" for this category on the flowsheet and score as described in step 2.

Best Verbal Response

7. The patient's best verbal response is assessed as follows:
   a. Score 5—Oriented and converses: The patient is aware of himself or herself and the environment (i.e., the patient is oriented to person, place, and time).
   b. Score 4—Disoriented and converses: The patient's conversation is confused. If you can hold the patient's attention, and the person responds to questions in a conversational manner but the responses indicate varying degrees of disorientation or confusion, use verbatim charting of the responses to qualify for this rating.
   c. Score 3—Inappropriate words: The patient's articulations are intelligible, but the speech used is exclamatory or random (usually shouting or swearing). No sustained conversational exchange is possible.
   d. Score 2—Incomprehensible sounds: The patient moans and groans and does not produce recognizable words.
   e. Score 1—No response.
   f. Score V—Untestable. If the patient is intubated or mute or the verbal subscale is otherwise untestable, enter "V" for this category on the flowsheet and score as described in step 2.

4. **Pupillary response**
   a. Check the size of the pupils. Pupil size is measured in millimeters; the average size is 3 mm. When evaluating the pupils, compare the size. Also, assess the positions of the two eyelids; if abnormalities are noted in either or both, ask the patient (if possible) or the family whether the condition is normal for the patient. **Ptosis** of the eyelid and **anisocoria** (unequal pupil size) can be normal variants in some people. However, anisocoric pupils also can be an indicator of a pathologic condition, such as early **Horner's syndrome** (also called *herniation syndrome*). A difference of less than 1 mm is not considered indicative of a pathologic condition (Figures 5-22 to 5-24).

      A **miotic pupil** is constricted (often to 2 mm, or pinpoint) and can be the result of pontine lesions that destroy sympathetic pathways. Extremely small pupils also can indicate narcotic use and lower brain stem compression. A **mydriatic pupil** is dilated to greater than 6 mm and is the result of pupil-dilating drugs (atropine, scopolamine) and extreme stress. With sympathetic innervation, pupils may dilate.
   b. Evaluate the shape of the pupils. Pupils usually are round and regular. Look for ovoid, keyhole, irregular, or fixed and/or dilated pupils.
   c. Check the pupils' reaction to light. Each pupil has dual innervation, from both the sympathetic and parasympathetic nervous systems. Consequently, the normal resting pupil size is not a constant. Observe for direct and consensual (indirect) reaction. Record how quickly the pupil changed in reaction to light. Keep in mind that a reactive pupil, in association with the absence of

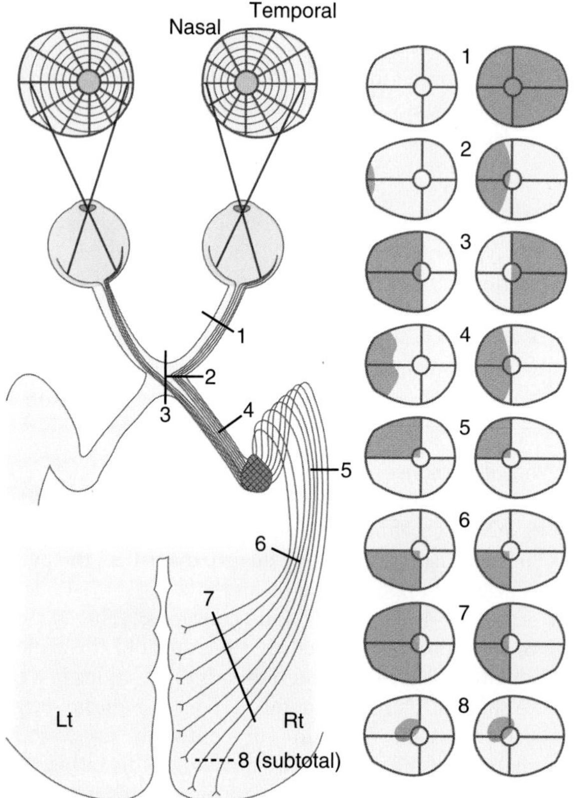

Figure 5-22

Visual fields affected by damage to the visual pathways. *1,* Optic nerve: unilateral amaurosis. *2,* Lateral optic chiasm: grossly incongruous, incomplete (contralateral) homonymous hemianopia. *3,* Central optic chiasm: bitemporal hemianopia. *4,* Optic tract: incongruous, incomplete homonymous hemianopia. *5,* Temporal (Meyer's) loop of the optic radiation: congruous partial or complete (contralateral) homonymous superior quadrantanopia. *6,* Parietal (superior) projection of the optic radiation: congruous partial or complete homonymous inferior quadrantanopia. *7,* Complete parieto-occipital interruption of the optic radiation: complete congruous homonymous hemianopia with psychophysical shift of the foveal point, often sparing central vision and resulting in "macular sparing." *8,* Incomplete damage to the visual cortex: congruous homonymous scotomas, usually encroaching at least acutely on central vision. (From Goldman L, Ausiello D: *Cecil medicine: expert consult,* ed 23, Philadelphia, 2007, Saunders.)

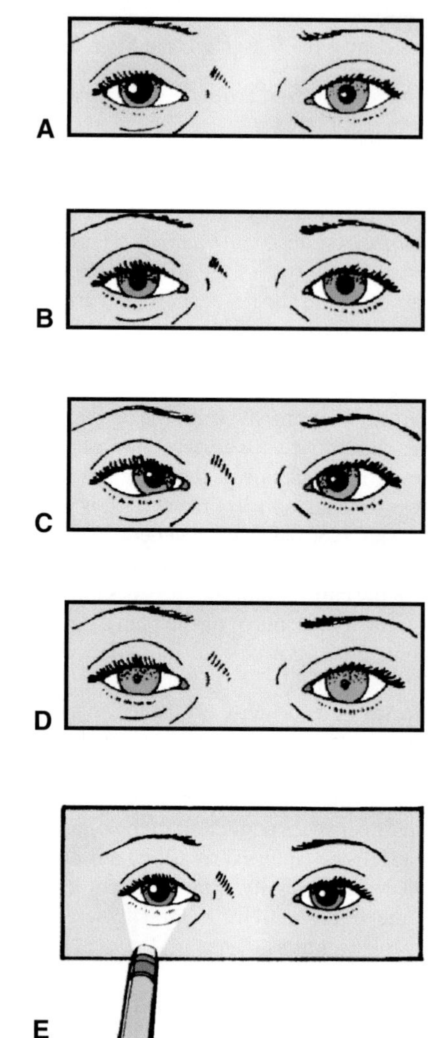

Figure 5-24

Abnormal pupillary responses. **A**, Oculomotor nerve compression. **B**, Bilateral diencephalon damage. **C**, Midbrain damage. **D,** Pontine damage. **E**, Dilated, nonreactive pupils. (From Urden LD, Stacy KM, Lough ME: *Thelan's critical care nursing: diagnosis and management,* ed 5, St Louis, 2006, Mosby.)

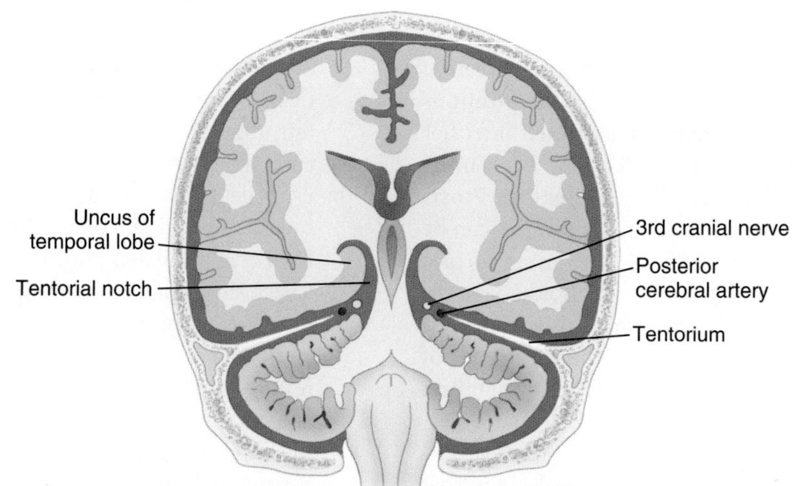

Figure 5-23

Note the location of cranial nerve III (the oculomotor nerve) and the relevance of unilateral pupil dilation when herniation threatens.

corneal reflexes and of an oculocephalic response, generally signifies a metabolic **encephalopathy** or drug overdose.

d. Assess for eye/pupil accommodation, constriction, and **convergence.** The **hippus phenomenon** demonstrates a state of physiologic pupillary unrest. The pupil constricts to direct light stimulus but cannot maintain the constriction and thus dilates (this response usually is diminished in the dark). This response is more prevalent in younger people. Coarse fluctuation in one or both eyes is seen with pathologic conditions.

   Photophobia (associated with cranial nerve V) is a sensitivity of the eyes to light. The cause is unclear, but the condition is noted in many patients with meningeal irritation and frequently is associated with meningitis, subarachnoid hemorrhage, and diseases such as migraine headaches.

e. Extraocular movements (EOMs): There are six cardinal directions of eye gaze, associated with various cranial nerves (Figure 5-25). These are assessed in the alert patient by asking them to follow your finger through the full range of eye motion. Symmetrical movement through the six directions is normal.

f. Evaluate for **nystagmus**, a repetitive, involuntary oscillation of one or both eyes in any plane of movement. Generally, three planes of movement are seen: horizontal, vertical, and rotary. Nystagmus can be caused by many factors, including toxins, retinal disease, vestibular disease, and lesions of the brain stem or cerebellum. However, it is not always an indicator of a pathologic condition.

g. Evaluate for conjugate eye movement (the two eyes working in unison). Normally the eyes move conjugately in the orbital sockets, blink periodically, and do not show abnormal eye movements. The eyeball neither protrudes (exophthalmos) nor is sunken in the orbits (enophthalmos), and the upper eyelid does not droop (ptosis).

   Disconjugate eye movement **(strabismus)** is an uncontrolled deviation of an eye. Normal horizontal disconjugate gaze is seen in drowsy or sedated patients. Vertical plane disconjugate gaze (skew deviation) results from pontine or cerebellar lesions. Sustained downward eye deviation occurs with several nonlocalizing neurologic disorders. Sustained upward gaze usually is the result of hypoxic encephalopathy.

h. Assess ocular movements in an unconscious patient (i.e., reflexive eye movements). The **doll's eyes response**, or oculocephalic reflex, is a test of cranial nerves III, VI, and VIII and an assessment of the integrity of the brain

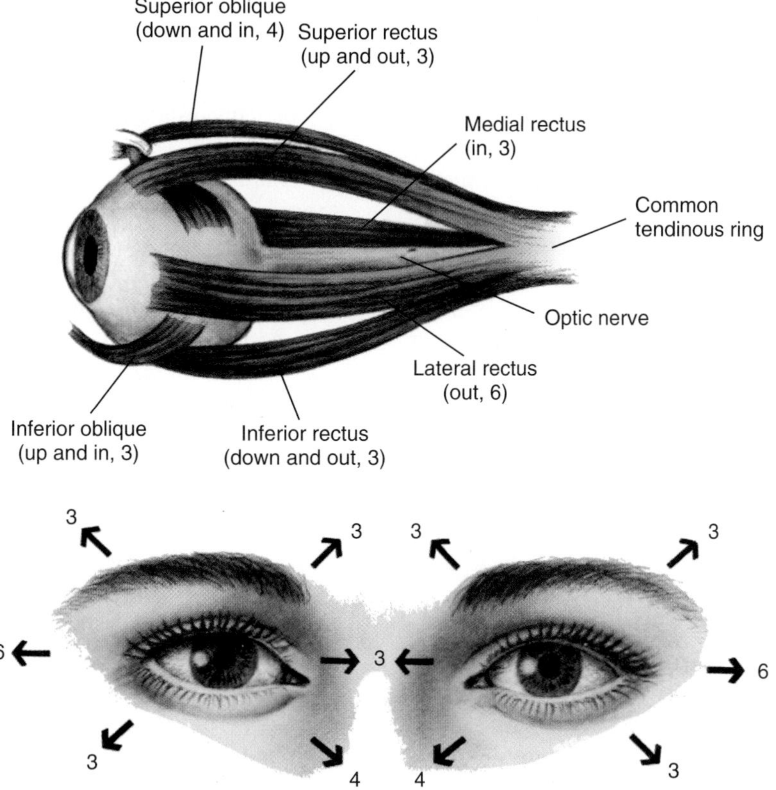

Figure 5-25

Extraocular movements. **A,** Extraocular muscles. **B,** Six cardinal directions of gaze and associated cranial nerve supply. (From Urden LD, Stacy KM, Lough ME: *Thelan's critical care nursing: diagnosis and management,* ed 5, St Louis, 2006, Mosby.)

stem. To perform the test, hold the patient's eyelids open and then quickly and gently turn the head side to side. The results are as follows:

- In an unconscious patient *with* an intact brain stem, the eyes deviate to the side opposite that to which the head is turned (this is recorded as, "Patient has doll's eyes response").
- In an unconscious patient *without* an intact brain stem, the eyes stay midposition, or fixed, or turn in the same direction the head is turned (recorded as, "Patient does not have doll's eyes response"). If vertebral column injury, this test cannot be performed.

    The doll's eyes response cannot be elicited in a normal, conscious individual, and the test cannot be performed if the patient has a vertebral column injury.

i. The **cold caloric examination** (or oculovestibular reflex test) can be performed in either a conscious or an unconscious patient to test cranial nerves III, VI, and VIII and brain stem integrity. This evaluation is performed by a physician, who first examines the patient to make sure the tympanic membrane is intact and that no cerumen impaction is present. The reflex is elicited by injecting 20 to 120 mL of water into each ear canal (allowing 5 minutes between ears) with the head of the bed elevated to 30 degrees. (Despite the exam's name, either cool water [30° C; 86° F] or warm water [44° C; 111.2° F] may be used for this test.)
    - In a normal, conscious patient, the test produces nausea and vomiting with conjugate, slow, tonic nystagmus toward the irrigated ear that lasts 30 to 120 seconds and a quick-phase nystagmus away from the irrigated ear. The helpful mnemonic is "cows": cold—opposite, warm—same. This means that if cold water is used, the quick-phase nystagmus moves the eyes away from the ear tested; if warm water is used, the quick-phase nystagmus moves to the same ear.
    - In an unconscious patient *with* an intact brain stem, the eyes move conjugately, and the quick-phase nystagmus may be lost.
    - In an unconscious patient *without* an intact brain stem there is no movement or disconjugate movement of the eye.

    NOTE: The cold caloric examination can be performed only if no neuromuscular blockade is in effect.

j. Evaluate the eye gaze. A sustained, conjugate eye deviation in the horizontal plane is normal. An abnormal eye gaze may indicate an irritative or destructive lesion.

k. Assess for **roving eye movements**, which are spontaneous, slow, random eye deviations that move in the horizontal plane, similar to the slow eye movements of sleep. Roving eye movements are normal in a comatose patient and suggest intact brain stem function.

5. **Motor and sensory function**
    a. Assess grip strength. Muscle strength in a responsive patient can be tested by grip. Note the equality of strength and the ability to release on command. Be sure to distinguish grip strength from the **grasp reflex** or postural adjustment. In an unconscious patient, muscle strength can be evaluated by observing the frequency and strength of spontaneous movement and comparing all extremities; or, you can watch for the response to pain stimuli, observing strength and comparing extremities.
    b. Test for the **pronation sign**. Ask the patient to hold the arms out straight, palms up, and eyes closed and to maintain this position for 20 to 30 seconds. With a normal response, the patient is well able to hold the position. With an abnormal response (pronator drift), one forearm pronates, and a downward drift with flexion of the fingers and elbow may be seen.
    c. Test for the plantar reflex (**Babinski's sign**). Use a hard object (e.g., pen or swab stick) to stroke the lateral surface of the sole, starting at the heel and swiping toward and across the ball of the foot (curved, continuous stroke). In individuals over 6 months of age, a normal reflex is flexion of all toes. A positive Babinski's sign is an abnormal response; that is, dorsiflexion of the great toe with fanning of the remaining toes (Figure 5-26). This indicates an upper motor neuron lesion in the brain, brain stem, or spinal cord. This reflex also may appear as **tentorial herniation** occurs.
    d. Test push-pull. Test the lower extremities by having the patient move the toes to show the ability to follow commands; bend the legs to check strength; and have the patient imitate the movement for pushing on the gas pedal.
    e. Evaluate muscle tone and size by flexing and extending the extremity to test resistance. Increased tone is marked by **paratonia** (spasticity); decreased tone is marked by flaccidity.
    f. Test gait with tandem walking heel to toe, heel walking, and toe walking (Table 5-3).

Signs of Meningeal Irritation

The following are signs of meningeal irritation, which may be seen with CNS infection and meningitis.

- Nuchal rigidity (stiff neck)
- **Kernig's sign**: This sign is present if the examiner is unable to passively extend the patient's knee fully because of hamstring resistance and pain. The patient must be supine, and the same hip and knee are flexed to 90 degrees to start.
- **Brudzinski's sign**: This sign is elicited by passive flexion of the neck and head on the chest. With a positive Brudzinski's sign, both the upper legs at the hips and the lower legs at the knee flex in response to passive flexion (Tables 5-4 and 5-5).

Boxes 5-5 and 5-6 provide additional information on rapid assessment of conscious and unconscious patients.

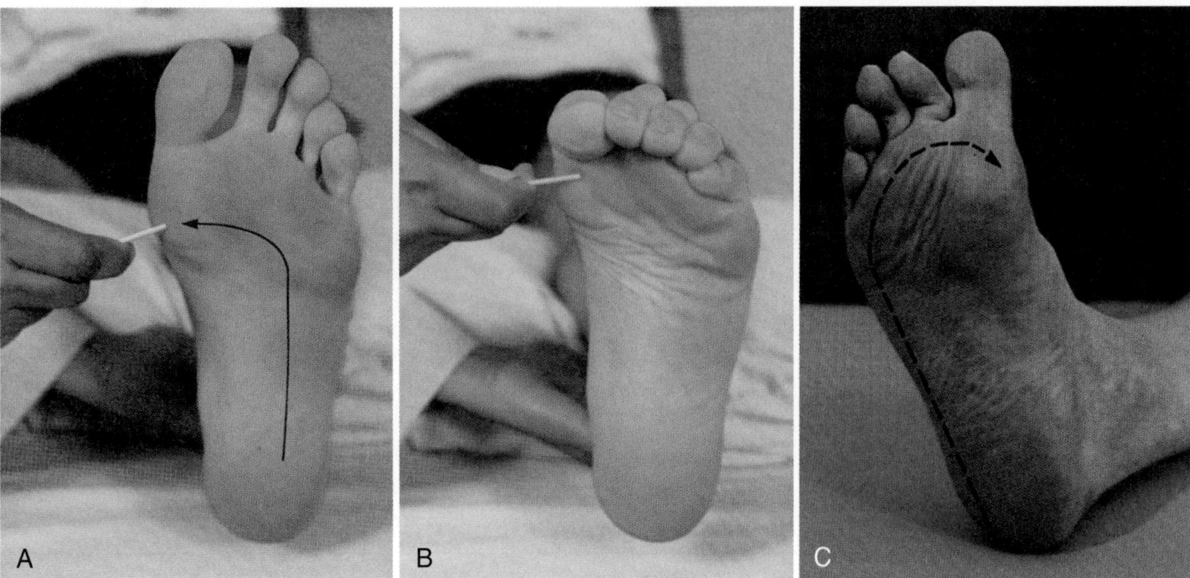

Figure 5-26

Elicitation of the plantar reflex. **A,** A hard object is applied to the lateral surface of the sole, starting at the heel, moving over the ball of the foot, and ending beneath the great toe. **B,** The normal response to plantar stimulation is flexion of all toes. **C,** Babinski's sign is characterized by dorsiflexion of the great toe and fanning of the other toes. (**A** and **B** from Barkauskas VH, Baumann LC, Darling-Fisher CS: *Health and physical assessment,* ed 3, St Louis, 2002, Mosby; **C** from Seidel HM, Ball JW, Dains JE: *Mosby's guide to physical examination,* ed 6, St Louis, 2007, Mosby.)

Table 5-3 Types of Gait

	Characteristics	**Possible Cause**
Ataxic	Staggering, unsteadiness, inability to remain steady with the feet together, tendency to reel to one side	Disease of the cerebellum or posterior columns
Dystonic	Irregular, nondirective movements	Disorder of muscle tone
Dystrophic	Waddling with the legs far apart, weight shifts from side to side, abdomen protrudes, lordosis possible	Weakness or wasting of pelvic girdle (muscular dystrophy), dislocated hip
Hemiplegic	Stiff movements, leg on affected side circles outward, foot drags on floor, arm on same side may be flexed and does not swing freely, person leans to affected side	Disorder of the corticospinal tract
Parkinsonian	Forward leaning (stooped) posture, head bent, hips and knees flexed; short, shuffling, rapidly accelerating steps, stiff turns, entire body rotating at once, difficulty starting and stopping	Basal ganglia defects of Parkinson's disease, extrapyramidal tract
Scissors	Short, slow steps with the legs alternately crossing over each other	Spastic paraplegia
Spastic	Short steps, dragging of the balls of the feet	Bilateral lesion of the corticospinal tract
Steppage	Exaggerated, high steps with the knees flexed and the feet brought down heavily	Footdrop secondary to lower motor neuron lesions

Modified from Hickey J: *The clinical practice of neurologic and neurosurgical nursing,* ed 5, Philadelphia, 2003, Lippincott Williams & Wilkins.

Table 5-4 Superficial Reflexes

Reflex	Involved Nerves	Normal Reaction
Corneal	Cranial nerves (CN) V and VII	Prompt closure of both eyelids when cornea is touched with a wisp of cotton
Pharyngeal	CN IX and X	Gagging response to pharyngeal stimulation
Abdominal	Epigastric (T6-T9); midabdominal (T9-T11); hypogastric (T11-L1)	Contraction of abdominal muscle when stroked, producing a brief, brisk movement of the umbilicus toward the stimulus
Cremasteric	L1, L2	Testicle elevation when inner aspect of thigh is stroked
Anal (anal wink; anocutaneous)	Inferior rectal branch of pudendal nerve, roots 2-4 sacral nerve roots	Contraction of anal ring as perineum is stroked or scratched
Bulbocavernous, bulbospongiosus	S2-S4	Contraction of anal sphincter when glans of penis is squeezed or Foley catheter is tugged
Plantar	L5, S1	Flexion of toes from stimulation of sole of foot

From Urden LD, Stacy KM, Lough ME: *Thelan's critical care nursing: diagnosis and management,* ed 5, St Louis, 2006, Mosby.

Box 5-5 Rapid Neurologic Assessment of a Conscious Patient

1. **Level of consciousness:** Ask the patient a variety of orientation questions (make sure you know the correct answers); focus the questions on recent and past events, people, and places in the patient's life, such as the spouse's name, the patient's home address, and what the patient ate at the previous meal.
2. **Facial movements:** When assessing the level of consciousness, observe the patient's facial movements for symmetry and listen to speech patterns for evidence of slurring.
3. **Pupillary function and eye movements:** Perform a pupil check and assess extraocular eye movements.
4. **Motor assessment:** Assess movement and strength in the upper and lower extremities.
5. **Sensory assessment:** Use your finger to stroke the patient bilaterally on the face, upper aspect of the arm, hand, leg, and foot; ask the patient to identify what is touched and whether the sensation is any different between the two sides.
6. **Vital signs:** Note any alterations in blood pressure, heart rate or rhythm, respiratory pattern, and temperature.
7. **Change in status:** At each subsequent evaluation, ask the patient whether he or she feels any differences between this and the previous examination.

From Urden LD, Stacy KM, Lough ME: *Thelan's critical care nursing: diagnosis and management,* ed 5, St Louis, 2006, Mosby.

Box 5-6 Rapid Neurologic Assessment of an Unconscious Patient

1. **Level of consciousness:** Perform the Glasgow Coma Scale assessment.
2. **Pupillary function:** Perform pupillary assessment, paying special attention to size, reactivity, and the shape of the pupil compared with the opposite eye.
3. **Motor examination:** Assess each extremity individually using a predetermined coding score for motor movement.
4. **Respiratory pattern:** If the patient is not receiving mechanical ventilation, observe the respiratory patterns for evidence of deteriorating function.
5. **Vital signs:** Include a comparison of preassessment and postassessment vital signs; pay special attention to the arterial blood pressure and intracranial pressure (ICP) if they are monitored.

From Urden LD, Stacy KM, Lough ME: *Thelan's critical care nursing: diagnosis and management,* ed 5, St Louis, 2006, Mosby.

DIAGNOSTIC EVALUATION OF NEUROLOGIC CONDITIONS

Every patient the critical care team transports is accompanied by the person's diagnostic studies or their results. A knowledge of these studies can help you with adjunct care that may be associated with the test result. Also, the critical care team sometimes assists with procedures in hospitals' imaging departments.

Head and Spine Radiographs

Skull radiographs have nearly become extinct, especially in trauma cases, because computed tomography (CT) has become the most commonly used diagnostic tool for cranial evaluation. In some areas, radiographs of the spine, which are used to identify fractures and other abnormalities, are still obtained as part of the secondary examination of a trauma patient; however, in many places, these, too, have been replaced by CT scans (see Chapter 7).

The five main views of the cervical spine are the atlas, axial, anterior-posterior, lateral, and oblique views. The thoracic and lumbar spines generally are radiographed in two views, the anterior-posterior and lateral views.

To see the entire cervical spine in the lateral view, the clinician must be able to view all seven vertebrae to the top of T1

Table 5-5 Classification of the Cranial Nerves

Cranial Nerve	Type	Location and Function	Evidence of Abnormality
CN I Olfactory nerve	Sensory	Receptors located in nasal mucosa; responsible for smell.	Inability to detect a specific odor
CN II Optic nerve	Sensory	Fibers originate from retina. At optic chiasm, fibers from nasal half cross; those from temporal half do not. Continue as optic tracts to lateral geniculate bodies and then to occipital cortex. Responsible for vision.	Gross defect in visual fields (e.g., loss of half of visual field)
CN III Oculomotor nerve	Motor	Nuclei located in midbrain. Parasympathetic fibers originate in or near Edinger-Westphal nucleus and cause pupillary constriction. Also responsible for accommodation, eye movement (up, down, and medial), and elevation of eyelid.	Lack of consensual pupillary response; improper eye movement and movement of the eyelid, including ptosis (drooping) of the eyelid
CN IV Trochlear nerve	Motor	Originates in lower midbrain and innervates superior oblique muscle, which controls movement of eye down and lateral.	Nystagmus (rapid, involuntary eye movements), wandering eye, unparallel gaze
CN V Trigeminal nerve	Motor	Originates in mid pons and innervates muscles of mastication; responsible for chewing movement.	Inability to clench teeth
	Sensory	Three divisions (ophthalmic, maxillary, and mandibular) transmit sensations of the face, teeth, and sinuses.	Inability to distinguish sensations on the cheeks; absence of blinking and tearing
CN VI Abducens	Motor	Originates in lower pons and innervates lateral rectus muscle for lateral eye movement.	Diplopia on lateral gaze
CN VII Facial nerve	Motor	Originates from pontomedullary region; innervates all muscles of facial expression, as well as salivary and lacrimal glands; also responsible for ability to close eyes.	Asymmetric facial movement (e.g., tics or drooping smile), inability to frown or to hold eyes shut against resistance
	Sensory	Input from anterior two thirds of tongue (taste)	Inability to detect salty, sour, or sweet taste
CN VIII Acoustic nerve	Sensory	Originates from pontomedullary region and has two divisions: cochlear provides auditory information; vestibular conducts information about equilibrium and mediates nystagmus.	Loss of hearing and balance
CN IX Glossopharyngeal nerve	Motor	Exits the medulla and innervates parotid salivary glands and pharyngeal muscles; responsible for secretion of saliva, swallowing, gag reflex, and reflex control of blood pressure and respirations.	Increased mucus in mouth, impaired gag reflex, nasal speech
	Sensory	Conducts information from pharynx and posterior one third of tongue; responsible for taste and sensations of tongue.	Inability to detect bitter taste, impaired gag reflex
CN X Vagus nerve	Motor and sensory	Exits medulla; responsible for swallowing, voice production, slowed heartbeat, accelerated peristalsis, and sensation of the larynx and pharynx.	Difficulty swallowing, loss of voice, hunger sensation, orthostatic hypotension
CN XI Spinal accessory nerve	Motor	Originates from medulla and upper cord and supplies trapezius and sternocleidomastoid muscles. Responsible for shoulder movements, neck rotation, movements of the head and viscera, and voice production.	Trapezius or sternocleidomastoid muscle weakness
CN XII Hypoglossal nerve	Motor	Originates in medulla and innervates muscles of the tongue, allowing tongue movement, swallowing, and phonation.	Wrinkling of tongue's surface, twitching of tongue, dysphagia, inability to protrude tongue and maintain it in a midline position

Modified from Hickey J: *The clinical practice of neurologic and neurosurgical nursing*, ed 5, Philadelphia, 2003, Lippincott Williams & Wilkins.

(sometimes called *C8*). Occasionally, transport team members are asked to help position patients during these radiographic examinations. Care must be taken to avoid pulling on the patient's arms and to prevent other untoward manipulations just to achieve a perfect radiograph. If obtaining these radiographs is delaying transport, it should be strongly recommended that the patient be immobilized and transport allowed to proceed, leaving the radiographs to be obtained on arrival at the higher level trauma center.

Computed Tomography

CT scans provide the clinician with a reconstructed view of multiple sections of an organ. As mentioned previously, in some areas this diagnostic tool has nearly replaced most plain radiographs, at least of the cervical spine. At many trauma centers, when a CT scan of the head is performed, the scan is continued down through the cervical spine. On a CT scan, bone appears white; blood is off-white; brain and spinal cord tissue are shaded gray; air is black; and CSF (fluid) is off-black (Figures 5-27 and 5-28).

For some CT scans, a contrast medium is injected intravenously (IV) to enhance the view of the blood vessels. However, if the patient is over 50 to 60 years of age or diabetic (or both), a recent creatinine level should be checked before administration of the contrast, because contrast media can cause acute contrast nephropathy, similar to **acute tubular necrosis (ATN)**, with resulting renal failure. If a contrast medium is used, the clinician may want you to infuse IV fluid boluses after the scan to facilitate removal of the agent. Using a contrast agent during CT despite an elevated creatinine level is a risk the clinician may choose to take based on the risk/benefit ratio.

Magnetic Resonance Imaging

Neurologists and neurosurgeons may prefer magnetic resonance imaging (MRI) to CT, especially for medical patients. MRI can provide greater detail and better views, which allows abnormalities to be identified more quickly than with other diagnostic tools. A contrast medium that is not iodine based usually is used for MRI scans. If your critical care team will be assisting with this procedure, you need to know the following:

1. The patient is required to lie still for long periods, in some cases as long as 90 minutes. Some patients require mild sedation to tolerate this.
2. The enclosed tunnel used with some MRI machines is confining, which may make the patient feel anxious. Mild sedation may be warranted if the patient can tolerate it. The tunnels have girth and weight limitations; however, newer MRI devices use a more open table, which is much better tolerated.
3. If the patient has been intubated, timely sedation and long-term paralysis may be indicated, because a patient who is neurologically impaired is unable to follow commands. If the patient has not already been intubated, the clinician must decide whether the need for MRI outweighs the process of intubation. Nonmetal ventilators must be used during the procedure.

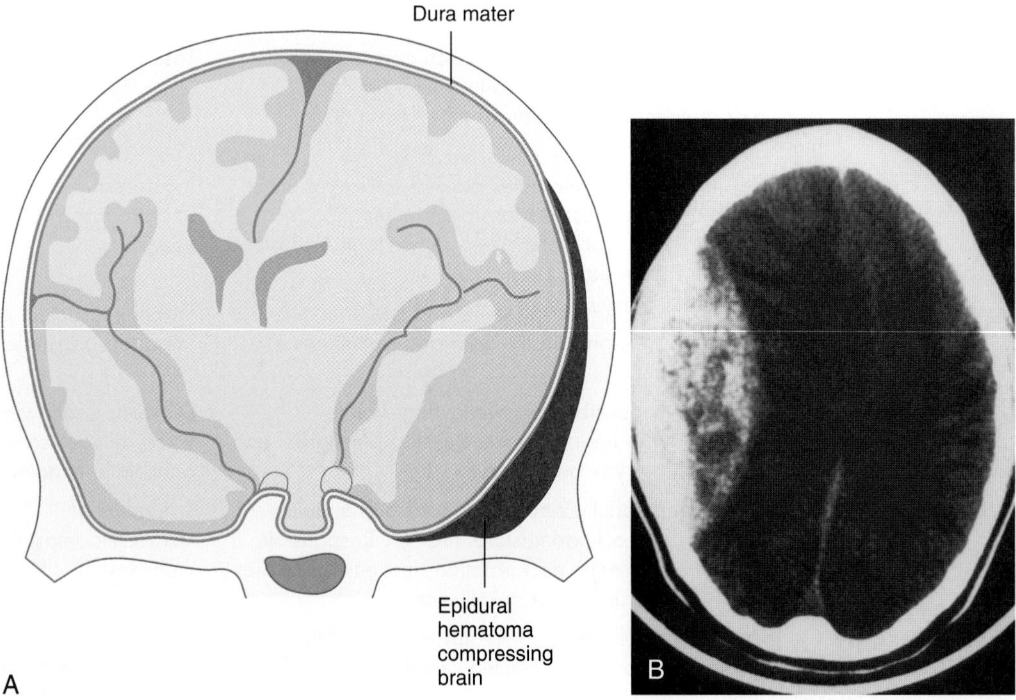

Figure 5-27

A, Epidural hematoma. **B**, Computed tomography (CT) scan of the hematoma. (**A** from the National Association of Emergency Medical Technicians: *PHTLS: prehospital trauma life support*, ed 6, St Louis, 2007, Mosby; **B** from Cruz J: *Neurologic and neurosurgical emergencies*, Philadelphia, 1998, Saunders.)

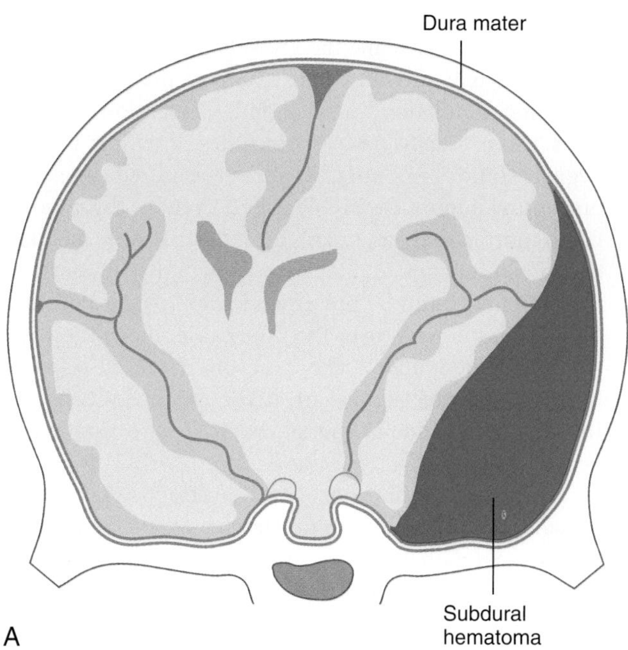

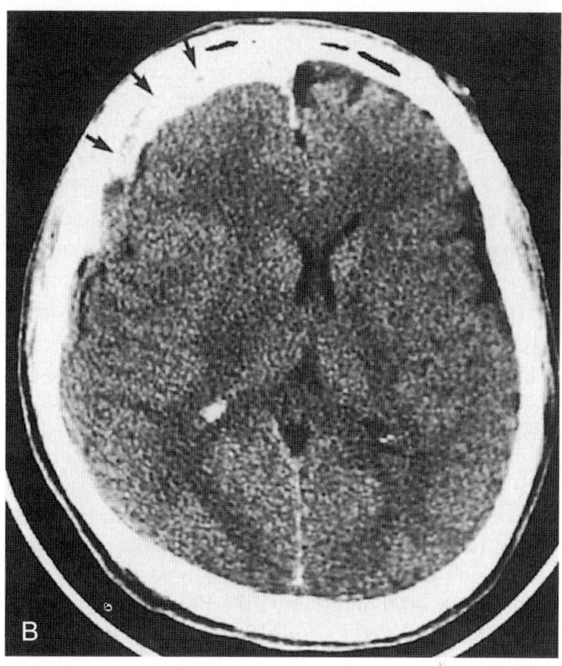

Figure 5-28

A, Subdural hematoma. **B**, CT scan of the hematoma. (**A** from the National Association of Emergency Medical Technicians: *PHTLS: prehospital trauma life support*, ed 6, St Louis, 2007, Mosby; **B** from Cruz J: *Neurologic and neurosurgical emergencies*, Philadelphia, 1998, Saunders.)

4. Most metals are not allowed near the magnet area. Implanted devices must be evaluated by the radiology department before the patient is allowed into the magnet. In addition, before entering the restricted area, you must remove any IV poles from the cart, as well as all pagers, radios, and keys from your personal clothing.

Cerebral Angiography

The angiography procedure begins with injection of a radiopaque contrast medium into the central circulation (via femoral access) to highlight the tissue vessels. The radiology technician then records a series of films that trace blood flow. The same treatment used to prevent contrast-induced nephrotoxicity is instituted for this procedure. Injection of the contrast medium into the subarachnoid space at L2-L3 provides a view of the spinal cord (called a *myelograph*). CT myelographs or MRI studies of the spine are preferred. CT is preferred for bony abnormalities.

Doppler Studies and Positron Emission Tomography

Ultrasonography can be used to evaluate the blood flow velocity through the carotid or cranial windows. The cranial windows include the thin temporal bone, the eyes, and the foramen magnum.

Positron emission tomography (PET) and related tomographic studies are nuclear medicine scans used to evaluate the cerebral blood flow.

Electrophysiology Studies

Electroencephalography and evoked potentials (EPs) are used to evaluate the electrical impulses of the brain. An electroencephalogram (EEG) is a very old test performed to diagnose seizure, stroke, or encephalopathy or to confirm brain death. In the EP examination, a stimulus is applied and the brain's electrical activity is then monitored; this test is used to evaluate the brain stem or as a sensory examination for a patient with a spinal cord injury.

Lumbar Puncture

A lumbar puncture is performed to obtain CSF for laboratory analysis. Also, the clinician may measure the CSF pressure immediately after the puncture. For this procedure, a hollow needle is inserted into the subarachnoid space at L3-L4 or L4-L5. A second (but higher risk) puncture site is C1-C2 (cisternal puncture). The patient may be in the side-lying position with the back arched (hyperflexed), or the person may be sitting with the head and upper body draped over a bedside table. Brain stem herniation is a risk if the ICP is high and too much CSF is drained. Another major risk factor is respiratory failure or arrest as a result of positioning and inhibition of chest muscle movement. Continuous respiratory and cardiac monitoring should be done during this procedure.

Cerebral Oxygenation Monitoring

Within the past few years, more modern techniques of determining whether the brain is meeting its metabolic needs, based on the cerebral blood flow, have been introduced. These techniques include PET imaging and measurement of the jugular venous oxygen saturation ($SjvO_2$) or the brain tissue oxygen pressure ($PbTO_2$). Internal jugular catheters and brain monitoring catheters may be used to determine these parameters.

DISEASE PROCESSES OF THE NEUROLOGIC SYSTEM

A discussion of all the acute and chronic diseases that affect the neurologic system is beyond the scope of this text. The focus here is on common, acute disorders, such as coma, head trauma, stroke, intracranial lesions, intracranial hypertension, and spinal cord injury; the management of these conditions; and on the complications the critical care transport team is most likely to encounter.

Coma

Coma is a very broad term used to indicate that a patient's level of consciousness is diminished. In a true sense, coma means that the ascending reticular activating system is not allowing the patient to be aroused when stimulated. Because use of the term *coma* can be quite confusing, the patient's LOC should be described according to the Glasgow Coma Scale.

The causes of coma can be categorized into two general types:

1. Structural and surgical causes: Structural or surgical causes of coma include trauma and **neoplasms**. The most common reason for a severely diminished LOC is intracranial hypertension.
2. Toxic and metabolic causes: Drug overdose, exposure to toxins, infectious diseases, electrolyte and endocrine disorders, and global encephalopathy after cardiac arrest are common toxic and metabolic causes of coma. These conditions are the most common reasons for coma in the ICU.

Whether the cause is surgical or medical, the pathologic condition affects the RAS fibers that control arousal and the cerebral cortex for awareness. Generally, if a patient has at least one functioning cerebral hemisphere and an intact RAS, consciousness is maintained.

In the ICU, management of a patient in a coma is mostly supportive; however, the overriding goal is to determine the cause of the coma. A detailed neurologic examination, along with a thorough history and diagnostic testing, are the keys to finding the cause. While the investigation goes on, the emergency and ICU providers must support the patient's airway, breathing, circulation, and vital signs. Prevention of complications also is a daily goal; this includes providing pulmonary hygiene (and preventing ventilator-acquired pneumonia), preventing immobility problems (e.g., venous thromboembolism, contractures, and skin breakdown), and maintaining end-organ function and adequate nutritional support.

Eye damage can be prevented by applying a polyethylene film or plastic wrap over the upper face, including the eyes, and instillation of eye drops or ointments also can help. Removal of contact lenses early in the assessment is important. Instillation of saline or special eye drops also aids in corneal health.

Reperfusion brain injury after cardiac arrest has received considerable attention from researchers and clinicians. Many cardiac centers have added aggressive postarrest intentional hypothermia protocols to help reduce neuronal injury after reperfusion. As always, follow your institution's protocols for this condition.

Traumatic Brain Injury

Head injury is defined as any injury to the scalp, skull (cranium or facial bones or both), or brain severe enough to interfere with normal function and require treatment. *Craniocerebral trauma* is traumatic injury to the cranial vault or to the brain. A term that more accurately describes the major traumatic event is *traumatic brain injury* (TBI) (Figure 5-29).

More than 2 million brain injuries occur each year in the United States. Of these, 500,000 to 750,000 are severe enough to require hospitalization. Head injury is the leading cause of trauma-related deaths; 75,000 to 100,000 patients die as a result of their injuries. The incidence of head trauma is highest in people 15 to 24 years of age, and males are two to three times more likely than females to suffer a TBI. Survivors of head injury can have lifelong, serious functional loss; about 5000 develop epilepsy, and 2000 remain in a persistent vegetative state. Treatment and rehabilitation of a single patient with a severe brain injury are estimated to cost $410,000 (based on 1996 costs); this does not reflect the cost of lifetime care.

TBI can be classified in many ways. The admission Glasgow Coma Scale score allows for classification according to the

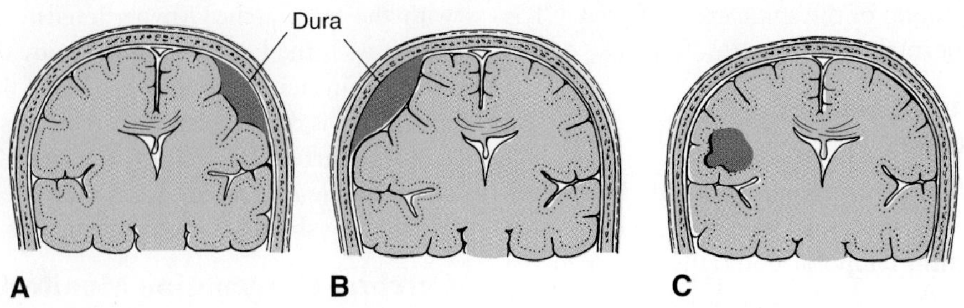

Figure 5-29

Types of hematomas. **A,** Subdural hematoma. **B,** Epidural hematoma. **C,** Intracerebral hematoma. (From Urden LD, Stacy KM, Lough ME: *Thelan's critical care nursing: diagnosis and management*, ed 5, St Louis, 2006, Mosby.)

Box 5-7 Glasgow Coma Scale (GCS) Classification of Brain Injury

Classification	GCS Score
Mild brain injury	13-15
Moderate brain injury	9-12
Severe brain injury	3-8

Modified from Hickey J: *The clinical practice of neurologic and neurosurgical nursing,* ed 5, Philadelphia, 2003, Lippincott Williams & Wilkins.

severity of the injury. Whether the injury is blunt or penetrating and **diffuse** or **focal** are further determinations that help define the TBI (Box 5-7).

Diffuse Traumatic Brain Injury

Concussion and diffuse axonal injury are examples of injuries that cause diffuse injury to brain cells. In concussion, the presentation may include a brief loss of consciousness (i.e., moments to hours) with subsequent disorientation, antegrade or retrograde amnesia, headache, dizziness, irritability, fatigue, and nausea. The severity of the concussion correlates with the duration of amnesia.

Diffuse axonal injury (DAI) formerly was known as a shearing lesion because of the mechanism of blunt trauma within the brain; this type of injury is seen with high-speed acceleration-deceleration, such as occurs with motor vehicle crashes, shaken baby syndrome, or high-impact blunt trauma. DAI usually is a serious injury, with a 30% fatality rate. Widespread damage occurs to the axons in the white matter. Clinically, DAI presents with immediate coma and no lucid period. Monitoring shows a low ICP initially.

Focal Traumatic Brain Injury

Direct or penetrating injuries can have a focal effect on brain tissue. All layers, from the scalp to the brain cells, may suffer a local bruise, laceration, or bleeding. Scalp injuries can be severe enough to cause exsanguination, especially in children. Skull fractures may be benign, but some occur in areas of the cranium where serious consequences can result; for example, fractures in the temporal area (which is thin and has an underlying artery), the occipital area (which is near the foramen magnum), and the basilar skull allow leakage of CSF and pose a risk for infection.

Contusion to the brain causes bruising without puncture of the pia mater, although the underlying cortical tissue and white matter may be hemorrhagic. Laceration involves tearing of the cortical surface of the brain. The circumstances surrounding a contusion and a laceration are similar, and the two injuries may be found together. Primary sites for these injuries are the frontal, temporal, and occipital lobes.

Intracranial hematomas include epidural (extradural) hematomas (bleeding into the potential space between the skull and the dura mater) and subdural hematomas (bleeding between the dura mater and the arachnoid layer).

Epidural Hematoma

Epidural clots occur in as many as 6% of patients with a TBI. This phenomenon may have a classic presentation: an initial period of diminished consciousness or loss of consciousness which, in 33% of patients, is followed by a lucid period, and then, within 6 hours, deterioration of consciousness. This type of arterial bleeding usually arises in the temporal bone (80% of cases) with a tear to the middle meningeal artery. It occurs predominantly in children and teenagers, because the dura mater is less firmly attached in these age groups. With prompt diagnosis and early surgical intervention, patients with an epidural hematoma and no other significant injury can expect a good outcome.

Subdural Hematoma

A subdural hematoma (SDH) is further classified as acute, subacute, or chronic based on the time between injury and the manifestation of signs and symptoms.

- Acute subdural hematomas tend to occur more commonly after age 1 year. Acute changes in the neurologic examination and decreased mental status may be seen, often after a blow to the head.
- A subacute SDH presents with neurologic signs 2 days to 2 weeks after a TBI.
- A chronic SDH is marked by signs that appear gradually, days to months after the injury. This condition is seen more often in people in later life, because as the brain mass shrinks, more space becomes available for the accumulation of blood. Individuals at risk for chronic SDH are the elderly, those on antiplatelet therapy, and those with clotting disorders. The clinical signs and symptoms of chronic SDH are subtle, because autoregulation and accommodation allow adaptation to a slow-growing blood mass. Treatment usually is nonsurgical in nature and includes management of intracranial pressure with maintenance of cerebral perfusion, and treatment of any complications (pneumonia, infection).

Traumatic Subarachnoid Hemorrhage

Tearing of small subarachnoid vessels causes blood to accumulate within the CSF and meningeal intima. Traumatic subarachnoid hemorrhage (TSAH) occurs in as many as 44% of patients with TBI and is the most common CT scan abnormality seen. The amount of blood that accumulates correlates with the outcome, especially if the patient also has some other cerebral injury. The patient may have a headache and photophobia, and vasospasm may occur 48 hours to 2 weeks after the injury.

Intracerebral Hemorrhage and Hematomas

Intracerebral hemorrhage and hematomas result when a significant acceleration-deceleration force is applied to the cranium, with subsequent shear injury of the deeper white matter, lacerations of deep veins, and hemorrhage. Most believe that these types of injuries rarely cause an increase in ICP, but a rapidly expanding hematoma can develop. Surgical intervention is unwarranted, because the blood eventually reabsorbs, but the ICP must be monitored and any abnormalities managed. A severe head injury accompanied by intracerebral hemorrhage usually indicates a poor neurologic outcome and significant neurologic handicaps (see Figure 5-29).

Penetrating Injuries

A TBI that penetrates the skull, causing significant focal injury, usually is the result of bullets, knives, teeth, darts, pencils, pellets, or skull fragments from a depressed fracture. These objects usually are classified as low- or high-velocity missiles (a knife is a low-velocity missile; a bullet is a high-velocity missile). A perforating injury in which a high-velocity object enters and exits the cranium is a further description of this type of TBI. Obviously, these injuries can cause extensive damage to the brain and intracranial vessels; however, the severity of the injury depends on the location and extent of the injury and the velocity of the missile.

Management is guided by whether missile fragments remain, the risk of subsequent infection, and whether secondary trauma to nonpenetrating tissue has occurred.

Seizures Secondary to Traumatic Brain Injury

About 5% of patients with a TBI subsequently have a seizure as a result of the injury. In the period immediately after injury and resuscitation, a seizure can dramatically increase the ICP, causing severe secondary brain cell injury. Some clinicians routinely prescribe antiseizure medications for a time for all patients with a moderate to severe TBI to reduce the likelihood of seizures. These medications include phenytoin, phenobarbital, divalproex, fosphenytoin, and levetiracetam. The critical care transport team should also have access to benzodiazepines; lorazepam is the drug of choice for control of active seizures.

Secondary Head Injury

When mechanical forces transfer energy to the head, a primary head injury is said to occur; the only answer for these events is prevention. Secondary head injury is the pathophysiologic consequences of the initial damage, as the body responds to the primary injury. The critical care paramedic's job is to minimize this secondary injury to the brain, which arises from biochemical and cellular changes that lead to additional brain tissue damage. The two leading causes of secondary brain injury are hypoxia and hypotension.

Without timely, aggressive management, secondary TBI contributes to a poor patient outcome or death. Some examples of secondary TBI include cerebral hypoxia, systemic hypotension (with decreased CBF and CPP), a sustained increase in the ICP, cerebral edema, expanding intracranial hematomas, infection, respiratory complications, electrolyte imbalance, and seizures.

General Management of Traumatic Brain Injury

Airway patency with cervical spine precautions are always the priorities in trauma cases. A patient with a moderate to severe TBI probably will require airway management, including intubation. Rapid sequence intubation (or medication-assisted intubation) and use of a neuromuscular blocking agent and a potent sedative can aid endotracheal intubation and help prevent sharp increases in the ICP during the procedure. The use of lidocaine to blunt the effect of succinylcholine may be considered, but this can be controversial. Oral intubation is preferred.

Breathing (respiratory rate, rhythm, and quality) with supplemental oxygen is the next priority. Provide controlled ventilation, if needed, to maintain the pH within the normal range, the $PaCO_2$ at 32 to 35 mm Hg, and the PaO_2 above 80 mm Hg.

Chronic prolonged hyperventilation ($PaCO_2$<25 mm Hg) should not be allowed after a TBI. Use of prophylactic hyperventilation ($PaCO_2$<35 mm Hg) should be avoided the first 24 to 48 hours after a TBI. Hyperventilation may be considered (but usually is not helpful) for brief periods for acute changes or for a prolonged increase in the ICP when other measures fail. (Measures to treat a rise in the ICP are discussed in the section on intracranial hypertension.)

Circulation and perfusion management are also high priorities. Maintain the systolic BP at 100 to 160 mm Hg (MAP over 90 mm Hg) or high enough to support a CPP of 70 mm Hg or higher. Monitor for an appropriate rate and for arrhythmias. Maintain a euvolemic state if possible. Do not administer IV free water (D_5W), because it will enter the cells, causing edema. Isotonic fluids are preferred. Some regions use hypertonic saline (which is controversial) for a high ICP.

An indwelling urinary catheter is necessary to achieve an adequate fluid balance (minimum of 0.5 mL/kg/hour of urine in adults). Insertion of a gastric tube to reduce intragastric pressure, prevent aspiration of gastric contents, and facilitate gastrointestinal (GI) function also is important.

Administer medications as prescribed and follow your protocols for intracranial hypertension, including elevation of the head of the bed. Continue to ask yourself the assessment question posed earlier: Is this patient with a TBI getting better or worse (and what are you doing about it)?

Stroke

A sudden loss of perfusion to a portion of the CNS tissue can be caused by any vascular disruption, including clots (thrombotic or embolic) or hemorrhage. By definition, stroke is diagnosed when the signs and symptoms of the vascular disruption last longer than 24 hours.

Stroke generally is classified as either ischemic or hemorrhagic. Ischemia causes 80% to 85% of cerebrovascular attacks (CVAs). Regardless of the origin, stroke is a major cause of acute neurologic symptoms and admission into the critical care system.

Ischemic Stroke

As a blood vessel becomes occluded by a thrombotic or an embolic clot, the area of the brain perfused by that vessel becomes ischemic. Major risk factors for the development of this type of stroke include valvular heart disease, a patent atrial foramen, atrial fibrillation, myocardial infarction, and cardiomyopathy. Thrombotic stroke, the most common type, arises from atherosclerotic disease in the vessels of the brain. These strokes are caused by plaque disruption and, commonly, vessel obstruction, similar to acute coronary syndromes.

Three other phenomena are associated with an ischemic event and classified as stroke:

- Transient ischemic attack (TIA), a focal neurologic event that resolves within 1 hour.
- **Reversible ischemic neurologic deficit (RIND)**, a focal event that resolves within 24 hours.
- Hypoperfusion stroke, or cardiac global brain infarction, caused by hypoperfusion or an anoxic event (e.g., cardiac arrest).

As the CNS vessels become obstructed and the **ischemic cascade** develops, an area of ischemic neurons undergoes dramatic chemical changes. Around this focus is an area of marginal blood flow, where some ischemia is occurring; this is called the **ischemic penumbra**. If the ischemia continues, infarction results; this area of infarction softens the brain, turning what was earlier described as custard into liquid.

The clinical presentation of ischemic stroke (Box 5-8) and the prognosis depend on the location of the stroke and whether collateral blood flow is available. If the anterior circulation (carotid artery) is affected, the cerebral hemispheres usually are affected. If the posterior circulation (vertebrobasilar artery) is involved, the brain stem or cerebellum (or both) are affected.

Hemorrhagic Stroke

Sudden rupture of a diseased blood vessel allows bleeding into tissue in the area and disrupts perfusion to the cells. The blood vessel disease can have many causes, including trauma, neoplasm, vasospasm, or congenital anomalies, such as aneurysms. The two types of hemorrhagic stroke are intracerebral strokes and subarachnoid strokes.

Intracerebral Hemorrhage

Often with intracerebral hemorrhage (ICH), a small intracerebral arteriole, damaged by chronic hypertension, ruptures and leaks blood onto the **parenchyma** of the brain. **Cerebral amyloid angiopathy** is a common cause of ICH in elderly patients. Intracerebral hemorrhage accounts for 10% of all strokes.

Subarachnoid Hemorrhage

Subarachnoid hemorrhage (SAH) accounts for 3% of all strokes. SAH results when blood from a cerebral vessel leaks into the subarachnoid space; this causes global vasospasm with resulting ischemia, which may be accompanied by obstruction of CSF outflow and a rise in the ICP. Because the bleeding typically is from an artery, SAH causes sudden and dramatic signs and symptoms, including acute unconsciousness, vomiting and severe headache with a rise in ICP. It is most commonly caused by an aneurysm, but arteriovenous malformations (AVMs) also can cause this type of CVA (Box 5-9).

Secondary Issues with Stroke

Keep in mind the following facts about secondary issues with stroke:

- Significant cerebral edema may develop in 10% to 20% of patients, possibly requiring management of intracranial hypertension.
- An ischemic stroke can become a hemorrhagic stroke if the leaking vessel breaks.
- Seizures may occur in 2% to 23% of patients in the first 24 hours or first few days.

Box 5-8 Neurologic Abnormalities in Acute Ischemic Strokes

- *Left (dominant) hemisphere:* Aphasia, right hemiparesis, right-sided sensory loss, right visual field defect, poor right conjugate gaze, dysarthria, difficulty reading, writing, or calculating.
- *Right (nondominant) hemisphere:* Neglect of the left visual space, left visual field defect, left hemiparesis, left-sided sensory loss, poor left conjugate gaze, extinction of left-sided stimuli, dysarthria, spatial disorientation.
- *Brain stem/cerebellum/posterior hemisphere:* Motor or sensory loss in all four limbs, ipsilateral facial dysfunction with contralateral body involvement (crossed signs), limb or gait ataxia, dysarthria, disconjugate gaze, nystagmus, amnesia, bilateral visual field defects.
- *Small subcortical hemisphere or brain stem (pure motor stroke):* Weakness of the face and limbs on one side of the body without abnormalities of higher brain function, sensation, or vision.
- *Small subcortical hemisphere or brain stem (pure sensory stroke):* Decreased sensation of the face and limbs on one side of the body without abnormalities of higher brain function, motor function, or vision.

From Urden LD, Stacy KM, Lough ME: *Thelan's critical care nursing: diagnosis and management,* ed 5, St Louis, 2006, Mosby.

Box 5-9 Classification of Subarachnoid Hemorrhage

Grade I	Asymptomatic or minimal headache and slight nuchal rigidity
Grade II	Moderate to severe headache, nuchal rigidity, no neurologic deficit other than cranial nerve palsy
Grade III	Drowsiness, confusion, or mild focal deficit
Grade IV	Stupor, moderate to severe hemiparesis, possible early decerebrate rigidity, and vegetative disturbances
Grade V	Deep coma, decerebrate rigidity, moribund appearance

From Urden LD, Stacy KM, Lough ME: *Thelan's critical care nursing: diagnosis and management,* ed 5, St Louis, 2006, Mosby.

Assessment, Diagnosis, and Management of Strokes

The National Institutes of Health (NIH) and the American Heart Association have established some practical guidelines for the care of stroke patients. The NIH stroke assessment, explanation, and scoring scale is available at www.ninds.nih.gov/doctors/NIH_Stroke_Scale_Booklet.pdf.

Along with evaluation using the stroke scale, additional assessment and diagnostic tests must be performed in a timely fashion. Your emergency medical system (EMS), emergency department (ED), and critical care protocols are likely to facilitate the necessary laboratory, electrocardiography, and radiologic studies, along with the decision making necessary for administration of fibrinolytic therapy and/or transfer of the patient to a stroke center (Table 5-6).

Did You Know?

Administration of tissue plasminogen activator (tPA, alteplase) for stroke is different from administration for acute coronary syndromes. The dosing scheme for stroke is as follows[6]:

1. **Calculate a dosage of 0.9 mg/kg of the patient's body weight, to a maximum of 90 mg. (Because this is considered a "high alert" medication pharmaceutically, a second provider should calculate the dose independently and check the administration.)**
2. **Reconstitute the drug with normal saline to a concentration of 1 mg/mL.**
3. **Draw up 10% of the total dose into a syringe for bolus administration. Administer the bolus over 1 minute.**
4. **Immediately begin a 1-hour infusion of the rest of the dosage.**
5. **If some of the drug is left over at the end of the 1-hour infusion, draw it out of the reconstituted IV line (before administration) and label the bag appropriately.**
6. **Do not leave all the drug hanging, because this creates an opportunity for drug error. You are likely to pass off the patient to other healthcare providers, and if this is done during the infusion without correction of the amount to be infused, the next healthcare provider may mistakenly allow infusion of the amount left in the bottle at the end of the hour.**

Management Unique to Ischemic Stroke

Determining the time from the onset of symptoms, ruling out the mimickers of stroke, and ruling out a hemorrhagic event are just the beginning of the management regimen for this common type of stroke. Determining whether the patient is a candidate for fibrinolytic therapy with tPA is a major decision, one that is likely to undergo some changes. The results of Safe Implementation of Treatments in Stroke (SITS) study, a prospective audit of the International Stroke Thrombolysis Registry (ISRT), and the findings of the European Cooperative Acute Stroke Study (ECASS 3), both published in 2008, showed that extending the original 3-hour window for tPA to 4.5 hours offered modest but significant improvement in clinical outcomes compared with placebo; however, providers should consult institutional guidelines or the neurology service before changing this protocol. Both of the previously mentioned studies cautioned that tPA should be administered as soon as possible in ischemic stroke.

Management Unique to Subarachnoid Hemorrhage

Intracerebral hypertension, surgery, rebleeding, hyponatremia, hydrocephalus, and vasospasm are common complications during the management of SAH. Rebleeding associated with aneurysm has a high mortality rate (70%); measures in the ICU to prevent this have included BP control (site-specific protocols) and anticonvulsant therapy.

Neurosurgical "clipping" of the aneurysm (if present in SAH) is likely within 1 or 2 days of the original event and prevents rebleeding, especially with a grade I or grade II aneurysm. Vasospasm is a problem in both nonoperative and operative cases.

Surgical AVM repair depends on the site of the malformation and the patient's overall status. Repeat procedures may need to be done in stages for overall management. A cerebral aneurysm or AVM that is surgically inaccessible may benefit from embolization. **Embolization** may be done in two ways but begins with femoral access, similar to cardiac catheterization. For one technique, beads or glue is embolized from the catheter and floats to the distal vessels that feed the AVM; this may be followed up with a craniotomy. In the other technique, balloons (inflated) or coils (electrical charge) are placed to clot off distal vessels that feed the AVM or aneurysm.

Cerebral vasospasm is a major complication after SAH involving an aneurysm. The literature shows that vasospasm subsequently occurs in up to 70% of SAHs involving an aneurysm. The patient may show improvement after repair of the aneurysm and then deteriorate neurologically when the vessel goes into spasms approximately 1 to 2 weeks later.

Many different combinations of therapy, including the following, are undergoing trials in attempts to find the regimen with the best outcome.

- Hypertensive, hypervolemic, hemodilution (HHH) therapy: Vasoactive medications are administered to increase the BP and cardiac output, along with fluid and volume expanders to dilute the blood. The premise is that pushing blood through the newly repaired aneurysm under high pressure, along with blood that moves through with less viscosity, reduces the risk of spasm in the vessel. Possible complications of HHH therapy

Table 5-6 Management of Hypertension Associated with Stroke

Blood Pressure*	Treatment
Patients Not Candidates for Thrombolysis	
DBP >140 mm Hg	Sodium nitroprusside (0.5 mcg/kg/min); aim for 10% to 20% reduction in DBP.
SBP >220 mm Hg, DBP = 121-140 mm Hg, or MAP[†] >130 mm Hg	10-20 mg labetalol[‡] IV push over 1-2 min; may repeat or double labetalol dose every 20 min to a maximum dose of 300 mg. Nicardipine (Cardene): For gradual reduction in BP, initiate therapy at 50 mL/hr (5 mg/hr). The infusion rate may be increased by 25 mL/hr (2.5 mg/hr) every 15 minutes up to a maximum of 150 mL/hr (15 mg/hr), until desired BP reduction is achieved. For more rapid BP reduction, initiate therapy at 50 mL/hr (5 mg/hr).The infusion rate may be increased by 25 mL/hr (2.5 mg/hr) every 5 minutes up to a maximum of 150 mL/hr (15 mg/hr) until desired BP reduction is achieved.
SBP <220 mm Hg, DBP = 120 mm Hg, or MAP <130 mm Hg	Emergency antihypertensive therapy is deferred in the absence of aortic dissection, acute myocardial infarction, severe congestive heart failure, or hypertensive encephalopathy.
Candidates for Thrombolysis	
Pretreatment	
SBP >185 mm Hg or DBP >110 mm Hg	1-2 inches of nitroglycerin paste (Nitropaste) or 1-2 doses of 10-20 mg labetalol[‡] IV push; if BP is not reduced and maintained <185/110 mm Hg, the patient should not be treated with tPA.
During and After Treatment	
Monitoring of BP	BP should be checked every 15 minutes for 2 hours, then every 30 minutes for 6 hours, and then hourly for 16 hours.
DBP >140 mm Hg	Sodium nitroprusside (0.5 mcg/kg/min).
SBP >230 mm Hg or DBP = 121-140 mm Hg	10 mg labetalol[‡] IV push over 1-2 min; may repeat or double labetalol dose every 10 minutes to a maximum dose of 300 mg or give initial labetalol bolus and then start a labetalol drip at 2-8 mg/min. If BP is not controlled by labetalol, consider sodium nitroprusside.
SBP = 180-230 mm Hg or DBP = 105-120 mm Hg	10 mg labetalol[‡] IV push; may repeat or double labetalol dose every 10-20 minutes to a maximum dose of 300 mg or give initial labetalol bolus and then start a labetalol drip at 2-8 mg/min.

From Urden LD, Stacy KM, Lough ME: *Thelan's critical care nursing: diagnosis and management*, ed 5, St Louis, 2006, Mosby.
BP, Blood pressure; *DBP*, diastolic blood pressure; *IV*, intravenous; *MAP*, mean arterial pressure; *SBP*, systolic blood pressure; *tPA*, tissue plasminogen activator.
*All initial blood pressures should be verified before treatment by repeating the measurement in 5 minutes.
[†]As estimated by one third the sum of the systolic and double diastolic pressure.
[‡]Labetalol should not be used in the following patients: asthmatic patients who are wheezing, those in cardiac failure, those who are abusers of cocaine or methamphetamines, or those with severe cardiac conduction abnormalities. For refractory hypertension, alternative therapy with sodium nitroprusside or fenoldopam may be considered.

include intracranial hypertension, cerebral edema, rebleeding, congestive heart failure (CHF), and electrolyte disturbances, among others.

- Nimodipine: Administration of this calcium channel blocker (60 mg doses given every 4 hours for 21 days) seems to reduce the ill effects of vasospasms through an unknown mechanism.
- Cerebral angioplasty: This procedure may be considered when drug therapy is not working and spasms are occurring, but an infarct has not yet evolved. The procedure is performed by an interventional neuroradiologist in a special stroke center.

Management Unique to Intracerebral Hypertension

Coma, intracerebral hypertension, and stimulation control are major management issues for patients with ICH. Because of the dramatic presentation and progression of intracerebral hemorrhage, aggressive airway management (intubation) usually is indicated. The other major management issue is the balance between the blood pressure and the cerebral perfusion pressure. Maintaining a narrow MAP window is essential for preventing further bleeding and a decline in the CPP. Because the ICP rises, the MAP should be kept below 130 mm Hg in a hypertensive patient (below 110 mm Hg in the postoperative period).

Euvolemia, an occlusion pressure (pulmonary artery occlusion pressure [PAOP], or pulmonary capillary wedge pressure [PCWP]) of 10 to 14 mm Hg, euthermia, sedation, and other regional protocols all are part of the treatment regimen for ICH. Neurosurgical intervention with craniotomy may be warranted for young patients and for patients with a large cerebral hemorrhage and neurologic deterioration or hydrocephalus.

Intracranial Masses

The causes of brain tumors (neoplasms) are not fully understood. Metastatic types usually are spread to the brain through the arterial circulation. These tumors are classified by their features, cell type, and degree of malignancy (grades I through IV) (Table 5-7). The prognosis depends on those factors and the size and location of the lesion.

Given the simplicity of the space within the intracranial cavity, rapidly growing tissue that takes up that space, encroaching on normal brain tissue, obviously becomes a concern. If the abnormal tissue grows slowly, the brain tissue can more easily accommodate it, producing only minor signs and symptoms. Often the neoplasm has its own blood supply and can present with hemorrhagic stroke. The tumor tissue may cause an overall cerebral edema or hydrocephalus (or both) and intracranial hypertension. The tumor itself rarely causes symptoms; however, by occupying space or by causing edema or hydrocephalus, it may cause a seizure or new-onset neurologic symptoms related to the tissue being destroyed.

Craniotomy

Craniotomy is a surgical procedure that can be performed to remove space-occupying lesions in the cranium or, in cases of diffuse edema, to allow for swelling. Space-occupying lesions may include neoplasms, aneurysms, AVMs, hematomas, and abscesses. Many surgical approaches (**transcranial, transsphenoidal**) and techniques can be used, depending on the site of the lesion. New, minimally invasive surgical techniques can help reduce collateral tissue damage.

Occasionally, critical care transport teams are asked to move postoperative craniotomy patients for specialized care. A number of complications may be seen in these patients, such as intracranial hypertension, hypertension, hemorrhage from the surgical site, fluid and electrolyte imbalance, CSF leakage, and problems arising from immobility (e.g., deep vein thrombosis [DVT], skin breakdown, corneal irritation, and VAP).

- Postoperative edema usually peaks within 72 hours, and intracranial hypertension may develop if the cranium is intact. In some patients, a bone flap may be removed (and preserved for later replacement); this allows for expansion caused by the expected edema and prevents the closed cranial vault from causing the hypertension. In other patients, a **ventriculostomy** is performed for intermittent or continuous CSF drainage. Both types of patients are managed with the standard therapy for intracranial hypertension.
- With the transcranial craniotomy approach, postoperative hemorrhage produces signs and symptoms that mimic those of a hemorrhagic stroke. The sphenoid craniotomy approach may result in a bloody external or throat drainage that warrants investigation. Another troublesome sign of internal hemorrhage is a sudden loss of vision, especially for lesions around the pituitary.
- As with any basilar skull fracture in acute trauma, CSF leakage may be apparent. Evaluate any clear drainage for CSF by performing a bedside glucose test on the fluid (standard procedure). Leakage is confirmed if the glucose level is over 30 mg/dL; this patient is at risk for infection.

Table 5-7 Tumor Types and Characteristics

Tumor	Clinical Features	Treatment and Prognosis
Glioblastoma multiforme	Often presents with nonspecific complaints and increased ICP; as tumor grows, focal deficits develop.	Rapidly progressive with a poor prognosis. Total surgical removal usually is not possible; response to radiation therapy is poor.
Astrocytoma	Presentation is similar to that of glioblastoma multiforme, but course is more protracted, often over several years; cerebellar astrocytoma, especially in children, may have more benign course.	Variable prognosis. By diagnosis, total excision usually is impossible (although it often is possible for cerebellar astrocytoma); tumor often is not radiosensitive.
Medulloblastoma	Glioma most often seen in children. Generally arises from roof of fourth ventricle and leads to increased ICP, with brain stem and cerebellar signs; may seed subarachnoid space.	Treatment consists of surgery with radiation therapy and chemotherapy.

Table 5-7 Tumor Types and Characteristics—cont'd

Tumor	Clinical Features	Treatment and Prognosis
Ependymoma	Glioma arising from ependyma of ventricle, especially fourth; leads early to signs of increased ICP; arises also from central canal of spinal cord.	Tumor not radiosensitive and best treated surgically, if possible.
Oligodendroglioma	Slow-growing glioma, usually arises in cerebral hemisphere in adults.	Treatment is surgical and usually successful.
Brain stem glioma	Presents in childhood with cranial nerve palsies, then long-tract signs in limbs; signs of increased ICP occur late in course.	Tumor is inoperable. Treatment involves irradiation and shunt for increased ICP.
Cerebellar hemangioblastoma	Presents with dysequilibrium, ataxia of trunk or limbs, and signs of increased ICP; at times familial may be associated with retinal and spinal lesions, polycythemia, and hypernephroma.	Treatment is surgical.
Pineal tumor	Presents with increased ICP, at times associated with impaired upward gaze (Parinaud's syndrome) and other deficits indicating midbrain lesion.	Treatment involves ventricular decompression by shunting, followed by surgical approach to tumor. Irradiation if tumor is malignant. Prognosis depends on histopathologic findings and tumor extent.
Craniopharyngioma	Originates from remnants of Rathke's pouch above sella turcica and depresses optic chiasm. May present at any age but usually appears in childhood with endocrine dysfunction and bitemporal field deficit.	Treatment is surgical, but total removal may not be possible.
Acoustic neuroma	Ipsilateral hearing loss is the most common initial symptom; subsequent symptoms may include tinnitus, headache, vertigo, facial weakness or numbness, and long-tract signs. May be familial and bilateral when related to neurofibromatosis. Most sensitive screening tests are MRI and brain stem AEP.	Treatment involves tumor excision by translabyrinthine approach, craniectomy, or a combination of these. Prognosis usually is good.
Meningioma	Originates from dura mater or arachnoid; compresses rather than invades adjacent neural structures. Increasingly common with advancing age. Tumor size varies greatly; symptoms vary with tumor site (e.g., unilateral exophthalmos [sphenoidal ridge], anosmia and optic nerve compression [olfactory groove]). Tumor usually is benign and can be readily detected by CT; may lead to calcification and bone erosion, which are visible on plain skull radiographs.	Treatment is surgical. Tumor may recur if removal is incomplete; patient may receive radiation therapy with incomplete excision to reduce risk of recurrence.
Primary central lymphoma	Associated with AIDS and other immunodeficiency states; may present with focal deficits or disturbances of cognition and consciousness; may be indistinguishable from cerebral toxoplasmosis.	Treatment involves whole-brain irradiation; chemotherapy may have adjunctive role. Prognosis depends on CD4 cell count at diagnosis.

From Gawlinski A, Hamwi D, editors: *Acute care nurse practitioner: clinical curriculum and certification review*, Philadelphia, 1999, Saunders.
AEP, Auditory-evoked potential; *AIDS*, acquired immunodeficiency syndrome; *CT*, computed tomography; *ICP*, intracranial pressure; *MRI*, magnetic resonance imaging.

Box 5-10 Classification of Intracranial Pressure

The intracranial pressure (ICP) is the pressure within the intracranial space. It is classified as follows:

- Normal: <10 mm Hg (0 to 10 mm Hg)
- Mild intracranial hypertension: 10 to 15 mm Hg
- Moderate intracranial hypertension: 15 to 20 mm Hg
- Severe intracranial hypertension: >20 mm Hg

Box 5-11 Cerebral Perfusion Pressure

The cerebral perfusion pressure (CPP) is a calculated value that represents the pressure available to perfuse the brain. The CPP is the difference between the mean arterial blood pressure and the intracranial pressure (CPP = MAP – ICP).

The formula for determining the MAP is:

$$\text{MAP} = \text{Diastolic BP} + \tfrac{1}{3}(\text{Systolic BP} - \text{Diastolic BP})$$

Example

A patient's BP is 140/80 mm Hg, and the ICP is 10 mm Hg. First, the MAP is calculated:

$$\text{MAP} = 80 + \tfrac{1}{3}(140 - 80)$$
$$= 80 + \tfrac{1}{3}(60)$$
$$\text{MAP} = 100 \text{ mm Hg}$$

According to the formula, then (CPP = MAP – ICP):

$$\text{CPP} = 100 - 10$$
$$\text{CPP} = 90 \text{ mm Hg}$$

A normal CPP is 80 to 90 mm Hg in adults (maintained ≥70 mm Hg) and 60 to 70 mm Hg in infants and young children. Lower than normal values indicate the following:

CPP <60 mm Hg: 90% increase in mortality from traumatic brain injury
CPP <50 mm Hg: Ischemia of the brain tissue
CPP <40 mm Hg: Extreme compromise of cerebral blood flow
CPP <30 mm Hg: Irreversible hypoxia

Syndrome of Inappropriate Antidiuretic Hormone and Diabetes Insipidus

Antidiuretic hormone (ADH) is secreted by the posterior pituitary gland. This hormone stimulates the renal tubules to retain water, usually when the serum osmolality increases or shock (hypovolemia) occurs. Hypothalamic or pituitary disease or trauma (surgical or otherwise) may result in low levels of ADH, which in turn results in large amounts of urination and fluid with electrolyte loss; this is called **diabetes insipidus (DI)**. DI may be central (lack of ADH secretion from the pituitary) or nephrogenic (lack of circulating ADH). The urine output may be as high as 200 mL/hour, resulting in hypotension and a low CPP; this may be a short-term complication of head trauma or a postoperative development with a craniotomy. Management includes volume and electrolyte replacement. Occasionally, desmopressin, a synthetic analog of ADH, or vasopressin (pituitary hormone) must be given intravenously to signal the body to constrict vessels and conserve water at the kidney tubules.

Syndrome of inappropriate antidiuretic hormone (SIADH) is a common complication with head trauma (surgery or blunt or penetrating trauma). SIADH is marked by a low sodium level and an inappropriately concentrated urine despite low serum osmolality and a normal blood volume. Before this diagnosis can be confirmed, the clinician must rule out other causes of euvolemic hyponatremia, such as hypothyroidism, hypoadrenalism, and renal failure. This complication also may be self-limiting, but fluid restriction is the primary management tool.

Intracranial Hypertension

As was discussed previously, the essentially closed cranial vault has three components: brain tissue, blood, and fluid (CSF). The brain can regulate itself within certain parameters; however, as stated by the Monro-Kellie doctrine, if any one component increases in volume, another component must decrease for the overall volume and pressure to remain constant; otherwise, the ICP rises (Boxes 5-10 and 5-11).

Cerebral Edema

Cerebral edema is an abnormal accumulation of water in the intracellular space, the extracellular space, or both; this causes an increase in the brain tissue volume, a development that usually is associated with a rise in the ICP. A number of mechanisms can lead to cerebral edema.

- *Vasogenic edema* is an extracellular edema. It is caused by a breakdown of the blood-brain barrier, which results in an increase in the capillary permeability of the arterial walls. This type of edema usually involves the white matter. Disruption of the blood-brain barrier allows plasmalike filtrate to leak into the extracellular space. Vasogenic edema sometimes is seen with tumors, cerebral infarcts, or abscesses.
- *Generalized vasogenic edema* may occur with trauma or meningitis. Use of corticosteroids (dexamethasone) is effective in treating this common complication, generally seen with brain tumors. The osmotic diuretic, mannitol may be helpful in the acute phase of this phenomenon.
- *Cytotoxic edema* is associated with a hypoxic or an anoxic episode and involves the gray and white matter. It also may be seen with hypo-osmolarity conditions (e.g., water intoxication, hyponatremia, and SIADH). With cytotoxic edema, the blood-brain barrier remains intact, but fluid in the intracellular space increases as a result of ATP-dependent, sodium-potassium pump failure. Sodium and fluid accumulate in the cells, and diffuse brain swelling results. Steroids are not effective for treating this disorder. Controversial treatment may include the use of furosemide or mannitol in the acute phase. Vasogenic and cytotoxic edema may be seen

together. Cytotoxic shock usually reaches its maximum level in 72 hours and can persist for several months.

- *Hydrocephalic edema* develops as the result of another obstructing pathologic condition in the brain. Circulation of CSF may be obstructed by masses or secretions (infection), causing dilation of the ventricles and subsequent compression of brain tissue. Nonobstructive hydrocephalus occurs when CSF is not reabsorbed by the arachnoid villi as quickly as it is produced. The clinical presentation depends on the speed with which the edema develops.
- *Hydrostatic and osmotic edema* occurs as water is pushed or pulled because of pressure gradients. An example of this form of cerebral edema may involve diabetic ketoacidosis (DKA) and the resuscitation process; it should be suspected if the patient remains in a coma despite reversal of the acidosis. The onset usually occurs 6 to 12 hours after DKA resuscitation, and the mortality rate is high once the cerebral edema begins. The formation of edema in this situation is associated with a low $PaCO_2$, a high blood urea nitrogen (BUN), and the use of bicarbonate (Box 5-12).

Management of Intracranial Hypertension

Once ICH is recognized, aggressive management must be implemented to salvage brain tissue and maintain the cerebral perfusion pressure. From the simple to the complex, these management protocols might include positioning, reduction of stimuli, ventilator settings, temperature and blood pressure control, prevention and treatment of seizure activity, and reduction of cerebral edema through CSF drainage systems or pharmacologic means.

Box 5-12 Signs and Symptoms of Increased Intracranial Pressure

Early Signs and Symptoms

- Deterioration of the level of consciousness (LOC) (confusion, restlessness, lethargy)
- Pupillary dysfunction
- Motor weakness
- Sensory deficits
- Cranial nerve palsies and dysfunction of extraocular eye movements
- Headache
- Seizures (possible)

Later Findings

- Continued deterioration of LOC (coma)
- Vomiting (possible)
- Papilledema (possible)
- Headache
- Hemiplegia, abnormal flexion (decortication) or extension (decerebration)
- Changes in vital signs
- Impaired brain stem reflexes (corneal, gag reflexes)

Factors That Can Affect Intracranial Pressure

- *Patient positioning:* Keep the head of the bed at 30 to 45 degrees, as long as the BP is not affected. Keep the head and neck in neutral position to allow for venous return.
- *Turning:* Keep pressure off the thorax and abdomen. Do not put the patient in the prone position, and avoid extreme flexion of the hips and knees.
- *Respiratory care:* Use optimal positive end-expiratory pressure (PEEP) cautiously, without increasing intrathoracic pressure. Cluster care (i.e., organize all bedside activities into one session). Coughing and suctioning increase the ICP. Use normal ventilation parameters.
- *ICU rest periods/cumulative activities:* Cluster care. Allow long rest periods.
- *Neuroassessment:* Incorporate stimulation with neurologic assessment into the clustered care routine if possible.
- *Oral and body hygiene in the ICU:* These activities overstimulate the patient; cluster them with other stimulating activities.
- *Touch:* Soothing touch from family members can be beneficial.
- *Bedside voices:* Screen conversation within the patient's hearing. Family members' voices can be helpful.
- *Family presence:* With education, family members can provide significant benefits to the patient with intracranial hypertension. Soothing voices and touch are important.

Treatment and Prevention of Increased ICP and/or Decreased CPP

ICP Monitoring

ICP monitoring is a useful tool, because it provides an objective assessment, allowing early diagnosis. It also enables the practitioner to evaluate autoregulation and compliance and to provide aggressive treatment (Figure 5-30).

There are many indications for ICP monitoring, including head trauma, a ruptured intracerebral aneurysm, known or suspected hydrocephalus, a space-occupying lesion, and sedation in a patient with a neurologic condition (who therefore is difficult to examine). ICP measurements help practitioners accurately assess the intracranial environment and the patient's ability to compensate for changes in that closed box.

Intracranial compliance is an expression of the relationship between the change in the ICP as a result of a change in the intracranial volume. It is a measure of how much "give" is present in the closed box of the skull and how much the intracranial contents can expand before the fit becomes so tight that the CPP is compromised. Intracranial compliance is described in the volume-pressure relationship curve (Figure 5-31). Skill 5-1 reviews ICP monitoring, and Box 5-13 provides a transport checklist for ICP monitoring.

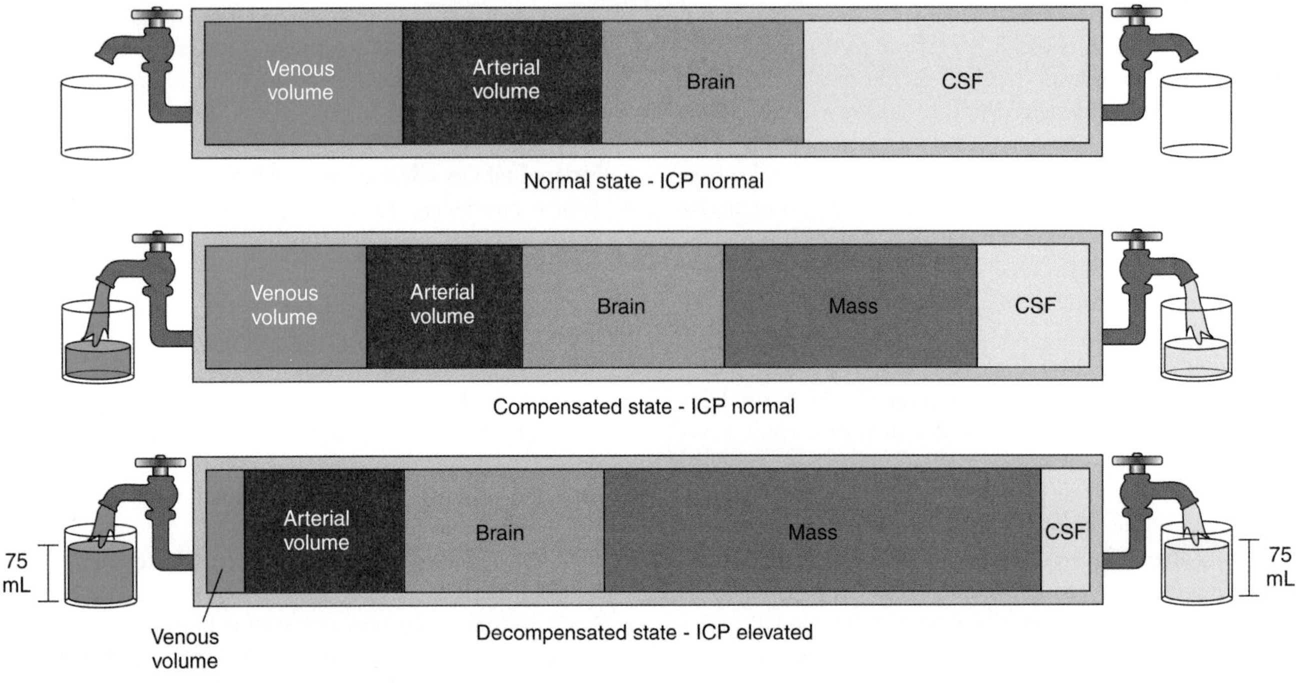

Figure 5-30

Monro-Kellie doctrine: intracranial compensation for expanding mass. The volume of the intracranial contents remains constant. If the addition of a mass (e.g., a hematoma) results in the squeezing out of an equal volume of cerebrospinal fluid (CSF) and venous blood, the intracranial pressure (ICP) remains normal. However, when this compensatory mechanism is exhausted, an exponential increase in ICP occurs for even a small additional increase in the volume of the hematoma. (From McSwain NE, Paturel JL: *The basic EMT: comprehensive prehospital patient care,* ed 2, St Louis, 2003, Mosby.)

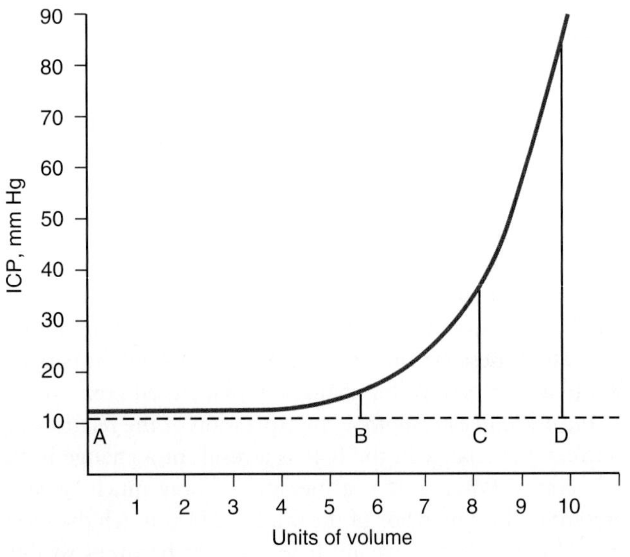

Figure 5-31

Volume-pressure relationship curve. *1,* Intracranial volume and pressure are normal. *2,* Intracranial volume has increased; the pressure is normal as a result of compensation. *3,* A further increase in volume and a slight increase in ICP have occurred; the patient's condition is extremely unstable. *4,* ICP is severely increased. Autoregulation is lost, and decompensation occurs. (From Sole ML, Klein DG, Moseley MJ: *Introduction to critical care nursing,* ed 4, Philadelphia, 2006, Saunders.)

Box 5-13 Transport Checklist for ICP Monitoring System

	Yes	No
1. Critical care transport monitor with ICP monitoring capabilities?		
2. Cable connections compatible with your transport monitor?		
3. Monitoring device secure and dressing intact?		
4. Connections and cable secure?		
5. Patient moved to transport cot and secured for transport?		
6. ICP monitoring system level with foramen of Monro?		
7. System zeroed once level?		
8. Waveforms consistent with neurologic condition?		
9. Stopcock closed for positioning (continuous drainage system)?		

Skill 5-1

INTRACRANIAL PRESSURE MONITORING

Methods and Sites of Monitoring

The four sites used to monitor the intracranial pressure (ICP) are the intraventricular space, subarachnoid space, epidural space and parenchyma. The method and site used depend on the patient's condition and the physician's preference.

1. *Intraventricular space:* A small catheter is inserted on the nondominant side through a burr hole into the ventricular system (ventriculostomy). The advantage of this method is that cerebrospinal fluid (CSF) can be drained if necessary.
2. *Subarachnoid space:* A small, hollow bolt or screw is inserted through a burr hole into the subarachnoid space. The device usually can be seen at the patient's frontal lobe, just behind the hair line. This method has a lower risk of infection, and the device can be quickly placed; however, the results are less accurate than with a ventriculostomy.
3. *Epidural space:* A small fiberoptic sensor is inserted into the epidural space through a burr hole (the dura must be scraped from the inner table of the cranium before insertion). This method is the least invasive of the four procedures, and the sensor is easy to insert; however, the results are less accurate than with ventriculostomy.
4. Intraparenchymal site: A subarachnoid bolt is placed, through which a small fiberoptic catheter is inserted into the brain tissue. This method requires only one zeroing event (insertion) for monitoring and is easily transported. However, this technique does not provide access to the CSF (see illustrations).

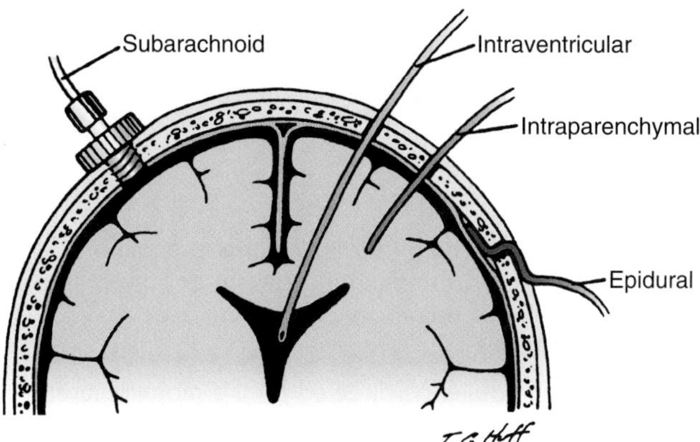

Intracranial pressure monitoring sites. (From Lee KR, Hoff JT: *Youman's neurologic surgery*, ed 4, Philadelphia, 1996, Saunders.)

Most ICP monitoring is done on the nondominant side of the cranium (right). The transducer is maintained at the level of the external auditory meatus (EAM), a landmark that correlates with the third ventricle. To find this landmark, first draw an imaginary line from the outer canthus of the eye toward the ear, and then draw another imaginary line in front of the ear; the EAM is located at the point where the two lines intersect.

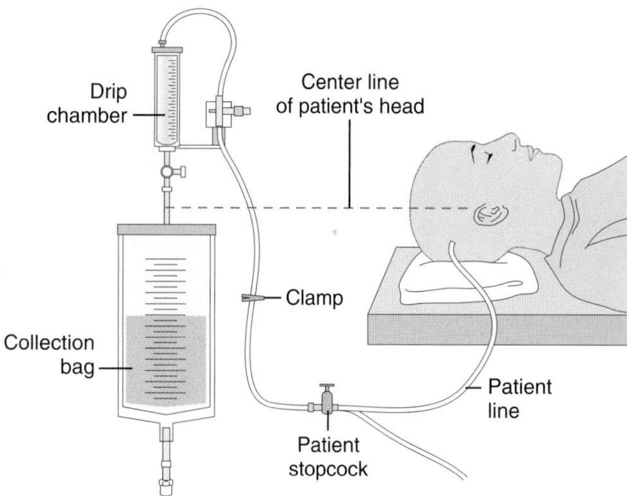

Continuous drainage system. Continuous drainage involves placing the drop chamber of the drainage system at a specified level (usually 15 cm) above the foramen of Monro. The system is left open to allow continuous drainage of cerebrospinal fluid into the chamber (which drains into a collection bag) against a pressure gradient that prevents excessive drainage and ventricular collapse. (Courtesy Codman/Johnson & Johnson Professional, Raynham, Mass.)

Note that this procedure for measuring the ICP is similar to that for measuring the arterial blood pressure. The ICP device must be leveled and zeroed before a pressure reading is obtained.

INDICATIONS

Establish continuous ICP monitoring

Obtain data for a treatment plan for a patient with elevated ICP

Drain excess CSF when the ICP is high

CONTRAINDICATIONS

Intracranial infection

Coagulopathies

An ICP bolt is contraindicated if CSF drainage is intended.

Excessive cerebral edema with collapsed ventricles may preclude placement of an intraventricular catheter.

EQUIPMENT

Skin cleansing agent (chlorhexidine-based solution)
Sterile gloves, hair cover, mask with facial cover, and cover gown
Sterile towels and draping
Local anesthetic
5 and 10 mL Luer-Lok syringes
18-gauge and 25-gauge needles
Twist drill and bits
Sutures (2-0 nylon, 3-0 silk, 4-0 Vicryl)
Scalp retractor
4 × 4 sterile gauze (sterile dressing tray)
Razor
External ventricular drain (EVD) system: 250 mL sterile saline and EVD tubing

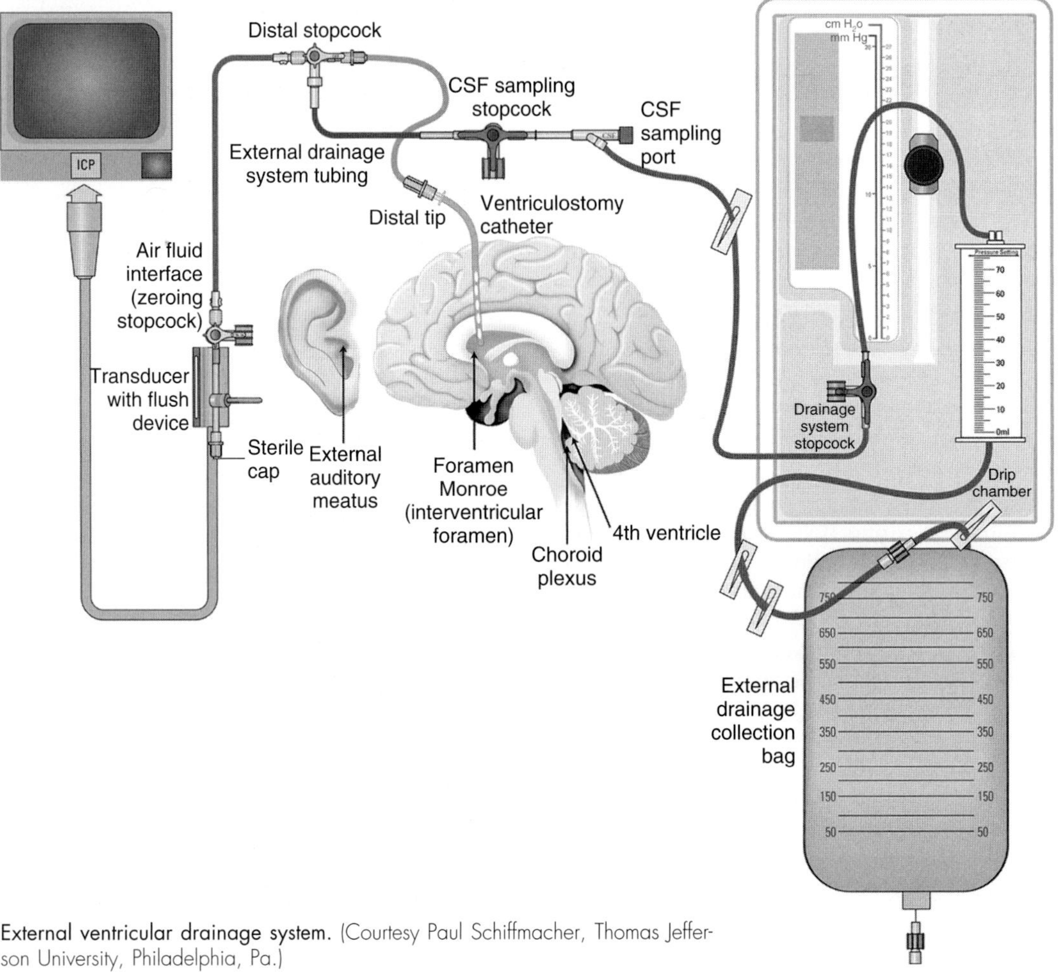

External ventricular drainage system. (Courtesy Paul Schiffmacher, Thomas Jefferson University, Philadelphia, Pa.)

ICP bolt or catheter setup:

- Fluid-coupled system: Transducer cable, external strain gauge transducer, pressure tubing, three-way stopcock, 0.9% sodium chloride flush.
- Fiberoptic system: Microprocessor monitor, preamp connector cable, monitor cable (monitor-to-monitor cable), fiberoptic ICP bolt catheter with calibration screwdriver.
- Sensor system: Microprocessor, cable, monitor cable (monitor-to-monitor cable), ICP bolt sensor catheter with calibration tool.

PREPARATION

Follow these steps if you will be assisting the physician specialist in the insertion procedure.

1. Gather the necessary equipment. The clinician will obtain informed consent from the family.
2. Explain the procedure to the family members. Also explain their role in reducing the patient's ICP. Obtain a history of right-sided or left-sided dominance from the family.
3. Perform a baseline neurologic assessment. Observe, document, and communicate any changes in the assessment, along with any signs of increased ICP.
4. Review the patient's laboratory studies pertinent to blood clotting.
5. Administer analgesics, sedatives, and a paralytic as needed.
6. Position the patient supine with the head and neck neutral. Elevate the head of the bed to 30 to 45 degrees. If spinal precautions are still being observed (post trauma), use the reverse Trendelenburg position and with head up 30 to 45 degrees.

PROCEDURE

1. Wash your hands and follow sterile precautions. Assemble the ICP monitoring device and flush it with saline if recommended by the manufacturer.
2. Plug in all cables as directed by the manufacturer.
3. Assemble and prepare the suction or cautery device at the bedside.
4. The nondominant hemisphere is used for monitoring. The assistant or clinician may cleanse the skin and shave the site.
5. Facilitate and assist with proper draping and sterile set-up.
6. Zero and level the monitoring device; the reference point is the foramen of Monro (the top of the external auditory canal).

7. When the ICP monitoring device has been positioned and secured, rinse any skin cleansing agent from the area and apply dressings (occlusive, Tegaderm).
8. Obtain the first ICP reading and document it. Monitor the waveforms and print them for the patient care record. Calculate and document the cerebral profusion pressure (CPP).
9. Set the alarm limits on the system.
10. Assess the ICP and CPP hourly, and also perform a full neurologic assessment. Perform these assessments more frequently if deterioration occurs or the clinician orders them.
11. Rezero the system if any cable or connections are dislodged or whenever the waveform appears dampened or does not fit the neurologic assessment.
12. Perform dressing changes according to hospital policy or as needed.

INTERPRETING ICP WAVEFORMS

Pulsations from the choroid plexus are transmitted to the CSF in the ventricles and subarachnoid space; this produces a waveform similar to the arterial pressure waveform, but of lower amplitude. A normal ICP waveform has three or more defined peaks, P1, P2, and P3 (see illustration in next section).

Normal Waveforms

1. P1 is the percussion wave, which represents the blood being ejected from the heart. Extremes of hypotension or hypertension change this waveform.
2. P2 is the tidal wave, which represents the intracranial brain bulk. This wave is more variable in size and shape and ends on the dicrotic notch. It is most closely linked with decreased compliance. A P2 that is equal to P1 shows decreased compliance. It also is used to predict when the ICP will elevate.
3. P3, which follows the dicrotic notch, represents closure of the aortic valve (see illustration).

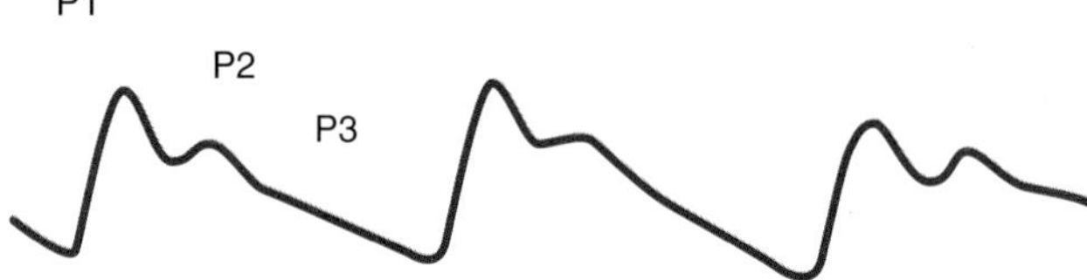

Normal ICP waveform. P1, Percussion wave. P2, Tidal wave with variable amplitude and shape; ends on dicrotic notch. P3, Dicrotic wave immediately after dicrotic notch; this wave slopes into the diastolic baseline position. (From Bader MK, Littlejohns LR: *AANN core curriculum for neuroscience nursing*, ed 4, St Louis, 2004, Elsevier.)

Abnormal Waveforms

1. A waves (plateau waves): These plateau-shaped waves form a clinically significant pattern. This pattern usually is seen when the ICP is high (>20 mm Hg), and sharp increases of 30 to 70 mm Hg occur and plateau for as long as 20 minutes. Often, the plateau is preceded by B waves, and this may indicate a decreased CPP with elevated ICP.
2. B waves (sawtooth waves): These sharp, rhythmic waves that appear in a sawtooth pattern indicate fluctuations in cerebral blood flow and poor compliance in a patient with a high ICP.
3. C waves (small rhythmic waves): These small, rhythmic patterns that occur every 10 minutes within the normal ICP levels are clinically insignificant (see illustration).

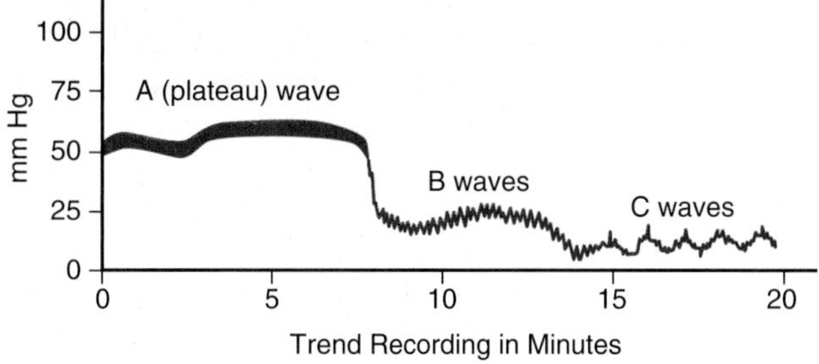

Intracranial pressure waves. Composite diagram of plateau waves (A waves), sawtooth waves (B waves), and small rhythmic waves (C waves). (From Barker E: *Neuroscience nursing: a spectrum of care*, ed 2, St Louis, 2002, Mosby.)

TROUBLESHOOTING THE ICP MONITORING DEVICE

1. If a dampened or aberrant waveform is seen, tissue or blood may be occluding the device.
   a. Check the tubing for air bubbles. The tubing may need to be changed by the clinician.
   b. With a fiberoptic or sensor system, the clinician may need to replace the catheter. Check the manufacturer's recommendations.
   c. Assess the monitoring system. Check for loose cables or connecting devices. Rezero the device at the correct reference level.
2. Compliant and noncompliant ICP monitoring systems.
   a. In a compliant ICP monitoring system, volume may be added to the closed system, and this addition has very little effect on the ICP.
   b. In a noncompliant system, the closed box is so tight that any tiny increase in any of the intracranial contents results in a massive increase in ICP. A procedure such as suctioning or turning the patient produces a sustained increase in ICP greater than 10 mm Hg for longer than 3 minutes. You also may note that P2 (the tidal wave) is equal to or greater in amplitude than P1 (see earlier illustration).

When the patient's monitoring system shows noncompliance, the healthcare team must keep stimuli to a minimum and institute measures to reduce the ICP.

CEREBROSPINAL FLUID DRAINAGE

Excess CSF can be drained from a closed system during periods of intracranial hypertension. A catheter is placed for ventriculostomy for 3 to 5 days, and the team must follow strict aseptic technique in handling the device. Extreme care must be taken when manipulating stopcocks to prevent fluid from being flushed into the brain *and* to prevent excessive drainage from the system, which could cause ventricular collapse and subsequent tissue damage.

Pharmacologic Measures for Controlling the Intracranial Pressure

You have reviewed several tactics for reducing a rising ICP, thereby maintaining the CPP to prevent secondary brain injury. Those tactics have included patient positioning, reduction of stimuli, maintaining the $PaCO_2$ and the PaO_2 within appropriate ranges, euthermia, euvolemia, CSF monitoring and drainage, and seizure and BP control. Diuretics and barbiturates also may have a role in controlling intracranial hypertension.

Diuretics

Both osmotic and nonosmotic agents, along with volume control (restriction), can assist the brain in managing the fluids within the brain and vasculature. If the blood-brain barrier is intact, mannitol can help pull fluids from the healthy areas of the brain; however, it may cause electrolyte disturbances and should not be used in patients with hypovolemia. Loop diuretics (furosemide) also may be used, because they pull sodium and water from edematous areas.

Barbiturates

Barbiturates have been used in a long-standing protocol that may assist with uncontrolled intracranial hypertension. The two most commonly used drugs in this category are phenobarbital and thiopental, both given in high doses. The goal is an ICP of 15 to 20 mm Hg and an MAP of 70 to 80 mm Hg. This therapy usually is tapered slowly, over 4 to 5 days (Box 5-14).

Herniation Syndromes

When cerebral edema or a mass develops in the semisolid brain within the essentially closed compartment, the pressure exerted by the lesion is not evenly distributed. This results in shifting or herniation of the brain tissue from one compartment to the other. Major patterns of herniation include uncal (tentorial), cingulate, central, and **tonsillar [medullary] herniation** (see Figure 5-23; also Table 5-8 and Figure 5-32).

Uncal Herniation

In **uncal herniation**, the most common herniation syndrome, a one-sided, rapidly expanding mass (usually temporal) displaces the tip of the temporal lobe (uncus). Pressure is applied at the edge of the tentorium over both the oculomotor nerve (cranial nerve III) and the posterior cerebral artery. The clinical signs are those of a classic herniation syndrome: ipsilateral pupil dilation with decreased level of consciousness, respiratory pattern changes, and contralateral hemiplegia. Without intervention, the uncus is pushed over the edge of the tentorium, causing bilaterally dilated pupils and a flaccid patient.

Table 5-8 Mechanisms of Intracranial Pressure (ICP) Elevation

Pathophysiology	Possible Causes	Treatment
Disorders of Cerebrospinal Fluid (CSF) Space		
Overproduction of CSF	Choroid plexus papilloma	Diuretics, surgical removal
Communicating hydrocephalus from obstructed arachnoid	Old subarachnoid hemorrhage	Surgical drainage from lumbar drain
Noncommunicative hydrocephalus	Posterior fossa tumor obstructing aqueduct	Surgical drainage by ventricular drain
Interstitial edema	Any of the above	Surgical drainage of CSF
Disorders of Intracranial Blood Flow		
Intracranial hemorrhage	Epidural hematoma	Surgical drainage
Vasospasm	Subarachnoid hemorrhage	Hypervolemia and hypertensive therapy
Vasodilation	Elevated arterial carbon dioxide ($PaCO_2$)	Hyperventilation
Increasing cerebral blood volume and ICP	Hypoxia	Adequate oxygenation
Disorders of Brain Substance		
Expanding mass lesion with local vasogenic edema	Brain tumor	Steroids, surgical removal
Ischemic brain injury with cytotoxic edema	Anoxic brain injury from cardiac or respiratory arrest	Resistant to therapy
Increased cerebral metabolic rate, which increases cerebral blood flow	Seizures, hyperthermia	Anticonvulsant medications to control fever

Modified from Urden LD, Stacy KM, Lough ME: *Thelan's critical care nursing: diagnosis and management,* ed 5, St Louis, 2006, Mosby.

Box 5-14 Collaborative Management Priorities for Intracranial Hypertension

- Position the patient to achieve maximum reduction of intracranial pressure (ICP).
- Reduce environmental stimulation.
- Maintain normothermia.
- Control ventilation to ensure a normal arterial carbon dioxide ($Paco_2$) level (35 ±2 mm Hg).
- Administer diuretic agents, anticonvulsants, sedation, analgesia, paralytic agents, and vasoactive medications to ensure a cerebral perfusion pressure (CPP) > 70 mm Hg.
- Drain cerebrospinal fluid for ICP > 20 mm Hg.

From Urden LD, Stacy KM, Lough ME: *Thelan's critical care nursing: diagnosis and management,* ed 5, St Louis, 2006, Mosby.

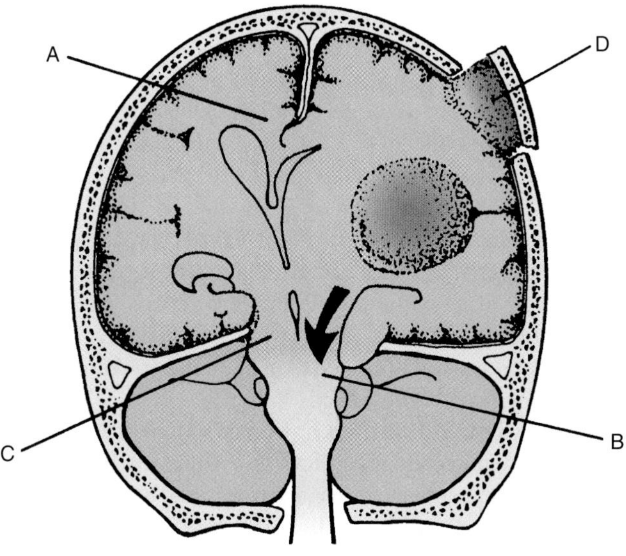

Figure 5-32

Supratentorial herniation. *A,* Cingulate. *B,* Uncal. *C,* Central. *D,* Transcalvarial. (From Urden LD, Stacy KM, Lough ME: *Thelan's critical care nursing: diagnosis and management,* ed 5, St Louis, 2006, Mosby.)

Cingulate Herniation

With cingulate herniation, an expanding lesion of one hemisphere shifts laterally and forces the cingulated gyrus under the falx cerebri. By itself this shift is not life-threatening; it happens often and is seen on CT as a shift of the midline. If no treatment is provided, uncal or central herniation follows.

Central Herniation

With central herniation, both hemispheres, the basal ganglia, and the diencephalon are pushed down toward the tentorial notch. Uncal and cingulated herniation usually precede this development. The patient loses consciousness; the pupils are small and reactive and progress to fixed and dilated.

Tonsillar (Medullary) Herniation

Tonsillar, or medullary, herniation sometimes is called a downward cerebellar herniation. It occurs when an expanding lesion of the cerebellum presses downward, pushing the tonsils through the foramen magnum. Because the medulla is displaced, respiratory and cardiac arrest ensue.

Other Neurologic Disorders

A comprehensive discussion of the many chronic neuromuscular and degenerative brain disorders is beyond the scope of this text. This section focuses on the those that affect consciousness and the ABCDs.

Guillain-Barré Syndrome

Guillain-Barré syndrome has a number of clinical presentations, including **acute inflammatory demyelinating polyradiculoneuropathy (AIDP)**. The cause of AIDP, which was first reported in the late 1970s, still is not known; however, the disease is associated with an immune response triggered by viral or bacterial sources and vaccines. The motor and sensory pathways of the peripheral and the autonomic nervous systems undergo segmental demyelination, which presents with ascending paralysis or weakness. As the disease affects the respiratory system and airway mechanics, admission to the ICU and supportive measures become necessary. Limited treatment is available for AIDP and involves diligent monitoring for complications (airway compromise, respiratory failure). In recent years, **plasmapheresis** and administration of IV immune globulins have shown some promise.

Seizure Disorders

Epilepsy is a brain disorder in which normal neuronal activity becomes disturbed. Epilepsy can arise from congenital malformations, critical medical illness, and TBI. The primary mechanism may be the neuronal wiring or a neurotransmitter imbalance. Nearly 70% of epilepsy seizures do not have an identifiable cause (idiopathic), but 30% have a treatable cause.

Typically, two types of seizures are seen in epilepsy, partial seizures and generalized seizures. These seizures generally are categorized according to whether loss of consciousness occurs.

- *Simple partial seizures* cause no impairment of consciousness; a single body part begins the seizure. Symptoms include:
  - Somatosensory: Tingling; hallucinations of sight, sound, or taste
  - Autonomic: Sweating, flushing, abnormal epigastric sensations
  - Psychological: Personality changes
- *Complex partial seizures* are marked by impaired consciousness in the beginning; they are essentially simple partial seizures followed by impaired consciousness.
- *Generalized seizures (convulsive and nonconvulsive)* can be categorized as follows:
  - Absence seizure: Brief loss of consciousness for seconds
  - Myoclonic seizure: Altered consciousness with isolated clonic movement
  - Clonic seizure: Various dysrhythmic body contractions

- Tonic seizure: Sustained contractions of large muscle groups
- Generalized tonic-clonic seizure: Alternating tonic-clonic movement
- Atonic seizure: Brief, generalized seizures in which the patient's head drops or the person falls to the ground (i.e., epileptic drop attacks)

The general treatment for epilepsy is to prevent seizures with drugs and to limit the side effects of those medications. The choice of drug is based on the underlying cause and the type of seizure the patient experiences. In general, antiepileptic drugs work by stabilizing the cell membrane through alteration of cation transport (ion channels).

Status epilepticus is a state of prolonged (or recurrent) seizure activity that lasts at least 30 minutes without an interval of consciousness. About 10% to 20% of patients who experience this emergency suffer from secondary anoxia; in such cases, prevention and treatment are the same as for seizures in a patient with intracranial hypertension.

Vertebral Column and Spinal Cord Injury

Each year, 10,000 to 12,000 traumatic spinal cord injuries (SCIs) are predicted to occur in the United States. The incidence is relatively low (approximately 40.1 per 1 million people), but the cost of overall management and long-term disability is high. These injuries primarily occur in young men 15 to 30 years of age.

The most common cause of SCI is trauma, predominantly motor vehicle crashes, falls, contact sports, diving or skiing incidents, and penetrating trauma with knives and guns. Medical causes include tumors, arthritis (which causes cord compression), and anterior spinal artery thrombosis. In oncology patients with neurologic deficits, the malignancy may cause spinal cord compromise; patients with myeloma and lymphoma are most at risk. This phenomenon usually begins with back pain and increasing signs of spinal cord disease. Treatment is aimed at **debulking** the tumor and IV steroids.

Mechanisms of SCI

The injury to the column or cord generally is caused by one of three mechanisms of energy transfer: hypertension/flexion, compression, or rotation. When the heavy head is quickly forced backward or forward, the whipping injury causes the cervical column to become hyperextended or hyperflexed, creating a high potential for cord damage. This is particularly risky in elderly individuals because of the arthritic changes in the cervical spinal column that occur with age.

Compression energy transfer creates a loading of one vertebra on top of another. This compression usually causes trauma to the anterior portion of the bony vertebra and can shatter the tissue. Axial loading injuries are compression-type energy transfers. Diving (head versus object) or landing in a standing or seated position loads the body weight on the column and can cause trauma throughout the body, but the most vulnerable areas are those with the greatest curves.

Rotation or lateral bending of the column allows for much less "give." Dislocations and fractures often occur when the heavy head and torso move in opposite directions.

When these types of energy patterns are applied to the unique spinal bones, fractures occur. The same types of injuries can occur in any bone (comminuted, compression, or simple), but because of the delicate neurologic tissue in the spinal cord, clinicians prefer to categorize these injuries as either stable or unstable fractures.

Ten percent of those who suffer a cervical spine injury have additional spinal column fractures. Some cervical spine fractures have special names; for example, a Jefferson fracture is an unstable injury to C1 (atlas) where it articulates with the cranium and C2 (Figure 5-33). A hangman's fracture extends through the pedicles of the axis (C2).

As with TBI, SCI involves a primary injury to neurologic cells and then secondary injury as a result of biochemical processes. The primary injury is irreversible, but the secondary process can be minimized.

Types of Cord Injury

Complete Transsection of the Spinal Cord

Complete transsection of the spinal cord is rare. The patient may incur a complete cord injury (primary and secondary tissue damage) but not with the primary insult. These injuries are described as complete or incomplete, depending on distal signs and symptoms. A complete injury is characterized by total loss of sensory and motor function distal to the primary

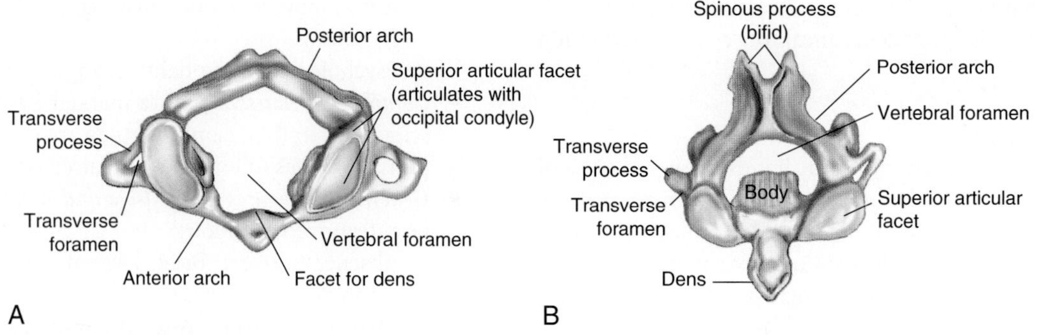

Figure 5-33

The first **(A)** and second **(B)** cervical vertebrae are shaped differently from the rest of the vertebrae of the spine. Their function is to support the skull and allow rotation and anterior-posterior motion of the head. (From the National Association of Emergency Medical Technicians: *PHTLS: prehospital trauma life support,* ed 6, St Louis, 2007, Mosby.)

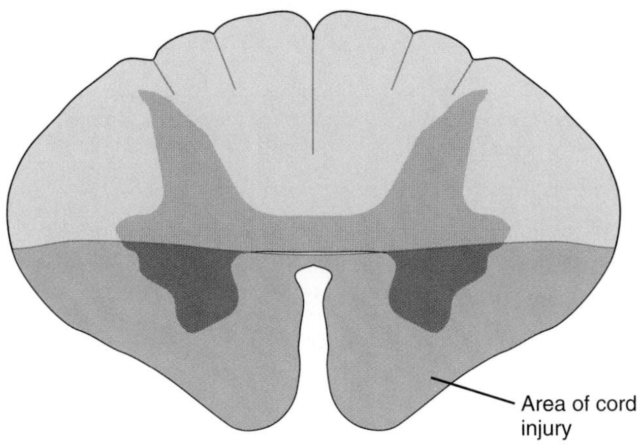

Figure 5-34

Anterior cord syndrome. (From the National Association of Emergency Medical Technicians: *PHTLS: prehospital trauma life support,* ed 6, St Louis, 2007, Mosby.)

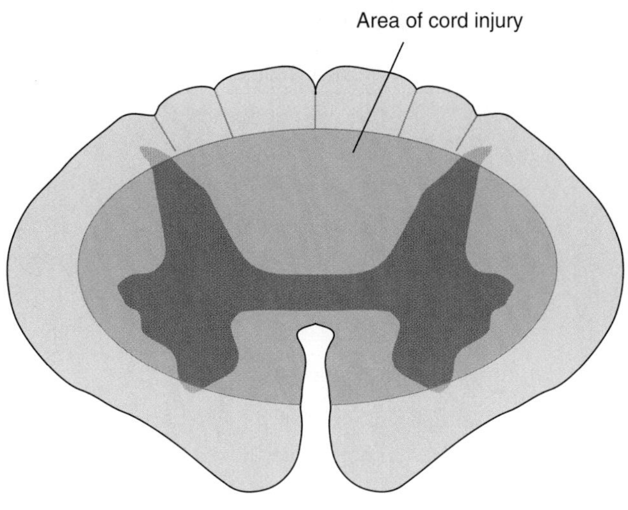

Figure 5-35

Central cord syndrome. (From the National Association of Emergency Medical Technicians: *PHTLS: prehospital trauma life support,* ed 6, St Louis, 2007, Mosby.)

injury. Complete injuries are further described as quadriplegia (C1 to T1) or paraplegia (T2 to L1).

Incomplete Transsection of the Spinal Cord

An incomplete SCI may present with a mixed loss of motor and/or sensory function distal to the lesion. If the injury is predominantly toward the dorsal side, sensory function is affected. If the ventral side is injured, motor function usually is affected distally. Various other syndromes also may present with incomplete injury.

- *Anterior cord syndrome:* Spinal arteries are injured, resulting in loss of motor function and of pain, temperature, and some light touch sensations. Some other light touch, motion, position, and vibration sensations are retained (Figure 5-34).
- *Central cord syndrome:* This syndrome usually occurs with hyperextension of the cervical spine. Its symptoms include weakness or **paresthesia** in the upper extremities but normal strength in the lower extremities. It often is seen in elderly individuals with cervical spine stenosis or spondylosis (Figure 5-35).
- *Brown-Séquard syndrome:* This syndrome usually results from a penetrating injury that partly transects the cord (one side). Symptoms include those of complete cord damage on one side only: loss of motor, vibration, motion, and position on one side (**ipsilateral**) and loss of pain, temperature, and sensation on the other side (**contralateral**) (Figure 5-36).
- *Posterior cord syndrome:* This syndrome is associated with a hyperextension injury to the cervical spine. It produces a group of symptoms that includes loss of position, pressure, and vibration senses distal to the injury.

Assessment and Management of Spinal Injury

The ABCDs of trauma care include maintaining a neutral, in-line stabilization of the head and neck with spinal column immobilization throughout (see Chapter 7 for information on ruling out spinal cord injury). In order to clinically clear the patient of spinal cord injury (and not immobilize), the patient must be able to communicate, alert and oriented, free of drugs or alcohol, and have no distracting injuries.

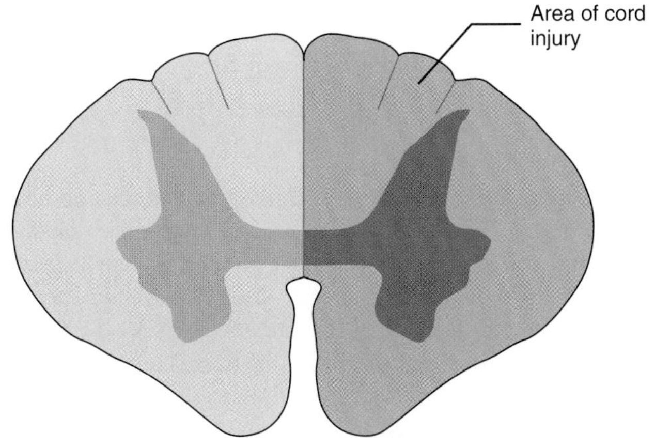

Figure 5-36

Brown-Séquard syndrome. (From the National Association of Emergency Medical Technicians: *PHTLS: prehospital trauma life support,* ed 6, St Louis, 2007, Mosby.)

When you arrive at a hospital in the middle of trauma resuscitation, the long spine board may have been removed, because it is generally considered to be an immobilization device for EMS transport. Follow your protocols for immobilization of trauma patients in transport.

The trauma physician has been trained to follow the same alphabet (ABCDs) as every other trauma team member. This includes "a finger or tube in every orifice" (see Chapter 7). One tube to which the team must pay particular attention is the gastric tube. Whether this tube is inserted orally or nasally, suctioning of gastric contents before or during transport is one of the keys to good airway management in a patient bound to a spine board.

Table 5-9 Spinal Nerve Innervation of Major Muscle Groups

Spinal Nerve	Muscle Group Movement	Assessment
C4-C5	Shoulder abduction	Arms are moved away from body against downward pressure from examiner's hands.
C5	Elbow flexion (biceps)	Arm is pulled up from resting position against resistance.
C7	Elbow extension (triceps) Thumb-index pinch	From flexed position, arm is straightened out against resistance. Index finger is held firmly to thumb against resistance to pull apart.
C8	Hand grasp	Examiner evaluates hand grasp strength.
L2	Hip flexion	Leg is lifted from bed against resistance.
L3	Knee extension	From flexed position, knee is extended against resistance.
L4	Foot dorsiflexion	Foot is pulled up toward nose against resistance.
S1	Foot plantar flexion	Foot is pushed down (e.g., stepping on the gas) against resistance.

From Sole ML, Klein DG, Moseley MJ: *Introduction to critical care nursing*, ed 4, Philadelphia, 2006, Saunders.

Your secondary assessment includes the dermatomes previously mentioned to determine current spinal cord function. Assessing for high thoracic or cervical spine injuries and being prepared for the two complications common with that area of trauma—neurogenic shock and ventilatory insufficiency—can help you provide good patient care (Table 5-9).

Neurogenic Shock

Two terms need to be differentiated, spinal shock and neurogenic shock. Spinal shock is a temporary condition involving complete loss of tone and reflexes but not necessarily tissue injury. Neurogenic shock is a form of distributive hypoperfusion in which the descending sympathetic tracts are disrupted. Any patient with a spinal cord injury from T6 superiorly to C1 can suffer from this serious complication.

A balance is supposed to exist between sympathetic and parasympathetic control of the heart rate and blood vessel size. When the sympathetic nervous system is suppressed, the parasympathetic system takes control, reducing the heart rate and dilating the blood vessels. This results in an unusual presentation of shock in which the patient has a good color and skin temperature, but also bradycardia and an extremely low BP. This type of shock can continue for up to 1 month after the primary injury to the cord, and vasoactive drugs usually are required to maintain the blood pressure.

Poikilothermy

Interruption of the sympathetic pathways also can cause **poikilothermy**, a result of suppression of the temperature-regulating centers in the hypothalamus. The patient's core temperature approaches the ambient temperature, and the individual will become hypothermic or hyperthermic, depending on the temperature of the room.

Hypoventilation

Complete injuries above C3 result in paralysis of the diaphragm; as this occurs, the patient shows diaphragmatic (seesaw) respirations with a decrease in the tidal volume and vital capacity. Paralysis of the abdominal and intercostal muscles also leads to ineffective cough and retention of secretions. Injuries from C6 through T11 may impair the intercostal and abdominal muscles.

Early recognition and prompt support of ventilatory status is important with cervical spine and high thoracic spine injuries. Medication-assisted intubation and in-line spinal immobilization techniques are important.

Management of Spinal Cord Injury

Unstable fractures of the vertebral column may require surgical repair of bony and connective tissues to stabilize the alignment and structure of the segments. For a stable fracture, nonsurgical management may include skeletal traction, for which tongs are placed in the sides of the cranium and weights are attached. The tongs usually are placed at the bedside in the ED or ICU for patients with some cervical and high thoracic alignment derangement or locked facets. If the patient is to be transported, ask whether the procedure can be delayed until arrival at the receiving hospital. If the device needs to be placed first, have the surgeon place it while the patient is positioned on your cart so that traction adjustment can be done with input from you on the position of the cot while in transit. Once situated in a hospital, these patients often are placed in a kinetic bed, where immobilization can continue while the patient is constantly turned to help prevent complications of stasis (e.g., DVT, decubitus ulcers, and pneumonia).

When cervical traction is discontinued, a halo brace usually is applied. This device has four tongs that are placed in the cranium, but a body vest is used to help immobilize the cervical spine while the patient is ambulatory.

Pharmacologic Management

Methylprednisolone

Administration of high-dose methylprednisolone within 8 hours of spinal cord injury has been recommended since 1990. Three studies done since then have provided various recommendations for and against use of the drug and have questioned its timing. According to the National Acute Spinal Cord Injury Studies (NASCIS I, II, III), along with follow-up studies that extended into early 2000, methylprednisolone should be administered in SCI as follows: a 30 mg/kg bolus is given over 15 minutes within 8 hours of injury; after 45 minutes, the drug is again administered at a dosage of 5.4 mg/kg/hour for the next 23 hours.

In nonpenetrating SCI, methylprednisolone is thought to significantly improve both complete and incomplete injuries. One study found that in patients treated earlier than 3 hours after injury, administration of methylprednisolone for 24 hours was best; however, in patients in whom treatment began 3 to 8 hours after injury, continuous infusion for 48 hours provided the best results.

Injury to the spinal cord begins a cascade of secondary events that include ischemia, inflammation, and calcium-mediated cell injury. Along with antiinflammatory effects, methylprednisolone is thought to have a neuroprotective effect by inhibiting lipid peroxidation and calcium influx.

The use of this drug at these dosages continues to be controversial. Many experts believe that the clinical gains are questionable, and the risks of steroid therapy are not inconsequential. In a recent survey, 91% of the spinal surgeons surveyed used steroids in SCI, but only 24% believed they were of any clinical benefit.

Consequently, a debate has arisen among experts, some of whom claim that this standard of care was established through questionable statistical procedures in research and that the NASCIS II study showed little if any benefits. Another survey of participants at the 2001 Canadian Spine Society meeting indicated that 75% of the respondents used the drug because everyone else was or out of fear of the consequences of failing to do so. The Canadian Spine Society and the Canadian Neurosurgical Society concluded that insufficient evidence was available to support the use of methylprednisolone as a treatment standard or guideline.

Autonomic Dysreflexia

Autonomic dysreflexia, or hyperreflexia, is a syndrome that sometimes occurs after the acute phase of SCI in patients with lesions at or above T6. This syndrome is more commonly seen in patients with a complete SCI than in those with incomplete spinal cord syndromes. It is seen only after recovery from spinal shock, when reflex activity returns.

Noxious stimuli, such as bladder or intestinal distention; pressure on the glans penis; renal calculi; cystitis; sudden, severe abdominal pain; and pressure sores may produce a sympathetic discharge that causes reflex vasoconstriction of blood vessels in the skin and **splanchnic bed** below the level of the injury. The vasoconstriction in the splanchnic bed distends baroreceptors in the carotid sinus and aortic arch, and the body attempts to lower hypertension by superficial dilation of vessels above the level of injury. The patient has severe hypertension and bradycardia and is in severe distress and discomfort. The head and neck are flushed, but the lower extremities are pale. The pupils are dilated, and nasal congestion is common. Sweating is noted above the level of the lesion, and goose bumps are seen above or below this level. Interventions for dysreflexia are as follows:

- Elevate the head of the bed.
- Establish IV access for administration of crystalloid fluids and medications as needed.
- Monitor cardiac values and pulse oximetry.
- Relieve the trigger.
  - Check the patency of the urinary drainage system or insert a urinary catheter.
  - Check for fecal impaction, lubricate the rectum, or use a local anesthetic
  - Eliminate pressure on the skin.
- Administer ganglionic blocking agents for hypertension.

Scenario Conclusion

During transport, you opt to decrease the ventilator rate to 10 breaths/min, and the $PETCO_2$ remains within a range of 38 to 42 mm Hg. An additional 2 L of lactated Ringer's solution had been infused, per your medical control physician's request; the patient's BP ranges from 100/80 mm Hg to 110/72 mm Hg, with a heart rate of 90 to 110 beats/min. A urinary catheter and gastric tube were inserted before transport. On arrival at your level I hospital, the urinary collection bag holds 200 mL of yellow urine.

The neurosurgeon at the level I hospital immediately inserts an ICP bolt into the subarachnoid space; the opening pressure is 42 mm Hg, and first B waves and then A (plateau) waves are recorded. A CT scan of the head shows DAI with edema formation.

SUMMARY

Acute neurologic conditions can be particularly challenging. Thorough assessment of these patients, along with the use of diagnostic and therapeutic tools and an in-depth knowledge of the workings of this unique system, help the critical care team provide the correct management and ongoing evaluation.

KEY TERMS

acute inflammatory demyelinating polyradiculoneuropathy (AIDP) A form of Guillain-Barré syndrome marked by inflammation of several peripheral nerves at once; also called *acute idiopathic polyneuritis.*

acute tubular necrosis (ATN) Acute renal failure with mild to severe damage or necrosis of tubule cells; it usually occurs secondary to nephrotoxicity, ischemia after major surgery, trauma (crush syndrome), severe hypovolemia, sepsis, or burns.

afferent A descriptive term meaning conveying or conducting toward a center.

amygdala The part of the limbic system that mediates emotions and is involved in primitive behavioral responses.

anisocoria Inequality in the diameter of the pupils.

apneustic center One of the respiratory centers near the pons (brain stem); it controls normal respirations. Disease in the apneustic center results in an abnormal respiratory pattern characterized by sustained inspiratory effort (less exhalation).

aqueduct of Sylvius A narrow passage or channel in the brain for cerebrospinal fluid that connects the third and fourth ventricles; also called the *cerebral aqueduct* or *aqueductus mesencephali.*

arachnoid mater Resembles a spider's web, this is the middle layer of the meninges that cover the brain. Cerebrospinal fluid flows freely beneath this layer in the space called subarachnoid. Called the *arachnoidea mater encephali* for the brain and the *arachnoidea mater spinalis* for the spinal cord covering.

arachnoid villi Numerous microscopic projections of the arachnoid mater into some of the venous sinuses.

Babinski's sign Dorsiflexion of the big toe with fanning of the other toes on stimulation of the sole of the foot. It is normal in infants but otherwise is a sign of a lesion in the central nervous system, particularly the pyramidal tract. Also called the *Babinski phenomenon, Babinski reflex,* or *plantar reflex.*

Broca's speech area An area comprising parts of the opercular portion of the inferior frontal gyrus; injury to this area may result in a minor form of motor aphasia.

Brudzinski's sign A sign seen with meningitis; because of severe neck stiffness, flexion of the neck usually results in flexion of the hip and knee; also called the *neck sign.*

cancellous bone A reticular, spongy, or latticelike structure usually found near bone marrow and at the epiphyses of bones; usually refers to bony tissue.

canthus The angle at either end of the fissure between the eyelids.

cerebral perfusion pressure (CPP) The difference between the mean arterial pressure and the intracranial pressure, normally 70 to 95 mm Hg.

cerebral amyloid angiopathy A vascular amyloidosis (a condition in which a starchlike substance accumulates in the brain) that affects the small and medium arteries of the leptomeninges and cerebral cortex, resulting in microinfarcts or hemorrhage. The condition occurs most often in the elderly, usually sporadically, and it may be asymptomatic or may result in hemorrhagic stroke or dementia. A hereditary form occurs with autosomal-dominant inheritance.

cholinergic A descriptive term for the sympathetic and parasympathetic nerve fibers that release acetylcholine at a synapse when a nerve impulse passes.

choroid plexuses The infoldings of blood vessels of the pia mater, which are covered by a thin coat of ependymal cells and which form tufted projections into the third, fourth, and lateral ventricles of the brain. The choroid plexus, which is supplied by the choroidal arteries, secretes cerebrospinal fluid.

circle of Willis The union of the anterior and posterior cerebral arteries (branches of the carotid artery), which form an anastomosis at the base of the brain.

cisterns Closed spaces that serve as reservoirs for lymph or other body fluids; the term frequently refers to the enlarged subarachnoid spaces that contain cerebrospinal fluid.

cold caloric examination A test of cranial nerves III, VI, and VIII and of brain stem integrity. The head of the patient's bed is elevated up to 30 degrees, and the physician injects 20 to 120 mL of water into each ear canal (allowing 5 minutes between the two tests). The physician watches for eye movement, known as the oculovestibular response, including conjugate or dysconjugate movement towards the tested ear.

conjugate Paired or equally coupled; working in unison.

contralateral Situated on, pertaining to, or affecting the opposite side.

conus medullaris The cone-shaped, lower end of the spinal cord, at the level of the upper lumbar vertebrae.

convergence The coordinated inclination of the two lines of sight toward their common point of fixation, or the point of fixation itself.

corneal reflexes The automatic closure of the eyelids in response to irritation of the cornea; also called the *blink* or *lid reflex.*

corpus callosum An arched mass of white matter in the depths of the longitudinal fissure. Including layers of fibers: the central layer, which consists primarily of transverse fibers connecting the cerebral hemispheres; the subsections, from anterior to posterior, are called the *rostrum, genu, trunk,* and *splenium.*

Cushing's triad A set of three signs (bradycardia, systolic hypertension, and irregular respirations) that indicates a rise in systemic blood pressure as a result of increased intracranial pressure. It also may indicate herniation syndrome.

debulking The removal of a major portion of the material that comprises a lesion (e.g., removal of most of a tumor so that less tumor is present, requiring subsequent treatment, such as chemotherapy or radiotherapy); also called *cytoreduction* and *cytoreductive surgery.*

dermatomes Areas of the skin supplied with afferent nerve fibers by individual posterior spinal roots.

descending transtentorial herniation Herniation caused by a supratentorial mass; it is marked by downward displacement of the most medial cerebral structures through the tentorial notch and compression of parts of the cerebrum and structures below the notch; the most common transtentorial herniation.

diabetes insipidus (DI) Any of several types of polyuria in which the volume of urine exceeds 3 L a day, causing dehydration, great thirst, and sometimes emaciation and great hunger. The underlying cause may be hormonal (central DI) or renal (nephrogenic DI).

diencephalon The caudal part of the prosencephalon, which mostly surrounds the third ventricle and connects the mesencephalon to the cerebral hemispheres; each lateral half is divided by the hypothalamic sulcus into a dorsal part (comprising the epithalamus, dorsal thalamus, and metathalamus) and a ventral part (comprising the ventral thalamus and hypothalamus). Also called the *interbrain.*

diffuse Not localized; widely distributed.

doll's eyes response A reflex in which rotation of the head laterally causes the eyes to deviate synergistically in the opposite direction. This reflex is assessed in premature infants and comatose patients to test for integrity of function of the oculomotor nerves and brain stem. Also called the *oculocephalic* or *oculocephalogyric reflex.*

dura mater The outermost, toughest, and most fibrous of the three membranes (meninges) covering the brain and spinal cord; also called the *pachymeninx.* (In Latin, *dura* means "hard" and *mater* means "mother.")

disconjugate With regard to gaze, a term that indicates that the eyes are not working in unison.

efferent A descriptive term meaning conveying away from a center.

embolization Therapeutic introduction of a substance into a vessel to occlude it.

encephalopathy Any degenerative disease of the brain.

epidural space The space that separates the dura mater from the bones in the vertebral canal; it contains fat, small veins, and the large meningeal arteries

exteroception The perception of stimuli originating outside or at a distance from the body.

extrapyramidal system Outside of the pyramidal tracts; an imprecise term referring to a functional system, rather than an anatomic part of the central nervous system, that controls motor activities and is not part of the pyramidal tract. It includes the corpus stratum, subthalamic nucleus, substantia nigra, and red nucleus, along with their interconnections with the reticular formation, cerebrum, and cerebellum. These structures control and coordinate especially the postural, static, supporting, and locomotor mechanisms.

falx cerebri A fold of the dura mater that extends downward in the longitudinal cerebral fissure and separates the two cerebral hemispheres. (In anatomic nomenclature, *falx* is a general term for a sickle-shaped organ or structure.)

focal Pertaining to a focus; the chief center of a morbid process.

foramen magnum The large opening in the anterior and inferior part of the occipital bone that connects the vertebral canal and the cranial cavity.

fossa A trench, channel, or hollow place.

galea aponeurotica The aponeurotic structure of the scalp; it connects the frontal and occipital bellies of the occipitofrontalis muscle.

ganglion A group of nerve cell bodies located outside the central nervous system. The term occasionally is applied to certain nuclear groups in the brain or spinal cord (e.g., the basal ganglia).

glia A word termination denoting the neuroglia.

grasp reflex A reflex in which stimulation produces a grasping motion of the fingers or toes; it is normal in infancy but pathologic in later life.

herniation syndrome The abnormal protrusion of an organ or other body structure through a defect or natural opening in a covering, a membrane, muscle, or bone. In this chapter, this refers to the protrusion of brain tissue through the foramen magnum.

hippocampus A curved elevation of gray matter extending the entire length of the floor of the temporal horn of the lateral ventricle. Starting on its ventricular aspect, the hippocampus usually is considered to comprise seven sublayers: the ependyma, alveus, stratum oriens, stratum pyramidale, stratum radiatum, stratum lacunosum, and stratum moleculare. This is part of the limbic system that controls emotional states, reflex movements, and memory.

hippus phenomenon Exaggerated, rhythmic contraction and dilation of the pupil, independent of changes in illumination or in fixation of the eyes; called also *papillary athetosis.*

Horner's syndrome Sinking in of the eyeball, ptosis of the upper eyelid, slight elevation of the lower lid, constriction of the pupil, narrowing of the palpebral fissure, and anhidrosis and flushing of the affected side of the face. It is caused by a brain stem lesion on the ipsilateral side that interrupts sympathetic nerve fibers.

ipsilateral Situated on, pertaining to, or affecting the same side.

ischemic cascade A series of steps or stages (physiologic process) that once initiated continues to the final step by virtue of each step being triggered by the preceding one, sometimes with cumulative effect. In this process, a deficiency of blood flow is caused by an obstruction of a vessel in an organ or the body.

ischemic penumbra An area of moderately ischemic brain tissue surrounding an area of more severe ischemia; blood flow to this area may be enhanced to prevent the spread of a cerebral infarction.

Kernig's sign A sign of meningeal irritation; the patient has pain and resistance while the knee is slowly extended when in dorsal decubitus position.

kinesthetic sense A muscular sense; an awareness of movement, weight, tension, and the position of body parts, which depends on input from joint and muscle receptors and hair cells; movement sense.

medullary respiratory center The part of the respiratory centers in the medulla oblongata, divided between the dorsal respiratory group and the ventral respiratory group.

miotic pupil A pupil that is constricted or contracted.

mydriatic pupil A pupil that is dilated.

myelin sheath A cylindric covering on the axons of some neurons that consists of concentric layers of myelin, formed in the peripheral nervous system by the plasma membrane of Schwann cells and in the central nervous system by oligodendrocytes. It is interrupted at intervals along its length by gaps known as the *nodes of Ranvier.* Myelin is an electrical insulator that speeds the conduction of nerve impulses.

myotomes A group of muscles innervated from a single spinal segment.

neoplasms Any new or abnormal growths, specifically those in which the growth is uncontrolled and progressive. Malignant neoplasms are distinguished from benign neoplasms by their greater degree of anaplasia (loss of differentiation) and the properties of invasion and metastasis. Also called *tumors.*

neurites The axis-cylinder processes of neurons. Both axons and dendrites are neurites.

neuroglia The supporting structure of nervous tissue. It consists of a fine web of tissue made up of modified ectodermal elements in which are enclosed peculiar branched cells known as *neuroglial* or *glial* cells. The neuroglial cells are of three types: astrocytes and oligodendrocytes, which appear to play a role in myelin formation, transport of material to neurons, and maintenance of the ionic environment of neurons, and microcytes, which phagocytize waste products of nerve tissue.

neurons The conducting cells of the nervous system. A typical neuron consists of a cell body, containing the nucleus and the surrounding cytoplasm; several short, radiating processes (dendrites); and one long process (the axon), which terminates in twiglike branches and may have branches projecting along its course.

neurotransmitter Any of a group of substances released on excitation from the axon terminal of a presynaptic neuron of the central or peripheral nervous system. Neurotransmitters travel across the synaptic cleft to excite or inhibit the target cell. Among the many substances with the properties of a neurotransmitter are acetylcholine, norepinephrine, epinephrine, dopamine, glycine, gamma-aminobutyrate, glutamic acid, substance P, enkephalins, endorphins, and serotonin.

nodes of Ranvier Constrictions on myelinated nerve fibers that appear at 1 mm intervals; at these sites, the myelin sheath is absent, and the axon is enclosed only by Schwann cell processes.

nystagmus An involuntary, rapid, rhythmic movement of the eyeball that may be horizontal, vertical, rotatory, or mixed.

paratonia Involuntary resistance to passive movement, as may occur with cerebral cortical disorders.

parenchyma The essential elements of an organ (i.e., the functional elements rather than the framework).

paresthesia An abnormal touch sensation, such as burning, prickling, or formication (tactile hallucination, such as a feeling of bugs crawling), often in the absence of an external stimulus.

photophobia Abnormal visual intolerance of light.

pia mater The innermost layer of the meninges.

plasmapheresis The removal of plasma from withdrawn blood, with retransfusion of the formed elements into the donor. Generally, type-specific fresh frozen plasma or albumin is used to replace the withdrawn plasma. The procedure may be done to collect plasma components or for therapeutic purposes.

pneumotaxic center A center in the upper part of the pons that rhythmically inhibits inhalation independently of the vagus nerve.

poikilothermy Variation of the body temperature according to the environmental temperature.

preganglionic fibers Autonomic nerve fibers anterior or proximal to a ganglion.

pronation sign Pronation of the forearm caused by passive flexion, as is seen in hemiplegia.

proprioception Perception mediated by proprioceptors or proprioceptive tissues. Proprioceptors are sensory nerve terminals found in muscles, tendons, and joint capsules that transmit information about movements and the position of the body.

ptosis Drooping of the upper eyelid from paralysis of the third nerve or from sympathetic innervation; also called *blepharoptosis.*

pyramidal A term referring to the pyramidal tract of the nervous system. The pyramids of the medulla oblongata are two rounded masses, one on either side of the anterior median fissure of the medulla oblongata, composed of motor fibers (pyramidal tract) that extend from the cerebral cortex to the spinal cord and medulla oblongata. Also called *pyramidal bulbi.*

reticular activating system (RAS) The system of cells of the reticular formation of the medulla oblongata that receives collaterals from the ascending sensory pathways and projects them to higher centers; the RAS controls the overall degree of CNS activity, including wakefulness, attentiveness, and sleep.

reversible ischemic neurologic deficit (RIND) Any focal neurologic deficit that resolves completely within 24 hours; previously called a *transient ischemic attack (TIA).*

roving eye movements Spontaneous, slow, random eye deviation that moves in the horizontal plane, similar to the slow eye movements of sleep. Roving eye movements are normal in a comatose patient and suggest intact brain stem functioning.

splanchnic bed Pertaining to the splanchnic nerves which are the nerves of blood vessels and viscera, especially the visceral branches of the thoracic, abdominal and pelvic parts of the sympathetic trunks..

squamous bone Flattened, platelike, or scalelike bone.

strabismus Deviation of the eye that the patient cannot overcome. The visual axes assume a position relative to each other that is different from that required by the physiologic conditions. The various forms of strabismus are called *tropias,* and the direction is indicated by the appropriate prefix; for example, cyclotropia, esotropia, exotropia, hypertropia, and hypotropia.

striatum In anatomy, a sheetlike mass of a substance.

subarachnoid space The potential space between the arachnoid mater and the pia mater.

subdural space The potential space between the dura mater and the arachnoid.

sutures In the skull, this is a fibrous joint of connective tissue between the various bones of the skull, named generally for the specific components of their formation.

syndrome of inappropriate antidiuretic hormone (SIADH) Persistent hyponatremia, hypovolemia, and inappropriately elevated urine osmolality, a condition associated with the release of vasopressin (antidiuretic hormone) in amounts excessive for the individual's state of hydration. Causes include vasopressin-secreting tumor cells, neoplasms, pulmonary disorders, and CNS diseases, including head trauma.

tactile sense Pertaining to the sense of touch.

tentorial herniation Protrusion of the brain structures through the tentorial notch.

tentorium cerebelli The process of the dura mater that supports the occipital lobes and covers the cerebellum. Its internal border is free and bounds the tentorial notch; its external border is attached to the skull and encloses the transverse sinus behind.

tonsillar (medullary) herniation Protrusion of the cerebellar tonsils through the foramen magnum, thereby exerting pressure on the medulla oblongata.

transcranial Performed through the cranium.

transsphenoidal Performed through the sphenoid bone.

uncal herniation Descending transtentorial herniation in which the uncus protrudes through the notch.

ventriculostomy Surgical creation of a free communication, or shunt, between the floor of the third ventricle and the underlying cisterna interpeduncularis; the procedure may be performed to treat hydrocephalus.

Wernicke's speech area Originally a term denoting a language center thought to be confined to the posterior part of the superior temporal gyrus adjacent to the transverse temporal gyri; the term now includes a wider zone that also encompasses the supramarginal and angular gyri. Also called the *Wernicke area* or the *Wernicke second motor speech area.*

REFERENCES

1. Urden LD, Stacy KM, Lough ME: *Thelan's critical care nursing: diagnosis and management,* ed 5, St Louis, 2006, Mosby.
2. Leach JL: *Scalp reconstruction.* Web MD, eMedicine. http://emedicine.medscape.com. Accessed May 19, 2008.
3. Danis DM, Blansfield JS, Gervasini AA: *Handbook of clinical trauma care: the first hour,* ed 4, St Louis, 2007, Mosby.
4. Hickey J: *The clinical practice of neurologic and neurosurgical nursing,* ed 5, Philadelphia, 2003, Lippincott Williams & Wilkins.
5. Marion DW, Darby J, Yonas H, et al: Acute regional cerebral blood flow changes caused by severe head injuries, *J Neurosurg* 74:407-414, 1991.
6. Field JM: ACLS resource text for instructors and experienced providers, Dallas, 2008, American Heart Association.

Bibliography

Alspach JG: *AACN core curriculum for critical care nursing,* ed 6, St Louis, 2006, Saunders.

Bhardwaj A, Mirski MA, Ultatowski JA: *Handbook of neurocritical care,* Totowa, NJ, 2004, Humana Press.

Bracken MB, Freeman DH Jr, Hellenbrand K, et al: A randomized, controlled trial of methylprednisolone or naloxone in the treatment of acute spinal cord injury: results of the Second National Acute Spinal Cord Injury Study, *N Engl J Med* 322:1405-1411, 1990.

Brain Trauma Foundation: *Guidelines for the management of severe traumatic brain injury,* ed 3 (2007). www.braintrauma.org/pdf/protected/Guidelines_Management_2007w_bookmarks.pdf. Accessed May 6, 2010.

Buechler CM, Blostein PA, Koestner A, et al: Variation among trauma centers' calculation of Glasgow Coma Scale score: results of a national survey, *Journal of Trauma (Injury, Infection and Critical Care)* 45:429-432, 1998.

Chestnut RM: Management of brain and spine injuries, *Crit Care Clin* 20:25-56, 2004.

Cho DY, Wang YC: Comparison of the APACHE III and Glasgow Coma Scale in acute head injury for prediction of mortality and functional outcome, *Intensive Care Med* 23:77-84, 1997.

Colen F: Oncologic emergencies: superior vena cava syndrome, tumor lysis syndrome, and spinal cord compression, *J Emerg Nurs* 34:535-537, 2008.

Cummins RO: *Advanced cardiac life support,* Dallas, 2006, American Heart Association.

Danis DM, Blansfield JS, Gervasini AA: *Handbook of clinical trauma care: the first hour,* ed 4, St Louis, 2007, Mosby.

Dorland NW: *Dorland's illustrated medical dictionary,* ed 31, Philadelphia, 2007, Saunders.

Dunn K: Identification and management of autonomic dysreflexia in the emergency department, *Top Emerg Med* 26:254-260, 2004.

Field JM: *ACLS resource text for instructors and experienced providers,* Dallas, 2008, American Heart Association.

Hansebout RR, Kachur E: *Acute traumatic spinal cord injury.* 2007 UpToDate. www.uptodate.com. Accessed September 10, 2007.

Harrahil M: Glasgow Coma Scale: a quick review, *J Emerg Nurs* 22:81-83, 1996.

Hugenholtz H: Methylprednisolone for acute spinal cord injury: not a standard of care, *Can Med Assoc J* 168:1145-1146, 2003.

Hickey J: *The clinical practice of neurologic and neurosurgical nursing*, ed 5, Philadelphia, 2003, Lippincott Williams & Wilkins.

Hoyt KS, Selfridge-Thomas J: *Emergency nursing core curriculum*, ed 6, St Louis, 2007, Saunders.

Irwin RS, Rippe JM: *Irwin and Rippe's intensive care medicine*, ed 5, Philadelphia, 2003, Lippincott Williams & Wilkins.

Jennett B, Bond M: Assessment of outcome after severe brain damage: a practical scale, *Lancet* 1:480-485, 1975.

Jennett B, Teasdale G: Aspects of coma after head injury, *Lancet* 1:878-881, 1977.

Jennett B, Teasdale G, Braakman R, et al: Prognosis of patients with severe head injuries, *Neurosurgery* 4:283-289, 1979.

Juarez VM, Lyons M: Interrater reliability of the Glasgow Coma Scale, *J Neurosci Nurs* 27:283-286, 1995.

Lin VW, Cardenas DD, Frost F, et al: *Spinal cord medicine: principles and practice*, New York, 2003, Demos.

Macrina D, Macrina N, Horvath C, et al: An educational intervention to increase use of the Glasgow Coma Scale by emergency department personnel, *Int J Trauma Nurs* 2:7-12, 1996.

Marshall LF, Gautille T, Klauber MR, et al: The outcome of severe closed head injury, *J Neurosurg* 75:S28-S36, 1991.

McKenry L, Tessier E, Hogan MA: *Mosby's pharmacology in nursing*, ed 22, St Louis, 2006, Mosby.

McQuillan KA, Flynn MB, Hartsock RL, et al: *Trauma nursing: from resuscitation through rehabilitation*, ed 3, Philadelphia, 2001, Saunders.

Meredith W, Rutledge R, Fakhry SM, et al: The conundrum of the Glasgow Coma Scale in intubated patients: a linear regression prediction of the Glasgow verbal score from the Glasgow eye and motor scores, *Journal of Trauma (Injury, Infection and Critical Care)* 44:839-845, 1998.

Mohr JP, Choi DW, Grotta JC, et al: *Stroke: pathophysiology, diagnosis and management*, ed 4, Philadelphia, 2004, Churchill Livingstone.

Morton PG, Fontaine DK, Hudak CM: *Critical care nursing: a holistic approach*, ed 8, Philadelphia, 2005, Lippincott Williams & Wilkins.

National Association of Emergency Medical Technicians: *PHTLS: prehospital trauma life support*, ed 6, St Louis, 2007, Mosby.

Parsons PE, Wiener-Kronish JP: *Critical care secrets*, ed 3, Philadelphia, 2003, Hanley & Belfus.

Plum F, Posner JB: *The diagnosis of stupor and coma*, ed 3, Philadelphia, 1980, FA Davis.

Proehl JA: The Glasgow Coma Scale: do it and do it right, *J Emerg Nurs* 18:421-423, 1992.

Schell HM, Puntillow KA: *Critical care nursing secrets*, ed 2, St Louis, 2006, Mosby.

Schreiber D: *Spinal cord injuries.* eMedicine. http://emedicine.medscape.com/article/793582. Accessed August 8, 2006.

Sole ML, Klein DG, Moseley MJ: *Introduction to critical care nursing*, ed 4, Philadelphia, 2005, Saunders.

Southard P: Recommended: in-service programs for applying the Glasgow Coma Scale, *Trauma Nurs Core Course News* 3:2, 1993.

Teasdale G: Acute impairment of brain function. Part 1. Assessing "conscious level," *Nurs Times* 71:914-917, 1975.

Teasdale G, Jennett B: Assessment of coma and impaired consciousness: a practical scale, *Lancet* 2:81-86, 1974.

Teasdale G, Knill-Jones R, VanDer Sande J: Observer variability in assessing impaired consciousness and coma, *J Neurol Neurosurg Psychiatry* 41:603-619, 1978.

Thompson SW: *Emergency care of children*, Boston, 1990, Jones & Bartlett.

Urden LD, Stacy KM, Lough ME: *Thelan's critical care nursing: diagnosis and management*, ed 5, St Louis, 2006, Mosby.

Vernberg K, Jagger J, Jane JA: The Glasgow Coma Scale: How do you rate? *Nurse Educ* 8:33-37, 1983.

Waxman SG, DeGroot J: *Correlative neuroanatomy*, ed 22, Norwalk, Conn, 1995, Appleton & Lange.

Weiner WJ, Goetz CG, editors: *Neurology for the non-neurologist*, ed 5, Philadelphia, 2004, Lippincott Williams & Wilkins.

Wiegand DL, Carlson KK: *AACN procedure manual for critical care*, ed 5, St Louis, 2005, Saunders.

Winkler JV, Rosen P, Alfry EJ: Prehospital use of the Glasgow Coma Scale in severe head injury, *J Emerg Med* 2:1-6, 1984.

REVIEW QUESTIONS

1. In the case study, the patient has a BP of 92/60 mm Hg. What is the patient's MAP?
2. In the case study, the patient's Glasgow Coma Scale score was 3; the opening ICP was 42 mm Hg.
   A. What is the patient's CPP?
   B. What type of perfusion to this patient's brain is occurring?
   C. Was your treatment appropriate with the goal of improving the CPP?
   D. Was the patient's autoregulation compliant or noncompliant?
3. In the case study, an ICP bolt was inserted. With the head of the patient's bed elevated to 30 degrees, to what should the device be leveled and zeroed?
4. A Hispanic patient who does not speak English is involved in an automobile accident. He is taken by private car to a local hospital. When you arrive, you find that spinal immobilization has not yet been applied. The patient appears disoriented, and his eyes remain closed despite verbal stimuli.
   A. How would you score this patient on the GCS?
   B. Is spinal immobilization warranted for this patient? Why or Why not?

5. In a healthy individual with no congenital anomalies, unequal pupils may be present with no signs of intracranial hypertension.
   A. True
   B. False
6. When CSF pressure in the subarachnoid space is high and the patient's blood volume is high with hypertension, what condition may result?
7. A patient recently diagnosed with an ischemic stroke has aspirated gastric contents while lying on the bedroom floor. The clinician suggests that he has intracranial hypertension. Findings for this patient are: pulse, 78 beats/min; respirations, 22 breaths/min; BP, 210/118 mm Hg; temperature, is 38.8° C (101.8° F); GCS score, 10. What treatment plan may help you reduce this patient's ICP?
8. A patient with a subarachnoid hemorrhage is deteriorating neurologically. Blood gas values are: pH, 7.44; $PaCO_2$, 28 mm Hg; HCO_3, 28 mEq/L; BE, +2 mEq/L. The lungs are clear, and the tidal volume seems slightly high. The patient is attempting to regulate his intracranial pressure. Can you explain how the patient is accomplishing this?
9. A patient who had had a serious TBI recently was released from the rehabilitation center. Her family is concerned, because she seems fearless, she continuously performs daring feats, and she is emotionally flat. What area of the brain may have been damaged?
10. An ICU staff member is trying to determine the gravity of the head trauma in a comatose patient. The staff member decides to evaluate the oculocephalic reflex. When the patient's head is turned to the side, the eyes stay midposition and then drop to the dependent side.
    A. Is this a positive or negative examination finding?
    B. What is the common name for this finding?
    C. Does the patient have a functioning brain stem?
11. The most common site for epidural hematoma formation is ______________.
12. The most common age group for the development of an epidural hematoma is ______________.
13. Those at greatest risk for the development of a chronic subdural hematoma are ____________________.
14. Aneurysm is a common cause of subarachnoid hemorrhage and "clipping" is a common treatment.
    A. The most common complication after this procedure is ______________.
    B. What types of therapy are used to prevent this common complication?
15. You are about to transfer a patient 24 hours after he suffered an isolated head injury. He is intubated, ventilated, and has been relatively stable. The local physician in charge is going on vacation and is concerned that the patient's BP is falling. You note that the Foley bag holds 1000 mL of urine, and the ICU nurse reports that the total output for the past 8 hours is 2500 mL. What may be happening to this patient? Why is this complication occurring?

CHAPTER 6

Gastrointestinal and Renal Systems

OBJECTIVES

1. Explain the anatomy and physiology of the gastrointestinal and renal systems.
2. Discuss the clinical disorders of the gastrointestinal and renal systems.
3. Integrate pathophysiologic principles and assessment findings to implement a treatment plan for a critical care patient with gastrointestinal and renal problems.

When dealing with critically ill patients, healthcare providers seem to gravitate to the cardiovascular and respiratory systems. We all know those ABCs (airway, breathing, circulation) by heart. Who can deny that an open airway, adequate breathing, an acceptable pulse and blood pressure are of absolute importance to life? However, do you feel the same way about the renal and gastrointestinal (GI) system? You should, because a person cannot have a good quality of life (or, in fact, cannot survive) unless these systems are working well. When the renal and GI systems malfunction, all cells in the body are affected. Changes in fluid status, electrolytes, nutrition, and waste product removal are only a few of the alterations that occur. Disorders of the renal and GI systems account for many admissions to the critical care unit and cause a large percentage of the life-threatening complications seen in critically ill patients. This chapter focuses on conditions of the GI tract and kidneys that occur in critically ill patients.

GASTROINTESTINAL SYSTEM

Scenario: GI Tract

Your transport service has been asked to care for a "sick medical patient." On arrival at the 100-bed hospital, you are directed to the medical floor, where a physician reports that the person is a "really sick" liver patient. He is a 50-year-old male with a history of nonalcoholic cirrhosis with chronic liver failure. He has been fairly noncompliant with his medical care and was brought in today with altered mental status and GI bleeding. The physician gives a quick report and ends by saying that the medical team has been debating whether to intubate the patient because of his condition.

Your bedside examination reveals a 6-foot-tall man with skinny arms and legs but a fairly large, shiny abdomen. He has jaundiced eyes and skin. He looks up at you and asks to go out in the sunshine (although it is night right now). He speaks in two- and three-word sentences. He shows no use of accessory muscles, but he is tachypneic.

Pulses are palpable, and the skin is dry and cool to the touch. Two peripheral intravenous (IV) lines are in place, and normal saline (NS) is running at 100 mL/hour per both with 1500 mL infused. The Foley catheter seems patent, and there is 250 mL of dark urine in the bag. A 1 L canister next to the patient is nearly full of bright red blood. The patient is wearing what appears to be a football helmet. A triple-lumen tube has been pulled through the face guard and secured. The nurse reports that this is a Sengstaken-Blakemore (SB) tube, which has slowed the GI bleeding.

The nurse gives you the report and states that there is concern the patient has upper GI bleeding from esophageal varices. The patient was due to have a transjugular intrahepatic portosystemic shunt (TIPS) procedure done, but he cancelled his last appointment. She hands you the copy of the laboratory results from this visit, and you note that the ammonia level, liver enzymes, and bilirubin are high and the prothrombin time (PT)/international normalized ratio (INR) is elevated. The arterial blood gas (ABG) results show metabolic acidosis with respiratory alkalosis.

As you move the patient onto the transport cot, you notice that he is trying to remove the helmet and special tube.

ANATOMY AND PHYSIOLOGY

The gastrointestinal tract (alimentary canal) is a hollow tube formed by the organs of the digestive system; the mouth, oropharynx, esophagus, stomach, small intestine, large intestine, and rectum (Figure 6-1). The liver, gallbladder, and pancreas are considered accessory organs, because they help with the digestive process and with maintaining the glucose, fat, and protein levels in the body. The main functions of the GI tract are the breakdown and absorption of food. Let's

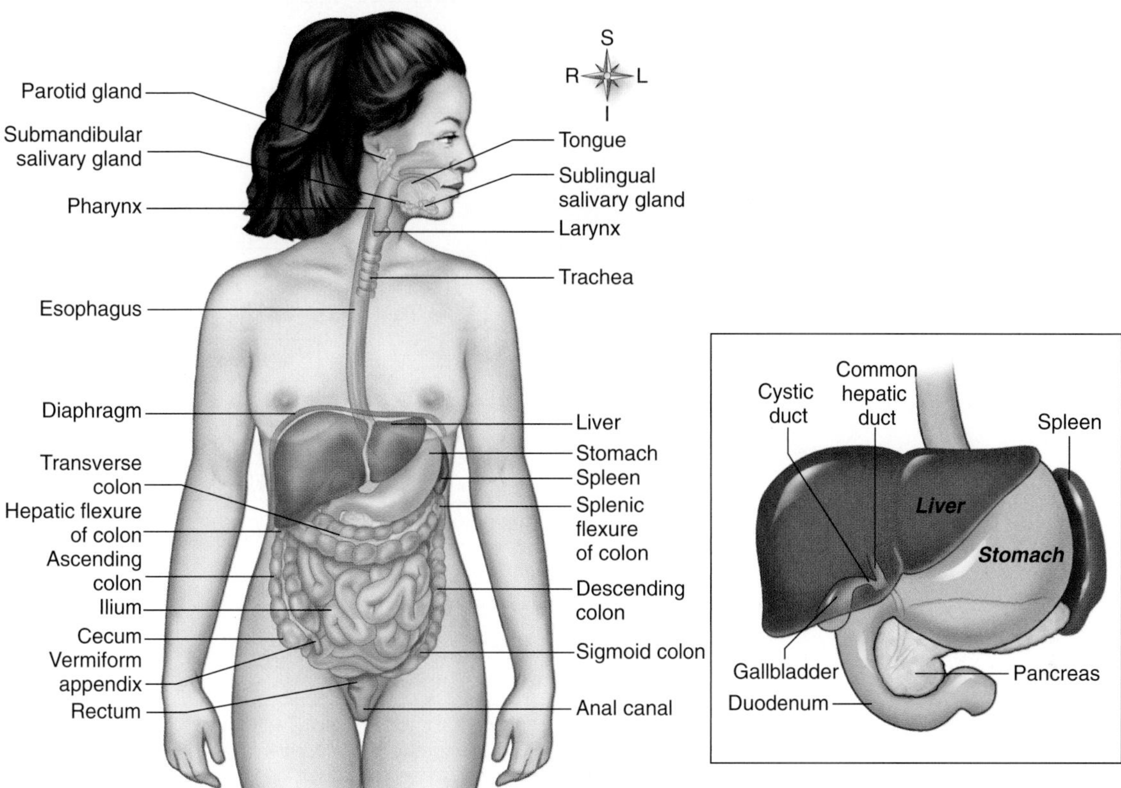

Figure 6-1

Location of the digestive organs. (From Patton KT, Thibodeau GA: *Anatomy and physiology*, ed 7, St Louis, 2009, Mosby.)

follow this process from beginning, ingestion of food, through the absorption of nutrients and elimination of the waste products.

The portion of the GI tract from the esophagus to the rectum has four distinct layers; from innermost to outermost, they are the mucosa, submucosa, **muscularis**, and serosa (Figure 6-2). The layers vary in thickness, and each layer has sublayers. Nerve fibers in the layers control the muscle contractions of peristalsis, and digestive glands in the layers secrete into the lumen of the GI tract through ducts. The layers are reviewed here as they relate to some of the patient conditions discussed later in the chapter.

Mouth

The mouth, with the assistance of the lips, cheeks, tongue, teeth, and salivary glands, aids the initial stage of digestion, which includes ingestion, mastication, and salivation. When food is put into the mouth, chewing begins to breakdown the food and mix it with saliva. Saliva is secreted by three pairs of major salivary glands: the submandibular, sublingual, and parotid glands. The parotid glands secrete enzymes that begin the chemical breakdown of polysaccharides into dextrins and sugars. Saliva contains mostly water, bicarbonate, potassium, chloride, the enzyme alpha amylase, and immunoglobulin A, an essential component in the destruction of oral bacteria and mucus. The body produces a large amount of saliva, about 1 L a day. The salivary glands are regulated by the autonomic nervous system. The teeth cut, tear, and grind the food into smaller particles. The muscular tongue allows a person to taste food, to place the food between the teeth, and to move the food bolus into the oropharynx; it also helps with speech. The tongue should appear slightly rough, pink, and moist.

Pharynx

The pharynx is the connection between the mouth and the esophagus, but it also is the connection between the mouth, nose, and trachea. For the food bolus to be moved from the mouth into the esophagus, the larynx, mouth, and nasopharynx must be closed. Many conditions that affect nerves or muscle, such as a stroke, can cause problems with this phase of swallowing, leading to the aspiration of food and water into the lungs.

Esophagus

The esophagus, the narrowest part of the digestive tube, lies behind the trachea and the heart. It is hollow, collapsible, and approximately 10 inches (25.4 cm) long. It enters the abdomen through the diaphragm and ends at the stomach. The thick inner layer of the esophageal wall protects this passageway from abrasion during swallowing.

The esophagus has two **sphincters**. The **hypopharyngeal sphincter** prevents air from entering the esophagus during

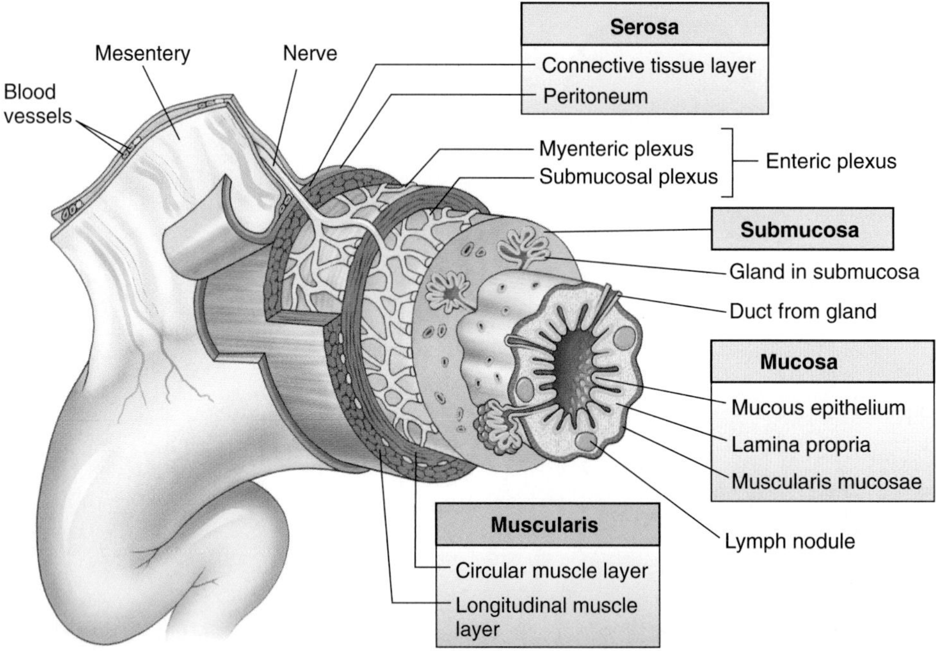

Figure 6-2

The wall of the gastrointestinal (GI) tract is composed of four layers with a network of nerves between the layers. In this general diagram of a segment of the GI tract, note that the serosa is continuous with a fold of serous membrane (the *mesentery*). Also note that digestive glands may empty their products into the lumen of the GI tract by way of ducts. (From McCance KL, Huether SE: *Pathophysiology: the biological basis for disease in adults and children,* ed 6, St Louis, 2009, Mosby.)

respiration. The **cardioesophageal (gastroesophageal) sphincter** allows food to be transferred into the stomach and prevents the reflux of gastric contents. The food bolus moves down the esophagus with the involuntary contraction of the muscle in the wall of the esophagus, a process called *peristalsis.*

Stomach

The stomach is a hollow organ that lies beneath the diaphragm in the epigastric area and left upper abdomen. It has three main areas: the fundus, the body, and the pyloric areas. The opening of the stomach is guarded by the gastroesophageal sphincter, which protects against regurgitation of stomach contents back into the esophagus. The **pyloric sphincter**, at the end of the stomach, opens into the proximal portion of the small intestine, the *duodenum.* Find all of these areas and structures of the stomach in Figure 6-3. The muscles in the lining of the stomach contract in waves to churn the food and mix it with gastric acids. Both of these mechanisms start breaking down the food into smaller particles (Box 6-1).

Large volumes of gastric juices are secreted into the stomach even before the food enters the mouth. The smell and sight of food causes the initial secretion into the stomach. As food is chewed and swallowed into the esophagus, more secretion occurs. The gastric secretions are made up of mucus, water, and significant amounts of potassium, acid, enzymes, and hormone (Box 6-2).

Box 6-1 Functions of the Stomach

- Serve as storage for food until it can be partially digested
- Secrete gastric juice, which includes hydrochloric acid and digestive enzymes
- Mix food (stomach muscles) with gastric juice to start digestion
- Secrete intrinsic factor, which protects vitamin B_{12} until it reaches the small intestine and then aids its absorption
- Secrete gastrin hormone, which helps regulate digestion
- Absorb some water and fatty acids
- Absorb some drugs and alcohol
- Help kill bacteria in food

Did You Know?

Placing a patient with a gastric tube for suctioning (lavage) on continuous suction can cause metabolic alkalosis as a result of removal of hydrochloric acid; it also can cause electrolyte disturbances, especially hypokalemia. In addition, continuous irritation of the gastric mucosa can lead to stress ulcers. For these reasons, intermittent suction is used for patients with a lavage tube.[1]

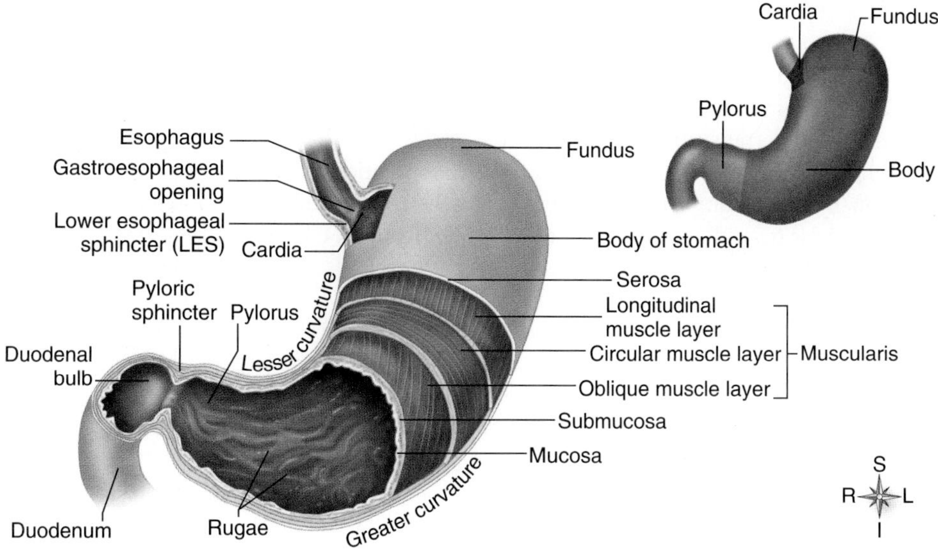

Figure 6-3

A portion of the anterior wall of the stomach has been cut away to show the muscle layers of the stomach wall. Note that the mucosa lining the stomach forms folds, which are called *rugae*. (From Patton KT, Thibodeau GA: *Anatomy and physiology*, ed 7, St Louis, 2009, Mosby.)

Box 6-2 Secretions of the Stomach

- Mucus (lines the stomach and protects the stomach wall from acid and enzymes)
- Enzymes (gastric lipase, pepsinogen, pepsin)
- Acid
  - Dissolves food fibers
  - Kills organisms
  - Converts pepsinogen to pepsin
  - Excessive loss could result in metabolic alkalosis
- Hormones (gastrin and histamine stimulate production of hydrochloric acid)
- Potassium (because the stomach level is higher than the plasma level, vomiting and suctioning can cause significant drops in body potassium)
- Intrinsic factor

Mucus lines the entire stomach and helps protect the stomach from the high level of acid secreted. The parietal cells secrete hydrochloric acid (HCl) and intrinsic factor. The acidic fluid helps dissolve food, denature proteins, and kill ingested bacteria. Intrinsic factor helps protect vitamin B_{12} from the digestive enzymes until it can be absorbed in the small intestine at the terminal ileum. The main gastric enzyme secreted by the stomach is **pepsinogen**, which is converted into pepsin by HCl. Pepsin helps digest proteins. The stomach also secretes hormones such as **gastrin** and histamine. Gastrin helps the stomach secrete gastric juice. Histamine increases the release of hydrochloric acid. The gastric juices also have a high level of potassium; therefore, prolonged vomiting or nasogastric suctioning can cause a significant potassium loss. Limited absorption takes place in the stomach, but some drugs, such as aspirin, can be absorbed along with some water and alcohol.

Small Intestine

The small intestine receives the partly digested food, called **chyme**, from the stomach by way of the pyloric sphincter. The small intestine is approximately 22 to 23 feet long and has three divisions, starting with the duodenum, then the jejunum, and finally the ileum. The ileocecal sphincter is the junction between the ileum and the large intestine. Most nutrients, minerals, and vitamins are absorbed in the small intestine, mostly in the duodenum and jejunum. The small intestine also absorbs most of the water that enters the GI tract.

The movement of chyme into the small intestine starts the intestinal phase of digestion, and gastric secretion decreases. Chyme stimulates the pancreas to secrete an extremely alkaline fluid into the duodenum. Because the pancreatic enzymes work better in an alkaline environment, sodium bicarbonate is secreted into the small intestine. In the duodenum, pancreatic juices are secreted to continue digestion. Carbohydrates are broken down by the pancreatic enzyme amylase. Proteins are broken down further into amino acids and peptides by the enzymes **trypsin, chymotrypsin**, and **carboxypeptidase**.

Bile is secreted by the liver and stored in the gallbladder. When the gallbladder is stimulated the bile enters the duodenum to aid the digestion of fats. Bile contains many substances, but bile salts and **lecithin** break down large drops of fat into smaller droplets and cover the droplets, a process called *emulsification*. Emulsification allows the fat droplets to become water-soluble so that the fat can be broken down by lipase and absorbed in the duodenum. The peristaltic waves and circular movements mix the contents and provide extensive contact with the lining of the small intestine to increase absorption.

Large Intestine

The large intestine is approximately 5 to 6 feet (1.8 meters) long and 2 inches (5.1 cm) in diameter. It is divided into the ascending colon, hepatic flexure, transverse colon, splenic flexure, descending colon, sigmoid colon, rectum, and anal canal. The cecum is a pouch in the right lower quadrant of the abdomen that receives chyme from the ileum. Close to the cecum is a small, narrow tube, the vermiform appendix, which serves as part of the gut barrier. Inflammation of this appendix may cause acute abdominal pain in the right lower quadrant, an indication of appendicitis. The cecum opens into the ascending portion of the colon, which moves toward the liver on the right side of the abdomen. The ascending portion turns, forming the transverse portion of the colon as it crosses to the left side of the abdomen. The transverse colon turns downward, forming the descending colon, which leads into the sigmoid colon (Figure 6-4). Water and electrolytes are absorbed from the chyme in the large intestine. As the chyme enters the sigmoid colon, it is entirely waste products, called *feces,* which include food residue, GI secretions, shredded epithelial cells, and bacteria (Figure 6-4).

Rectum

The rectum is the last 7 to 8 inches (20.3 cm) of the GI tract (the last 1 inch is called the *anal canal*). The walls of the anal canal have vertical folds of tissue, each of which contains an artery and a vein. Hemorrhoids, which are enlargements of the veins in the anal canal, are a common problem. The opening of the canal, the anus, is guarded by two sphincter muscles.

Accessory Organs

As mentioned, the accessory organs of the digestive system are the liver, gallbladder, and pancreas. Figure 6-5 shows the relationships of the accessory organs to each other and to the stomach.

Liver

The liver, the largest organ in the abdomen, weighs about 4 pounds (1.8 kg). It is located under the diaphragm and reaches from the right side over to the epigastric area. The liver has two major lobes, the right lobe and the left lobe (Figure 6-6). Each lobe is divided into lobules, which are hexagonal cylinders that contain the liver cells (hepatocytes). A branch of the hepatic vein extends through the center of each lobule; this is called the *central vein.* On the corners of the lobule are small branches of the hepatic artery, portal vein, and hepatic ducts. The portal vein collects blood from the abdominal organs and dumps the blood into the small branches of the portal vein, called *sinusoids,* which are located between the rows of hepatocytes. Sinusoids also receive arterial blood from branches of the hepatic artery providing oxygen to the liver cells. Venous blood from the sinusoids drains into the central vein. The venous blood from all the central veins flows into the hepatic vein and then back into the main venous supply,

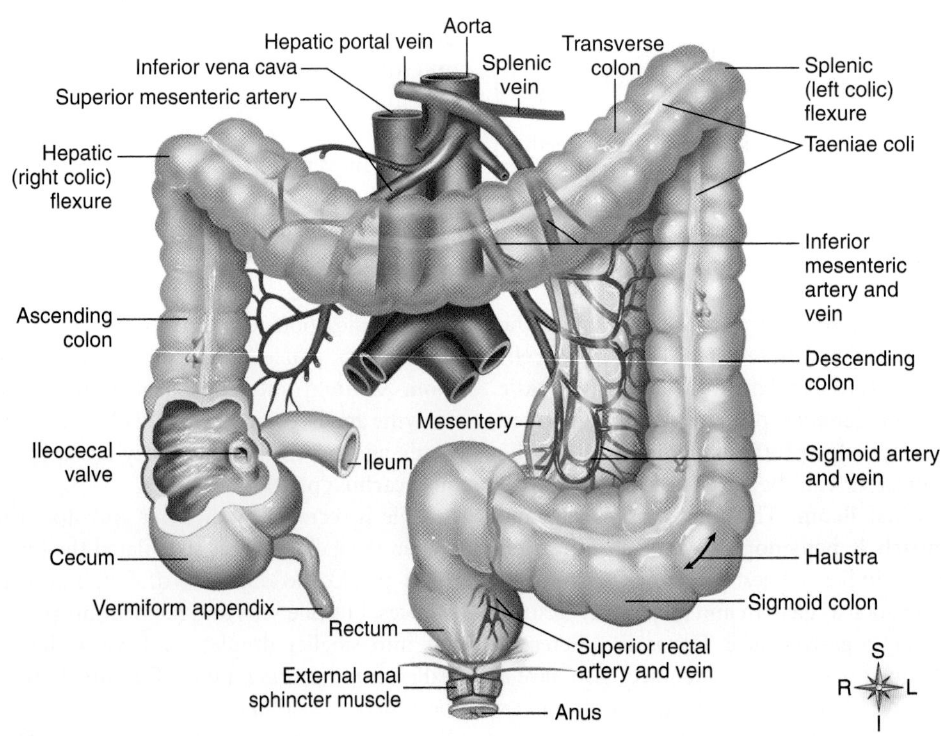

Figure 6-4

Divisions of the large intestine and adjacent vascular structures. (From Patton KT, Thibodeau GA: *Anatomy and physiology,* ed 7, St Louis, 2009, Mosby.)

the inferior vena cava. The sinusoids are lined with **Kupffer cells**, which cleanse the blood of bacteria. The shape of the lobules is extremely important to liver function. Review Figure 6-7 and pay close attention to the structure of the lobule and the configuration of its blood supply.

The liver performs multiple important functions (Box 6-3). It plays a key role in the metabolism of carbohydrates, fats, and proteins and the storage of vitamins and minerals. It also helps maintain the blood sugar level by secreting glucose into the circulation in response to low blood sugar levels. The liver converts monosaccharides to glycogen, which it stores for later use. It also makes glucose from amino acids. The liver affects all nutrients, protein, and fats, not just glucose. It produces albumin, the main plasma protein that helps maintain the intravascular volume. Albumin, which is an *oncotic protein,* keeps fluid in the intravascular space through oncotic pressure gradients. The liver also produces many clotting factors, including prothrombin, which is measured in laboratory tests as the prothrombin time (PT).

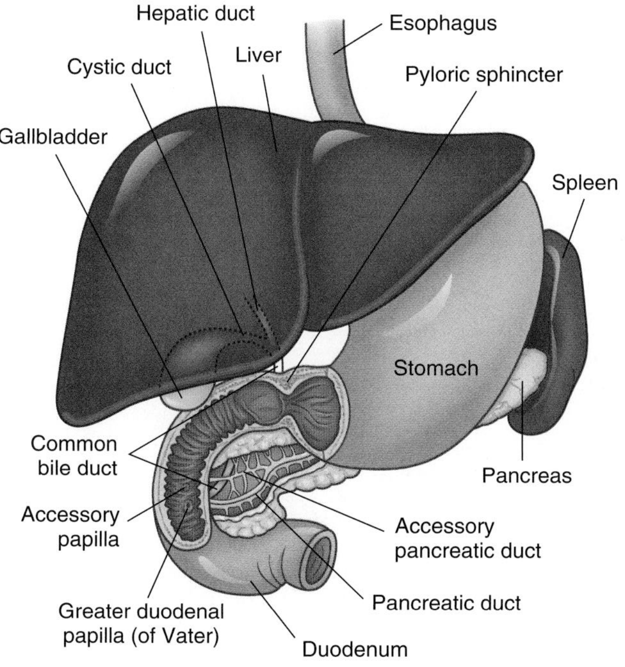

Figure 6-5

Location of the liver, gallbladder, and exocrine pancreas, the accessory organs of digestion. (From McCance KL, Huether SE: *Pathophysiology: the biological basis for disease in adults and children,* ed 6, St Louis, 2009, Mosby.)

Gallbladder

The gallbladder is a saclike organ tucked under the liver. Bile produced by the liver enters the gallbladder through a network of ducts and is stored for future use. The gallbladder opens into the cystic duct, which leads into the common bile duct. The two hepatic ducts from the liver also lead into the common bile duct. Bile passes from the liver through the hepatic ducts into the common bile duct and back up the cystic duct into the gallbladder. The gallbladder stores and concentrates the bile until it is needed for digestion. Approximately 30 minutes after a meal, the gallbladder is stimulated to release bile into the cystic duct, from which it passes into the common bile duct and eventually flows into the duodenum. A sphincter prevents the duodenal contents from entering the bile system. A common problem in the gallbladder is gallstones, which may remain in the cavity of the gallbladder or lodge in the ducts (e.g., cystic duct or common bile duct).

Box 6-3 Functions of the Liver

- Form and excrete bile
- Metabolize carbohydrate, protein, and fat
- Store fat-soluble vitamins A, D, E, and K and minerals
- Inactivate some endocrine hormones (e.g., glucocorticoids)
- Detoxify medications
- Filter the blood (to prevent infections)
- Synthesize many clotting factors
- Synthesize albumin and most globulin proteins
- Synthesize serum enzymes
- Convert ammonia to urea

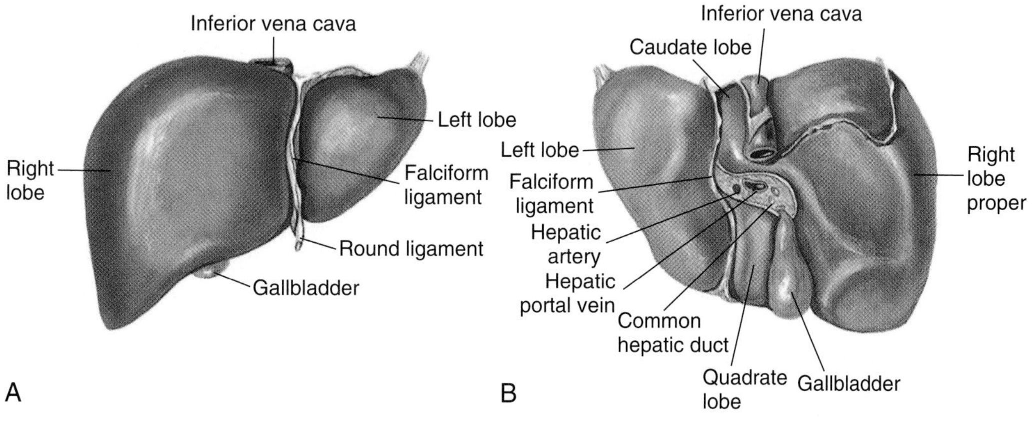

Figure 6-6

Gross structure of the liver. **A,** Anterior view. **B,** Posterior view. (From Carlson KK: *Advanced critical care nursing,* Philadelphia, 2009, Saunders.)

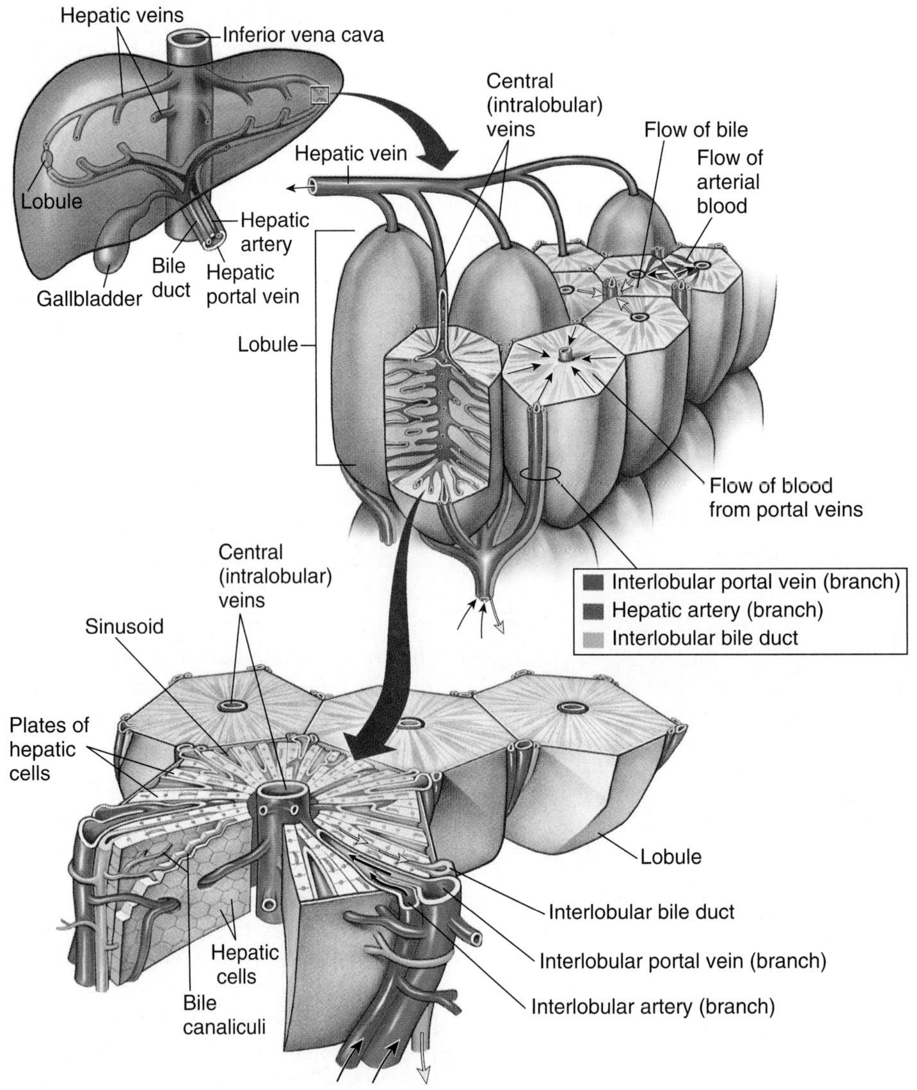

Figure 6-7

Structure of the lobule, the functional unit of the liver. (From Carlson KK: *Advanced critical care nursing*, Philadelphia, 2009, Saunders.)

Pancreas

The pancreas is an eel-like organ located behind the stomach. The head of the pancreas is by the duodenum, and the tail reaches the spleen (Figure 6-8). Most of the pancreatic tissue produces and releases digestive enzymes into the small intestine through the pancreatic duct, which merges with the common bile duct used by the gallbladder; this is considered the exocrine function of the pancreas. The endocrine portion of the pancreas releases insulin, glucagon, and **somatostatin** hormones.

Structural Support and Arterial Blood Supply to the GI Tract

The abdominal organs are loosely held in place by a large, continuous membrane called the *peritoneum* or *peritoneal membrane.* This membrane lines the entire abdominal cavity (parietal layer). The membrane also coats most of the organs in the abdomen (visceral layer). The parietal and visceral layers allow the formation of the peritoneal cavity, the basis for peritoneal dialysis used in patients with renal failure.

The GI tract receives a rich supply of arterial blood from the aorta. The blood supply is greatest during active digestion and decreases dramatically between meals. Because most organs have at least two sources of arterial blood, problems usually develop only when both arteries are impaired. In a critically ill patient, especially a patient with hypovolemia or low cardiac output from other causes, a decrease in the blood supply to the GI tract sets the patient up for potential complications. The mesenteric arteries that feed the small intestine are the most common sites of diminished blood flow, which may result in ischemia or necrosis.

ASSESSMENT OF THE GI TRACT

History

When taking a patient's history, pay special attention to the current symptoms. Common symptoms related to the GI tract

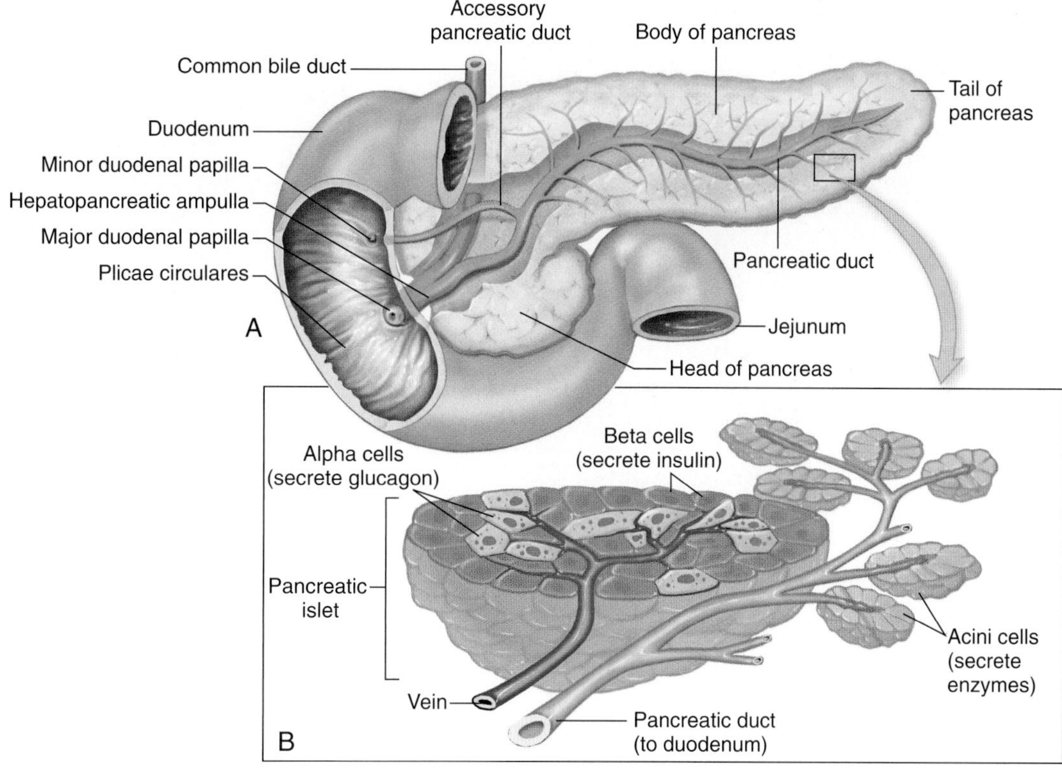

Figure 6-8

A, Pancreas dissected to show the main and accessory ducts. The main duct may join the common bile duct, as shown here, to enter the duodenum by a single opening at the major duodenal papilla, or the two ducts may have separate openings. The accessory pancreatic duct usually is present and has a separate opening into the duodenum. **B,** Exocrine glandular cells (around the small pancreatic ducts) and endocrine glandular cells of the pancreatic islets (adjacent to the blood capillaries). Exocrine pancreatic cells secrete pancreatic juice, alpha endocrine cells secrete glucagon, and beta cells secrete insulin. (From Patton KT, Thibodeau GA: *Anatomy and physiology*, ed 7, St Louis, 2009, Mosby.)

include nausea, vomiting, burning, pain, and diarrhea or constipation. Patients do not always complain the loudest about the most significant symptom. In many cases the patient has had a similar episode, and you can compare the present symptoms to past symptoms.

As you know, the patient's medication history is important. Patients use many over-the-counter (OTC) medications for GI symptoms. Ask directly about these nonprescription medications. For example, in one case a patient who was diagnosed with a life-threatening electrolyte and metabolic disorder failed to report his use of nonprescription medications. After some time, the clinician discovered that the cause of the disorder was an overdose of an antacid. Another serious example of the significance of OTC medications is the use (or misuse) of acetaminophen (e.g., Tylenol), which is a major cause of liver toxicity and failure. As you attend your patients, let the person's history, current symptoms, and vital signs guide the care you provide.

Inspection

After assessing the ABCDs and determining that no emergency interventions are required for those processes, evaluate the patient's overall appearance. The color of the skin, mucous membranes, and sclerae of the eye can provide information about the GI system. For example, jaundice caused by a pathologic liver condition gives the skin and sclerae a yellow-orange color. Observe the patient's posture. Patients with abdominal pain may try to position the body to reduce the pain, which can be a clue to the origin of the pain. Assessing the moistness of the tongue and surrounding mucous membranes provides information about the patient's hydration status. If the patient has signs of hypovolemia, inspect for signs of bleeding. If possible, inspect the abdomen for obvious scars, recent wounds, or suture lines. Check for **Cullen's sign** (a bluish tint around the umbilicus) or **Grey Turner's sign** (discoloration and induration of the skin of the costovertebral angle), which may indicate intraperitoneal bleeding. Also look for an abnormal abdominal contour, which might indicate a mass or hernia.

The abdomen usually is divided into quadrants, with the umbilicus as the center point (Figure 6-9). The organs in each quadrant can serve as a guide to an underlying pathologic condition. The right upper quadrant (RUQ) includes the liver, gallbladder, duodenum, pancreas, right kidney, right adrenal gland, and part of the ascending and transverse colon. The left upper quadrant (LUQ) includes the stomach, spleen, left lobe of the liver, left kidney, left adrenal gland, and part of the transverse and descending colon. The right lower quadrant (RLQ) contains the cecum, appendix, right ovary, and right ureter. The left lower quadrant (LLQ) contains the

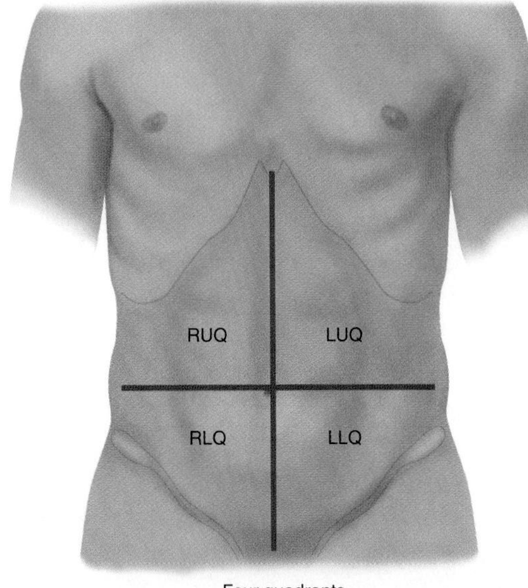

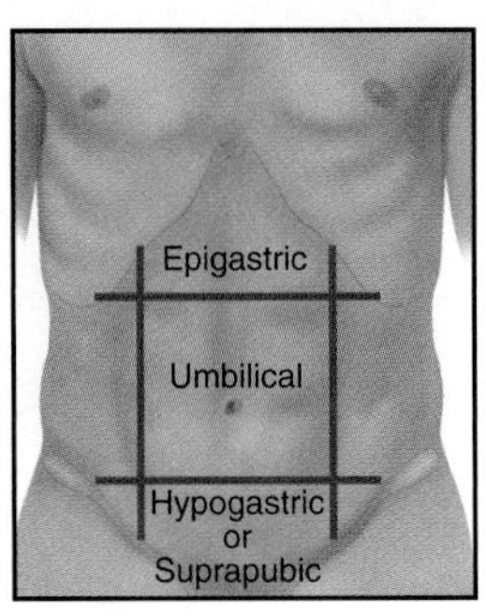

Figure 6-9

Abdominal quadrants. (From Jarvis C, Thomas P: *Physical examination and health assessment,* ed 5, St Louis, 2008, Mosby.)

left ovary, left ureter, sigmoid colon, and part of the descending colon.

Auscultation

Normal bowel sounds are high-pitched, gurgling, irregular sounds that occur approximately five to 30 times a minute. All quadrants of the abdomen should have bowel sounds. Hyperactive bowel sounds are louder and occur more frequently than normal; hypoactive sounds are more difficult to hear and much less common over several minutes (Table 6-1). Hypoactive or absent bowel sounds indicate decreased motility of the GI tract. When listening to bowel sounds, you should use the diaphragm of the stethoscope, applying it with light pressure; start below and to the right of the umbilicus and work your way systematically through all quadrants.

Percussion

In the prehospital environment, we have always heard that using percussion to assist with our assessments is difficult. However, with critical care patients, it is imperative to obtain as much information as possible during the assessment. Percussion can provide information about the deep organs in the abdomen, such as the size and position of the liver and spleen; it also can help detect fluid, distention, and masses. Percussion should be performed before palpation. Because the abdomen is sensitive, muscle tensing is common during assessment, and percussion often helps relax the tense muscles. Using a light touch, follow an organized approach through all four regions. Normal sounds include **tympany** over the stomach, **hyperresonance** over the intestines, and dullness over the liver. Abnormal sounds include dullness in the areas of both flanks, which may indicate ascites; other areas of dullness may be caused by masses, a distended bladder, or enlarged organs.

Palpation

Light palpation of the abdomen should not cause any pain if the patient is in the proper position (i.e., knees and hips flexed). Tenderness on palpation usually indicates inflammation. The patient also may have rebound tenderness if the peritoneal membrane is inflamed. Rebound tenderness is assessed by applying pressure to the abdominal wall and then quickly releasing the pressure; pain after the release is an indication of rebound tenderness. Palpate the abdomen for firmness, which may indicate fluid or blood in the abdomen. Areas the patient indicates are tender should be palpated last.

Did You Know?

The assessment sequence for the abdominal area is:

1. **First, look**
2. **Then listen**
3. **Then feel**

Palpation of the abdomen can actually quiet bowel sounds for several minutes; it also can cause pain, which may distort the rest of the examination.[2]

DIAGNOSTICS AND LABORATORY VALUES

Laboratory Tests for the GI Tract

Two laboratory tests commonly used for diagnosis of the GI tract and for continuing assessment are the complete blood

Table 6-1 Abnormal Abdominal Sounds

Sound	Possible Cause
Hyperactive bowel sounds (borborygmi), loud and prolonged: High pitched, tinkling sounds	Hunger, gastroenteritis, or early intestinal obstruction
	Intestinal air and fluid under pressure; characteristic of early intestinal obstruction
Decreased (hypoactive) bowel sounds: Infrequent and abnormally faint	Possible peritonitis or ileus
Absence of bowel sounds (confirmed only after auscultation of all four quadrants and continuous auscultation for 5 min)	Temporary loss of intestinal motility, as occurs with complete ileus
Friction rubs: High-pitched sounds heard over liver and spleen (RUQ and LUQ), synchronous with respiration	Pathologic conditions (e.g., tumors, infection) that cause inflammation of organ's peritoneal covering
Bruits: Audible swishing sounds that may be heard over aortic, iliac, renal, and femoral arteries	Abnormality of blood flow (requires additional evaluation to determine specific disorder)
Venous hum: Low-pitched, continuous sound	Increased collateral circulation between portal and systemic venous systems

Doughty DB, Jackson DB: *Gastrointestinal disorders,* St Louis, 1993, Mosby.
RUQ, Right upper quadrant; *LUQ,* left upper quadrant.

count (CBC) and the serum electrolyte levels. The hematocrit (Hct), which measures the volume of red blood cells in relation to the volume of plasma, is affected by changes in volume status; it increases with severe dehydration and decreases with severe hemorrhage or overhydration. Men have a slightly higher Hct (40% to 54%) than women (37% to 46%).

Many GI disorders can cause electrolyte disturbances. Patients with diarrhea and vomiting are at risk for potassium and sodium losses, and patients with bowel obstructions may have a low sodium level. The normal levels for the electrolytes and the symptoms of electrolyte disorders are presented in Boxes 6-9 to 6-12 later in the chapter.

Laboratory tests required for the diagnosis of individual disorders may include liver enzyme levels, coagulation studies, and albumin levels for liver disorders; blood urea nitrogen (BUN) and creatinine levels for volume status and renal function; and lipase levels for conditions of the pancreas. Table 6-2 lists some laboratory tests that may be used for the GI tract.

Did You Know?

A patient may appear to have GI bleeding when in fact oral or nasal bleeding or trauma is the source of the blood. The patient may swallow blood from an oral source (or, for example, from a nosebleed 6 hours earlier) and vomit it up later; this can mimic GI bleeding. It is important to check for any such circumstances and to ask the patient about them when possible.[3]

DISORDERS AND MANAGEMENT OF THE GI SYSTEM

Gastrointestinal Bleeding

GI bleeding is a common complaint in the emergency department and is frequently seen in critically ill patients. According to Thelan's critical care book, GI bleeding results in approximately 300,000 hospital admissions a year. The mortality rate is 7% to 10%, and despite the medical advances that continually occur, the rate has not changed in more than 50 years

The main functions of the GI tract are digestion and the absorption of nutrients. To accomplish these purposes, the GI tract has a vast network of blood vessels, where bleeding can occur at any point. Upper GI bleeding occurs from the esophagus to the duodenum. Lower GI bleeding occurs from the jejunum to the rectum. The anatomic division between the upper and lower GI tracts is the **ligament of Treitz**, a suspensory ligament at the juncture of the duodenum and the jejunum.

The patient may have chronic bleeding in small amounts daily or massive hemorrhage. The appearance of the blood and the area where it is observed may help differentiate upper GI bleeding from lower GI bleeding (Box 6-4). If the patient vomits bright red blood, this usually is a sign that the blood is coming from the upper GI tract and the bleeding started recently. If blood has been in the stomach for a time, the vomited blood will be partly digested and have the appearance of coffee grounds. If the stool looks black and tarry (i.e., melanotic stool), the blood has undergone extensive digestion and is probably from the upper GI tract. Bright red blood in the stool usually is from the lower part of the colon or rectum, because no digestion occurs in the colon. However, keep in mind that larger amounts of upper GI bleeding can increase peristalsis, which pushes large amounts of GI blood through to the colon in a short time, making it appear bright red.

Assessment of GI Bleeding

The patient's response to bleeding is based on the amount of blood lost, the duration of the blood loss, and other co-morbidities. The patient's and family members' perceptions of the amount of blood lost before your arrival often are inaccurate and overestimated. To estimate blood loss, pay

Table 6-2 Laboratory Tests for the Gastrointestinal System

Parameter	Description	Normal Values*	Abnormal Findings†
Albumin	Main protein of plasma; maintains oncotic pressure	3.5-5.5 g/dL	*Increased:* Peptic ulcer, nephrosis, dehydration *Decreased:* Liver injury, cirrhosis, ascites, malnutrition
Alkaline phosphatase (ALT)	Enzyme found in bone, liver, intestine, and placental tissue	13-39 units/L	*Increased:* Biliary obstruction, hepatitis from gallbladder disease, intestinal ischemia or infarction, cirrhosis *Decreased:* Malnutrition
Ammonia	Waste product from nitrogen breakdown during protein metabolism	9.5-49 mcg/dL	*Increased:* Liver disease, encephalopathy, gastrointestinal bleeding
Amylase	Enzyme produced by the pancreas to digest carbohydrates	30-110 units/L	*Increased:* Acute pancreatitis, penetrating/perforating peptic ulcer, necrotic bowel, acute cholecystitis, bowel obstruction
Aspartate aminotransferase (AST)	Enzyme found in the heart, liver, and muscle tissue	5-40 units/L	*Increased:* Cirrhosis, hepatitis, pancreatitis, intestinal injury, alcoholism, trauma *Decreased:* Total liver failure
Bilirubin	Produced in the liver, spleen and bone marrow, by product of hemoglobin breakdown	Total bilirubin: <1 mg/dL Indirect (unconjugated): <0.8 mg/dL Direct (conjugated)	*Increased indirect (unconjugated):* Hepatitis, cirrhosis, sepsis, hemolysis *Increased direct (conjugated):* Gallstones, extrahepatic duct obstruction, extensive liver metastasis, cholestasis
C-reactive protein	Abnormal glycoprotein produced by the liver during acute inflammation		*Increased:* Pancreatitis (best indicator of pancreatitis but can be elevated with other types of acute inflammation)
Globulins	Plasma proteins formed in the liver; lymphatic: alpha, beta, gamma	2-5.2 g/dL	*Increased:* Hepatitis
Helicobacter pylori	Bacterium	Negative	*Positive:* Infection of the stomach; cause of most peptic ulcers
Hematocrit	Percentage of red blood cells in a volume of blood	Males: 41%-53% Females: 36%-48%	*Increased:* Dehydration, severe diarrhea *Decreased:* Anemia, renal disease, hemorrhage
Hemoglobin	Oxygen-carrying protein in the red blood cells	Males: 13.5-17.5 g/dL Females: 12-16 g/dL	*Increased:* Hemoconcentration late in bowel obstruction *Decreased:* Anemia, renal disease, liver disease
Lactate dehydrogenase (LDH)	Enzyme found in almost all body tissues; isoenzymes can be measured to differentiate which tissue released LDH	135-225 units/L	*Increased:* Liver, renal disease, pancreatitis, hemolysis
Lactic acid	Byproduct of carbohydrate metabolism during anaerobic metabolism	0.5-2.2 mmol/L	*Increased:* Shock, sepsis, heart failure, tissue ischemia, severe liver disease
Lipase	Pancreatic enzyme for fats	31-141 units/L	*Increased: Acute* and chronic pancreatitis, pancreatic cancer, acute cholecystitis, renal failure, bowel obstruction, peptic ulcers
Partial thromboplastin time (PTT)	Evaluates coagulation system	26-39 sec	*Increased:* Liver disease, disseminated intravascular coagulation (DIC), heparin
Prothrombin time (PT)	Evaluates coagulation system	12.5-14.5 sec	*Increased:* Liver disease, warfarin, DIC, bile duct obstruction, vitamin K deficiency
Gamma glutamyltransferase	Enzyme found in the liver, bile ducts, and kidney	Males: 7-40 units/L Females: 4-25 units/L	*Increased:* Acetaminophen toxicity, biliary disease, liver disease

*Many laboratory tests can be processed by different methods, which have different normal values; use the normal value specified by your laboratory.
†The causes of abnormal findings included in this table indicate a gastrointestinal or genitourinary problem; consult a laboratory manual for other causes.

Box 6-4 Causes of Gastrointestinal Bleeding

Esophagus

Varices
Inflammation
Gastritis, gastroesophageal reflux
Ulcers
Tumors
Mallory-Weiss tears

Stomach

Ulcers
Gastritis
Tumors
Angiodysplasia
Varices

Small Intestine

Ulcers
Angiodysplasia
Crohn's disease
Diverticulitis

Large Intestine

Tumors
Polyps
Ulcerative colitis
Crohn's disease
Diverticulosis
Escherichia coli and other enteroinvasive bacterial infections
Anal or rectal fissures
Hemorrhoids

Table 6-3 Clinical Classification of Hemorrhage

Class	Blood Loss (%)	Clinical Signs and Symptoms
1	≤15	Pulse rate: Normal or <100 beats/min (supine) Capillary refill: <3 sec Urine output: Adequate (30-35 mL/hour) Orthostatic hypotension Apprehensive
2	15-30	Pulse rate: Increased (>100 beats/min) Capillary refill: Sluggish Pulse pressure: Decreased Blood pressure: Normal (supine) Urine output: Low (25-30 mL/hour) Tachypnea
3	30-40	Pulse rate: >120 beats/min (supine) Hypotension Skin: Cool, pale Confused Hyperventilating Urine output: Low (5-15 mL/hour)
4	≥40	Pulse rate: >140+ beats/min Profoundly hypotensive Confused, lethargic Urine output minimal

From Klein DG: *AACN Clin Issues Crit Care Nurs* a:508, 1990.

careful attention to the clinical picture, laboratory findings, and vital signs. Outright hypotension in a supine patient usually indicates loss of about 40% of the total blood volume. Blood loss activates the compensatory mechanism for shock. In most patients who have not been medicated, the sympathetic nervous system increases the heart rate and constricts the arteries to maintain perfusion. Constriction of arteries to shunt blood to critical organs may result in cold, clammy skin, decreased urinary output, and changes in the patient's level of consciousness (LOC).

The Hct does not immediately decline as the patient is losing whole blood; rather a decreased Hct reflects the degree of blood loss after 24 hours. The Hct also can be decreased as a result of hemodilution from emergency fluid resuscitation. Therefore, the initial Hct measurements are not reliable indicators for guiding blood replacement. The patient also requires coagulation studies and measurement of the electrolyte levels, BUN, and creatinine. The BUN may be increased as a result of digestion of blood, and the BUN to creatinine ratio may be increased to 20:1 (Normal ratio is 10-20:1). (More information about the BUN and creatinine is presented in the renal section later in this chapter.)

Clinical Presentation of GI Bleeding

The clinical presentation of patients with GI bleeding depends very much on the amount of blood lost. Clinical classifications of hemorrhage are used to describe the degrees of blood loss and their signs and symptoms (Table 6-3).

Management of the Bleeding Patient

Some patients with GI bleeding may stop bleeding on their own; however, these patients still require support until the bleeding stops. In the initial phases, the management of a patient with GI bleeding is similar to the treatment given to any bleeding patient. We are trained to look for any bleeding that can be compressed and stopped. Because compression of the GI tract is difficult, the initial management in these cases is resuscitation.

As always, you first assess the ABCDs. Does the patient need intubation? A patient who is vomiting blood is at risk for aspiration and inability to protect the airway. With massive bleeding, volume loss may be great enough to impair the LOC, leaving the patient unable to maintain the airway. Assess the breathing effort. Most emergency patients breathe rapidly out of anxiety and fear, but a shock state also can increase the respiratory rate. If the patient is in shock, the peripheral circulation may be severely vasoconstricted, and pulse oximetry may not be as accurate. Assess the patient for other signs of respiratory distress and hypoxia. Administer the level of oxygen appropriate to your assessment of the patient's breathing status. Even if breathing is adequate and pulse oximetry is normal, always give the patient low flow oxygen.

Circulation is assessed by checking the pulse and blood pressure and evaluating the peripheral circulation. Vascular access must be obtained, and aggressive fluid resuscitation is performed in certain circumstances using NS or lactated Ringer's solution (LRS) and guided by hemodynamic monitoring. With active bleeding, a bolus of 500 mL should be administered quickly and the patient's hemodynamic status then reassessed. Patients who continue to bleed, requiring more than 4 to 5 units of packed red blood cells, may also need other blood products, such as platelets and fresh frozen plasma. The goal usually is to maintain the patient with IV fluids until typing and cross-matching can be completed.

Ulcers

An ulcer is a break into the mucosa of the GI tract that may extend through multiple layers of the GI wall. The two most common types of ulcers are peptic ulcers and stress ulcers. Peptic ulcers are the most common ulcers, and stress ulcers are a complication seen in critically ill patients. Ulcers are caused by the action of acid and peptic juices on the mucosal lining of the GI tract; they are the result of an imbalance between the **gastroduodenal mucosal defense mechanism** and the level of gastric acid and pepsin.

In the United States, about 5 million people have peptic ulcer disease (PUD). Peptic ulcers occur most often in the duodenum but may also develop in the stomach. The ulcer typically presents as an individual lesion less than 4 cm in diameter that may penetrate all layers of the GI wall (Figure 6-10). Almost all patients with a duodenal ulcer have a ***Helicobacter pylori*** infection. This infection also causes about 70% of gastric ulcers. *H. pylori* infections occur in a large percentage of the population, but only 10% to 20% of those infected develop peptic ulcers. The bacterium does not invade the tissues, but rather causes increased inflammation and immune response in the area. Hyperacidity along with the infection increases the risk of ulceration. Conditions that may increase acidity include excessive secretion of gastrin, chronic use of nonsteroidal antiinflammatory drugs (NSAIDs), alcohol abuse, smoking, and high-dose corticosteroid or long-term steroid use. Conditions closely associated with the development of duodenal peptic ulcers include cirrhosis, chronic obstructive pulmonary disease (COPD), renal failure, and hyperparathyroidism. Peptic ulcers often heal without treatment but frequently recur, eventually requiring treatment.

Peptic ulcers may cause a gnawing, burning pain in the epigastric area. If the ulcer perforates the entire GI wall, the

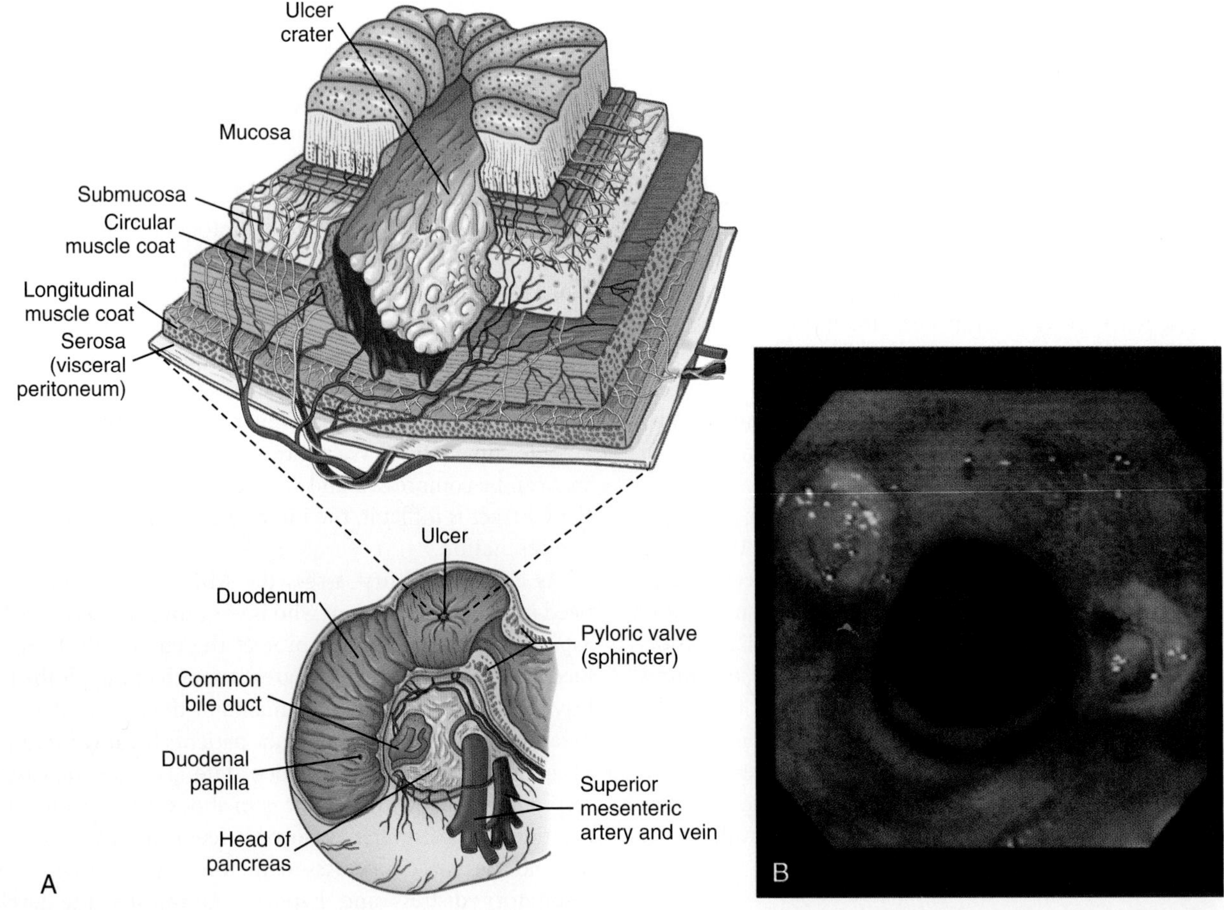

Figure 6-10

Duodenal ulcer. **A,** A deep ulceration in the duodenal wall extends as a crater through the entire mucosa and into the muscle layers. **B,** Endoscopic view of a duodenal ulcer. (From Carlson KK: *Advanced critical care nursing*, Philadelphia, 2009, Saunders.)

pain may radiate to the back, left upper abdominal quadrant, or chest; it has been known to mimic the pain of a myocardial infarction. Peptic ulcer pain frequently is felt between meals, during meals, or at night. Pain from ulcers in the stomach often is relieved by antacids and occurs during eating, although these are not absolute findings. The pain of duodenal ulcers may be relieved by food. Patients with gastric ulcers usually have more anorexia, vomiting, and weight loss. Table 6-4 presents the characteristics of gastric and duodenal peptic ulcers.

A stress ulcer is also known as *stress-related erosive syndrome* (SRES) (a **syndrome** is a set of symptoms that occur together) or *hemorrhagic gastritis.* It occurs as a result of physiologic and psychological stress that disrupts the balance between a healthy mucosal lining and increased gastric acid secretion. Stress ulcers tend to occur at multiple sites and are distributed mainly in the stomach, with some in the duodenum. They are irregular erosions into one or two layers of the GI wall and usually do not perforate the entire wall. A reduction in the mucosal blood flow is a common contributing event in a critically ill patient. All patients in the critical care unit should be considered at high risk for the development of stress ulcers. Some conditions that pose a very high risk include trauma; cerebral injury, especially with increased intracranial pressure; all forms of shock; severe burns; heart failure; and sepsis. A patient with a low risk initially has an increased risk if placed on a mechanical ventilator. Although fewer than 4% of patients with a stress ulcer have a large hemorrhage requiring transfusion, the mortality rate rises dramatically with massive hemorrhage. A prophylactic regimen of proton pump inhibitors or histamine 2 (H_2) blockers has reduced the incidence of stress ulcers in critical care patients.

Did You Know?

The top five causes of both upper and lower GI bleeding are as follows[4]:

Upper GI Bleeding
Duodenal ulcers (50%)
Gastric erosions (23%)
Varices (10%)
Mallory-Weiss tears (7%)
Esophagitis (6%)

Lower GI Bleeding
Diverticulosis (43%)
Angiodysplasia (20%)
Undetermined (12%)
Neoplasms (9%)
Colitis (9%)

Management of a Patient with Ulcers

In addition to fluid resuscitation for bleeding (discussed earlier), a patient with a bleeding ulcer requires treatment aimed at stopping the bleeding and treating the ulcer to prevent rebleeding. During active bleeding, lavage of the stomach through a nasogastric tube may be tried. Years ago, the accepted treatment for GI bleeding was gastric lavage with iced saline or tap water. It has now been determined that iced

Table 6-4 Characteristics of Gastric and Duodenal Ulcers

Characteristics	Gastric Ulcer	Duodenal Ulcer
Incidence		
Age at onset	50-70 yr	20-50 yr
Family history	Usually negative	Positive
Gender (prevalence)	Equal in women and men	Equal in women and men
Stress factors	Increased	Average
Ulcerogenic drugs	Normal use	Increased use
Cancer risk	Increased	Not increased
Pathophysiology		
Abnormal mucus	May be present	May be present
Parietal cell mass	Normal or decreased	Increased
Acid production	Normal or decreased	Increased
Serum gastrin	Increased	Normal
Serum pepsinogen	Normal	Increased
Associated gastritis	More common	Usually not present
Helicobacter pylori	May be present (60%-80%)	Often present (95%-100%)
Clinical Manifestations		
Pain	Located in upper abdomen	Located in upper abdomen
	Intermittent	Intermittent
	Pain–antacid relief pattern	Pain–antacid or –food relief pattern
	Food-pain pattern	Nocturnal pain common
Clinical course	Chronic ulcer without pattern of remission and exacerbation	Pattern of remission and exacerbation for years

From McCance K, Huether SE: *Pathophysiology: the biological basis for disease in adults and children,* ed 6, St Louis, 2009, Mosby.

lavage is not effective in controlling the bleeding; in addition, it may increase mucosal damage and drop the patient's core body temperature. Gastric lavage remains a controversial treatment; therefore, the question is whether to lavage or not to lavage. Some experts believe that lavage does not have any benefit. Others believe that it may be beneficial for clearing out blood and clots before endoscopic procedures. If large volumes are to be used, the lavage solution should be warmed slightly to avoid lowering the body temperature. The recommended solution for large-volume lavage is NS or LRS, rather than tap water, to reduce the movement of electrolytes out of the stomach. If only small amounts of fluid will be used, room-temperature tap water is acceptable. Skill 6-1 reviews the steps of gastric lavage.

Skill 6-1

GASTRIC LAVAGE

The process of passing a gastric tube into the stomach or duodenum to wash out toxic substances or control hemorrhage has been used for nearly two centuries, yet little evidence supports its continued widespread use, especially for cases of gastrointestinal (GI) decontamination.

Considerations for this therapy include the timing of the ingestion and the patient's state of consciousness and ability to cooperate and maintain the airway. Clinical studies have not confirmed the benefit of gastric lavage overall for victims of toxic ingestion, and the procedure should not be considered unless it can be performed within 60 minutes of ingestion in an alert, oriented patient. In patients with GI hemorrhage, isotonic fluid (saline) can be administered and then drained; this cleanses the stomach of clots and blood, allowing a GI specialist to identify the source of the bleeding endoscopically.

INDICATIONS

Ingestion of a life-threatening amount of toxin (within 1 hour of ingestion)

Active upper GI bleeding

CONTRAINDICATIONS

Patient with a diminished level of consciousness or diminished ability to maintain the airway (unless intubated)

Ingestion of corrosive substances (acid, alkali)

Ingestion of a hydrocarbon with high aspiration potential

Patient at risk of hemorrhage or GI perforation because of a pathologic condition or recent surgery, or who has some other medical condition that could be further compromised by gastric lavage

Combative patient (may be at greater risk of complications)

COMPLICATIONS

Aspiration pneumonia

Laryngospasm

Hypoxia and hypercapnia

Mechanical injury to the throat, esophagus, and stomach

Fluid and electrolyte imbalance

PROCEDURE

1. The patient should be thoroughly evaluated and well prepared for gastric lavage; perform preprocedural patient education. Monitors, oxygen, suction equipment, and IV access (two lines), along with good patient positioning, help facilitate the procedure.
2. Facilitate intubation if the patient may not be able to follow commands, cooperate, or maintain the airway during the procedure. Place an oral airway or bite block between the patient's teeth.
3. Wash your hands and follow full standard precautions.
4. Use a large-bore tube: 36 to 40 Fr (30 English gauge) for adults; 24 to 28 Fr for children. The tube should have a rounded end and should be firm enough to pass into the stomach through the mouth, yet flexible enough not to damage the mucosa.
5. Assemble and pretest the suction equipment. Gather the appropriate fluids and syringes.
6. Measure the distance from the bridge of the patient's nose to the earlobe and then to the tip of the xiphoid process. Note this distance on the gastric tube for proper positioning after insertion.
7. Position the patient in the left lateral decubitus position with the head of the bed elevated 10 to 20 degrees and the bed adjusted to a slight reverse Trendelenburg position. This facilitates entry of the tube into the stomach. As an alternative, high Fowler's position may be used.
8. Lubricate 6 to 10 cm of the distal end of the tube with hydroxyethylcellulose jelly. Follow your protocols for use of a topical anesthetic in the oropharynx.
9. Aiming the tube back and down, insert it into the oral cavity over the tongue. When the tube is positioned against the pharynx, flex the patient's head forward to facilitate passage. (If the patient is conscious, having the person swallow sips of water can help the tube pass.) If the patient has been intubated, use capnography to make sure the endotracheal tube (ETT) is in the proper position.

10. If you meet resistance while passing the tube, rotating the tube may help. Continue to advance the tube until the predetermined depth (see step 6) is achieved.
11. Attach a syringe to the suction tip, aspirate fluid, and evaluate the pH of the fluid. Normal values are <5.5 for gastric fluid and >6 for intestinal fluid; if the tube was placed incorrectly into the respiratory tree, the fluid will be alkaline (>7).
12. Ask the patient to speak; phonation indicates that the tube has not entered the vocal cords.
13. Secure the properly positioned tube with tape or another device.
14. Aspirate the gastric contents and note the amount and color.

Gastric Decontamination

15. In an adult patient, use 200 to 300 mL of warm fluid (normal saline [NS]) or water. In children, instill 10 mL/kg of body weight of warmed saline. Avoid water intoxication and/or hyponatremia with large amounts of absorbed tap water.
16. Aspirate fluid at low suction (80 mm Hg) or with an attached syringe. Continue until the fluid is clear of particulate matter.

Gastric Hemorrhage

17. Nasogastric or orogastric lavage can be performed in patients with upper GI bleeding (see illustration). Most causes of upper GI bleeding can be identified by esophagogastroduodenoscopy (EGD) and subsequently treated with coagulation, injection, embolization, or banding.

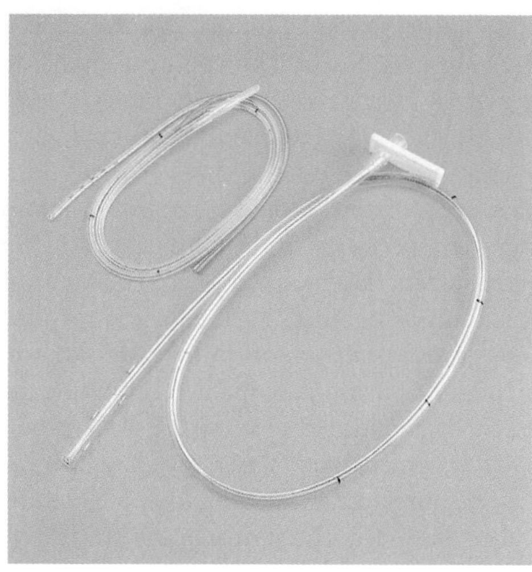

Top, Nasogastric/orogastric tube. *Bottom,* Oral gastric lavage tube. Sanders M: *Mosby's paramedic textbook*, ed 3, St Louis, 2007, Mosby.

18. Confirm radiographically that no free air is present in the abdomen.
19. Use of an aspiration syringe, rather than continuous suction, is preferable.
20. When the procedure is finished, clamp the tube and remove it slowly and steadily. If esophageal spasm is detected (i.e., you have difficulty removing the tube), glucagon may be given subcutaneously or intramuscularly.

Endoscopic Examination and Treatment

Endoscopy is used to diagnose the cause of GI bleeding and, in many patients, also to treat the ulcer. For **esophagogastroduodenoscopy (EGD)**, the endoscope is inserted through the mouth and down to the duodenum. EGD can be done during active bleeding or after the bleeding stops to prevent recurrence. During EGD, the mucosal wall of all the structures is examined and may be photographed, biopsied, or cultured for *H. pylori.*

If a lesion is found during EGD, the clinician has several therapy options. Endoscopic treatment to stop bleeding or prevent recurrent bleeding of the same lesion has a very high success rate. The bleeding can be stopped with a heater probe or laser coagulation. Many physicians use injection of a substance into the ulcer (e.g., ethanol, epinephrine, saline, or sclerosing agents) to stop the bleeding. Epinephrine injection into a bleeding ulcer constricts the vessels and frequently stops the bleeding. A **sclerosing agent** causes scarring over the area, preventing future bleeding.

The endoscope also can be used to attach a band or clip that pulls the sides of the ulcer together, allowing the tissue to fuse over time. This technique is not used as much as injection therapy, and it usually is not attempted during active bleeding.

During the endoscopic procedure, the patient must be continually assessed for airway compromise and hemodynamic stability. The patient usually is given some form of sedation if the blood pressure is acceptable. You must watch the patient's vital signs and respiratory status and continue fluid resuscitation as needed. Follow the guidelines for a conscious sedation procedure. If the bleeding cannot be stopped, the patient may be considered for surgical intervention, but surgery is rarely needed. Elective surgery has been used to reduce the recurrence of an ulcer after the bleeding has been controlled. Such treatment may involve a partial resection of the stomach or a procedure to reduce the secretion of gastric juices (e.g., severing of the vagal nerve). The gastric opening at the pylorus can be expanded to speed up gastric emptying, thereby shortening the time the highly acidic contents are in the stomach.

Patients diagnosed with *H. pylori* infection are treated with antibiotics. The infection can be detected by a urea breath test or other laboratory tests, including culture of a specimen obtained during an endoscopic procedure. Prophylactic use of antibiotics for all patients with *H. pylori* infection is not recommended, because only a small number of patients with the infection actually develop ulcers.

Antacids, H_2 receptor blockers, and proton pump inhibitors may prevent ulceration of the GI mucosa and are used to treat current ulcers. H_2 receptor blockers (e.g., famotidine [Pepcid]) inhibit histamines at the H_2 receptor on the cells that secrete gastric acid. Proton pump inhibitors block the formation of gastric acid by competitively binding the surface of the cells that produce gastric acid. Use of proton pump inhibitors (e.g., omeprazole [Prilosec]) has been shown to reduce the rate of rebleeding after endoscopic therapy. Antacids neutralize the pH in the stomach, inactivate pepsin, and relieve pain by coating the stomach.

Many patients self-medicate with OTC preparations before the ulcer is diagnosed. When you ask about the patient's medication history, pay close attention to the type and amount of antacids used. Antacids contain different electrolytes and base products, depending on their formulation, and taking these medications in large quantities can affect the electrolyte and acid-base status.

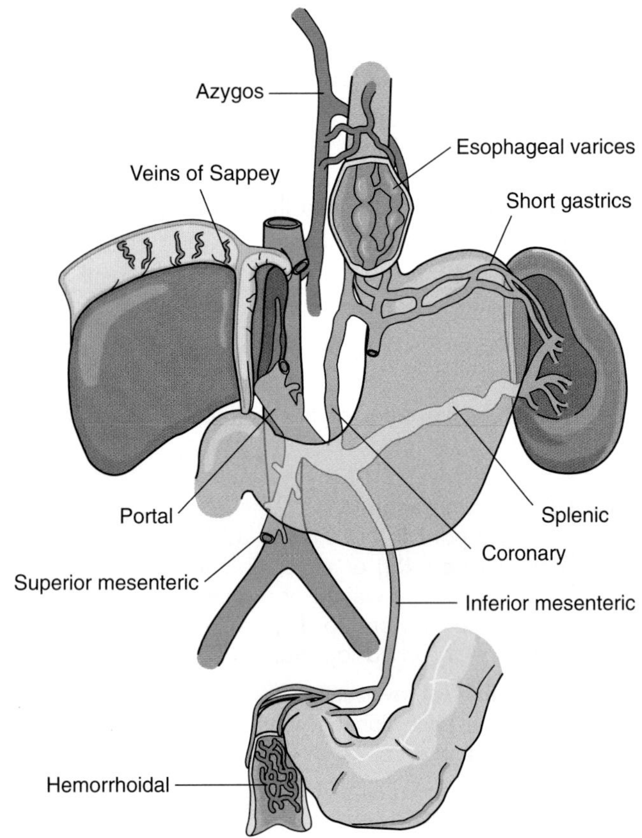

Figure 6-11

Varices caused by portal hypertension. (From Carlson KK: *Advanced critical care nursing*, Philadelphia, 2009, Saunders.)

Esophageal and Gastric Varices

Varices are collateral veins that become tortuous and distended over time in the esophagus, stomach, and rectum and in rare cases on the abdomen. Remember, the collateral veins develop as a result of the increased pressure in the portal circulation. High pressure in the portal veins causes vessels to open between the portal circulation and the lower pressured systemic veins, allowing blood to bypass the obstructed portal vessels and engorge the collateral varices. Portal hypertension may be caused by hepatic failure, hepatic vein thrombosis, or right-sided heart failure, but it occurs most often in patients with liver cirrhosis (Figure 6-11). Esophageal varices are the most common result of portal hypertension.

The varices rupture spontaneously, with no warning, and each episode of bleeding increases mortality by as much as 20%. Esophageal varices rupture more commonly, but rupture of gastric varices usually results in greater blood loss. Seventy percent of patients have a recurrence of the bleeding within 1 year. A patient with ruptured varices requires emergency treatment for hemorrhage. Blood loss can be extreme, so fluid resuscitation and typing and cross-matching for blood products should be done immediately. Blood transfusions and fluid resuscitation must be carefully calculated to meet the patient's exact needs. Increasing the blood volume too much may cause more bleeding.

Management of Bleeding Varices

A vasoconstrictor, such as vasopressin (Pitressin) or octreotide (Sandostatin), may be used to reduce **splanchnic** blood flow and portal vein pressure. As blood flow decreases, coagulation may occur, stopping the bleeding. The drug is given by IV bolus and then by a continuous drip. Octreotide is used more often because it has fewer systemic effects than vasopressin. Octreotide stops bleeding in about 85% of patients.

Endoscopic treatment can be used during active bleeding, but it is more successful after the bleeding has stopped. Injection of sclerosing agents may stop the bleeding by causing a thrombosis in the varices. Once the bleeding has stopped, endoscopy probably will be repeated to determine whether further treatment is needed to prevent rebleeding. This treatment usually involves placing a band or clip around each individual varix. Sclerosing agents can be injected as a preventive measure.

Balloon tamponade tubes may be used for gastric or esophageal varices when other treatments have failed to stop the bleeding. Different tubes are available for this purpose; the **Sengstaken-Blakemore tube** and the Minnesota tube are the most used types. The Sengstaken-Blakemore tube has three lumens: one for the gastric balloon, one for the esophageal balloon, and one for gastric suction. The Minnesota tube has four lumens, which allows for balloons and suctioning for both the stomach and the esophagus. Balloon tamponade tubes are used if IV therapy or endoscopic treatment has failed. However, because these treatments are so successful, tamponade tubes are rarely needed.

The tubes first are inserted into the stomach. After placement has been confirmed, the gastric balloon is inflated. Tension is applied to the tube, which lets the inflated stomach balloon anchor the tube in place. The esophageal balloon then is inflated to provide the tamponade effect on the varices and stop the acute bleeding (Figure 6-12); this balloon is held in place by some kind of traction device. Balloon tamponade tubes can be used only for 24 to 48 hours. Their effectiveness rates are good, but some studies show a 50% incidence of rebleeding when the balloons are deflated. The major complications with the use of these tubes are pulmonary aspiration, balloon migration, and esophageal erosion and rupture.

Life-threatening airway obstruction can occur if the balloon migrates. If the gastric balloon deflates, the esophageal balloon quickly rises into the pharynx, occluding the airway. You must be prepared to cut the lumens, deflating all the balloons, and remove the tube immediately.

Before transport, review the patient care and care of the tube with the current healthcare provider. Endotracheal intubation is nearly always done before placement of a tamponade tube. Identify all the lumens of the tube. Also, some form of traction is required during transport of a patient with a balloon tamponade tube; traction must be maintained on the tube at all times to prevent migration of the balloons. Frequent suctioning above the esophageal balloon is required to prevent aspiration. Assess the patient's tolerance of the device regularly, watching for recurrence of bleeding. Assess the airway frequently. Keep your scissors handy in case the balloon obstructs the airway. Skill 6-2 reviews the steps for using an esophagogastric tamponade tube.

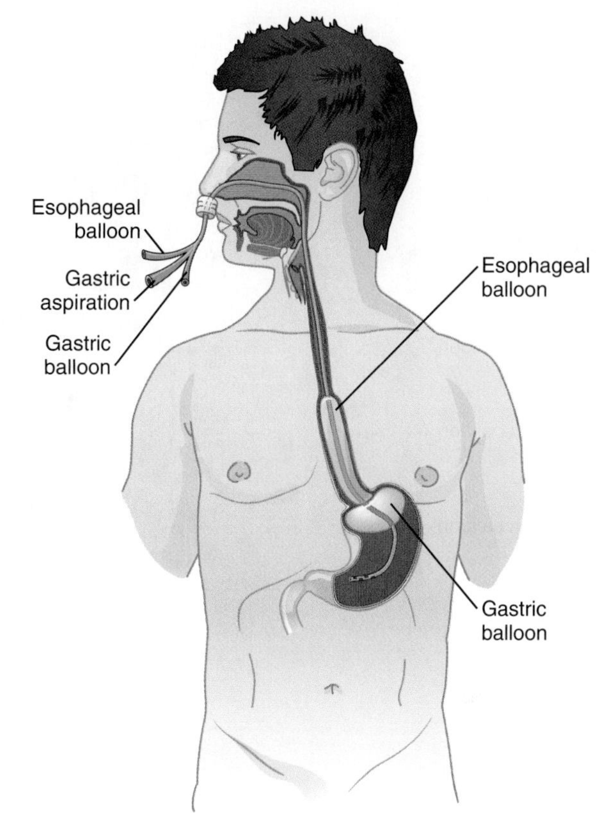

Figure 6-12

Balloon tamponade therapy. A Sengstaken-Blakemore tube is in place, and both the esophageal and gastric balloons have been inflated. (From Carlson KK: *Advanced critical care nursing*, Philadelphia, 2009, Saunders.)

Skill 6-2

ESOPHAGOGASTRIC TAMPONADE

Esophagogastric tamponade tubes, which are available in a wide variety, are used to control bleeding from gastric or esophageal varices. These tubes have separate lumens, which allow the healthcare provider to suction while applying pressure to bleeding sites with balloons. The tube is inserted by the oral or the nasal route, which can cause discomfort and pain for the patient and pose a risk of aspiration of gastric contents. Sedation policies and procedures may be used to aid placement and maintenance of the tube; if necessary, medication-assisted intubation may be done to reduce the likelihood of aspiration. The illustrations show the Sengstaken-Blakemore tube and the Minnesota four-lumen tube.

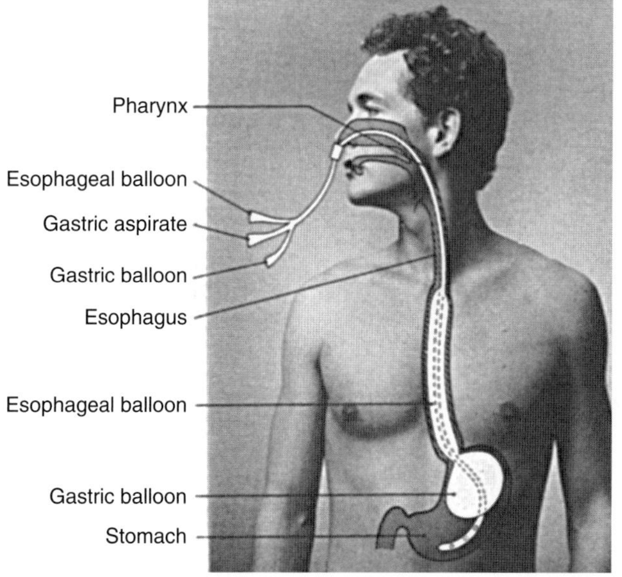

Sengstaken-Blakemore tube. Wiegand D, Carlson K: *AACN procedure manual for critical care*, ed 5, Philadelphia, 2005, Saunders.

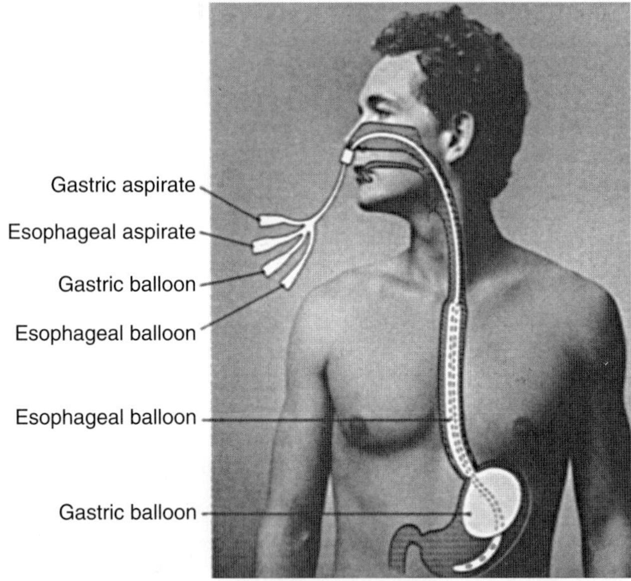

Minnesota four-lumen tube. Wiegand D, Carlson K: *AACN procedure manual for critical care,* ed 5, Philadelphia, 2005, Saunders.

INDICATIONS

Bleeding gastric varices

Bleeding esophageal varices

CONTRAINDICATIONS

Esophageal strictures

Recent esophageal surgery

Nasal insertion of the tube (if the patient has coagulopathies)

EQUIPMENT

Three- or four-lumen tube
Bulb syringe and basin
Saline for irrigation
One or two nasogastric (NG) tubes
Lubricant
Topical anesthetic
Cuff pressure gauge
Four tine-protected clamps
Tape
Bite block
Two suction setups
Balanced-suspension traction or football helmet with padding
Intubation cart or equipment

PROCEDURE

1. Gather the equipment.
   - Attach the pressure gauge to the gastric balloon port.
   - Set up both suction units.
   - Apply cardiac and respiratory monitors to the patient.
2. Pretest the tube system.
   a. Refer to the manufacturer's recommendations for balloon inflation amounts. Inflate the esophageal balloon as indicated. Check for proper function. Deflate the balloon for insertion.
   b. Inflate the gastric balloon while watching and making notes on the pressure manometer for inflation levels of 100, 200, 300, 400, and 500 mL of air.
   c. Immerse inflated balloons in water to check for air leaks.
   d. Deflate the balloons entirely and clamp.
3. Wash your hands and follow standard precautions.
4. Some recommend a preprocedural gastric lavage to help reduce the likelihood of gastric aspiration during the tamponade procedure. If the clinician chooses to do this, follow the procedure for NG tube insertion and gastric lavage (see Skill 6-1). Remove the NG tube.
5. Lubricate the esophagogastric tamponade tube thoroughly (balloons and distal to the balloons).
6. Apply the topical anesthetic to the tube or directly to the oropharynx and/or nasopharynx. Follow your institution's protocols for nasogastric or orogastric tube insertion and the use of topical anesthetics.
7. Prepare the patient. Provide patient education, position the patient, remove any false teeth, and insert a bite block. If the patient has been intubated, insert an oral airway. Prevent the patient from biting the tube.
   - Position the patient in mid or high Fowler's position if the person is conscious.
   - Use the head-down, left lateral position if the patient has been intubated.
8. Premeasure the tube from the bridge of the nose to the earlobe to the tip of the xiphoid. Note the distance for comparison during insertion.
9. Insert the tube into the mouth or the selected nostril. Advance it until it is 10 cm past the noted premeasured depth or is at least at the 50 cm mark on the tube. (Follow the manufacturer's recommendation for depth of placement.)
10. Instill saline into the gastric suction port and suction (lavage) until all large clots have been removed.
11. Connect the gastric suction port to intermittent suction at 60 to 120 mm Hg. Note the amount of blood in the suction container and report it to the clinician.
12. Connect the esophageal suction port (Minnesota tube) to intermittent suction at 120 to 200 mm Hg and note the amount of blood.
13. Confirm correct tube placement by testing the pH of the aspirate from the gastric suction port. Normal values are <5.5 for stomach aspirate and >6 for intestinal aspirate; pulmonary secretions have an alkaline pH (>7).

Did You Know?

Techniques to confirm correct placement of a gastric tube include the simplest method: assume that if gastric-looking secretions (e.g., yellow, green, cloudy) come out of the tube, it is in the right place. This type of fluid can be aspirated from the respiratory tree even after intubation.[5]

Did You Know?

Other techniques to confirm gastric tube placement have included the air bubble method. After insertion of the tube, a bulb syringe is attached to the port; a rapid insufflation of air with simultaneous auscultation of the bubble sound at the epigastrium should verify that the tube is in place. However, recent studies have shown false-positive results with this technique.[5]

14. Inflate the gastric balloon, taking care to prevent accidental inflation of this larger balloon in the esophagus. Slowly inflate the balloon in increments of 100 mL while observing the pressure in the tube at each increment up to 500 mL. If the pressure increases by more than 15 mm Hg, withdraw all the air from the balloon and advance the tube approximately 10 cm. Begin the inflation process again in the same manner.
    - Once the balloon has been inflated, clamp this lumen with a tine-protected clamp.
    - Obtain an anterior-posterior (AP) flat plate radiography of the abdomen
15. When the tube's position has been confirmed radiographically, withdraw the tube slightly until resistance is felt and then double-clamp the gastric balloon port to prevent air leakage. Pulling the balloon onto the leaking varices creates the tamponade effect.
16. Mark a reference point on the tube where it exits the mouth or nose.
17. Inflate the esophageal balloon *only if* the bleeding is not controlled by the gastric balloon alone.
    - Clamp the gastric balloon port and disconnect the pressure manometer.
    - Attach the pressure manometer to the esophageal balloon port
    - Follow the manufacturer's recommendations for balloon inflation. Gradually inflate this balloon to 25 to 45 mm Hg and then double clamp this port with tine-protected clamps. Esophageal pressure from the balloon may cause the patient to complain of chest pressure.
18. If the bleeding continues, apply gentle traction to the tube so that both the esophageal and gastric balloons are exerting direct pressure on the varices.
    - One- to 3-pound weights can be added to a balanced suspension traction.
    - If the tube was inserted through a naris, add a bulky dressing beneath the nose and tape the tube to it.
    - If the tube was passed nasally or orally, place a football helmet on the patient and secure the tube to the face guard (see illustration).

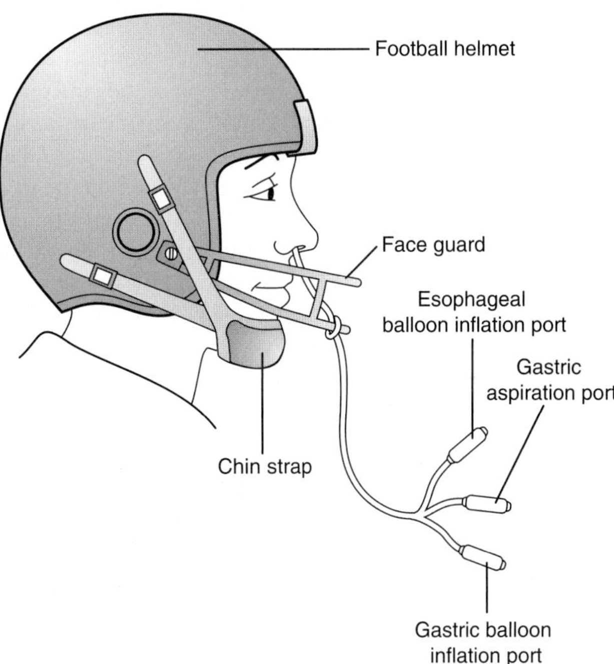

Tamponade tube secured in position with helmet. Wiegand D, Carlson K: *AACN procedure manual for critical care*, ed 5, Philadelphia, 2005, Saunders.

19. Maintain mid to high Fowler's position.
20. If a Sengstaken-Blakemore tube was used, insert an NG tube with the distal tip positioned above the esophageal balloon. Secure the two tubes together at the mouth and connect the NG tube to intermittent suction at 120 to 200 mm Hg.

Pancreatitis

Pancreatitis is an inflammation of the pancreas that results in premature activation of digestive enzymes (Box 6-5). Acute pancreatitis can be classified as mild edematous or hemorrhagic; the most severe form is pancreatic necrosis with multiple organ failure. About 300,000 cases of pancreatitis are seen in the United States each year; 80% of these are associated with alcoholism or obstructive biliary disease, such as gallstones. The combined mortality rate for all types is about 7%, but pancreatitis with necrosis has a high mortality rate.

Normally, the digestive enzymes produced by the pancreas are activated after they enter the GI tract. The most common theory for the development of pancreatitis is an injury to the pancreatic cells that causes leakage of the enzymes into the pancreatic tissue, leading to autodigestion of the pancreas. The pancreas develops edema and possibly hemorrhage and necrosis. In the mild edematous form, the patient maintains hemodynamic stability, and few complications develop. In the hemorrhagic form, bleeding into the pancreatic tissue occurs, but hemodynamic stability usually is maintained. However, in some cases the patient may bleed into the abdominal cavity and suffer significant blood loss. If necrosis of the pancreatic tissue occurs, more enzymes and inflammatory mediators are absorbed into the bloodstream, damaging vessels and other organs. As vessels are damaged, the membranes become permeable, allowing fluid to leave the intravascular system and move into the tissues. Loss of intravascular volume may cause hypovolemic shock. The heart muscle may suffer myocardial depression, further reducing the perfusion of the tissues. This may lead to multiple organ damage, including further necrosis of the pancreas. The mortality rate for this severe form of pancreatitis can be very high.

Box 6-5 Causes of Pancreatitis

- Alcohol
- Gallbladder disease
- Drugs
  - Diuretics
  - Acetaminophen
  - Oral contraceptives
  - Tetracycline
  - Sulfonamides
  - Angiotensin-converting enzyme (ACE) inhibitors
  - Human immunodeficiency virus (HIV) infection, antiretroviral medications
  - Many others
- High triglyceride level
- Trauma
- Pregnancy
- Infections
- Insecticides
- High calcium level
- Surgery

Clinical Presentation

The patient usually presents with severe midepigastric or LUQ pain, which the person describes as excruciating or rates as maximum intensity. The abdominal pain may radiate to the back, flank, or even the left shoulder and is described as twisting or knifelike. The pain may diminish in intensity if the patient lies in a fetal position, which reduces the stretch on the pancreas. The intensity of the pain correlates well with the degree of pancreatitis. The patient usually is nauseated and may have significant vomiting. The respiratory rate may be fast and shallow in response to the severe pain. Patients also may present with hypotension, tachycardia, tachypnea, anxiety, fever, weakness, and diaphoresis.

Fluid usually pools inside the inflamed pancreas, but in some cases it may collect in the abdominal cavity. Because this fluid is from the intravascular space, the patient may develop hypotension, resulting in an extremely unstable condition. Complicating the hypovolemia that may occur as a result of the fluid shifts into the abdomen, the patient also may have hemorrhage into the pancreas or abdomen. Assess the patient for signs of intraabdominal bleeding, such as a firm, distended abdomen and bruising of the abdomen, along with a change in vital signs.

As the pancreatitis evolves, the patient may develop numerous complications involving multiple organs, which in turn complicates the clinical picture (Figure 6-13). Some of the more common problems are hypovolemic shock, dysrhythmias, renal failure, pneumonia, hypoxia, and acute respiratory distress syndrome (ARDS). Although these complications usually occur in only a small percentage of cases, they put the patient in an extremely unstable condition that requires a high level of care.

Diagnosis

The diagnosis of pancreatitis is based on the patient's clinical presentation, laboratory test results, and imaging studies. Several other disorders can have a similar presentation, but pancreatitis should be suspected in all patients with severe epigastric or LUQ pain. Lipase (and sometimes amylase) testing should be added to the routine blood tests. Amylase is released from the pancreas 2 to 12 hours after the onset of the abdominal pain. In mild cases the amylase level may not rise significantly; or, if the patient has had symptoms for a few days, the amylase level may already be back to normal. A number of disorders can cause elevation of the amylase level, which makes diagnosis based on these results alone impossible; however, an amylase value two to three times the normal level is highly indicative of pancreatitis.

Lipase levels rise 4 to 8 hours after the onset of symptoms, peak in 24 hours, and return to normal in 2 weeks. Newer tests, such as **C-reactive protein** and urinary **trypsinogen**, may be better indicators of pancreatitis and are becoming more widely available. The C-reactive protein level rises during inflammation, but it also is elevated by other causes of acute inflammation. Trypsinogen is released by the pancreas, absorbed by the bloodstream, and filtered into the urine by the kidneys.

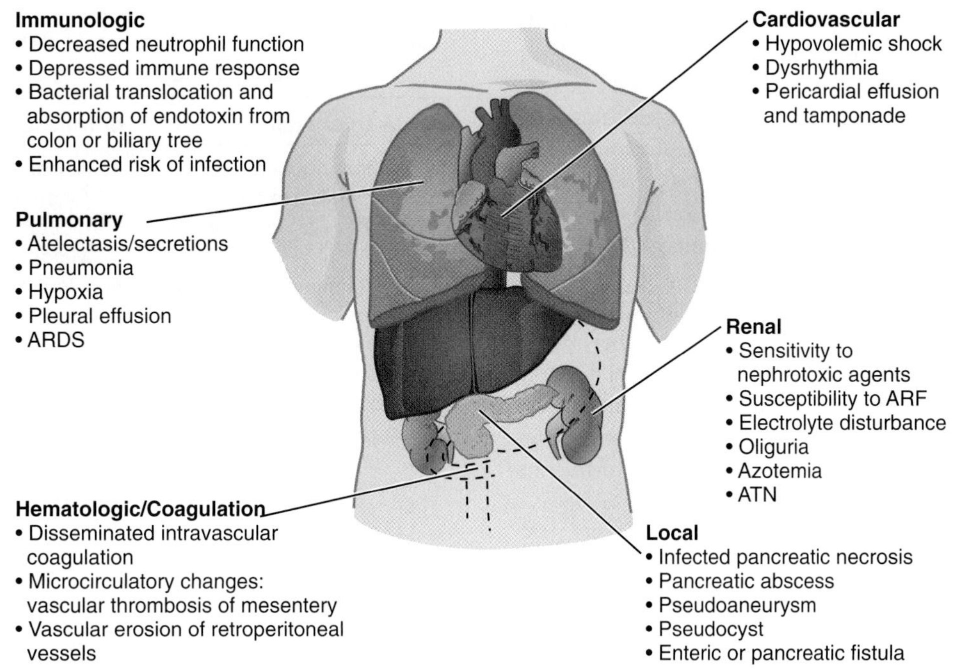

Figure 6-13

Local and systemic complications of acute pancreatitis. (From Carlson KK: *Advanced critical care nursing,* Philadelphia, 2009, Saunders.)

The imaging study most often used in the diagnosis of pancreatitis is a contrast-enhanced computed tomography (CT) scan, which can help determine the presence and severity of some complications. Magnetic resonance imaging (MRI) and **magnetic resonance cholangiopancreatography (MRCP)** can aid the diagnosis of pancreatitis and provide better images of the biliary tree; however, these techniques usually are reserved for patients who cannot have a contrast CT scan. Ultrasound does not visualize the pancreas well but can determine whether the patient has gallbladder disease or pseudocysts.

Did You Know?

A mnemonic for the common causes of pancreatitis is "bad time."[4]

- **B Biliary (gallstones [40% to 60%], parasites, malignancy)**
- **A Alcohol (35% to 70%)**
- **D Drugs**
- **T Trauma, toxins**
- **I Idiopathic, ischemic, infectious, inherited**
- **M Metabolic (hyperlipidemia, hypercalcemia)**
- **E Endoscopic retrograde cholangiopancreatography**

Management

Management goals for pancreatitis include adequate pain control, maintenance of hemodynamic stability, and removal of the causative agent if possible. Pain management is very important. In the past, the preferred narcotic for this purpose was meperidine (Demerol). Some believe that morphine actually increased the pain because it stimulated the sphincters that control the flow of bile and digestive juices into the duodenum. Meperidine causes less stimulation of those sphincters, but all narcotics cause it to some extent. Because meperidine may cause neuromuscular irritation and seizures, it should not be used for longer than 48 hours, and it should not be used at all in patients with renal disease. Morphine and other narcotics (e.g., fentanyl [Sublimaze] and hydromorphone [Dilaudid]) have not been shown to affect patient outcomes negatively and are often used.

Antiemetics may help the patient's nausea. If the patient is vomiting, a nasogastric (NG) tube may be used to keep the stomach empty. Besides reducing nausea and vomiting, keeping the stomach empty may help limit the release of pancreatic hormones, which in turn may help reduce the patient's pain. Whether the patient should be kept on nothing by mouth (NPO) status or maintained on some form of enteral nutrition is the subject of debate. Recent studies have shown that a patient with a mild case of pancreatitis may be able to continue oral fluids and food. A patient with severe pancreatitis frequently has severe nausea and vomiting and usually is kept NPO for at least 24 hours.

The patient is monitored continually for hypovolemia. Large amounts of fluids may be pulled from the intravascular space into the tissues and abdominal cavity. Volume resuscitation with IV solutions, colloids, and blood may be needed to keep the patient's condition stable. The goal of fluid resuscitation is a central venous pressure (CVP) of at least 8 mm Hg or a pulmonary artery catheter (PAC) wedge pressure of 15 to 18 mm Hg; a systolic blood pressure above 90 mm Hg; and a urine output greater than 0.5 mL/kg/hour. Perfusion is maintained in the hopes of reducing complications and preventing organ failure.

Respiratory distress may result if the large, fluid-filled abdomen limits movement of the diaphragm. Other mechanisms include fluid movement from the abdominal lymphatics into the pleural lymphatics, causing a pleural effusion, and leakage of fluid out of the pulmonary capillary bed, causing pulmonary edema. Hypoxia damages the pancreas further and speeds the process of multiple organ failure. ARDS is a common complication of necrotizing pancreatitis.

Hypovolemia causes low perfusion pressures, but the myocardial muscle also is affected by the inflammatory mediators released; the result of all this is myocardial depression and lower cardiac output. Decreased perfusion occurs in all organs, but the kidneys are particularly susceptible to low perfusion, which may cause acute renal failure. In addition, low perfusion further insults the pancreas, increasing the necrosis of the pancreatitis. Pay attention to the patient's electrolytes, especially calcium. In severe cases of pancreatitis, calcium may deposit into areas of fat necrosis, causing hypocalcemia. Remember that low calcium can cause tetany. Calcium levels are maintained with IV calcium replacement. The patient also may need potassium and magnesium replacement.

Some patients develop hyperglycemia, because the pancreas releases glucagon as the endocrine cells are damaged. The insulin output of the pancreas is reduced or absent, and insulin administration usually is required to maintain the glucose level. Because the blood glucose level is very volatile, the insulin must be given carefully. Most patients receive small amounts of insulin continuously by an IV drip; this allows the blood sugar level to be checked hourly, and appropriate adjustments in the insulin dosage can be made as needed.

Liver Failure

Acute liver failure (ALF) and **chronic liver failure** (CLF) lead to overwhelming metabolic and systemic complications in all organs of the body. Liver failure is devastating because of this organ's multiple, complex functions, which include the metabolism of carbohydrates, fats, and proteins; the development of clotting factors; and the cleaning processes performed by a healthy liver. Imagine what would happen to the body if all these functions were lost.

The liver can maintain homeostasis until approximately 80% of the liver cells are damaged. Depending on the cause, liver function can deteriorate rapidly or over a lengthy period (Table 6-5). Acute liver failure is identified by presenting symptoms of jaundice (yellow pigmentation) and mental alteration with an illness of less than 26 weeks' duration that also involves massive necrosis of the liver cells. The patient also must have had no preexisting liver disease. With chronic liver failure, liver function decreases over a period of at least 6 months; patients with CLF also may have an acute episode that rapidly diminishes liver function. The most common cause of ALF that complicates chronic liver failure is significant infection or bleeding, such as GI bleeding.

Table 6-5 Common Causes of Acute and Chronic Liver Failure

Acute Liver Failure	Chronic Liver Failure
• Acetaminophen toxicity	• Hepatitis C
• Other drug reactions	• Alcoholism
• Hepatitis D with hepatitis B	• Gallbladder disease
• Autoimmune liver disease	• Metabolic disease
• Shock, hypoperfusion	• Tumors
• **Wilson's disease** (defect of copper metabolism)	
• Mushroom poisoning	

Acetaminophen toxicity causes almost 40% of ALF cases in the United States, and other drug reactions account for 13%. The short-term survival rate for ALF is less than 15%, but if the patient receives a liver transplant, the survival rate rises to about 65%.

Patients with ALF and CLF have some similar and dissimilar clinical presentations, which require several differences in the management of the patient.

Chronic Liver Failure

Cirrhosis

Cirrhosis is the end result of CLF of any cause. Chronic inflammation causes deposition of fibrotic tissue in the liver lobule, which disrupts the layout of the hepatic cells as they relate to the circulatory system of the liver (Figure 6-14). Liver cells regenerate, but the new cells are not arranged in the normal pattern, which contributes to the disruption of the lobule. If the new cells are not close to the blood supply, they cannot perform liver functions. The fibrotic tissue also impairs blood flow through the liver. (Review the structure of the lobule in Figure 6-7.)

Remember that the portal veins carry blood from the GI tract, pancreas, and spleen to the liver. With impaired flow, blood backs up in the system, causing **portal hypertension**. Increased pressure in the portal veins causes the development of collateral connections to the systemic circulation. Early in the disease process, the development of collateral veins helps lower the portal pressure; however, the blood shunted into the systemic circulation does not pass through the liver for filtration. As the disease progresses, the back flow of blood affects the portal, splenic, and mesenteric circulations. As the pressure further increases, the thin veins become engorged with high blood volumes and pressures (i.e., they become varices; see Figure 6-11); this occurs mainly in the esophagus, but also

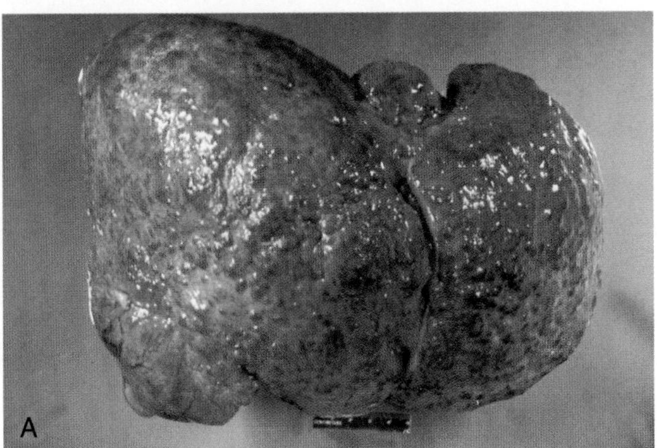

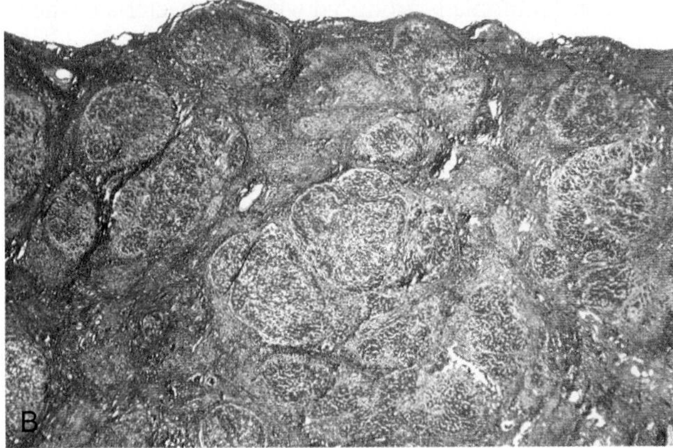

Figure 6-14

Alcoholic cirrhosis. **A,** The characteristic diffuse nodularity of the surface reflects the processes of nodular regeneration and scarring. The greenish tint of some nodules is due to bile stasis. A hepatocellular carcinoma can be seen as a budding mass at the lower edge of the right lobe *(lower left)*. **B,** Microscopic view shows nodules of varying size entrapped in blue-staining fibrous tissue. The liver capsule is at the top. (Masson trichrome.) (From Kumar V, Abbas AK, Fausto N et al: *Robbins and Cotran pathologic basis of disease,* ed 8, Philadelphia, 2009, Saunders.)

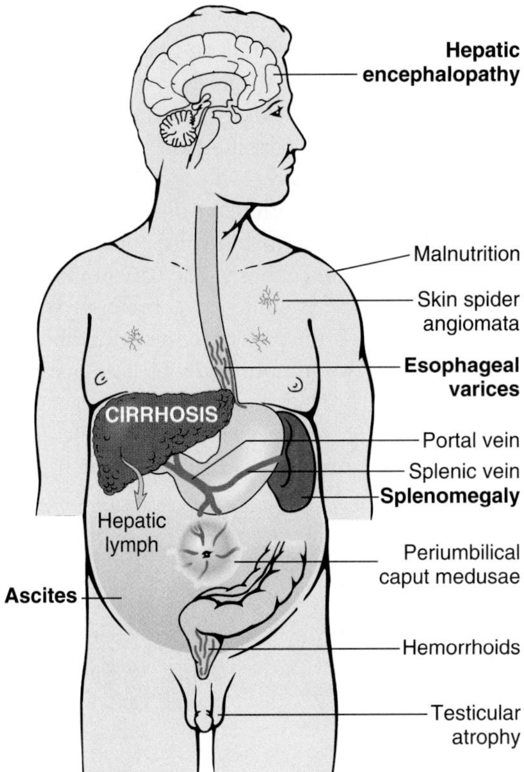

Figure 6-15

The major clinical consequences of portal hypertension with cirrhosis, shown for the male. In women, oligomenorrhea, amenorrhea, and sterility are commonly seen as a result of hypogonadism. (From Kumar V, Abbas AK, Fausto N et al: *Robbins and Cotran pathologic basis of disease,* ed 8, Philadelphia, 2009, Saunders.)

in the stomach, duodenum, and rectum. The varices are prone to abrupt rupture, causing massive GI bleeding. (The care of these patients is discussed in the section on GI bleeding later in the chapter.) Umbilical and abdominal veins can become enlarged, and the patient may develop ascites. In addition, portal hypertension can have multiple effects on the rest of the body (Figure 6-15).

Therapy with beta blockers and long-acting nitrates may be used to try to reduce the problems associated with portal hypertension. These drugs decrease the vascular pressure, which reduces the portal pressure; however, they also affect the systemic circulation and may cause systemic hypotension. An invasive procedure, **transjugular intrahepatic portosystemic shunt (TIPS)**, shunts portal blood into the inferior vena cava (Figure 6-16). Surgery also can be performed to shunt blood from the portal circulation, but these procedures have a fairly high mortality rate.

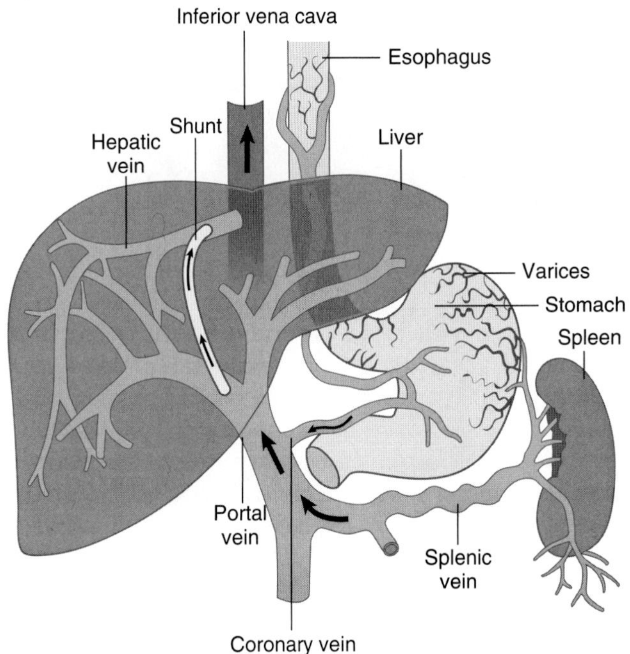

Figure 6-16

Transjugular intrahepatic portosystemic shunt (TIPS). (From Fink MP, Vincent JL, Kochanek PM: *Textbook of critical care,* ed 4, Philadelphia, 2005, Saunders.)

Ascites

Ascites is the collection of fluid and protein in the peritoneal cavity (Figure 6-17). It is the most common complication of cirrhosis, and 25% of patients die less than 18 months after the development of ascites. The fluid and protein accumulate from the intravascular space, which reduces intravascular volume. Ascites can occur with other disorders, such as heart failure, tumors, and even malnutrition; however, 80% of patients with ascites have cirrhosis. The patient may have significant hemodynamic instability as a result of the loss of intravascular volume. If the patient requires fluid boluses, NS should be used. LRS would not usually be used because of its lactate content; a cirrhotic liver cannot process lactate.

Another major problem for a patient with ascites is respiratory compromise, because the enlarged abdomen limits the movement of the diaphragm. In addition, high abdominal pressures can push fluid into the pleural space, causing a pleural effusion; therefore, patients with ascites should be watched for dyspnea, shallow breathing, and hypoxia.

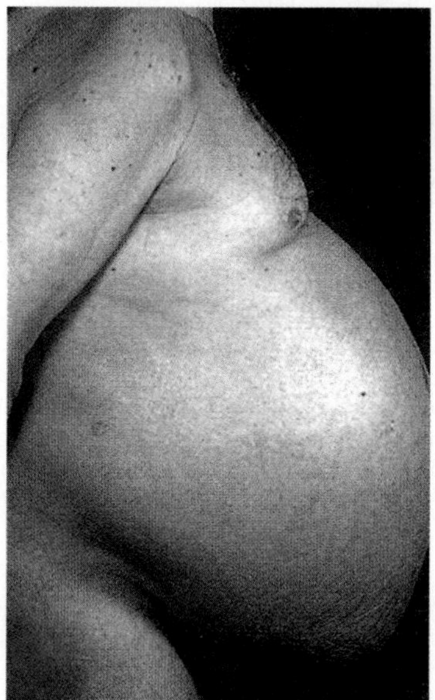

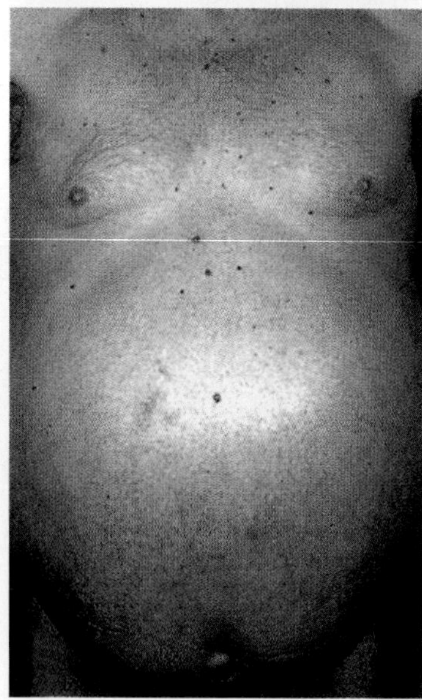

Figure 6-17

Massive ascites. (From Sanders M: *Mosby's paramedic textbook*, ed 3, St Louis, 2007, Mosby.)

Treatment for ascites involves reducing the patient's fluid intake while keeping a careful eye on the intravascular volume. Diuretics may help control the overall body water, and **paracentesis** may be performed to reduce the existing fluid.

Hepatic Encephalopathy

Hepatic encephalopathy is a disturbance in brain function that occurs when the liver fails. The mechanism is poorly understood, but the condition is probably the result of the accumulation of many toxic substances, one of which is ammonia. Ammonia is produced when the bacteria of the GI tract act on nitrogenous waste products. The increased levels of toxic substances cause altered nerve transmission in the central nervous system. Early symptoms may involve speech, concentration, and cognitive abilities; as the encephalopathy progresses, all cognitive function is lost. The patient may flap the arms (asterixis) or have rapid, jerky movements of the pupils (hippus). Reflexes decrease, including the gag reflex, and the patient eventually falls into a coma (Box 6-6). When caring for a patient with hepatic encephalopathy, assess the patient carefully for LOC changes. These patients are at high risk for aspiration and may need emergency intubation to protect the airway.

Several factors may speed the progression of the encephalopathy, such as infection, fluid and electrolyte disorders, hypoxia, and medications. GI bleeding rapidly increases symptoms, because digestion of the blood in the GI tract increases ammonia levels significantly. The progression of the encephalopathy may be slowed with treatment, but patients progress though all stages. Treatment includes reducing the animal protein in the diet, avoiding sedation, and bowel cleansing. **Lactulose** is used to increase the movement of ammonia from the blood into the gut, but it also increases the peristalsis of the colon, resulting in quicker excretion of ammonia and other waste products. Other medications can be used if the patient is unable to take lactulose. Rifaximin (Salix) is considered an orphan drug for this use, but it seems to be well tolerated by patients. Side effects to watch for

Box 6-6 West Haven Criteria of Altered Mental State

Stage 0	Normal personality and behavior
Stage 1	Short attention span, impaired addition and subtraction, hypersomnia, insomnia, euphoria or depression, asterixis
Stage 2	Lethargy or apathy, disorientation, slurred speech, asterixis, inappropriate behavior
Stage 3	Gross disorientation, bizarre behavior, semistuporous to stupor, no asterixis usually
Stage 4	Coma

include abdominal distention, fluid and electrolyte loss through diarrhea, and hypernatremia. Antibiotics such as neomycin are used to reduce the normal bacteria in the GI tract, which slows the production of ammonia.

Bleeding

Clotting factors diminish with cirrhosis, which increases the risk for bleeding. Absorption and utilization of vitamin K also decline. Therefore, the patient should be carefully assessed for occult or massive bleeding. Minimize invasive procedures and protect the patient from bleeding. If the patient has significant bleeding, packed red cells are transfused. Platelets and/or fresh frozen plasma (FFP) are given if the platelet count drops below 50,000 mcL, and clotting factors can be infused.

Infection

The patient with cirrhosis is at high risk for bacterial and fungal infections as a result of loss of the Kupffer cells, which clean the blood. Malnutrition and the increased levels of toxin also reduce the overall functioning of the immune system. Patients with ascites may develop a bacterial peritonitis that can be very painful. Early detection of any infections and antibiotic treatment are vital. A few experts recommend prophylactic antibiotics, because the patient could die of an overwhelming infection.

Hepatorenal and Hepatopulmonary Syndromes

Hepatorenal syndrome is renal failure caused by the liver failure. The main mechanism for the renal failure is low perfusion from low intravascular volume. The patient may need dialysis or any treatment discussed in the renal section of this chapter. **Hepatopulmonary syndrome** occurs when the pulmonary artery pressure increases; the increased pressure causes shortness of breath and symptoms of right-sided heart failure. This disorder is differentiated from a cardiac condition by the presence of a normal pulmonary wedge pressure.

Metabolic Derangements

Metabolic acidosis can occur if the buildup of toxins and low perfusion cause the development of lactic acid. Metabolic alkalosis could occur if a blood transfusion with citrate is given. The most common finding is metabolic acidosis with a respiratory alkalosis until the patient's respiratory status is compromised. As the respiratory compromise increases, the patient's condition changes to respiratory acidosis. Pleural effusion, pulmonary edema, and limited diaphragmatic movement result in carbon dioxide buildup and decreasing oxygen levels.

Replacement of potassium, magnesium, or phosphorus may be required, and electrolytes should be assessed frequently. Most patients have **dilutional hyponatremia**, and the sodium level should be raised slowly. Hyperglycemia usually is present early. Tight control of the blood glucose level is better for the patient. As the liver failure progresses, hypoglycemia can occur. Some electrolyte and glucose problems may be treated with enteral feeding. A high protein intake could increase the hepatic encephalopathy, but protein replacement is still needed.

Acute Liver Failure

Remember that ALF is identified by the presenting symptoms of jaundice (yellow pigmentation) and mental alteration in a patient with an illness of less than 26 weeks' duration marked by massive necrosis of the liver cells. ALF is caused by massive hepatic necrosis, and the mortality rate without transplantation can be as high as 90%. The condition of a patient with ALF usually changes rapidly. The patient is at high risk for many of the conditions discussed for patients with CLF. Metabolic problems, electrolyte disorders, bleeding, infection, and neurologic changes also occur in patients with ALF, but the care of these patients differs for some clinical problems.

Hemodynamic Stability

Patients with ALF have a **systemic inflammatory response syndrome (SIRS)** that affects cellular permeability. Fluid leaks out of the vascular space, leaving the patient hypovolemic. Decreased albumin levels also contribute to the loss of fluid from the intravascular space, and in a small percentage of patients with ALF, ascites can result. The patient usually requires albumin replacement. With severe hypotension, large volumes of crystalloids may be required to correct the hypovolemia. Adequate fluid resuscitation usually can be assessed by a CVP or pulmonary artery catheter. A patient with ALF requires rapid, early transport to a specialized liver transplant center. The patient's condition may be extremely unstable, making the transport process difficult and very challenging.

Hepatic Coma

The most alarming development for a patient with ALF may be the rapid loss of neurologic functioning. Interestingly, the faster the hepatic coma develops after the jaundice appears, the better the prognosis. Hepatic coma of ALF is different from the hepatic encephalopathy of the patient with CLF. A patient with ALF has a very fast decline in neurologic functioning, compared to the months or years required for a patient with cirrhosis. Patients with ALF have severe levels of cerebral edema and high intracranial pressures. Hepatic encephalopathy does not usually involve cerebral edema.

Another difference may be the ammonia level. Patients with CLF usually have a high ammonia level that requires considerable patient care to reduce it. In ALF, the ammonia level may be elevated in only a small percentage of patients, and it requires less treatment than in CLF patients.

Careful attention to the respiratory status and neurologic level of a patient with ALF is important. Intubation may be required quickly as the neurologic status deteriorates. Treatment of the increased intracranial pressure includes keeping the head in the midline position and elevated to at least 30 degrees to facilitate the drainage of blood. A response may be seen with administration of mannitol, an osmotic diuretic. If the intracranial pressure reaches a critical level, the patient may be placed in a barbiturate coma. While the patient awaits liver transplantation, it is imperative to keep the intracranial pressure low to prevent permanent brain damage or brain death from herniation of the brain stem. (Review Chapter 5 for more details on the care of a patient with elevated intracranial pressure.)

Bleeding

Patients with ALF have bleeding problems similar to those in patients with CLF. Circulating clotting factors are used and are not replaced by the diseased liver. The patient is at risk for bleeding from mucous membranes or IV sites or even for GI bleeding. Blood replacement is needed to maintain the hematocrit at an acceptable level. Platelets usually are not replaced unless the level drops extremely low (<100,000 per microliter) or the bleeding continues. Clotting factors may be administered in the form of FFP if bleeding continues or possibly before invasive procedures.

Glucose and Other Metabolic Derangements

Patients with ALF may have hyperglycemia or hypoglycemia, depending on the stage of liver failure. Hyperglycemia usually is seen early in ALF and requires insulin administration. As mentioned previously, tight control of the glucose level is better for the patient. The glucose level should be assessed frequently, because a rapid loss of blood glucose occurs as liver failure continues. Large amounts of glucose may be needed to maintain the blood sugar level. The patient also is at high risk for metabolic acidosis, because the liver has lost the ability to process lactate; this allows acids to accumulate. A number of electrolyte disorders can occur; therefore, continual assessment for electrolyte disturbances are necessary.

Care of a Patient with ALF and Acetaminophen Overdose

Acetaminophen overdose accounts for 40% of ALF cases in the United States, and more than 60,000 overdose cases are estimated to occur each year. Twenty percent of the deaths caused by excess acetaminophen are the result of unintentional overdose. Taking the drug with alcohol increases the risk of liver damage. Early treatment can help prevent damage to the liver. Treatment provided within 1 hour for an alert patient may include gastric lavage and then administration of activated charcoal. The drug level in the blood should be measured, along with a full toxicology screen and an alcohol level. The patient then is given **N-acetylcysteine (NAC)** based on the drug level. If the drug level is extremely high, the patient should be transported to a liver transplantation center for continued treatment and preparation for possible liver transplantation.

Acetaminophen-induced liver injury occurs in four stages.

Stage 1: *Pre–liver injury:* Up to 24 hours after ingestion. Nonspecific symptoms, including nausea, vomiting, diaphoresis, and malaise, occur in the first 8 hours and then subside. Some patients may not have symptoms.

Stage 2: *Liver injury:* 12-24 hours after ingestion. In some cases signs of liver damage develop within 8 hours. Nausea, vomiting, and RUQ or epigastric pain may be evident.

Stage 3: *Maximum liver injury:* 3 to 4 days after ingestion. Depending on the severity of the toxicity, the patient may have a wide variety of signs and symptoms, including hepatic encephalopathy, coma, and coagulopathy. Hypoglycemia and metabolic acidosis may occur. Death may be caused by hemorrhage, ARDS, or cerebral edema.

Stage 4: *Possible recovery period:* Hepatic enzymes may return to baseline within 5 to 7 days. Actual cell recovery may take months with complete liver regeneration.

Treatment with NAC is started if the acetaminophen concentration is on or above the nomogram treatment line; the acetaminophen concentration is greater than 10 mcg/mL and the time of ingestion is unknown; and/or the aspartate transaminase (AST) level is elevated. Liver failure and death are completely preventable if NAC is given early after ingestion. Circumstances that complicate the assessment and treatment decisions include an unknown time of ingestion; ingestion that occurred more than 24 hours previously; chronic excessive dosing; use of newer formulations of combination drugs with acetaminophen; age under 5 years; and pregnancy.

NAC usually is given orally in a dilute solution through a straw from a closed container (because of the smell). The loading dose is 140 mg/kg, followed by a maintenance dose of 70 mg/kg every 4 hours. Any dose vomited within 1 hour of administration is repeated, and antiemetics may be needed. IV administration of NAC must be done cautiously, because anaphylaxis can result if the drug is given rapidly in high concentrations. If given intravenously, NAC is infused in a 3% solution (30 g of NAC in D_5W to a total volume of 1 L). The initial IV bolus is 140 to 150 mg/kg over 1 hour, followed by continuous infusion of 15 mg/kg for 4 hours, then 7.5 mg/kg/hour for 16 hours.

Abdominal Surgery

Abdominal surgery has undergone dramatic changes. In most cases, open abdominal procedures requiring large incisions have given way to laparoscopic techniques. Laparoscopic surgery has a much lower rate of complications and a faster recovery time. However, despite these advances, some patients still require an open procedure. Both open and laparoscopic techniques have complications. Although the list of possible complications is quite long, the incidence of surgical complications is quite low.

Respiratory complications include pneumonia, atelectasis, and pulmonary embolism. Pain tends to cause patients with abdominal wounds to breathe less deeply on inspiration. Adequate pain control may help the patient breathe deeper, but the person still is at risk for decreasing respiratory effort because of the effects of narcotics. Another reason for depressed respiratory effort is immobility. Patients need to be ambulated and educated on the prevention of these complications during the hospital stay, and mobility at home also must be stressed.

The patient should be assessed for respiratory rate, pulse oximetry, signs of hypoxia, lung sounds, and signs of pulmonary embolism. Pulmonary emboli usually are caused by deep vein thrombosis. Preventive measures are used for most hospitalized patients, such as mechanical compression stockings and possibly heparin therapy.

Circulatory complications include hypovolemia, shock, hemorrhage, and thrombophlebitis. Patients can be hypovolemic as a result of hemorrhage or inadequate fluid administration during and after surgery. Fluid loss also may occur from the kidney as urine or from an NG tube or other drains. Watch the patient carefully for signs of hypovolemia, such as low blood pressure, tachycardia, and other signs of shock. A patient with mild to moderate hypovolemia may have increased thirst, dry mucous membranes, and a decreased urinary output; the blood pressure and heart rate may be normal. For all patients, intake and output should be carefully recorded in the postoperative period.

GI complications include nausea and vomiting, constipation, abdominal distention, hernia, bowel obstruction, and postoperative ileus. **Ileus** is paralysis of the bowel, which results in failure to pass bowel contents even though no bowel obstruction is present. Ileus can be caused by peritonitis, narcotic use, abdominal distention, and anesthesia. Bowel obstructions occur as a result of lesions that block passage of intestinal contents. The most common cause of bowel obstruction is **adhesions**, which can form after surgery or trauma that has caused peritoneal irritation. Adhesions essentially strangle the bowel. They may develop over a long period, causing a bowel obstruction even 20 years after the surgery. Bowel obstruction also can be caused by hernias. If the patient has an ileus or a small bowel obstruction, the initial treatment usually is NPO status. If the patient is vomiting, an NG tube is used for suctioning. Many small bowel obstructions resolve over a few days, but some require surgery.

Infections of the abdomen, such as peritonitis and abscess, also may occur. They are seen more often as a result of leakage of bowel contents during or after bowel surgery. These patients also are at risk for urinary retention and urinary tract infections. Use of a urinary (Foley) catheter increases the risk of infection.

Complications of the surgical incision include infection, wound dehiscence, and evisceration. The abdominal wound should be kept dry and assessed for any signs of infection, such as redness, warmth, and drainage. **Dehiscence** is the separation of the suture line; if the internal organs extrude through the open incision, evisceration has occurred.

Bariatric Surgery

Some of the most challenging circumstances of patient care can arise in individuals who have had bariatric surgery. Bariatric surgery can be loosely divided into two types, restrictive procedures and bypass procedures (Figure 6-18). Gastric bypass surgery creates a small gastric pouch that is connected to the jejunum of the small intestine; this results in a decreased ability to absorb nutrients. A drawback of bypass surgery is malnutrition, which can lead to multiple nutrient, vitamin, and mineral deficiencies. Metabolic derangements can be life-threatening. Also, the patient is at increased risk for all the surgical complications already discussed.

One life-threatening complication is leakage of bowel contents into the peritoneal cavity, which can result in sepsis. Leakage usually occurs in the immediate postoperative period or 7 to 10 days after the surgery. An obese patient may not always show the normal symptoms of peritonitis and sepsis. Presenting symptoms of peritonitis usually include fever and abdominal pain and tenderness. However, an obese patient may have very little abdominal pain and tenderness because of the large size of the abdomen. This patient has a very high risk of sepsis from leakage at the surgical site. Such patients may show only tachycardia, even with a significant

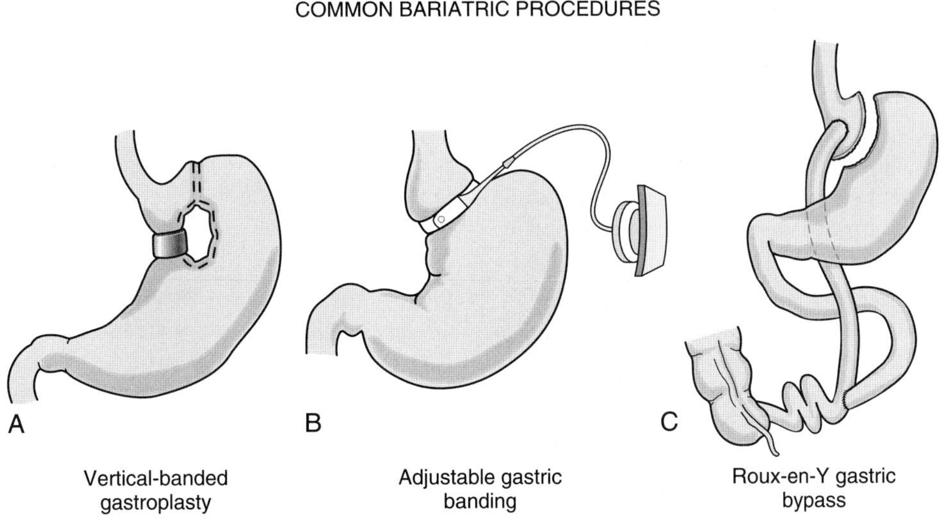

Figure 6-18

Common surgical techniques for the treatment of obesity. **A,** Vertical-banded gastroplasty. **B,** Adjustable laparoscopic band. **C,** Roux-en-Y gastric bypass. (From Bope ET, Rakel RE, Kellerman R: *Conn's current therapy 2010*, Philadelphia, 2009, Saunders.)

intraabdominal pathologic condition. If tachycardia greater than 120 beats/min is the only symptom noted in a patient who has had gastric bypass surgery, an abscess or leakage should be assumed until proven otherwise. Patients with bowel leaks usually should undergo immediate surgery so as to reduce the long-term recovery time and mortality. A patient who has had gastric bypass surgery and becomes septic usually progresses rapidly to multisystem organ failure.

A patient who has had gastric bypass must eat very small amounts of food; this can lead to low protein levels, along with other deficiencies of nutrients, minerals, and vitamins. Water also is ingested in frequent, small amounts. Patients may not take in enough water and become dehydrated. Electrolyte imbalances, anemia, deficiencies of vitamins and minerals, and dehydration are ongoing problems after the postoperative period.

Band surgery is a newer restrictive technique for weight loss. An inflatable band is applied around the stomach, and a port for saline insufflation is routed out to the surface, usually in the upper abdomen. When the band is tight enough, the patient feels full with a smaller food intake. The band may need to be adjusted several times to achieve the correct amount of restriction. This type of weight loss procedure is safer than gastric bypass, because a laparoscopic approach is used and no incision is made into the GI tract. Possible complications related to the procedure itself include port site infection, gastric prolapse, pouch dilation, and band erosion. Any of the general complications discussed earlier are possible, but the current technique has a very low complication rate. Weight loss is slower with gastric band surgery than with bypass surgery.

Transportation of patients who have had bariatric surgery is a challenge. Assessment of the patient, including getting accurate blood pressure readings, often is difficult. IV access may be impossible, especially if the patient is dehydrated. The patient may be difficult to intubate if an airway emergency arises. If you are transporting a patient from one hospital to another, evaluate the IV access before leaving to make sure it is likely to remain patent for the entire trip. If an IV line cannot be placed, always consider an intraosseous (IO) insertion. Make sure you are able to take the patient's blood pressure; if you do not have a cuff that fits the upper arm, a radial pressure reading usually can be taken with an adult cuff. Assessment of the patient's airway needs and respiratory status can help you plan the appropriate care to prevent problems during transportation.

Nutrition

Nutritional support is essential to the care of a critically ill patient. Proteins, for example, are not stored for later use; therefore, if a patient does not have regular protein intake, proteins in the muscle are used for energy. Muscle protein releases less energy than does ingested protein, and loss of muscle protein weakens the muscles, including the respiratory muscles. Albumin is essential for maintenance of the intravascular fluid volume. Many patients arrive in the critical care department with some form of malnutrition. Attention to early nutritional support is essential. Patients who become malnourished are prone to more complications and a higher mortality rate. Most of these patients are unable to eat a regular diet, so nutrition must be provided by enteral tube feedings or parenteral (intravenous) means.

Enteral feeding has proved to be a safe, effective way to provide nutritional support. Feeding the gut has multiple benefits; it increases GI blood flow, maintains the immune function of the GI mucosa, and provides needed nutrients. Improved wound healing and protection from gastritis are other benefits. For enteral feeding, the patient must have some GI function; if no GI function is present, the patient requires parenteral nutrition.

Enteral feedings are tailored to meet the patient's nutrient, vitamin, and mineral needs. If the patient has impaired digestion, a simple formula of partly digested nutrients can be used. Most patients are given a more complex formula of carbohydrates, fats, and proteins that is digested normally. Specialty formulas are available that can meet a patient's particular requirements. For example, a trauma patient usually needs a high-calorie, high-protein, high-potassium formula, whereas a patient with renal failure requires a low-protein, low-potassium formula. As the patient improves or suffers more complications, feeding requirements can change quickly. Common complications of enteral feeding include tube complications, aspiration, intolerance of the feedings, and diarrhea.

With total parenteral nutrition (TPN), patients can have a number of metabolic complications, including electrolyte disturbances. Hyperglycemia occurs in a high percentage of critically ill patients given TPN. High glucose levels diminish the immune response and may cause an osmotic diuresis. Tight glucose control is needed so that insulin can be added to the TPN formula. The insulin is given as a continuous separate drip or as sliding scale dosing.

The complications of enteral and parenteral feeding are presented in Boxes 6-7 and 6-8.

Box 6-7 Complications of Enteral Feedings

Tube Complications

Clogged feeding tube
Necrosis of nares
Sinusitis
Displacement
Otitis media
Skin irritation

Formula Complications

Overhydration
Underhydration
Intolerance
Metabolic derangements (hyperglycemia)
Aspiration
Diarrhea
Failure to provide ordered calories

Box 6-8 Complications of Parenteral Nutrition

Technical Complications

Pneumothorax
Air embolism
Subclavian vein thrombosis

Septic Complications

Infection
Septic shock

Metabolic Complications

Hyperglycemia
Hypoglycemia
Metabolic acidosis
Electrolyte disturbances
Underfeeding
Overfeeding

Other Complications

Atrophy of gastrointestinal mucosa
Impaired immune function

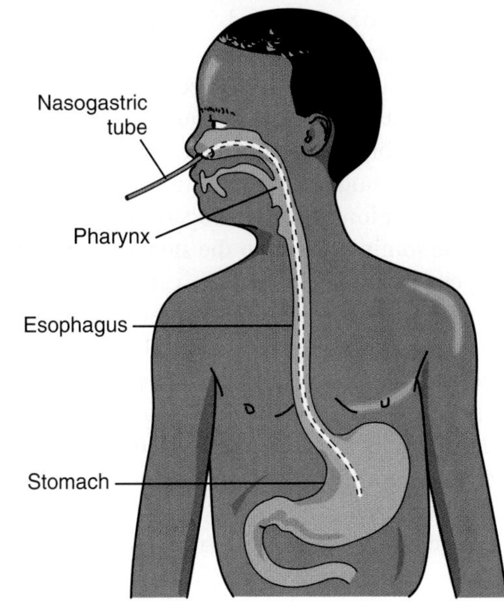

Figure 6-19

Nasogastric (NG) tube. (From Sanders M: *Mosby's paramedic textbook,* ed 3, St Louis, 2007, Mosby.)

Gastric Tubes

Nasogastric Tubes

Large-bore NG tubes usually are inserted to decompress the stomach by removing air and gastric contents. An NG tube also can be used to irrigate the stomach in cases of GI bleeding or overdose. The NG tube can be a single lumen tube that may be attached to low intermittent suction or a double lumen tube, which has an air vent. The air vent provides continuous flow of air through the tube, preventing excessive suction force on the gastric mucosa. Continuous suction may be applied when an air vent is present (Figure 6-19).

The NG tube must be inserted carefully and passed into the stomach without causing significant trauma. Before the tube can be used, its position must be verified. NG tubes have been inserted into the brain through the basilar skull and into the lungs. Patients with lung placement do not always have respiratory symptoms that indicate the problem. The position of the NG tube can be confirmed by auscultation of air in the stomach and by aspirating acidic gastric contents and measuring the pH. However, instillation of air into the stomach with concomitant auscultation can be misinterpreted. Also, the aspirate obtained from a tube in the lung looks like gastric contents, and the gastric aspirate of a patient who has been taking medications to lower the stomach pH will not have an acidic pH. Tube placement is best confirmed radiographically or with a carbon dioxide (CO_2) analyzer.

Tube placement should be reconfirmed before transport. Assess the amount and color of drainage and the level of suction used. Many patients with low aspiration totals can tolerate going without suction for short periods; however, when a large volume must be removed, suction or manual aspiration is required for long transport times. Allowing the volume of the stomach to increase without suctioning can lead to vomiting and aspiration around the tube. Make sure the tube is secure and will not be affected when you move or provide care for the patient.

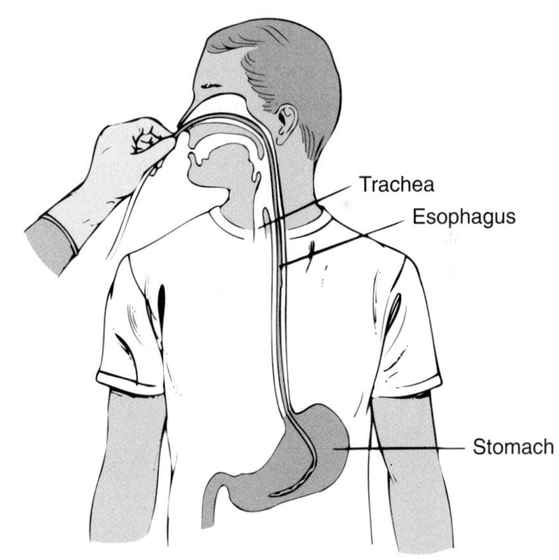

Figure 6-20

Nasoenteric feeding tube. (From Elkin MK, Perry AG, Potter PA: *Nursing interventions and clinical skills,* St Louis, 2007, Mosby.)

Feeding Tubes

A feeding tube may be inserted into the stomach or the small intestine (Figure 6-20). It should be a small-bore tube, which causes less discomfort for the patient and may reduce the risk of aspiration. Feeding tubes usually have a single lumen and are not designed to be attached to suction. Proper placement should be confirmed, usually radiographically, before feeding is started.

For patients with short-term needs, the feeding tube is inserted into the stomach or duodenum. Nasal tubes, which are more comfortable for most patients, require special attention to the skin around the tube and under the tape used to secure the tube. For long-term feeding, the tube can be placed through the abdominal wall into the stomach or small intestine at the level of the jejunum. This can be done surgically or percutaneously, much as a central catheter is placed, by **percutaneous endoscopic gastrostomy (PEG)** (Figure 6-21) or **percutaneous endoscopic jejunostomy (PEJ)**. Long-term feeding tubes also tend to be small, so clogging is still a major concern. Many tubes have internal balloons and outer, flat "bumpers" to secure them. However, even with this system, tubes can be dislodged.

Clogged feeding tubes are a major problem. The most common cause is inadequate irrigation after feedings have been stopped or after administration of medications. The tube should be irrigated with 30 to 60 mL of water every 4 to 8 hours and after bolus feedings or administration of medications. Feeding should never be stopped without irrigation. If the tube becomes blocked, try to irrigate with warm water. Do not use carbonated beverages or cranberry juice (which was recommended in the past), although some institutions have a protocol for digestive enzyme irrigation of a clogged tube. If the tube cannot be cleared, another tube must be inserted. If a G-tube or PEG tube is accidentally pulled out, EMS providers can place a Foley catheter in the hole to keep the stoma patent until definitive placement of a feeding tube.

Surgical Drains

A **T-tube** is used to collect bile from the gallbladder in patients who have undergone surgery of the common bile duct, cholecystectomy, or liver transplantation (Figure 6-22).

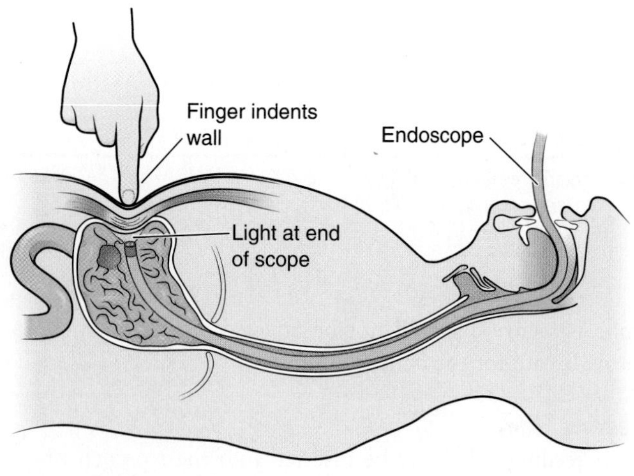

Figure 6-21

Placement of a percutaneous endoscopic gastrostomy (PEG) tube. (From Roberts JR, Hedges JR: *Clinical procedures in emergency medicine*, ed 5, Philadelphia, 2009, Saunders.)

The upper cross bar of the T-tube is inserted into the common bile duct, and the long portion is brought out of the abdomen through an incision. The tube, which is connected to a bag that allows gravity drainage, usually is secured to the abdominal wall with a suture. A T-tube can be left in place for weeks. The suture can become loose, so avoid any pull on the tube. A dressing may be placed on the abdomen around the tube to collect drainage.

A **Penrose drain** is a flat, single lumen tube that may be inserted into a surgical site to drain fluids (Figure 6-23). It is used when drainage of large amounts of fluid is expected, such as with an abscess. The fluid drains into absorbent dressings that may need frequent changing. Other, closed drainage systems can be used in which low pressure can be applied to aid drainage. The **Jackson Pratt drain** has a small bulb on the end (Figure 6-24). An air port is opened, and the bulb is compressed. While compression is maintained, the air port is closed, creating a low pressure system. The bulb is small, so this drain would be used when small amounts of drainage are expected. The Hemovac drainage system drains more fluid but still should be used for small amounts of drainage (Figure 6-25). As with the Jackson Pratt system, the collection system is compressed, creating a vacuum. Both the Jackson Pratt and Hemovac systems have gradations that facilitate measurement of the fluid output. In both drainage systems, the tubes may or may not be secured with a suture. When emptying the containers, make sure you do not pull on the drainage tubes.

Rectal Tubes

Rectal tubes are used to help control and collect liquid diarrhea stool. Continuous exposure to liquid stool and constant cleansing of the skin can cause skin breakdown. A straight tube may be used, but newer tubes have a balloon that is inflated to keep them in place. Some manufacturers recommend that the balloon be deflated every 2 hours and the patient assessed more frequently. Pressure from the balloon may cause necrosis.

General Care of Gastric Tubes and Drains

Before transport, learn as much about the tubes as you do about the patient's history, medications, and other care. Information you need includes the types of tubes, when they were inserted, and the reasons they were inserted. Make sure all tubes are patent and functioning appropriately, and check to make sure the tubes have been properly secured. Assess the insertion site for signs of infection and the condition of the dressings. Ask the current caregiver about the color, consistency, and amount of drainage from each tube. Also ask how often the drains have been emptied. If possible, all drains should be emptied before the patient is transported.

Determine whether tube feedings will continue during transport or will be stopped. If stopped, make sure the feeding tube is well irrigated. Most often, tube feeding is discontinued during transport. If it is to continue, determine what must be done to prevent complications such as aspiration, including how to run the feeding pump.

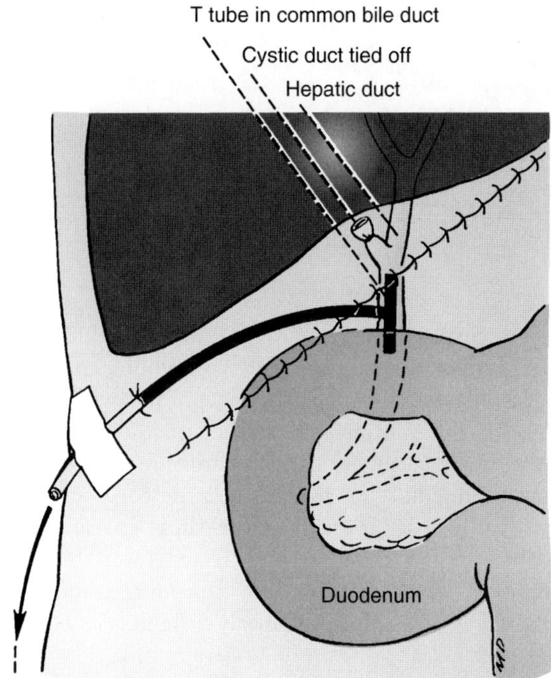

Figure 6-22

T-tube placement in the common bile duct. (From Drain CB. Odom-Forren J: *PeriAnesthesia nursing: a critical care approach,* ed 5. Philadelphia, 2008, Saunders.)

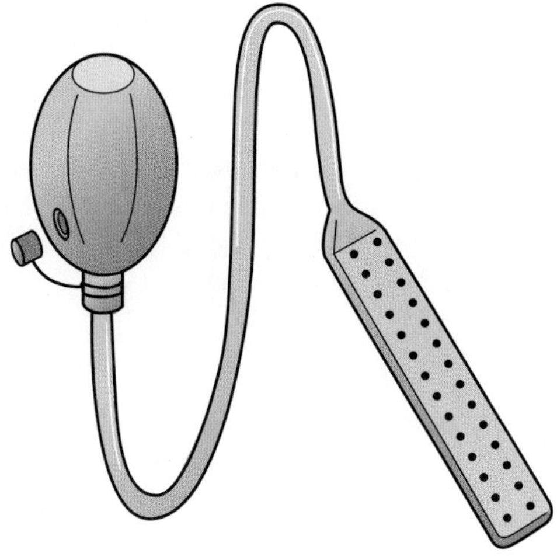

Figure 6-24

Jackson Pratt drainage system. (From Roberts JR, Hedges JR: *Clinical procedures in emergency medicine,* ed 5, Philadelphia, 2009, Saunders.)

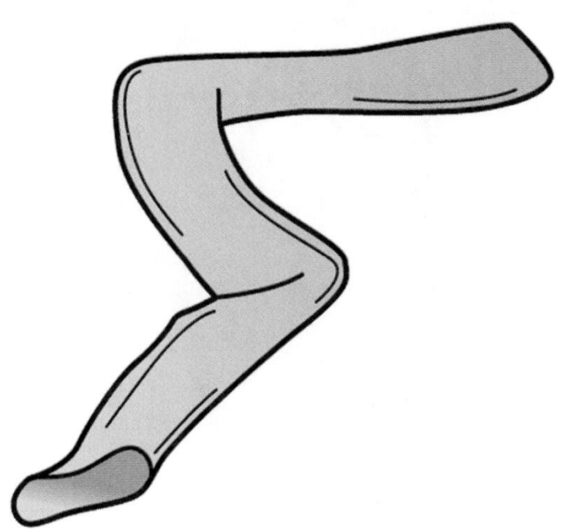

Figure 6-23

Penrose drain. (From Roberts JR, Hedges JR: *Clinical procedures in emergency medicine,* ed 5, Philadelphia, 2009, Saunders.)

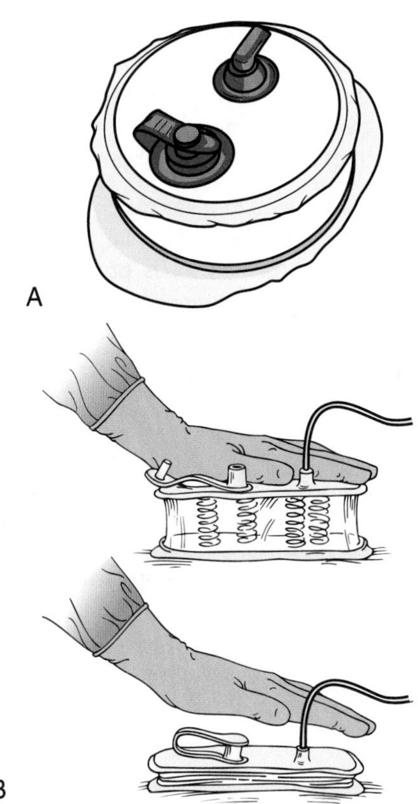

Figure 6-25

A, Hemovac drain reservoir. **B,** Activating a Hemovac drain reservoir. (From Phillips N: *Berry and Kohn's operating room technique,* ed 11, St Louis, 2007, Mosby.)

During transport, record the amount of fluids removed from the patient and add the amount to the patient's output during transport. Loss or gain of small amounts of fluids can be important in a critically ill patient, so keep a careful record of intake and output.

Scenario Conclusion: GI Tract

For the crew's and the patient's safety, you decided to perform a medication-assisted intubation. Octreotide was administered IV bolus and then as a continuous infusion during the transfer. The Sengstaken-Blakemore tube was repositioned after the ETT had been placed, and the combination therapy stopped the GI bleeding. After the airway was secured and the patient stopped moving around, the transport proceeded without mishap. At the receiving hospital, the GI bleeding was definitively treated, and the SB tube was removed 2 days later. The patient subsequently redeveloped esophageal bleeding and succumbed during the resuscitation.

RENAL SYSTEM

Scenario: Renal System

Your critical care transport team is called to assist a 42-year-old patient with diabetes who complains of generalized weakness and abdominal cramping. His admission vitals are: pulse, 128 beats/min; respirations, 36 breaths/min (and slightly labored with some crackles auscultated bilaterally in the lung fields); BP, 96/40 mm Hg; temperature, 36.1° C (96.9° F). As you are placing him on the cardiac monitor, he complains of chest pressure, and you note a wide complex tachycardia (rate, 138 beats/min). The patient admits to chronic renal failure and has missed his last dialysis run by 2 days. He reports about 30 to 50 mL of urine production per day, and his most recent creatinine level was about 9 mg/dl.

The physician wants you to give calcium gluconate empirically, followed by glucose and insulin with sodium bicarbonate. As you wonder why this patient needs such a cocktail of drugs, the patient moans with increasing chest pressure.

We all know the importance of fluids for the health of all cells in the body. The kidneys are responsible for a number of functions that are crucial for maintaining homeostasis. The main functions of the kidneys are to remove waste, maintain the water and electrolyte balance, and help maintain the acid-base balance. The kidneys also play key roles in red blood cell synthesis and blood pressure control.

ANATOMY AND PHYSIOLOGY

The kidneys sit in the abdominal retroperitoneal space on each side of the aorta. Each kidney is 11 to 12 cm (4.4 to 4.8 inches) long and 2.5 to 3 cm (1 to 1.2 inches) thick. The kidneys are similar in color and shape to the kidney bean. The medial surface of the kidney is concave. The ureters, blood supply, and nerves enter or exit the kidney in the concave area, called the *hilum.* Several layers of fat and connective tissue surround the kidney for support and protection. The outer layer, or capsule, of the kidney is made up of a tough, fibrous tissue that also helps protect the kidney (Figure 6-26).

Did You Know?

The right kidney is lower because of the large liver on the right side. The exact position of the kidneys depends on the position of the body. When a person is standing, the kidneys fall lower in the abdomen.[2]

The nephron is the functioning unit of the kidney. Each kidney is composed of approximately 1 million nephrons. The two types of nephrons are cortical nephrons, which account for 85% of all nephrons, and the juxtamedullary nephrons. The anatomic placement of the nephrons forms two distinct sections, the medullary pyramids and the cortex tissue. The cortex tissue forms an outer layer that dips between the pyramids. The tips of the pyramids are directed toward the concave portion of the kidney. The nephrons produce urine through the tips of the pyramids into the calyx, the first section of the

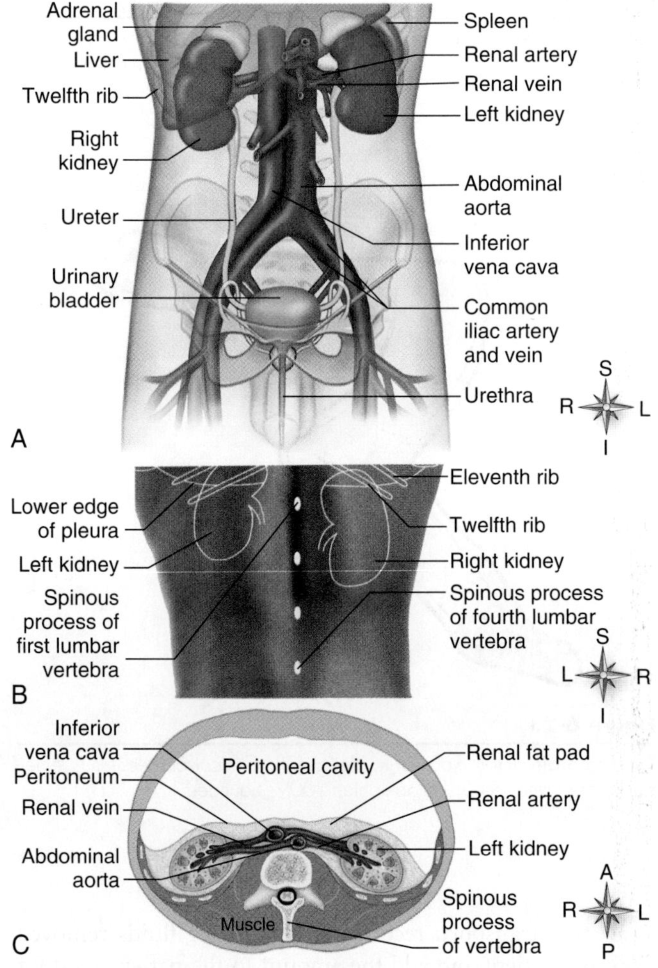

Figure 6-26

Urinary tract system. (From Patton KT, Thibodeau GA: *Anatomy and physiology,* ed 7, St Louis, 2009, Mosby.)

urine collection system. The calyces are cuplike structures that surround each pyramid tip. The calyces form the renal pelvis, which is outside the kidney tissue in the hilum area. The renal pelvis connects to the ureter, which goes to the bladder. (Locate the cortex, pyramids, and urine collection system in Figure 6-27.) The kidneys receive approximately 25% of the cardiac output (1200 mL/min) through the renal arteries, which supply blood to the kidney.

The ureters are muscular tubes with walls lined with smooth muscle, which contracts to propel urine into the bladder. The ureters are approximately 25 to 30 cm (10 to 12 inches) long. The bladder is located behind the symphysis pubis and below the parietal peritoneum. Smooth muscle and epithelial tissue in the bladder wall allow the bladder to distend to accommodate large amounts of urine. As many healthcare professionals can attest, the bladder can hold huge volumes of urine on a long, busy day. The bladder also can collapse when empty.

The bladder has three openings, the two ureters and the urethra, which form a triangle on the bladder floor. Right and left ureters enter the bladder from the posterior corners of the bladder floor, and the urethra leaves the bladder at the anterior corner of the triangle. The urethra is the small tube that passes urine from the bladder to the exterior of the body (see Figure 6-26).

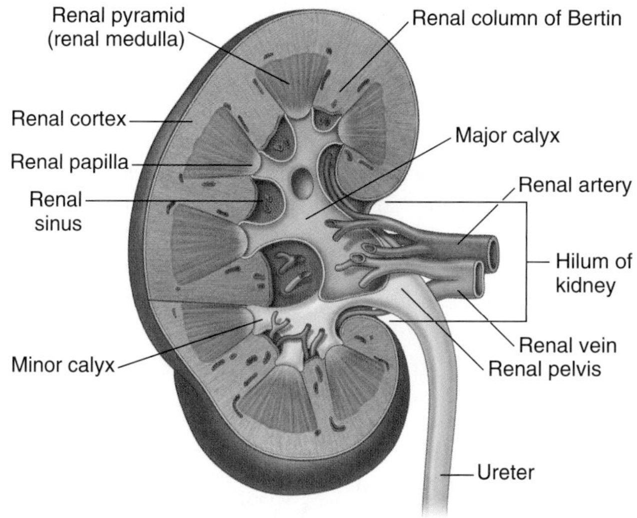

Figure 6-27

Structure of the kidney. (From Wein A, Kavoussi L, Novick A et al: *Campbell-Walsh urology*, ed 9, Philadelphia, 2007, Saunders.)

Structure of the Nephron

The nephron is made up of the glomerulus, the vascular system, and the tubule system. As mentioned previously, the kidneys receive about 1200 mL of blood per minute through the renal arteries (off the abdominal aorta), or about 25% of the cardiac output. Each renal artery divides into anterior and posterior branches, which then subdivide into lobar arteries. Within the lobes of each kidney, interlobar arteries direct blood to the glomerus, and arcuate arteries are near the pyramids. (Figure 6-28).

The interlobar arteries lead into the afferent arteriole, which helps form a capillary bed, called the *glomerulus*. The glomerulus has a semipermeable membrane that allows filtration of blood into the nephron tubule system. The membrane is permeable to small particles and water but not to large particles such as proteins and blood cells. Unlike with other capillaries in the body, not enough oxygen is given off to the tissues to convert the blood to venous blood. After the glomerulus, the efferent arteriole carries the arterial blood into

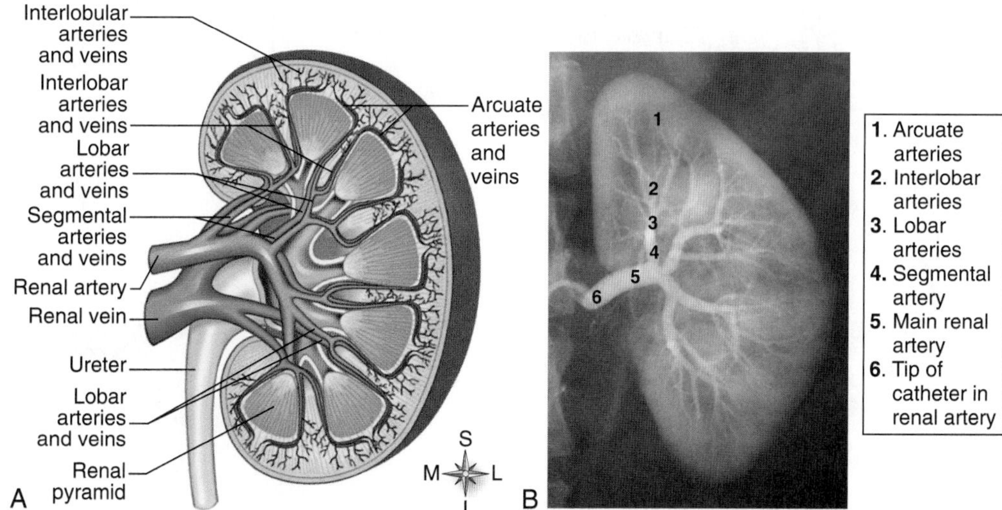

Figure 6-28

Circulation through the kidney. **A,** Major arteries and veins of the renal circulation. **B,** Renal arteriogram. (From Patton KT, Thibodeau GA: *Anatomy and physiology*, ed 7, St Louis, 2009, Mosby.)

another capillary bed, the vasa recta. The vasa recta (or peritubular capillaries) surrounds the renal tubule system; it reabsorbs needed substances and water back into the body and provides oxygen to the kidney tissue. The blood then becomes venous and returns to the body through a venous network similar to the arterial network, ending in the renal vein. The layout of the vascular system as it surrounds the nephron is shown in Figure 6-29; note how the vasa recta flows down to the tip of the pyramid and then back up. If you looked directly at a dissected kidney, the pyramids would appear darker red because of the blood supply in the pyramid (see Figure 6-28).

The glomerulus is surrounded by a saclike structure called *Bowman's capsule.* Look at Figure 6-30 and find the parts of the nephron as we discuss each one. Bowman's capsule collects the filtrate from the glomerulus and sends it into the proximal tubule. About 85% of the filtered water and substances are reabsorbed into the body from the proximal tubule. The proximal tubule leads into the loop of Henle, a hairpin-like structure that dips into the medullary pyramids. The loop of Henle provides the right conditions so that the kidney can concentrate or dilute the urine based on the body's current water needs. The loop of Henle leads into the distal convoluted tubule, which fine-tunes electrolyte and water reabsorption. Hundreds of distal convoluted tubules dump filtrate into each of the collecting ducts. A collecting duct runs from the outer cortex tissue to the tip of one of the medullary pyramids. The collecting duct is the system's last chance to reabsorb water from the filtrate. Filtrate then drips from the collecting tube through the end of the pyramid into the minor calyx; it now is considered urine. The urine travels from the minor calyx to the major calyx, into the renal pelvis, and down the ureter to the bladder. Now locate the two nephrons in Figure 6-29 and find all the sections of the nephron, paying attention to how the nephrons are positioned in relation to the blood supply.

Urine Formation

Urine formation is complex and involves three processes:

1. *Filtration* is the movement of water and particles from the plasma across the semipermeable membrane of the glomerulus into Bowman's capsule.
2. *Reabsorption* is the movement of water and particles out of the tubules and back into the body through the venous system.
3. *Secretion* is the movement of particles such as potassium and hydrogen ions from the tubule cells into the filtrate, allowing the kidney to maintain electrolyte and acid-base balance.

The first step, filtration, occurs at the glomerular capillary membrane. As mentioned, the glomerulus is a semipermeable membrane that allows all particles in the blood to be filtered into Bowman's capsule except most proteins and blood cells. After the fluid from the plasma crosses the membrane into Bowman's capsule, it is called *filtrate.* Because the glomerulus

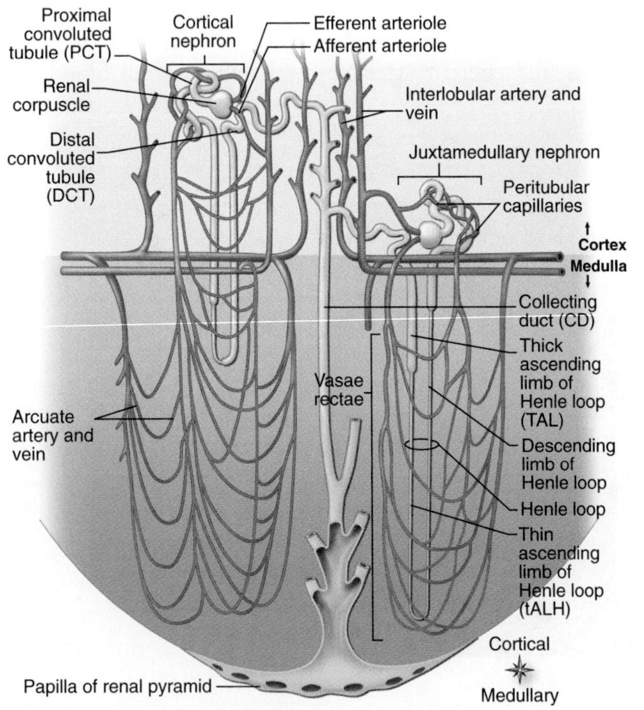

Figure 6-29

Nephron with blood vessels. (From Patton KT, Thibodeau GA: *Anatomy and physiology*, ed 7, St Louis, 2009, Mosby.)

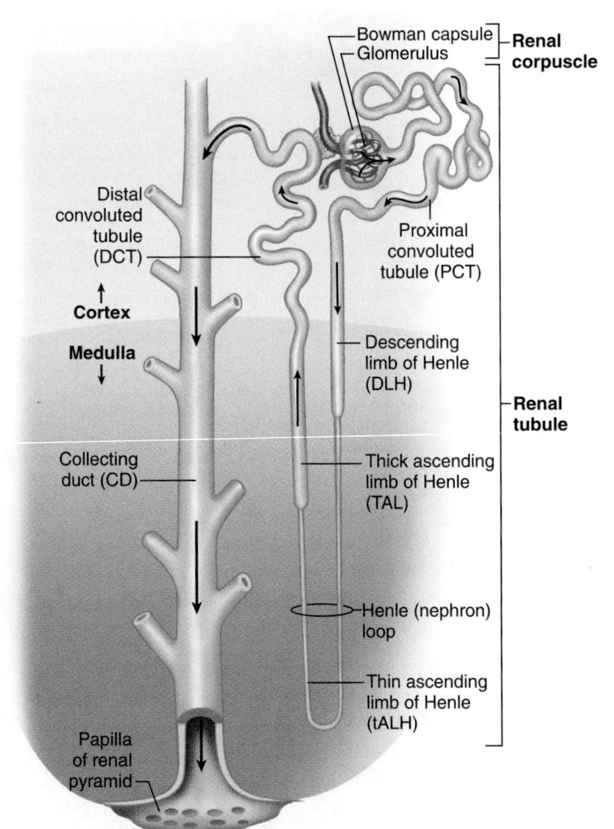

Figure 6-30

Components of the nephron. (From Patton KT, Thibodeau GA: *Anatomy and physiology*, ed 7, St Louis, 2009, Mosby.)

has no way to filter just the waste products, needed substances, such as water, electrolytes, and glucose, must be reabsorbed into the body. Of the renal blood flow (1200 mL/min), approximately 125 mL/min is filtered at the glomerulus; this is the glomerular filtration rate (GFR).

Understanding the process of glomerular filtration is vital to an understanding of renal problems in a critically ill patient. Filtration occurs because of a pressure gradient that pushes substances and water out of the glomerular capillary into Bowman's capsule. This pressure gradient is derived from three major forces, some of which oppose each other.

- **Capillary hydrostatic pressure** is the pressure of the blood itself inside the glomerulus. It depends mainly on the systemic pressure, the degree of dilation of the renal artery, and the volume of blood present. This pressure favors filtration.
- **Plasma colloid oncotic pressure** is the pressure, or the osmotic pull, of the plasma proteins in the bloodstream. Protein cannot cross the semipermeable membrane, so proteins act as an osmotic agent, pulling back into the glomerulus. This pressure opposes filtration.
- **Bowman's capsule pressure** is the pressure exerted by any filtrate in the epithelial sac that is Bowman's capsule. This pressure opposes filtration.

These three pressures cannot be measured at the bedside, but pressures taken from animal experiments can be used to demonstrate the filtration process. For example, assume the following pressures:

Capillary hydrostatic pressure: 60 mm Hg
Plasma colloid oncotic pressure: 32 mm Hg
Bowman's capsule pressure: 18 mm Hg

Add the two pressures that oppose filtration, the plasma colloid oncotic pressure and the Bowman's capsule pressure; the result is 50 mm Hg. Now subtract that value from the capillary hydrostatic pressure, or the pressure that pushes fluid out of the glomerulus: $60 - 50 = 10$ mm Hg. The result, 10 mm Hg, is the net filtration pressure that is pushing fluid out into Bowman's capsule. This filtration pressure allows the kidney to move water and solutes out of the plasma and into the nephron.

Theoretically, any change in the pressures changes the amount of filtration. See what would happen to filtration if the capillary hydrostatic pressure fell to 50 mm Hg because the patient's systemic blood pressure fell and all other pressures remained the same. What would be the net filtration pressure? What would be the effect on the urine output? The net filtration pressure would be 0 mm Hg, and no filtration would take place. If no filtration occurs, no urine is formed. How many of your patients have had low blood pressure?

Several factors affect the net filtration, which in turn affects the GFR. The glomerulus is a semipermeable membrane that can be affected by many conditions. If its permeability decreases, filtration decreases. Chronic glomerulonephritis causes decreased permeability. Over time the glomerulus scars because of the chronic inflammation. If permeability increases, filtration increases because more fluid and large particles can move across the membrane. Increased filtration could be caused by acute glomerulonephritis or by the severe sepsis that is seen in critically ill patients.

When renal blood flow decreases, the net filtration pressure decreases, leading to a decreased urine output. Blood flow can be affected by any shock state or by low cardiac output, both of which can cause low blood pressure. If the blood pressure falls too low, filtration can stop completely. Remember the net filtration pressure you calculated when the patient's systolic pressure decreased—0 mm Hg. Zero net filtration pressure results in no urine output.

On the other hand, when renal blood flow increases, filtration increases, increasing urine output. To protect renal function, the kidneys are able to autoregulate to accommodate changes in the systemic blood pressure. When the patient's blood pressure decreases, the afferent arteriole dilates and the efferent arteriole constricts to maintain a higher pressure in the glomerulus; this maintains the GFR near normal levels. Autoregulation works well for most decreases in blood pressure; however, when the pressure drops below a systolic pressure of 80 mm Hg, the GFR dramatically falls because of lack of hydrostatic capillary pressure. The kidney also regulates for higher blood pressures by dilating the efferent arteriole, which decreases the hydrostatic pressure in the glomerulus. When the patient's blood pressure increases above autoregulation limits, filtration increases, causing an increase in urine output. In most patients the upper autoregulation level is 50 to 150 mm Hg; hypertensive patients, therefore, may have a higher than normal urinary output. This is not life-threatening over a short period.

Stimulation of the sympathetic nervous system (SNS) also may affect the GFR. SNS stimulation causes vasoconstriction of the afferent and efferent arterioles, leading to decreased blood in the glomerulus and decreased filtration. This same effect occurs when a critically ill patient is given vasoconstrictors for hypotension. Renal blood flow to the glomerulus can be stopped completely. Decreasing filtration allows waste products to build up in the body; however, remember that the kidney cells get their oxygen supply from the blood flow after the glomerulus. Vasoconstriction of the afferent and efferent arterioles frequently causes renal ischemia and acute renal failure.

The last major determinant of filtration is the protein level of the plasma, which determines the oncotic pressure. When the plasma protein level is low, oncotic pressure in the blood is decreased; this leads to less resistance to filtration, and the GFR increases. Patients with low serum proteins may have a very high urinary output, which puts them at risk for significant water loss. Low plasma proteins may be seen in patients with severe malnutrition or burns. When the plasma protein level is too high, the oncotic pressure in the blood is increased, which reduces filtration and also urinary output.

Filtrate Processing

The filtrate in Bowman's capsule is almost exactly like the plasma except that no proteins are present. The filtrate flows into the proximal convoluted tubule, where 65% to 80% of it is reabsorbed into the body. As the filtrate enters the proximal tubule, many of the particles are absorbed through the tubule wall into the interstitial space and then into the peritubular capillaries. As the number of solutes (Na^+, glucose, K^+, amino acids, HCO_3^-, urea) is absorbed, the osmolarity of the fluid in the tubule lumen decreases. When the osmolarity of the fluid in the tubule lumen is less than that of the interstitial fluid around the tubule, water is drawn by osmosis into the peritubular capillaries. Most of the osmotic pull is related to the amount of sodium reabsorbed.

Some particles are absorbed using a carrier protein. Most carrier proteins transport only a specific particle. Because a limited number of carrier proteins is available for each particle, there is a transport maximum for that particle. Glucose is a substance that uses a carrier protein. When all carrier proteins for glucose are attached, the glucose that is not attached to a protein is not reabsorbed. The proximal tubule is the only area of the nephron in which proteins carry glucose. If the patient's plasma glucose level is normal, all the glucose is reabsorbed. If the patient has an elevated glucose level, all available proteins may be attached to glucose and the extra glucose molecules stay in the filtrate, moving through the rest of the nephron. Because there are no proteins for glucose transport in the rest of the nephron, the patient has glucose in the urine. In patients with diabetes, this is called "spilling sugar." If the patient spills a high level of glucose into the urine, the glucose acts as an osmotic agent, and urine output is extremely high. This is the main cause of dehydration in a diabetic individual with ketoacidosis (DKA).

The proximal tubule also can secrete substances the body does not need into the filtrate, such as hydrogen, potassium, and waste products of drugs that have been metabolized by the tubule cells. Many antibiotics are metabolized by the kidney. The filtrate leaves the proximal convoluted tubule and enters the loop of Henle. The major function of the loop of Henle is concentration or dilution of urine. The loop of Henle builds up a hyperosmolar interstitial fluid in the medullary pyramids with high concentrations of sodium and chloride. The collecting tube, which receives approximately 10% of the original filtrate volume, is responsible for the final concentration of the filtrate but is normally impermeable to water. If the patient's GFR is 125 mL/min and the collecting tube does not reabsorb any water, the patient's urinary output is 750 mL/hour. To allow absorption of water at the collecting tube, **antidiuretic hormone (ADH)** is released by the posterior pituitary. ADH changes the membrane of the collecting tube so that it is permeable to water. Water is reabsorbed by osmotic pull; therefore, the high osmolarity in the interstitial fluid provided by the loop of Henle allows water reabsorption across the collecting tube membrane. When the body needs to get rid of more water, less ADH is released, so less filtrate is reabsorbed at the collecting tube, and the patient has a higher urine output (Figure 6-31). If no ADH is present or if the loop of Henle does not maintain the hyperosmolar interstitial fluid, the kidney cannot concentrate urine.

The distal convoluted tubule acts as a fine tuner for electrolyte and acid-base balance. It functions under the direction

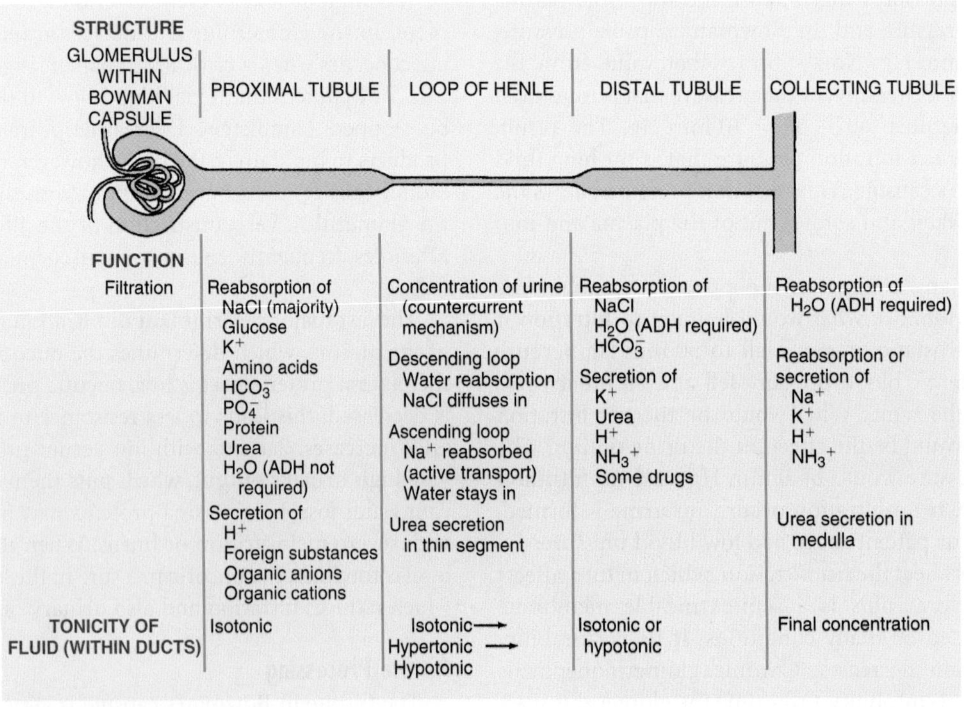

Figure 6-31

Major functions of the nephron segments. (From McCance KL, Huether SE: *Pathophysiology: the biological basis for disease in adults and children*, ed 6, St Louis, 2009, Mosby.)

of **aldosterone**, a hormone from the adrenal cortex. When aldosterone is present, sodium and water are reabsorbed and potassium and hydrogen are excreted. Once the filtrate hits the collecting tube, small adjustments are made in the electrolyte content and major amounts of water are reabsorbed. In a healthy adult, usually 99% of the filtrate is reabsorbed into the body and most of the waste products are eliminated in the urine. If the collecting tube does not absorb water, the urine output could be as high as 600 mL/hour. Review Figure 6-31 to see where substances are absorbed as the filtrate moves through the nephron.

Functions of the Kidneys

Maintenance of Body Water and Composition of the Extracellular Fluid

Maintenance of body water and composition of the extracellular fluid are probably the most important functions of the kidneys. Urea, creatinine, and uric acid are byproducts the kidneys filter out through the complex process of urine formation. Solutes, such as electrolytes, are absorbed or eliminated into the urine based on the body's needs for maintaining appropriate electrolyte levels. The regulation of sodium levels is extremely important to maintaining water levels in the extracellular fluid compartment. Water is eliminated in exact quantities, in the form of urine, to maintain homeostasis.

Elimination of Metabolic Wastes and Foreign Waste

Urea, uric acid, and creatinine, the byproducts of protein metabolism, must be eliminated from the body daily; a buildup of these substances can be life-threatening. Urea is measured as the BUN. It is the end product of protein metabolism resulting from the breakdown of ammonia in the liver. Creatinine is the end product of protein metabolism by the muscles. All creatinine is filtered by the kidneys; therefore, when the kidneys are not working correctly, increased creatinine levels in the blood may be a good indicator of the degree of decreased kidney function. (The BUN and creatinine are discussed later in the chapter.)

Most drugs are metabolized by the liver; however, some drugs are metabolized by the tubule cells, and the metabolites are then released into the urine. The kidney also filters inactive drug metabolites that the liver has deposited into the bloodstream.

Regulation of Blood Pressure

Blood pressure is regulated by three major components: blood volume, the **renin-angiotensin-aldosterone system (RAAS)** (Figure 6-32), and the autonomic nervous system. The kidney helps control blood volume and maintains intravascular volume by regulating sodium levels. Renin is released by the kidney in response to decreased renal blood flow; renin converts **angiotensin** into **angiotensin I**. Angiotensin I is converted to **angiotensin II** by angiotensin-converting enzyme (ACE) in the pulmonary vasculature. Angiotensin II is a powerful vasoconstrictor, and it also stimulates the release of aldosterone, which increases sodium reabsorption.

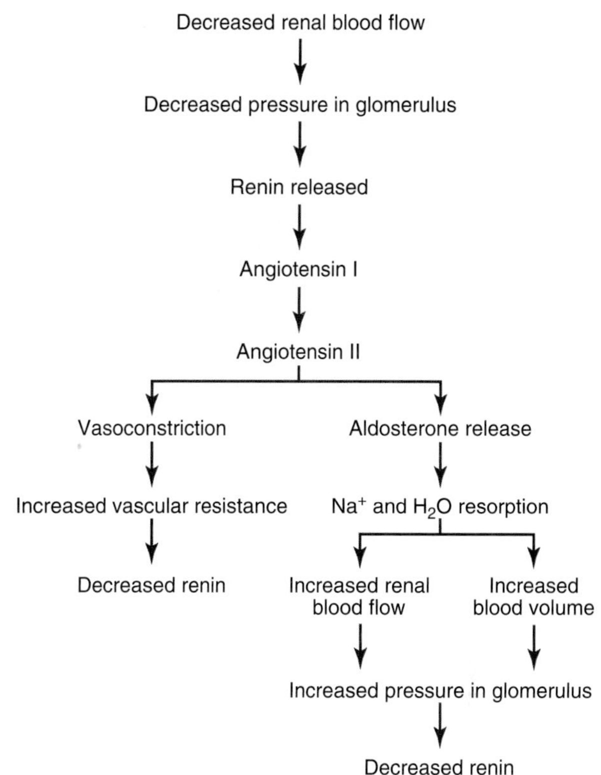

Figure 6-32

Renin-angiotensin-aldosterone system. (From Urden LD, Stacy KM, Lough ME: *Thelan's critical care nursing*, ed 5, St Louis, 2006, Mosby.)

Regulation of Acid-Base Balance

The kidneys regulate acid base balance through reabsorption or elimination of bicarbonate and hydrogen ions based on the pH. The kidney also can generate new bicarbonate into the plasma when a severe acidosis is present. Renal control of acid-base balance takes a few days to a week to maximize, but once activated, it is a very good buffering system.

Production of Erythropoietin

Erythropoietin is produced and released by the kidney to stimulate the bone marrow to produce red blood cells. The stimulus for its production is decreased oxygen levels in the renal blood supply. A patient with renal failure is at risk for anemia from loss of erythropoietin. In patients with chronic hypoxia (e.g., those with chronic obstructive pulmonary disease [COPD]), more erythropoietin is released. Extreme anemia is treated with blood transfusions or synthetic erythropoietin.

Synthesis of Vitamin D

Vitamin D is necessary for the absorption of calcium and phosphorus by the small intestine. Vitamin D can be obtained through the diet or synthesized by ultraviolet light in the skin. Vitamin D is in an inactive form until the kidneys activate it to vitamin D_3. Without the activated form of vitamin D, a patient's ability to absorb calcium from the GI tract decreases, making the person hypocalcemic.

Controlling Fluid Balance

Fluid balance is a crucial factor in the proper function of the kidneys. Three factors involved in the regulation of body fluids are ADH, aldosterone, and **atrial natriuretic peptide (ANP)**. ADH is secreted by the posterior pituitary and controls the extracellular fluid (ECF) volume. Osmoreceptors in the hypothalamus and liver send signals for the release of ADH. After it is released, ADH is carried through the circulation to the nephrons. With ADH present, water is reabsorbed, resulting in a high ECF volume. Of course, the opposite also is true; in the absence of ADH, the volume of the ECF is greatly diminished.

Aldosterone, once released by the RAAS, acts on the distal tubules to reabsorb sodium into the circulation; once sodium is retained, so is water. When the vascular fluid volume drops, renin is released, which converts angiotensin. The subsequent conversion to angiotensin II further constricts the renal vasculature. This reduces renal blood flow and any available glomerular filtrate, which sends the signal for the release of ADH. This process assists not only in the maintenance of fluid balance, but also in the maintenance of electrolyte balance.

ANP is secreted from cells in the atria of the heart secondary to cardiac muscle stretch and hypervolemia/hypernatremia. ANP blocks aldosterone and ADH production, which affects the sodium and water balance; this causes vasodilation and increases sodium and water excretion by the kidneys. Fluid overload is decreased through diuresis, which reduces preload and afterload and decreases the cardiac workload.

Electrolyte Balance

Fluid and Electrolytes

The body has two distinct fluid compartments, and fluids and electrolytes move between them. The largest compartment is the fluid inside the cells, the *intracellular compartment.* The other compartment, the *extracellular compartment,* includes the fluid in the blood vessels, the intravascular fluid, and the fluid between the blood vessels and the cells (i.e., the interstitial fluid). The intracellular fluid accounts for 40%, the intravascular compartment for 5%, and the interstitial fluid for 15% of the body's weight. Water, therefore, makes up about 60% of the body's weight. Water provides a means of moving oxygen, nutrients, and electrolytes, which are required by every cell in the body. Electrolytes are a major component of body fluids. They are compounds that dissociate into ions when in fluids. Ions, which are either positively charged or negatively charged, give fluid the ability to conduct an electrical current. Maintaining the balance of water and electrolytes in each compartment is extremely important for normal body functioning (Figure 6-33).

The movement of fluid and electrolytes between compartments is governed by osmosis, osmolality, diffusion, active transport, and filtration. To understand the physiology of the renal and GI systems, an understanding of these processes is important.

Osmosis is the movement of water through a semipermeable membrane from an area of low concentration of particles to an area with a higher concentration of particles (solute) (Figure 6-34). Essentially, water is pulled to the more concentrated side of the membrane. The concentration of particles is measured as the *osmolality,* the number of particles in a volume of water. Osmolality, or osmotic pull, is the main way water is moved from one compartment to another. The normal osmolality of the blood is 285 to 295 mOsm/L. All fluids given to a patient have a certain osmolality, which affects the way the patient's body handles the fluid. An *isotonic* fluid has an osmolality similar to that of plasma. Isotonic fluids do not cause significant movement of water into or out of the plasma.

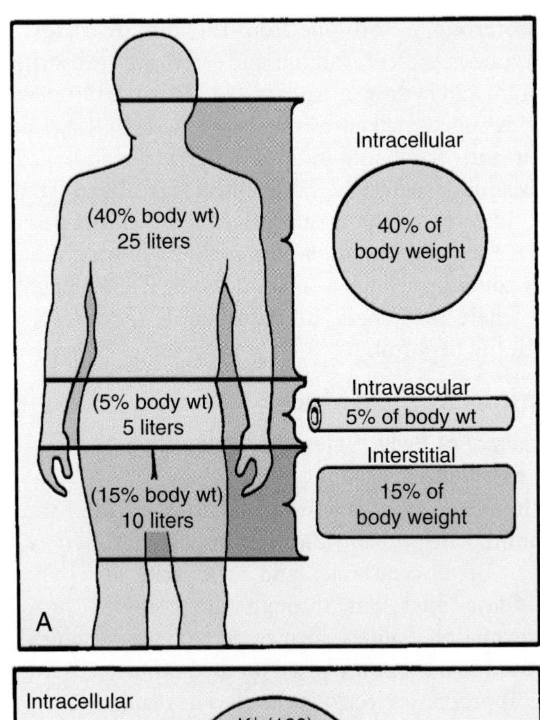

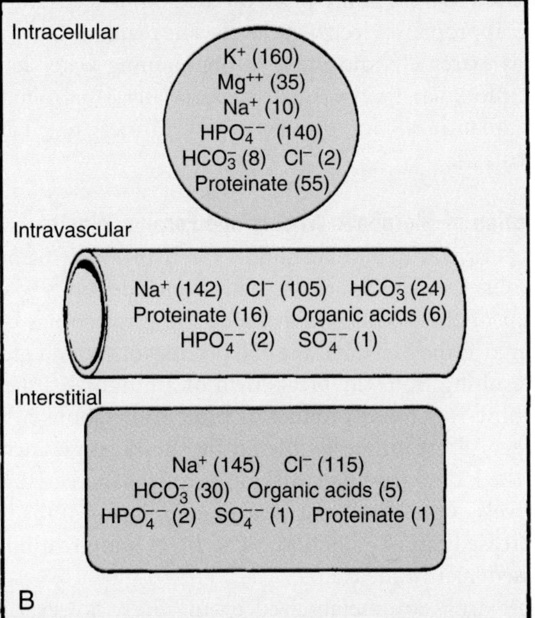

Figure 6-33

A, Fluid compartments. **B,** Electrolytes by fluid compartment. (From Urden LD, Stacy KM, Lough ME: *Thelan's critical care nursing,* ed 5, St Louis, 2006, Mosby.)

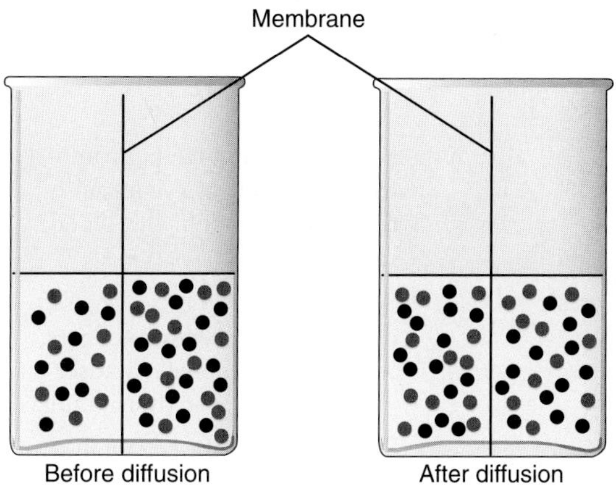

Figure 6-34

Osmosis through a semipermeable membrane. (From Lewis SL, Heitkemper MM, Dirksen SR et al: *Medical-surgical nursing: assessment and management of clinical problems,* St Louis, 2007, Mosby.)

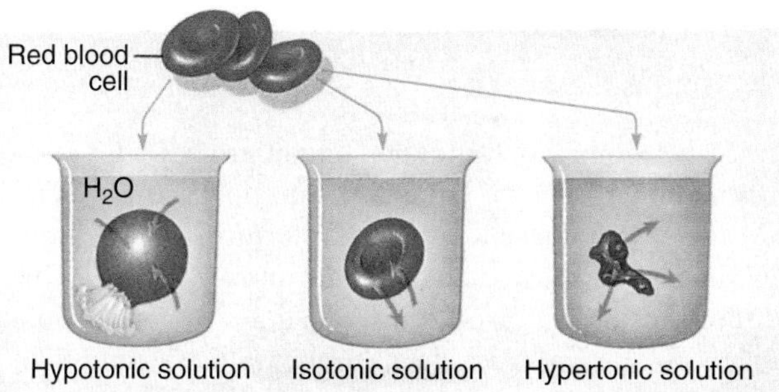

Figure 6-35

Effects of hypotonic, isotonic, and hypertonic solutions on red blood cells. **A,** A *hypotonic* solution, which has a low ion concentration, causes swelling and lysis of the cells. **B,** In an *isotonic* solution, which has a normal ion concentration, the cells keep their normal shape. **C,** A *hypertonic* solution, which has a high ion concentration, causes shrinkage (crenation) of the cells. (From Sanders M: *Mosby's paramedic textbook,* ed 3, St Louis, 2007, Mosby.)

Examples of isotonic IV fluids are normal saline and lactated Ringer's solutions. A *hypertonic* fluid contains a higher concentration of particles compared to the plasma. When a patient is given hypertonic fluids (e.g., 3% NS), water is pulled from the cells into the vascular space. This type of fluid might be used for a patient with intravascular dehydration or a patient with cellular edema. *Hypotonic* solutions have a lower concentration of particles compared to plasma; therefore, hypotonic fluids help move fluids from the plasma into the cells (Figure 6-35). An example of a hypotonic solution is 0.45% NS.

Diffusion and active transport involve the movement of particles across a membrane. *Diffusion* is the movement of particles across a semipermeable membrane from an area of high concentration to an area of low concentration. The particles move across the membrane until the number of particles is equal on both sides. Active transport allows the movement of a substance against a concentration gradient. This allows the movement of a substance from an area of low concentration into an area of high concentration. For example, potassium has a high concentration inside the cells compared to outside the cells, but potassium still needs to be replaced in the cells. Active transport moves the potassium into the cell against the gradient with the use of energy.

Filtration is the movement of fluids and substances through a semipermeable membrane using a pressure gradient. This is the process the glomerular membrane uses to filter the blood and start the process of urine formation.

Electrolytes are extremely important to all body functions. They provide nerve transmission and contractility of muscle, and they help maintain fluid compartments and a host of other functions. If electrolytes are not maintained at the proper level, loss of body functions and possibly death result. Sodium is responsible for maintaining the water content of the plasma and is the major electrolyte of the plasma. Potassium is the major electrolyte of the intracellular fluid. For a brief review of the major electrolytes and symptoms of electrolyte imbalances, see Boxes 6-9 to 6-12 before reading further.

Box 6-9 Sodium

Normal	135-150 mEq/L
Effects of sodium	Main electrolyte in plasma; body water movement; extracellular fluid osmolality; neuromuscular activity; enzymes activity; acid-base balance
Hypernatremia	*Symptoms:* Lethargy, weakness, irritability, agitation, mania, delirium, seizures, coma, increased deep tendon reflexes, nuchal rigidity, thirst, elevated body temperature, flushed skin, dry mucous membranes
Hyponatremia	*Symptoms:* Anorexia, impaired taste, muscle cramps, headache, personality changes, weakness, lethargy, nausea and vomiting, abdominal cramps, seizures and coma, absent or diminished reflexes, papilledema, fingerprinting edema over sternum

ASSESSMENT OF THE GENITOURINARY TRACT

History

If the patient reports having chronic renal failure, end-stage renal disease, or renal insufficiency, several more questions should be included in the history portion of your initial assessment. Ask the patient what type of renal failure has been diagnosed and whether he or she makes any urine. Is the patient on dialysis? If the answer is yes, what type of dialysis and access device is used? How much fluid typically is dialyzed off? Does the patient have a dialysis fistula or graft in an

Box 6-10 Potassium

Normal	3.5-5.3 mEq/L
Effects of potassium	Main electrolyte in cells; transmission of nerve impulses; intracellular osmolality; enzymatic reactions; acid-base balance; muscle contractility
Hyperkalemia	*Symptoms:* Weakness; flaccid paralysis; paresthesias of the face, tongue, feet, and hands; nausea and vomiting; intestinal colic; diarrhea; twitching; hyperreflexia proceeding to paresthesia and paralysis; bradycardia proceeding to cardiac arrest; ventricular fibrillation; oliguria; ECG changes (peaked T waves, widened QRS complex, prolonged PR interval, flattened or absent P waves, ST segment depression)
Hypokalemia	*Symptoms:* Fatigue, muscle weakness, leg cramps, nausea and vomiting, ileus, constipation, paresthesias, enhanced digitalis effect, decreased urine concentration (nephrogenic diabetes insipidus), decreased reflexes and muscle tone, ECG changes (ST segment depression, flattened T waves, presence of U waves, ventricular dysrhythmias) NOTE: Hypokalemia potentiates the effect of digitalis.

Box 6-11 Magnesium

Normal	1.5-2.5 mEq/L
Effects of magnesium	Promotes neuromuscular transmission and contraction of myocardium; activates enzymes; maintains active transport
Hypermagnesemia	*Symptoms:* Lethargy, nausea and vomiting, slurred speech
Hypomagnesemia	*Symptoms:* Weakness, irritability, tetany, delirium, convulsions, ventricular dysrhythmias, long QT interval, torsades de pointes

extremity? Does the patient have a fever (think graft infection)? How often does the patient have dialysis and when was the last dialysis session? Check to see whether the patient has had any problems with dialysis recently. Any signs of fluid overload or heart failure? Check not only the patient's medication list, but also compliance with blood pressure (BP) medications and so on.

Box 6-12 Calcium

Normal	9-10.5 mg/dL
Effects of calcium	Forms bone and teeth; promotes transmission of nerve impulses, muscle contraction, and blood clotting; activates enzymes
Hypercalcemia	*Symptoms:* Lethargy, weakness, decreased deep tendon reflexes, constipation, anorexia, nausea and vomiting, polyuria, dysrhythmias
Hypocalcemia	*Symptoms:* Numbness, tingling of the extremities and around the mouth, muscle tremors, cramps, tetany, convulsions, dysrhythmias, confusion, anxiety, psychosis, ECG changes (prolonged QT interval)

Physical Assessment

Physical examination techniques do not provide a lot of direct information about the kidneys. Inspection should focus on the flanks and the abdomen. Any bruising, distention, or guarding may indicate a hematoma around the kidney. During your overall inspection of the patient, note any signs of volume depletion or overload, which could be a warning sign of kidney problems. Skin turgor is a good indicator of fluid volume status, and inspection of the oral cavity also provides important clues (dry mouth, cracked lips and tongue).

The renal arteries can be auscultated for abnormal renal artery bruits, but bruits are very difficult to hear. Auscultate on either side of the umbilicus and listen for a swooshing sound similar to that of a cardiac murmur. The presence of this renal artery bruit normally indicates stenosis.

The kidneys are not easily palpated, although in a thin patient, you may be able to palpate the lower portion of the right kidney. Percussion is performed to detect pain and the accumulation of air, fluid, or solids around the kidney.

For the most part, the physical assessment relates to the effects of disease processes on other body organs. When assessing the patient, observe the person's general appearance. Note the color of the skin. For example, the skin of a patient with end-stage renal disease may be grayish yellow. What is the patient's level of responsiveness? A severe enough buildup of waste products can cause the patient to become confused or to decline into a coma. Does the person show any signs of distress?

The most common problem that requires transport of a patient to the emergency department is volume overload. Look for clues to the volume status, such as an increased heart rate, increased respiratory rate, edema, neck vein distention, and "wet" lungs. (Other problems that might occur are discussed in the section on renal failure.)

Terms commonly used to describe the level of urine production are *anuria* and *oliguria.* Oliguria is a urine output of less than 400 mL a day; anuria is a daily urine output below 50 mL. Remember, normal urine production is considered to be at least 0.5 mL per kilogram of body weight per hour for the adult (1-2 mL/kg/hr for infants and children).

DIAGNOSTICS AND LABORATORY VALUES

Laboratory Tests

Creatinine

Creatinine is a byproduct of creatine phosphate, which is used in skeletal muscle contraction. Creatinine is released from muscle at a fairly constant rate and is excreted by the kidneys. As the GFR decreases, the plasma creatinine level increases. In a steady state, the serum creatinine is a better marker of the GFR than is the BUN. Acute renal failure occurs in a non–steady state, which is marked by several patterns of change in the GFR. Changes in GFR are poorly reflected by daily changes in the creatinine level. Several other substances may be better assessments of the GFR on a daily basis, but these require further study and are not readily available.

The creatinine level can be elevated by acute or chronic renal impairment or hyperthyroidism, and a small increase can occur after a meal heavy on meat. The approximate normal value is 0.6 to 1.2 mg/dL, depending on the laboratory doing the test. In addition, laboratories often report different normal values for men and women; women typically have a lower value because of their lower muscle mass.

Did You Know?

A doubling of the creatinine suggests a 50% reduction in the GFR.[2]

Creatinine Clearance

Creatinine clearance is a measure of the GFR. Because creatinine is released from muscle at a steady state and filtered by the kidneys, the release of creatinine into the urine reflects the filtration rate. However, creatinine clearance is not a perfect measurement of the GFR. Because the kidney tubule cells secrete a small amount of creatinine into the urine, the creatine clearance value slightly overestimates the GFR. Other tests of the GFR can be done, but these require injection of a substance, so the creatinine clearance usually is used.

To calculate the creatinine clearance (CrC), a 4-, 12-, or 24-hour urine sample is collected, and one blood sample is drawn to determine the plasma creatinine (Cr) level. Most laboratories use a 24-hour urine collection. The formula for calculating the CrC is:

$$\text{CrC} = \frac{\text{Urine Cr} \times \text{Urine volume}}{\text{Plasma Cr}}$$

The creatinine clearance is a useful test in the early stages of chronic renal failure. However, collection of all the urine is vital to the accuracy of the test result. Consequently, in critically ill patients, whose condition changes rapidly, a test requiring a 24-hour urine sample is not very useful for assessing kidney function.

Blood Urea Nitrogen

Urea is formed in the liver as an end product of protein metabolism. Protein is broken down into amino acids, which are catabolized by the liver into free ammonia. The liver combines the ammonia into urea, which is excreted by the kidneys. An elevated blood urea nitrogen is referred to as **azotemia**, which is not specific for renal failure. In addition to chronic and acute renal failure, an increased protein intake, dehydration, and increased protein breakdown can elevate the BUN. It also is elevated by a decrease in renal perfusion, as may occur in patients with congestive heart failure, hemorrhage, or burns. The BUN decreases in patients who eat a low-protein, high-carbohydrate diet; in late pregnancy; and in patients who are receiving parenteral nutrition or who have severe liver disease or impaired absorption. The ratio of BUN to creatinine in the plasma normally is 10 : 1. This ratio can be used to differentiate the reasons for the increases in urea and creatinine. A normal BUN value is 10 to 20 mg/dL.

Potassium

Potassium is the major electrolyte inside the cell. Normally, the plasma potassium level is about 4 mEq/L, and minor changes in this level can significantly affect cell function. Potassium is balanced by the kidneys. Serious potassium imbalances are a common finding in the critical care unit. A critical degree of hyperkalemia (an excess of potassium) occurs when the potassium level exceeds 6.5 mEq/L. The electrocardiogram (ECG) of patents with hyperkalemia should be monitored for peaked, tall T waves, a widened QRS complex, or a decreased ST segment (Figure 6-36). A critical degree of hypokalemia (insufficient potassium) occurs when the potassium level is less than 2.5 mEq/L.

Osmolality

Osmolality is the measurement of the number of dissolved particles in a certain volume of blood or urine. As the amount of free water increases or the number of particles decreases, the osmolality decreases; conversely, as the amount of free water decreases or the number of particles increases, the osmolality increases. An increased serum osmolality is seen with uremia, azotemia, dehydration, and renal tubular acidosis. Hypervolemia causes a decrease in the serum osmolality. Serum and urine osmolality measurements are used to help assess fluid status in critically ill patients. The serum osmolality, in combination with the sodium, potassium, creatinine, and BUN levels, can aid in the diagnosis of the cause of acute renal failure.

Urinalysis can be used to differentiate multiple problems that affect the kidneys, in addition to other disorders the patient may have (Table 6-6).

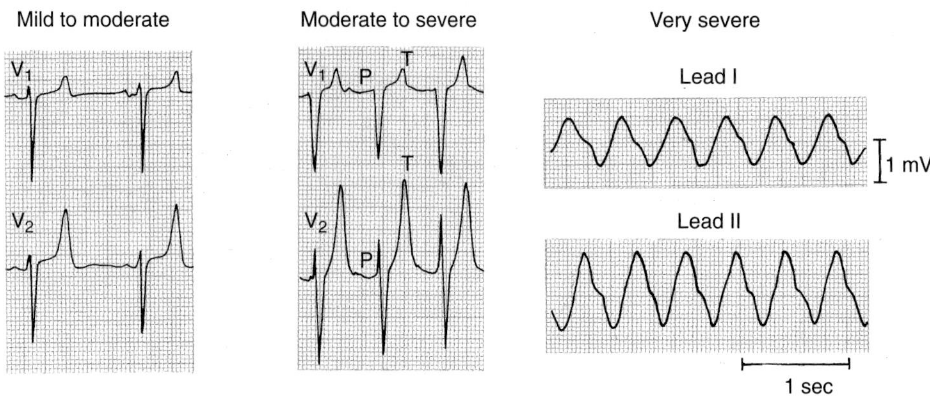

Figure 6-36

Electrocardiogram of a patient with hyperkalemia. (From Goldberger AL: *Clinical electrocardiography: a simplified approach,* St Louis, 2006, Mosby.)

Table 6-6 Urinalysis Findings

Parameter	Normal Findings*	Abnormal Findings†
Color	Clear, light yellow	Many medications and conditions can change the color of the urine. *Red:* Renal injury, blood *Black:* Dye for renal function tests *Blue:* Some diuretics, methylene blue *Brown:* Bile pigment, renal disease, some laxatives *Amber:* Bilirubin *Green:* Bacterial infection, some diuretics *Orange:* Bile pigment, dehydration, jaundice *Light colored:* Diuresis caused by alcohol ingestion, diuretics
pH	4.6-8	*Increased:* Metabolic alkalosis, diuretic therapy, gastric secretion *Decreased:* Metabolic acidosis, starvation, renal failure
Protein	None or up to 8 mg/dL	*Increased* (proteinuria): Renal disease
Specific gravity	1.005-1.030	*Increased:* Dehydration, decreased renal blood flow, vomiting, diarrhea *Decreased:* Overhydration, renal failure, diuresis
Leukocyte esterase	Negative	*Present:* Urinary tract infection (presence of white blood cells)
Nitrates	Negative	*Present:* Urinary tract infection (gram-negative bacteria convert nitrates to nitrites)
Ketones	Negative	*Present:* Hyperglycemia
Crystals	Negative	*Present:* Potential for kidney stones
Casts	None present	*Present:* Renal tubule damage
White blood cells (WBCs)	0-4	*Present:* Urinary tract infection
Red blood cells (RBCs)	<3	*Present:* Glomerulonephritis, kidney stones, acute renal necrosis, renal trauma

*Many laboratory tests can be processed by different methods, which have different normal values; use the normal value specified by your laboratory.
†The causes of abnormal findings included in this table indicate a gastrointestinal or genitourinary problem; consult a laboratory manual for other causes.

DISEASE PROCESSES AND MANAGEMENT OF THE RENAL SYSTEM

Acute Renal Failure

Acute renal failure (ARF) is a sudden, rapid deterioration of renal function marked by a drop in the GFR and rising blood levels of urea and other waste products (azotemia). A more quantified definition may be a decrease in the GFR by 50% or a doubling of the serum creatinine level over a short time; in some patients, however, just a modest increase in the creatinine level signals the start of renal failure. As many as 20% of critically ill patients and 50% of patients with septic shock develop ARF. Depending on the cause, ARF may be reversible, and many patients return to normal kidney function. However, the emergence of ARF as a complication of another condition significantly increases mortality among critically ill patients. Mortality increases even more among patients with ARF who do not need dialysis. The goals of therapy are to prevent further damage to the kidneys and to stabilize the patient's condition long enough to allow the kidneys to repair themselves.

Etiology

Identifying patients at higher risk of ARF is the first step in preventing the disorder. All critically ill patients should be considered high risk, and several factors are associated with an even greater risk (Box 6-13). Close attention must be paid to the patient's fluid balance, BP, and renal function to prevent damage to the kidneys. The dosages and blood levels of medications must be monitored closely, because many medications are toxic to the kidneys.

Box 6-13 Patients at Higher Risk for Acute Renal Failure

A greater risk of acute renal failure is seen with the following:

- Advanced age
- Preexisting renal insufficiency
- Diabetes
- Hypertension
- Hypotension
- Vasoactive drug therapy
- Heart failure
- Sepsis
- Surgery
- Trauma

The most common cause of ARF is poor perfusion of the kidneys. It is imperative that healthcare providers recognize and treat causes of reduced kidney perfusion; they also must monitor the patient's hemodynamic status and provide rapid transport to an appropriate facility.

The etiology of ARF can be divided into three broad categories: prerenal failure, intrarenal failure, and postrenal failure (Table 6-7).

Prerenal failure is caused by any condition that reduces renal perfusion; this accounts for 40% of all cases of hospital-acquired renal failure. Low perfusion of the kidneys reduces urinary output and the release of waste products. As mentioned previously, when perfusion starts to fall below autoregulation limits, the kidneys attempt to maintain function by stimulating the RAAS. Angiotensin II, a powerful vasoconstrictor, is released in an attempt to raise the systemic blood pressure. Aldosterone also is released to increase salt and water reabsorption, further reducing urinary output, and ADH causes even more water reabsorption. Waste products, especially urea, are reabsorbed as a result of the dynamics of the extra water reabsorption. This mechanism causes a rise in the BUN to creatinine ratio to greater than 20:1. If perfusion falls too far below autoregulation levels, filtration may stop completely.

Intrarenal failure is the result of damage to parts of the nephron. Inflammatory processes, such as glomerulonephritis, can damage the glomerulus; as a result, proteins and cell debris leak into the tubules and may obstruct filtrate flow. The most common cause of intrarenal failure is acute tubular necrosis (ATN), which accounts for 50% of cases of ARF. The tubule cells are damaged directly, either by an ischemic condition or by the presence of a toxin. The kidney cells become ischemic when perfusion or the oxygen available becomes

Table 6-7 Common Causes of Acute Renal Failure

Prerenal Causes	Intrarenal Causes	Postrenal Causes
Severe dehydration, caused by: • Hemorrhage • Severe GI losses • Urinary losses • Ketoacidosis • Diuretics • Burns • Third spacing • Sepsis • Neurogenic shock • Anaphylaxis • CHF • Myocardial infarction • Cardiogenic shock • Pericardial tamponade • Dysrhythmias • Renal artery disorders	• Glomerulonephritis and other immune disorders • ATN (ischemic causes) ○ All causes of prerenal failure ○ Sepsis ○ Cardiac or vascular surgery ○ Cardiopulmonary bypass ○ Hypotension, sepsis, hypovolemia ○ Severe hypoxemia ○ Renal artery stenosis or thrombus ○ Obstetric complications • ATN (toxic causes) ○ Rhabdomyolysis ○ Tumor lysis syndrome • Biologic substances • Radiographic contrast dye • Medications (especially antibiotics) • Environmental agents • Heavy metal (mercury)	Mechanical causes: • Stones (most common cause of obstruction) • Tumor • Benign prostatic hypertrophy • Urethral strictures • Edema • Indwelling catheter obstruction • Blood clots Functional causes: • Diabetic neuropathy • Pregnancy • Ganglionic blocking agents • Spinal cord disease

ATN, Acute tubular necrosis; *CHF*, congestive heart failure; *GI*, gastrointestinal.

extremely compromised. Low perfusion also is a cause of prerenal failure; however, the low perfusion in ATN causes necrosis of the nephron, not just loss of function, as in the prerenal form. Toxic injury leads to damage to the proximal tubule but does not usually interfere with the basement membrane; ischemic injury leads to damage to multiple areas of the tubule and the basement membrane. If enough of the basement membrane remains intact, the kidney tissue can regenerate and achieve full function; therefore, more patients with toxic injury return to full function.

Postrenal failure is caused by an obstruction to urine flow. The pressure created by the buildup of urine exceeds the glomerular filtration pressure, which reduces filtration. ARF from postrenal failure is not seen as often as ARF from prerenal or intrarenal causes.

Clinical Course and Treatment

The major clinical problems that occur in ARF are volume overload, hyperkalemia, and infection (Table 6-8).

Significant metabolic acidosis also is possible, and body water must be monitored closely. This requires careful measurement of intake and output and daily weights and possibly invasive hemodynamic monitoring, along with frequent physical assessment for fluid overload. Treatment for volume overload includes fluid restriction, diuretics, and possibly low-dose dopamine. To maintain fluid restrictions, intake should be measured frequently and precisely to determine the exact amount of fluids given. Many critically ill patients require multiple drug infusions, which can make meeting fluid restrictions difficult.

Many patients with ARF have conditions that require significant fluid resuscitation. If perfusion pressures are not maintained, the kidneys will be damaged further. Crystalloids, colloids, and blood products may be used to stabilize the patient's hemodynamic status. For example, a patient with ARF from septic shock is caught in a vicious cycle; fluid leaks from the extracellular space into the tissues, which reduces the intravascular volume and the perfusion of vital organs.

Table 6-8 Signs and Symptoms of Clinical Problems in Acute Renal Failure

Volume Overload	Hyperkalemia	Infection
Weight gain	Irritability	Fever
Edema	Restlessness	Increased white blood cells
Jugular venous distention	Anxiety	Decreased white blood cells
Crackles	Nausea and vomiting	
Dyspnea	Abdominal cramps	
Increased respiratory rate	Weakness	
Increased heart rate	Dysrhythmias	
	Peaked, tall T waves	
	Cardiac arrest	

Balancing fluid resuscitation in this situation is difficult. As waste products build up, the patient may need renal replacement therapy (dialysis) while still requiring large amounts of fluids.

Diuretics may be used in an attempt to keep the urine output at an acceptable level. Loop diuretics, such as furosemide (Lasix), are used with mixed results. To reduce the possibility of high-dose side effects, furosemide might be given as a continuous IV drip. Damaged renal tubule cells do not respond well to diuretics, especially in those with chronic renal failure. If urinary output does not increase with diuretics, mannitol (Osmitrol) may be tried. Mannitol is an osmotic diuretic, which causes less electrolyte disturbance than other diuretics. If no response is seen, trying mannitol again may only add significantly to the volume overload.

For many years, low-dose dopamine (1 to 3 mcg/kg/min) was used to increase renal blood flow in critically ill patients in hopes of improving kidney perfusion. Dopamine may increase urine output on the first day of treatment, but the effect does not last into the second day of treatment. Administration of low-dose dopamine is somewhat controversial, although many critical care departments still use it. If dopamine is used, watch for tachycardia, a common side effect.

Hyperkalemia can be a life-threatening complication of ARF. Treatment should be aimed at keeping the potassium level below 6.5 mEq/L. As soon as renal failure is determined, all potassium in IV fluids and any nutritional supplements should be reduced or eliminated. The treatment for extreme hyperkalemia includes stabilizing the cells with calcium and then removing the potassium from the cell with either glucose/insulin or continuous albuterol nebulization. Potassium exchange resins (e.g., Kayexalate enemas or dialysis) may then be done to remove potassium from the body.

A patient with ARF is very susceptible to serious infections, which are a common cause of death in critically ill patients. The normal clinical picture of infection, such as fever and changes in the white blood cell count, may not be seen in these patients. Pay close attention, therefore, to prevention: use aseptic technique, use invasive catheters as seldom as possible and, most important, follow good hand washing practices.

When renal function is reduced, acids accumulate, resulting in a metabolic acidosis. If the acidosis has no other cause, the patient may not have a critical drop in pH. Treatment usually is triggered by a drop in the pH below 7.0 to 7.2. The patient's dietary intake of protein should be limited, and a bicarbonate infusion may be ordered. Watch the patient carefully for cardiac instability, which is exacerbated by hyperkalemia and acidosis.

Other clinical conditions that can occur include anemia, mild bleeding tendencies, and low calcium and high uric acid levels. These conditions rarely cause serious symptoms or require significant treatment, but the patient should be watched closely. As renal function declines, control of the volume of body water, the potassium level, or metabolic acidosis may be lost, resulting in the need for some form of renal replacement (discussed later in the chapter). The point at which renal replacement therapy should be started is a matter of debate. Some clinicians advocate early use of renal replacement; others suggest that patients may have a better chance of survival if renal replacement is used later or, if the patient is lucky, not at all because renal function finally improves.

Acute Tubular Necrosis

Remember the three broad categories for causes of ARF: prerenal failure, intrarenal failure, and postrenal failure. As mentioned, ATN is the most common cause of intrarenal failure, and it ranks second to prerenal azotemia as the most common cause of all types of ARF in hospitalized patients. ATN is caused by an ischemic or a toxic incident, and it follows a clinical sequence divided into four phases: the initiation phase, the oliguric/anuric phase, the diuretic phase, and the recovery phase.

Initiation Phase

The initiation (or onset) phase is characterized by a drop in the GFR to critical levels, which occurs as a result of impaired renal blood flow and decreased glomerular ultrafiltration pressure. This phase lasts hours to days.

Oliguric/Anuric Phase

If the patient is not producing urine, the oliguric/anuric phase can last as long as 2 weeks; it lasts 1 week in patients with ATN who are producing urine. As dead tissue accumulates in the tubule, back flow of urine occurs, contaminating the renal tissue. Azotemia (elevated BUN and creatinine levels) begins, marked by electrolyte disturbances and acidosis.

Diuretic Phase

Over time, the kidney tissue can repair itself, resulting in improved renal function; this is called the *diuretic stage* because urine output increases. The kidney usually recovers the ability to process urine slowly; filtration resumes first, but the kidney is not yet able to concentrate the urine. This results in a high urine output and the washout of some electrolytes. Clinical problems in this phase include fluid deficit, hypokalemia, and hyponatremia. During this phase the patient needs fluids based on the hourly urinary output, which can reach 300 mL/hour or more. The high urine output washes out potassium and sodium until the kidney regains the ability to balance electrolytes. Normal saline is used for fluid replacement, with the addition of potassium. The patient must be watched carefully for signs of dehydration, hypokalemia, and hyponatremia. As mentioned, patients with ARF are at high risk for infection, and during the diuretic phase, the risk is even greater. The kidney usually recovers most of the ability to concentrate urine within 2 to 3 weeks.

Recovery Phase

Recovery can take up to a year, and any further insult to the kidney must be prevented during this time. Most patients, but not all, regain total function of the kidney. The patient may be left with renal insufficiency that does not involve a significant loss of function or in rare cases may be diagnosed with chronic renal failure. Careful attention must be paid to preventing infections. Renal function gradually improves over time.

Chronic Renal Failure

Chronic renal failure is the irreversible loss of renal function with a progressive slide into end-stage renal failure. CRF affects nearly all cells in the body, causing widespread clinical problems in all organ systems. The kidney has remarkable adaptive ability, and symptoms of the decline in renal function do not present until renal function is reduced to at least 25% of normal.

Etiology and Clinical Presentation

The two most common causes of CRF are hypertension and diabetes mellitus (Table 6-9). Forty percent of patients with end-stage renal disease have either type 1 or type 2 diabetes. A number of theories have been proposed to explain the causative factors of CRF, including a genetic predisposition, long-term exposure to metabolic waste products, and poor glucose control with high glucose levels. The beginning pathophysiology is very different among the various causes of CRF, but the end stage is very similar. In some cases, the patient may take years to slide into end-stage renal failure; many other patients retain some renal function and never need dialysis.

The early stages of renal failure are reduced renal reserve and renal insufficiency, for which the focus of care is preservation of renal function. An acute insult to the kidney speeds

Table 6-9 Causes of Chronic Renal Failure

Infections	Chronic Pyelonephritis
Inflammatory disease	Glomerulonephritis
Hypertensive vascular disease	Hypertension, benign nephrosclerosis, malignant nephrosclerosis, renal artery stenosis
Connective tissue disorders	Systemic lupus erythematosus, polyarteritis nodosa, progressive systemic sclerosis
Congenital and hereditary disorders	Polycystic kidney disease, renal tubular acidosis
Metabolic disorders	Diabetes mellitus, gout, hyperparathyroidism, amyloidosis
Toxic nephropathy	Analgesic abuse, lead nephropathy
Obstructive nephropathy	*Upper urinary tract:* Stones, neoplasm, retroperitoneal fibrosis *Lower urinary tract:* Prostatic hypertrophy, urethral stricture, congenital anomalies

the progression of CRF. At end-stage renal failure, the patient usually has less than 10% of the normal GFR and requires dialysis or renal transplantation.

The systemic effects of CRF (Box 6-14) are related to the deposition of waste products in most tissues of the body and to other biochemical disturbances, such as hyperkalemia and metabolic acidosis.

Treatment of Chronic Renal Failure

Nutrition and Fluids

Nutrition for patients with CRF must be individualized based on the type and extent of damage to the kidney. For most patients with CRF, the diet should be low in protein, sodium, potassium, and phosphorus. These patients require a high-caloric intake from carbohydrates and fats to combat tissue atrophy and the development of ketoacidosis.

Fluid restriction also is needed to control excess body water; less water than needs to be removed during dialysis, which makes the patient's condition more stable. Fluid restrictions are difficult, and a large percentage of patients do not follow the recommendations. As a result, the heart must pump large volumes of fluid, and the potential arises for pulmonary edema and problems with dialysis.

Drug Therapy

Most patients with renal failure require a variety of medications to improve their quality of life and to help maintain renal function. If the patient is in early renal failure, still producing some urine, some type of diuretic may be prescribed. Hypertension may lead to CRF, but CRF causes hypertension in many patients. Antihypertensives are used, and many patients require frequent changes in dosage or medication to keep the BP under control. Uncontrolled hypertension is a significant problem for patients with CRF. Most patients also receive some form of medication to prevent ulcers, such as proton pump inhibitors.

To deal with anemia, the patient usually receives synthetic erythropoietin to stimulate the bone marrow to produce red blood cells, iron, and folate supplements. Other supplements include vitamins, especially B and D, and essential amino acids. In late stages, the patient may suffer from severe itching and require **antipruritics**.

Dialysis

Dialysis usually is required when the patient reaches end-stage failure. Hemodialysis is the most common form of dialysis, but many patients prefer to do peritoneal dialysis at home. To do well on dialysis, the patient must follow medical and nutritional recommendations. Over time, dialysis becomes less effective, and the symptoms of uremic syndrome increase.

Cardiovascular disease is two to five times more prevalent and is the major cause of death in patients with CRF. Patients on dialysis have a cardiovascular mortality rate 10 to 20 times higher than that of the general population; for dialysis patients under age 45, the risk is 100 times that of the general population.

Common reasons the patient seeks acute care or requires transport are related to the effects of uremic syndrome or

Box 6-14 Systemic Effects of Uremic Syndrome and End-Stage Renal Failure

Cardiopulmonary Effects

- Hypertension
- Pericarditis
- Pulmonary edema
- Congestive heart failure
- Dysrhythmias
- Respiratory alkalosis

Neurologic Effects

- Peripheral neuropathy
  - Pain and burning in the legs
  - Restless leg syndrome
  - Loss of vibration
  - Decreased deep tendon reflexes
- Encephalopathy
  - Fatigue
  - Loss of attention, decision making
  - Confusion
  - Stupor and coma
- Loss of motor coordination
- Twitching
- Foot drops progressing to paraplegia

Gastrointestinal Effects

- Anorexia
- Nausea and vomiting
- Mouth ulcers, peptic ulcers
- Bleeding
- Pancreatitis
- Ammonia odor to the breath

Endocrine Effects

- Decreased growth in children
- Sexual and reproductive dysfunction

Hematologic Effects

- Anemia
- Platelet disorders
- Bleeding

Immunologic Effects

- Increased risk of infection

Skeletal Effects

- Bone inflammation
- Bone demineralization
- Spontaneous fractures
- Bone pain

Skin and Eyes

- Yellow-gray appearance
- Dry skin, itching
- Uremic frost
- Hypertensive retinopathy

acute elevations in fluid volume or potassium levels. High levels of waste products may diminish the level of consciousness. Most patients with CRF have hypertension, which may become out of control, but the patient also may have hypotension, especially after a dialysis session. If the patient presents in acute pulmonary edema, he or she may not respond to the normal therapies in your protocols. Diuretics will not increase urine output in most patients who are already on dialysis. Vasodilators may have the best effect if the patient's BP can tolerate them, but the patient needs emergency dialysis.

Hyperkalemia in patients with CRF is treated the same way as for patients with ARF. If the patient is in cardiac arrest, consider hyperkalemia, but remember that the patient has a high risk of cardiovascular problems, such as myocardial infarction and cardiac tamponade from a pleural effusion. If the patient presents with hypotension, the recommended fluid bolus is 200 to 250 mL, repeated if needed after another assessment. NS should be administered, not LR, because the latter has potassium and is acidic.

Renal Replacement Therapy

Renal replacement therapy is the process of removing fluid and waste products through a semipermeable membrane. This process can be intermittent or continuous, depending on which therapy is selected from the many now available. As mentioned, debate continues over when a patient with ARF should be placed on renal replacement therapy. The decision usually is based on factors such as volume overload unresponsive to diuretics or fluid restrictions, and inability to manage hyperkalemia, metabolic acidosis, or uremia effects. Early therapy has not proved any more effective than waiting until the patient has no other options. The type of replacement therapy used depends on the individual patient and the resources of the hospital. The four most common types of renal replacement for ARF are peritoneal dialysis, hemodialysis, sustained low-efficiency daily dialysis, and continuous renal replacement therapy.

Peritoneal Dialysis

In peritoneal dialysis (PD), the patient's peritoneal membrane is used as the semipermeable membrane. A sterile, hyperosmolar dialysate fluid is infused into the abdominal cavity through an abdominal catheter (Figure 6-37). The fluid remains in the cavity for a specified period, called the *dwell time.* The dwell time lasts 30 minutes or up to 6 hours and is individualized for each patient. After the dwell time, the fluid is drained out of the peritoneal catheter. The hyperosmolar dialysate fluid pulls water out of the patient by osmosis. The most frequently used dialysate has a large amount of glucose, which allows the osmolality to be increased or decreased based on how much fluid the patient needs to release. Waste products and electrolytes move across the membrane, using a diffusion gradient from a high concentration to a lower concentration. Peritoneal dialysis allows a patient with CRF to handle dialysis at home. Most patients have their dwell time at night while they are sleeping, using a machine called a cycler.

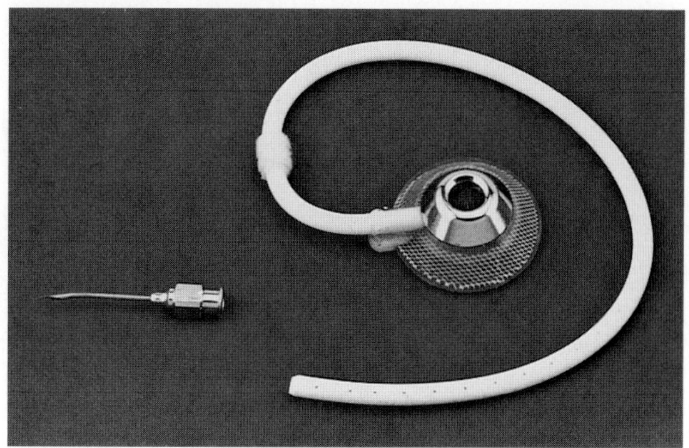

Figure 6-37

Abdominal catheter. (From Katz VL, Lentz GM, Lobo RA, et al: *Comprehensive gynecology,* St Louis, 2007, Mosby.)

In a critically ill patient, peritoneal dialysis may be continuous so that small amounts of fluid are removed slowly; this helps the patient maintain hemodynamic stability. This method of dialysis also does not require anticoagulation. However, even with these advantages, peritoneal dialysis is not used frequently in critically ill patients. This mode is effective but not as efficient as the other modes of renal replacement. Peritoneal dialysis cannot be used for a patient who has had abdominal trauma or surgery. Also, the extra volume in the abdomen may put pressure on the diaphragm, reducing respiratory function in many patients who already have respiratory compromise. Other risks for all patients on PD include peritonitis, hyperglycemia, and protein loss.

Did You Know?

Hyperkalemia, hypermagnesemia, and hypocalcemia are common electrolyte disturbances in acute renal failure. Hyperkalemia is common in the oliguric phase of ARF and can be life-threatening. Hypermagnesemia is common but usually not life-threatening unless healthcare providers overtreat the hyperkalemic patient with magnesium. Hypocalcemia also is common but usually not severe.[6]

Hemodialysis

Hemodialysis (HD) uses a dialysis filter with a semipermeable membrane. The most commonly used filter is a hollow fiber tube; the patient's blood runs through the hollow portion, and the dialysate runs on the outside of the filter in the opposite direction. This countercurrent flow makes filtration more efficient and provides significant fluid and solute removal. In addition, a positive hydrostatic pressure is applied to the blood compartment and a negative hydrostatic pressure is applied to the dialysate compartment, which pulls off more fluid from the patient. Hemodialysis allows a large amount of fluid and solute to be removed in a very short period. The large shifts in fluids, electrolytes, and waste products may be important in a critically ill patient with life-threatening pulmonary edema or hyperkalemia; however, in many patients they make the person's condition even more unstable.

A patient with a low mean arterial pressure may not be able to tolerate the initial priming with HD; therefore, other methods of dialysis may have to be used. During the initiation of HD, the patient must be monitored for hypotension and serious dysrhythmias, which occur most frequently in the first hour of dialysis. Bicarbonate-based dialysate, which most centers now use, has made HD safer for patients in unstable condition, but serious complications can still arise. Hemodialysis also requires significant anticoagulation, which increases the risk of bleeding. Patients with CRF usually undergo HD 3 or 4 days a week. In a critically ill patient, HD is performed daily or every other day. Daily dialysis has become popular, because the fluid and waste load does not build up as high between dialysis passes.

Sustained Low-Efficiency Daily Dialysis

Sustained low-efficiency daily dialysis (SLEDD) is a newer form of HD that allows filtration of fluids and waste products over a 6- to 12-hour session every day. Smaller amounts of fluid are removed every hour compared to a 3-hour hemodialysis session; therefore, the patient has a better chance of remaining hemodynamically stable. This mode is safer for the patient, because less anticoagulation usually is required. This mode requires significant time from the dialysis-trained healthcare providers, which increases the cost significantly in most centers. In 2007 approximately 2000 patients with CFR were doing home HD, most using a form of SLEDD. The patient dialyzes nightly, removing small amounts of fluid and waste products hourly, for 6 to 8 hours. Skill 6-3 outlines the steps for use of dialysis access in emergency situations.

Did You Know?

The mnemonic AEIOU can be used as a memory aid for the indications for renal replacement therapy[7]:

- **A Acidosis**
- **E Electrolyte imbalances**
- **I Ingestions (toxins such as aspirin, lithium, methanol)**
- **O Overload (volume or fluid overload)**
- **U Uremia**

Skill 6-3

USING DIALYSIS ACCESS IN EMERGENCY SITUATIONS

The arteriovenous (AV) access surgically created for hemodialysis in a patient's with end-stage renal disease (ESRD) is a specialized fistula that generally is used only for its intended purpose. The extremity in which the access is created is extremely vulnerable, and other healthcare providers are warned not to perform any procedures in that area. However, patients with these protected AV access sites are at high risk for emergencies in which vascular access is required. Also, these same patients can present some of the most challenging circumstances for attempting to establish a peripheral intravenous (IV) line. In a life-threatening situation, using the AV access site may be a viable option.

The two types of dialysis access are the AV fistula and the AV graft. The AV fistula, a common type of dialysis access, is created through union of an artery and a vein. This leaves one scar at the surgical union. For an AV graft, an artery and a vein are joined by the placement of an intervening synthetic graft. This produces two scars, one for the artery and one for the vein.

INDICATIONS

Life-threatening conditions in which vascular access cannot be postponed

Emergencies in which the benefits outweigh the risks

CONTRAINDICATIONS

Situations in which the risks outweigh the benefits (Box 6-15)

PROCEDURE

1. Gather the equipment for emergency peripheral IV access (butterfly needles are easier to secure). Assess the AV fistula or graft site for thrill and document.
2. Apply a standard tourniquet lightly to the high axillary area of the arm.
3. Wash your hands and follow standard precautions.
4. Cleanse the skin over the site according to policy. The cleansing procedure should include Betadine and then alcohol in a wet-to-dry technique.
5. Insert the needle into the site (at a 20- to 35-degree angle for an AV fistula; at a 45-degree angle for an AV graft) until flash is noted (see illustration).

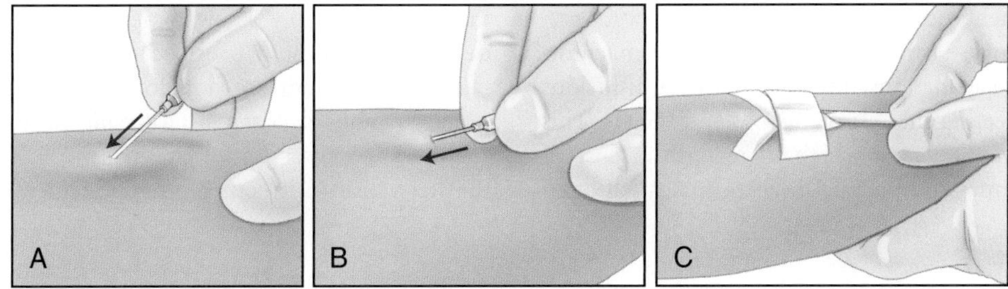

Accessing an AV fistula. **A** and **B,** A needle is inserted into the fistula. **C,** The needle or catheter is secured in place.

Box 6-15 Decision Tree for Accessing a Dialysis Graft or Fistula

1. Is CPR in progress? — No: Continue assessment
   Yes: Use dialysis access
2. Vital signs normal? — Yes: Continue assessment
   No: Can vascular access wait? — Yes: Continue assessment
   No: Use dialysis access
3. Is ECG normal? — Yes: Continue assessment
   No: Is patient symptomatic; is arrhythmia life-threatening?
   Yes: Use dialysis access
4. Is use of access likely to improve outcome? — No: Do not use!
   Yes: Use dialysis access

From Manning MA: Use of dialysis access in emergent situations, *J Emerg Nurs* 34:37-40, 2008.

6. Insert the needle approximately ⅛ inch as the angle is lowered to the skin surface. To prevent bleeding, advance the needle or catheter to the hub.
7. Be prepared to quickly attach flushed IV tubing and an infusion bag to the catheter or needle with a pressure bag inflated, because venous pressure at this site is high.
8. Secure the device to prevent accidental dislodgement at a high-pressure site.
9. Assess for and prevent infiltration of fluids or bleeding into the site, which would render the fistula or graft dysfunctional.
10. To discontinue use of the site, remove the needle or catheter and apply pressure for at least 10 minutes. Assess for and document thrill at the site.
11. Evaluate the extremity frequently for thrombosis, a major complication after use of an AV fistula or graft.
12. If the fistula has been accessed recently (within 24 hours), your insertion should be approximately 1 inch above or below the previous site.

Continuous Renal Replacement Therapy

Continuous renal replacement therapy (CRRT) is an umbrella term for several types of blood purification therapies that allow small amounts of fluid and waste products to be removed from the patient continuously 24 hours a day. These methods were designed for critically ill patients in unstable condition, because many of these patients were unable to tolerate normal hemodialysis. The first mode developed required arterial access; the patient's pressure was used to move the blood through a canister that contained the dialysis filter. The canister had a drainage bag that collected the removed fluid, and the blood was returned to the patient through a venous line. The amount of fluid filtered was regulated by the position of the drainage bag. If the bag hung lower, more fluid was filtered. A major complication of this system is clotting of the filter, which occurs when the patient's BP falls, a common event in patients in the critical care unit. To prevent clotting, anticoagulation is used in CRRT (Box 6-15).

Most clinicians today use a mode in which venous blood is pumped from a double or triple lumen central venous catheter into the CRRT machine and returns to the patient through a second venous port. The CRRT machine's filter is similar to that used for hemodialysis, and the machine can be programmed for the desired amount of fluid to be removed each hour. One of the more frequently used modes is continuous venovenous hemodiafiltration (CVVHD). This mode uses ultrafiltration and diffusion to remove fluid and waste products.

CRRT is used for patients in very unstable condition. It is especially good for a patient who requires a high fluid volume to maintain perfusion pressures but still needs to have potassium and waste products removed. This mode is highly labor-intensive, which is considered a disadvantage. Filtration and fluid replacement needs must be calculated hourly. A highly skilled ICU nurse is required to regulate the machine, perform the hourly calculations, and change the IV infusions as needed, while meeting the rest of the patient's needs. This patient should have 1:1 care, which increases the cost of CCRT. Small ICUs may not be able to keep nurses educated in this skill if only a few patients need CRRT. The risk of dehydration or fluid overload arises if the calculations and patient assessment are not done correctly. Other complications include bleeding as a result of the anticoagulation required and infection of the invasive line. Skill 6-4 reviews the steps for continuous renal replacement therapy.

Skill 6-4

CONTINUOUS RENAL REPLACEMENT THERAPY

Continuous renal replacement therapy (CRRT) is similar to standard hemodialysis in that it purifies the blood. However, CRRT can be done continuously in critically ill patients, who may not be able to tolerate large shifts of fluid in a shorter time span. Blood is circulated through a porous filter via a large catheter through one of two systems: pumped or nonpumped: Nonpumped arterial blood is propelled through the patient's mean arterial pressure (MAP). In the pumped system (for those with lower MAP), a mechanical roller "milks" the tubing to facilitate more forceful flow. There are four types of CRRT:

- *Slow continuous ultrafiltration (SCUF)*: 100 to 300 mL/hour is removed through both arterial and venous access, which poses a risk of clotting. This method is not often used.
- *Continuous venovenous hemofiltration (CVVH)*: 5 to 20 mL/min, up to 7 to 30 L/day, is removed. This method is usually chosen when significant amounts of fluid must be removed.
- *Continuous venovenous hemodialysis (CVVHD)*: Similar to traditional hemodialysis, this method uses countercurrent flow (blood one way, dialysate in the opposite direction). It is ideal for a critical care patient in unstable condition.
- *Continuous venovenous hemodiafiltration (CVVHDF)*: This method combines CVVH and CVVHD to remove the most fluid and solutes.

INDICATIONS

Removal of a large volume in a hemodynamically unstable patient

Hypervolemic or edematous patient unresponsive to diuretic therapy

Patient with multiple organ dysfunction syndrome

Fluid balance and management in patients requiring large-volume infusions

Contraindications to traditional peritoneal dialysis or hemodialysis

Inability to tolerate anticoagulation therapy

COMPLICATIONS

See Table 6-10 and Box 6-16.

CONTRAINDICATIONS

Hematocrit >45%

Terminal Illness

PROCEDURE: TERMINATING CRRT

This procedure applies to pumped systems (i.e., CVVH, CVVHD, and CVVHDF).

Box 6-16 Complications of Continuous Renal Replacement Therapy

Circuit

Air embolism
Clotted hemofilter
Poor ultrafiltration
Blood leaks
Broken filter
Recirculation/disconnection
Access failure
Catheter dislodgment

Pump

Circuit pressure alarm
- Decreased inflow pressure
- Decreased outflow pressure
- Increased outflow resistance

Air bubble detector alarm
Power failure
Mechanical dysfunction

Patient

Code/emergency situation
Dehydration
Hypotension
Electrolyte imbalances
Acid-base imbalances
Blood loss/hemorrhage
Hypothermia
Infection
Blood transfusion reaction

From Headrick CL: *Nurse Clin North Am* 10:197-207, 1998.

Table 6-10 Complications Associated with Continuous Renal Replacement Therapy

Problem	Cause	Clinical Manifestations	Management
Decreased ultrafiltration rate	Hypotension, dehydration, kinked lines, bent catheter, clotting of filter	Decreased ultrafiltration rate, minimal flow through blood lines	• Observe filter and arteriovenous system. • Control blood flow. • Control coagulation time. • Position patient on back. • Lower height of collection container.
Filter clotting	Obstruction, inadequate heparinization	Ultrafiltration rate decreased despite lowering of collection container	• Control anticoagulation (heparin/citrate). • Maintain continuous system anticoagulation. • Call physician. • Remove system. • Prime catheters with anticoagulant solution. • Prime and connect new system. • Start predilution at 1000 mL/hour of saline (0.9% solution). • Do not use three-way stopcocks.
Hypotension	Increased ultrafiltration rate; leakage of blood; disconnection of a line	Bleeding	• Control amount of ultrafiltration. • Control access sites. • Clamp lines. • Call physician.
Fluid and electrolyte changes	Too much or too little fluid removed; inappropriate replacement of electrolytes; inappropriate dialysate	Changes in mentation; increase or decrease in CVP, PAOP, ECG changes, BP, and heart rate; abnormal electrolyte levels	• Observe for: ○ Changes in CVP/PAOP ○ Changes in vital signs ○ ECG changes caused by electrolyte abnormalities • Monitor output values every hour. • Control ultrafiltration.
Bleeding	System disconnection; increased heparin dose	Oozing from catheter insertion site or connection	• Monitor ACT at least hourly (heparin). • Adjust heparin dose within specifications to maintain ACT. • Monitor serum calcium if using citrate as an anticoagulant. • Observe dressing on vascular access for blood loss. • Observe for blood in filtrate (filter leak).
Access dislodgment or infection	Catheter or connections not secured; break in sterile technique; excessive patient movement	Bleeding from catheter site or connections; inappropriate flow/ infusion; fever; drainage at catheter site	• Observe access site at least once every 2 hours. • Make sure clamps are within reach at all times. • Observe strict sterile technique when dressing vascular access.

From Urden LD, Stacy KM, Lough ME: *Thelan's critical care nursing: diagnosis and management,* ed 5, St Louis, 2006, Mosby.
ACT, Activated coagulation time; *BP,* blood pressure; *CVP,* central venous pressure; *ECG,* electrocardiograph; *PAOP,* pulmonary artery occlusion (or wedge) pressure.

1. Wash your hands and follow standard precautions.
2. Turn off infusions into the system.
3. Open the normal saline (NS) flush solution to the vascular access line and clamp the ultrafiltration line.
4. With certain pump systems, you must press END TREATMENT. If a blood pump is running, clamp the arterial line near the patient and open the NS flush with the hemofilter/arterial end up.
5. When the entire circuit is clear of blood, turn off the pump and clamp both ends of the lines.
6. The intensive care unit (ICU) must document the amount of NS infused and the ultrafiltrate (UF) remaining in the collection bag, along with the patient's weight and vital signs.
7. Reinstill heparin and citrate in the access ports per policy.

Access Devices and Tubes Used by Renal Patients

Fistulas and Grafts

Chronic dialysis patients need long-term access devices. Initially the patient may be given a central venous catheter while a fistula or graft is inserted. Arteriovenous fistulas are created by surgically pulling an artery and vein together, usually in the arm. The high arterial flow creates swelling, causing a pseudoaneurysm. Once the area has healed, a needle can be inserted into the aneurysm area to obtain outflow. Blood is returned to the body in a vein distal to the fistula. Because the development of enough flow to the fistula may require weeks to months, patients need a temporary access until the fistula is ready. An arteriovenous graft is a synthetic tube that is implanted into the patient with one end inserted into a vein and the other end inserted into an artery. Grafts usually form a U shape that can be palpated under the skin surface (Figure 6-38.)

Care must be taken never to measure the BP or to draw blood from the access limb. To assess patency, listen for a bruit and palpate for a thrill. A **thrill** is a vibration caused by the flow of blood through the fistula or graft. A **bruit** is the audible vibration heard with a stethoscope. Check the distal extremity for adequate circulation. Make sure the patient is not wearing tight-fitting clothing or jewelry around the extremity. If the patient requires restraints, be careful not to place a restraint over the graft or fistula site.

Central Venous Lines

Care of a central venous catheter used for dialysis is similar to the care of any central line. The lumens used for dialysis should be reserved for that purpose, if possible. The more the lines are accessed, the higher the rate of infection and the greater the chance of losing the line, which would require reinsertion. The catheter site should be kept clean and dry and should be covered with an occlusive dressing.

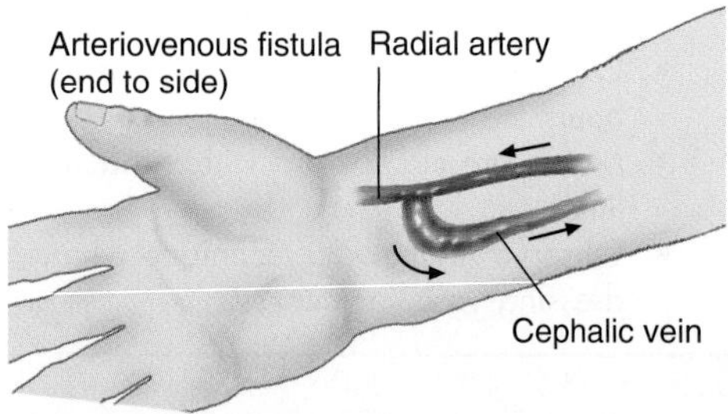

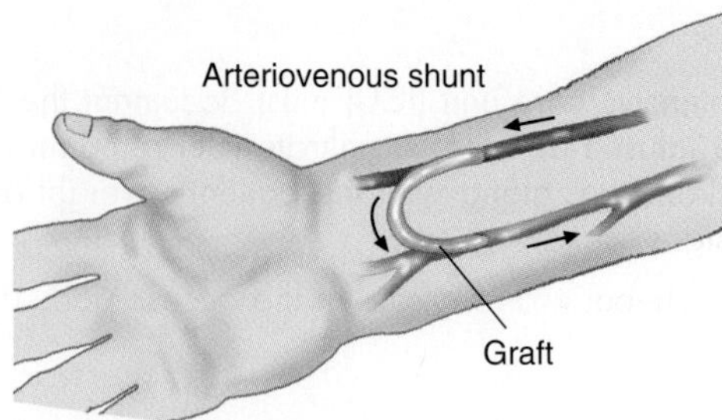

Figure 6-38

Arteriovenous shunts. (From Sanders M: *Mosby's paramedic textbook*, ed 3, St Louis, 2007, Mosby.)

Peritoneal Catheters

The PD catheter is placed into the abdominal cavity to allow administration and removal of dialysate solutions. The catheter most often used has a cuff that is placed into the subcutaneous layer of the skin; this helps anchor the catheter in place. Recently placed catheters can slip out of place easily, so be careful when transporting patients with these devices. Aseptic technique should be used whenever the catheter is accessed, and the catheter should be capped when not in use. These patients are at high risk for peritonitis. Do not confuse the PD catheter with feeding catheters of the abdomen (Figure 6-39).

Bladder Drainage Catheters

Indwelling catheters in the bladder are most commonly inserted through the urethra. However, in some patients a catheter may need to be inserted into the bladder through the abdominal wall; this is called a *suprapubic catheter.* Suprapubic catheters have a dressing around them initially, but most patients do not need the dressing after the site has healed. Over time a well-healed path develops, and the catheter usually can be changed easily. Both types of indwelling catheters are connected to a closed gravity drainage system.

For long-term use, some patients may have a collection bag that is attached to the leg, although most hospitalized patients have a larger drainage bag that hangs on the bed. Never pull on the catheter, and make sure no kinks or twists occur in the tubing. The collection bag should always be kept lower than the patient's bladder, even for short transports. These patients are at huge risk for a urinary tract infection, which in some can lead to urosepsis. Monitor the patient for signs of infection.

Scenario Conclusion: Renal System

When a diabetic patient with renal failure presents with fluid overload and cardiac dysrhythmia, you should assume (correctly) that the patient has a high potassium level, which can cause the clinical symptoms you saw. In fact, the potassium level can be predicted based on the ECG changes. Because obtaining laboratory test results may take valuable time, the condition is treated empirically with calcium (to stabilize the irritable cells), insulin and glucose (to move the potassium into the bloodstream), and then removal of wastes from the body with cation exchange resins or dialysis. Once the cardiac rhythm had stabilized and the potassium level had decreased, the patient was sent to the ICU for immediate dialysis.

SUMMARY

GI and renal disorders can cause life-threatening complications for critical care patients. Disorders of the GI tract can disrupt one or several functions. The renal system, particularly the kidneys, is responsible for the life-sustaining balance of water and solute transport and for maintaining and regulating acid-base balance and removing metabolic waste. The critical care team must provide in-depth assessments and aggressive treatment and management for patients with disorders of the GI and renal systems.

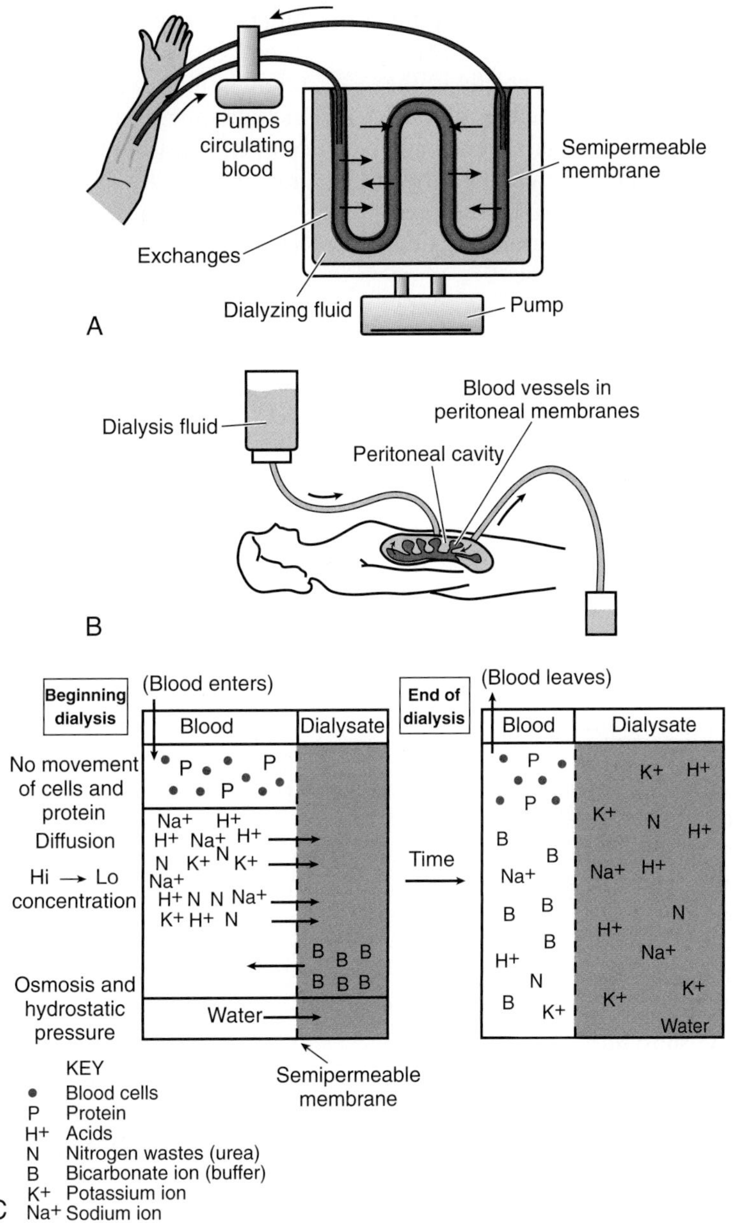

Figure 6-39

A, Hemodialysis. **B,** Peritoneal dialysis. **C,** Principles of dialysis. (From Aehlert B: *Paramedic practice today,* St Louis, 2009, Mosby.)

KEY TERMS

acute liver failure (ALF) A condition characterized by jaundice (yellow pigmentation), mental alteration, and massive necrosis of the liver cells in a patient with an illness of less than 26 weeks' duration. The patient also must have had no preexisting liver disease.

adhesion The stable joining of parts to each other, as in wound healing or some pathologic processes; a fibrous band or structure by which parts adhere abnormally.

aldosterone The major mineralocorticoid secreted by the adrenal cortex; it promotes retention of sodium and bicarbonate, excretion of potassium and hydrogen ions, and secondary retention of water. Large excesses can cause plasma volume expansion, edema, and hypertension. Secretion of aldosterone is stimulated by a low plasma potassium concentration and angiotensin II.

angiodysplasia Small abnormalities of the blood or lymphatic vessels.

angiotensin Any of a family of polypeptide vasopressor hormones formed by the catalytic action of renin on angiotensinogen; also called *angiotonin.*

angiotensin I A decapeptide cleaved from angiotensinogen by renin; it has some biologic activity but serves mainly as a precursor to angiotensin II.

angiotensin II An octapeptide hormone formed by the action of angiotensin-converting enzyme (ACE; peptidyl-dipeptidase A) on angiotensin I, chiefly in the lungs but also at other sites, including the blood vessel walls, uterus, and brain. It is a powerful vasopressor and stimulator of aldosterone secretion by the adrenal cortex, and it also functions as a neurotransmitter. Its vasopressor action raises the blood pressure and diminishes fluid loss in the kidney by restricting blood flow.

antidiuretic hormone (ADH) An agent that acts as a vasopressin, suppressing the rate of urine formation.

antipruritics Agents that relieve or prevent itching (e.g., diphenhydramine, hydroxyzine).

atrial natriuretic peptide (ANP) A hormone involved in natriuresis and the regulation of renal and cardiovascular homeostasis. It is synthesized as a prohormone in the granules of the atrial myocytes and is released into the circulation in response to atrial dilation or increased intravascular fluid volume. Besides causing natriuresis, it causes diuresis and renal vasodilation and reduces circulating concentrations of renin, aldosterone, and vasopressin, thereby normalizing blood pressure and the circulating blood volume. Also called *atriopeptin* and *atrial natriuretic factor.*

azotemia A condition characterized by an excess of urea or other nitrogenous compounds in the blood; called also *uremia.*

Bowman's capsule pressure The pressure exerted by any filtrate in the epithelial sac that is Bowman's capsule.

bruit A venous hum.

C-reactive protein A globulin that in the presence of calcium precipitates the C substance of pneumococcal cells. This is an abnormal protein detectable in the blood only during the acute phase of certain illnesses, such as rheumatic fever or *Streptococcus pneumoniae.*

capillary hydrostatic pressure The pressure of the blood itself inside the glomerulus.

carboxypeptidase Any exopeptidase that catalyzes the hydrolytic cleavage of the terminal or penultimate peptide bond at the C-terminal end of a peptide or polypeptide.

cardioesophageal (gastroesophageal) sphincter The lower esophageal sphincter.

chronic liver failure (CLF) A condition marked by decreasing liver function that has lasted at least 6 months.

chyme The semifluid, homogeneous, creamy or gruel-like material produced by digestion of food in the stomach; called also *chymus.*

chymotrypsin A serine endopeptidase that preferentially cleaves peptide bonds on the carboxyl side of amino acids with bulky hydrophobic residues, particularly tyrosine, tryptophan, phenylalanine, and leucine. It is secreted by the pancreas as the inactive proenzyme chymotrypsinogen.

Crohn's disease A chronic granulomatous disease of the gastrointestinal (GI) tract and a principal form of inflammatory bowel disease; the etiology is unknown. The disease can involve any part of the GI tract but most often is found in the terminal ileum. Characteristics include scarring and thickening of the bowel wall, which frequently lead to intestinal obstruction and the formation of abscesses and fistulas. Recurrence after treatment is common. The disease is also called *Crohn's colitis* and *regional* or *segmental enteritis.* When confined to the ileum, it is called *regional* or *terminal ileitis.*

Cullen's sign A bluish discoloration of the skin around the umbilicus, indicating intraperitoneal hemorrhage; it most often is seen with acute hemorrhagic pancreatitis or rupture of a fallopian tube as a result of an ectopic pregnancy.

dehiscence In regard to surgery, a separation of the layers of a surgical wound; it may be partial and superficial only or complete, with disruption of all layers.

dilutional hyponatremia A condition marked by a low plasma concentration of sodium as a result of loss of sodium from the body with nonosmotic retention of water, such as is induced by vasopressin; hypovolemia also may be present.

esophagogastroduodenoscopy (EGD) Endoscopic examination of the esophagus, stomach, and duodenum.

gastrin Any of the several polypeptide hormones released from peptidergic fibers in the vagus nerve and from G cells in the pyloric glands of the gastric antrum; forms include little gastrins, big gastrins, and minigastrins. Gastrin stimulates the secretion of gastric acid, causing contraction of the lower esophageal sphincter and modifying gastric and esophageal motility; it also increases the growth of acid-secreting mucosal cells and weakly stimulates the secretion of pancreatic enzymes and gallbladder contraction.

gastroduodenal mucosal defense mechanism An immune or defense mechanism arising from the communication between the stomach and the duodenum.

Grey Turner's sign Discoloration (bruising) and induration of the skin of the costovertebral angle caused by the extravasation of blood with acute hemorrhagic pancreatitis; also called *Turner's sign.*

Helicobacter pylori A gram-negative, microaerophilic bacterium that causes gastric and pyloric ulcers and also is associated with stomach cancer.

hepatopulmonary syndrome Arterial hypoxemia caused by pulmonary vasodilation in conjunction with chronic liver disease; it usually occurs as a result of portal hypertension in cirrhosis.

hepatorenal syndrome A condition characterized by functional renal failure, oliguria, and a low urinary sodium concentration without pathologic renal changes; it is associated with cirrhosis and ascites or with obstructive jaundice.

hyperresonance An exaggerated resonance. Resonance is the prolongation and intensification of sound produced by transmission of its vibrations to a cavity, especially a sound elicited by percussion.

hypopharyngeal sphincter The upper esophageal sphincter.

ileus Intestinal obstruction that has a nonmechanical cause, such as paralysis or failure of peristalsis.

Jackson Pratt drain A closed wound drainage system composed of a drainage tube and a collection vessel.

Kupffer cells A type of stellate cell found in the sinusoids of the liver; these cells have intense phagocytic activity and are part of the reticuloendothelial system.

lactulose A synthetic disaccharide that is used as a cathartic and also to enhance the excretion or formation of ammonia in the treatment of portosystemic encephalopathy, including the stages of hepatic precoma and coma.

lecithin (phosphatidylcholine) A phospholipid in which choline is attached to the phosphate group of phosphatidic acid by an ester linkage; it is a major component of cell membranes and is localized preferentially in the outer surface of the plasma membrane.

ligament of Treitz The ligament that suspends the fourth part of the duodenum from the retroperitoneal cavity. Also called the *musculus suspensorius duodeni.*

magnetic resonance cholangiopancreatography (MRCP) An MRI examination of the bile ducts and pancreas in which a contrast dye is used.

Mallory-Weiss tears Hematemesis or melena that typically follows many hours or days of severe vomiting and retching; it is traceable to one or several slitlike lacerations of the gastric mucosa, longitudinally placed at or slightly below the esophagogastric junction. Also called *Mallory-Weiss syndrome.*

muscularis With regard to the digestive tract, one of the four layers that compose the portion of the GI tract extending from the esophagus to the rectum.

N-acetylcysteine (NAC) An antidote to acetaminophen overdose; NAC interferes with the metabolic process that produces hepatotoxic metabolites of acetaminophen.

paracentesis Surgical puncture of a cavity with a needle or other hollow instrument for diagnostic or therapeutic aspiration of fluid. In the abdomen, a trocar is inserted through an incision into the peritoneal cavity so that a therapeutic agent can be injected or ascitic fluid removed.

Penrose drain A thin rubber tube, usually 0.5 to 1 inch in diameter.

pepsinogen A proenzyme secreted by chief cells, mucous neck cells, and pyloric gland cells that is converted into pepsin in the presence of gastric acid or of pepsin itself.

percutaneous endoscopic gastrostomy (PEG) Insertion of a feeding tube through the chest wall into the stomach under endoscopic guidance; it is used for long-term tube feeding.

percutaneous endoscopic jejunostomy (PEJ) Insertion of a feeding tube through the abdominal wall into the jejunum under endoscopic guidance; it is used for long-term tube feeding.

plasma colloid oncotic pressure The pressure or the osmotic pull of the plasma proteins in the bloodstream.

portal hypertension Increased pressure in the portal vein caused by obstruction of blood flow through the liver.

pyloric sphincter The part of the pylorus (the most distal part of the stomach) that helps move chyme through to the duodenum.

renin-angiotensin-aldosterone system (RAAS) The system that regulates sodium balance, fluid volume, and blood pressure by means of renal secretions. Reduced perfusion prompts the secretion of renin, which hydrolyzes a plasma globulin to convert angiotensinogen to angiotensin I, which in turn is converted to angiotensin II. This stimulates the secretion of aldosterone, resulting in sodium retention, a rise in blood pressure, and restoration of renal perfusion, which shuts off the signal for renin release.

Sengstaken-Blakemore tube A multilumen esophageal tube used for tamponade of bleeding esophageal varices. One lumen leads to a balloon that is inflated in the stomach to hold the instrument in place and compress the vessels around the cardia; a second lumen leads to a long, narrow balloon that is used to exert pressure against the varices in the esophageal wall; a third lumen allows aspiration of stomach contents.

sclerosing agent An agent administered to cause hardening (sclerosis).

somatostatin Any of several cyclic tetradecapeptides elaborated primarily by the median eminence of the hypothalamus and by the delta cells of the pancreatic islets. They inhibit the release of growth hormone, thyrotropin, and corticotrophin by the adenohypophysis; of insulin and glucagon by the pancreas; of gastrin by the gastric mucosa; of secretin by the intestinal mucosa; and of renin by the kidney.

sphincters Ringlike bands of muscle fibers that constrict a passage or close a natural orifice.

splanchnic Visceral; pertaining to one of the splanchnic nerves.

syndrome A set of symptoms that occur together; the sum of signs of any morbid state.

systemic inflammatory response syndrome (SIRS) A syndrome related to the immune system response to an antigenic stimulus, including antibody production, cell-mediated immunity, and immunologic tolerance. The response can cause tissue injury and may lead to multi-organ dysfunction syndrome.

T-tube A self-retaining, T-shaped drainage tube that often is used in the common bile duct.

thrill A sensation of vibration felt by the examiner on palpation of the body, such as over the heart, a murmur, or an aneurysm.

transjugular intrahepatic portosystemic shunt (TIPS) The creation of an artificial percutaneous shunt between the hepatic and portal veins in the liver to allow placement of an expandable stent; the procedure is performed by a transjugular route under radiologic guidance for the treatment of bleeding esophageal varices.

trypsin A serine endopeptidase that catalyzes cleavage of peptide bonds on the carboxyl side of either arginine or lysine. It is secreted by the pancreas as the proenzyme trypsinogen and converted to the active form in the small intestine by enteropeptidase. The active enzyme catalyzes the cleavage and activation of additional trypsinogen and other pancreatic proenzymes important to protein digestion.

trypsinogen The inactive proenzyme of trypsin; it is secreted by the pancreas and activated in the duodenum through cleavage by enteropeptidase.

tympany A tympanic, or bell-like, percussion note. Ruminal tympany is a kind of indigestion or bloat.

Wilson's disease A rare, progressive, autosomal recessive disease caused by a defect in the metabolism of copper. Accumulation of copper in the liver, brain, kidney, cornea, and other tissues results in copper poisoning, with cirrhosis in the liver and degenerative changes in the brain, particularly the basal ganglia. Liver disease is the usual presenting symptom in children, and neurologic disease is most common in young adults. A characteristic feature is a pigmented ring at the outer margin of the cornea.

REFERENCES

1. Wiegand D, Carlson K, editors: *AACN procedure manual for critical care*, ed 5, Philadelphia, 2005, Saunders.
2. Sole ML, Klein DG, Mosely MJ: *Introduction to critical care nursing*, ed 4, Philadelphia, 2005, Saunders.
3. Marx JA, Hockberger RS, Walls RM: *Rosen's emergency medicine concepts and clinical practice*, ed 6, St Louis, 2006, Mosby.
4. Parsons P: *Critical care secrets*, ed 4, St Louis, 2007, Mosby.
5. Carlson KK: *Advanced critical care nursing*, ed 5, St Louis, 2009, Saunders.
6. McCance K, Huether S: *Pathophysiology: the biological basis for disease in adults and children*, ed 5, St Louis, 2006, Mosby.
7. Modified from Palevsky PM: Renal replacement therapy: indications and timing, *Crit Care Clin* 21:347-356, 2005.

Bibliography

Carlson KK: *AACN advanced critical care nursing*, St Louis, 2009, Saunders.

Jarvis C: *Physical examination and health assessment*, ed 5, St Louis, 2007, Saunders.

Kozier B, Erb G, Berman A, et al: *Fundamentals of nursing: concepts, processes and practice*, ed 7, Upper Saddle River, NJ, 2004, Prentice Hall.

Kumar V, Abbas A, Fausto N, et al: *Robbins and Cotran pathologic basis of disease*, ed 7, Philadelphia, 2005, Saunders.

Lemone P, Burke K: *Medical surgical nursing: critical thinking in client care*, Upper Saddle River, NJ, 1996, Prentice Hall.

McCance K, Heutherer S: *Pathophysiology: the biologic basis for disease in adults and children*, ed 5, St Louis, 2006, Mosby.

Morton P, Fontaine D, Hudak C, et al: *Critical care nursing: a holistic approach*, ed 8, Philadelphia, 2005, Lippincott Williams & Wilkins.

Thibodeau G, Patton K: *Anatomy and physiology*, ed 4, St Louis, 1999, Mosby.

Urden LD, Stacy KM, Lough ME: *Thelan's critical care nursing: diagnosis and management*, ed 5, St Louis, 2006, Mosby.

Wolf DC: *Hepatic encephalopathy. eMedicine.* www.emedicine.com/med/TOPIC3185.HTM. Accessed May 3, 2010.

REVIEW QUESTIONS

1. In the first case study, the patient demonstrated both respiratory alkalosis and metabolic acidosis. Given his chronic and acute disease processes, why are these opposites appearing in the acid-base balance spectrum?
   A. Metabolic acidosis is the primary problem arising from liver failure, and the body attempts to compensate through the respiratory system.
   B. Respiratory alkalosis is the primary problem arising from liver failure, and the body attempts to compensate through the metabolic system.
   C. Patients with liver failure always breathe faster because of ascites and thus develop respiratory alkalosis.
   D. The metabolic acidosis is from hemorrhage only.

2. Use of balloon tamponade tubes for esophageal varices may be life-saving. Which statement about their use is correct?
   A. The esophageal balloon may migrate if the gastric balloon fails, and airway obstruction may occur.
   B. No traction or forward pressure may occur, or the tube will migrate.
   C. Placement of three lumen or four lumen tubes prevents aspiration.
   D. Use of these tubes has increased because of the incidence of liver failure.

3. To facilitate correct insertion of a nasogastric tube, you should:
   A. Elevate the head of the bed up 90 degrees and have the patient swallow the tube.
   B. Aim the tube straight back into the patient's throat and then flex the patient's head to facilitate passage at the pharynx.
   C. Position the patient in the left lateral decubitus position with the head of the bed elevated to 10 to 20 degrees.
   D. Both B and C
4. Portal hypertension occurs because:
   A. The veins to the kidneys become constricted.
   B. The liver becomes smaller and constricts the vessels.
   C. The portal vessels from the GI tract become constricted.
   D. The esophagus becomes twisted.
5. The diagnosis of pancreatitis may be aided by:
   A. A peak amylase level two to three times normal at 2 to 12 hours after the onset of midepigastric pain and vomiting.
   B. A peak lipase level 4 to 8 hours after the onset of knifelike pain in the upper abdomen and back.
   C. An elevated C-reactive protein level and the appearance of trypsinogen in the urine.
   D. All of the above
6. A major consequence of portal hypertension is the development of:
   A. Collateral blood flow that also becomes engorged in the GI tract
   B. Ascites and dyspnea
   C. Hepatic encephalopathy
   D. Engorged blood vessels in the urinary system
7. A patient in the ICU has known hepatic failure. The hemodynamic monitoring system shows a PA pressure of 52/34 mm Hg and an occlusion (wedge) pressure of 10 mm Hg. The patient's BUN and creatinine levels are severely elevated, and urinary output is 0.25 mL/kg/hour. What condition or complication may have developed?
   A. Right ventricular failure
   B. COPD
   C. Multisystem organ dysfunction syndrome
   D. Hepatorenal and hepatopulmonary syndromes
8. A 462-pound (210-kg) patient who had gastric bypass surgery 2 weeks ago comes to the emergency department complaining of a vague feeling of weakness. The vital signs are: pulse, 142 beats/min; respirations, 28 breaths/min; BP, 112/68 mm Hg; pulse oximetry, 94% on room air; and temperature, 35.4° C (95.7° F). The patient has already lost 30 pounds (13.5 kg). Choose the correct statement about the diagnosis and treatment of this patient.
   A. This may be a normal postoperative complaint.
   B. Obese patients may show only tachycardia, even with a significant abdominal pathologic condition.
   C. A thorough respiratory diagnostic workup should be performed, because the patient probably has pneumonia.
   D. A thorough cardiac diagnostic workup should be performed, because the patient probably has CHF.
9. A patient with multisystem trauma is taken to the ICU after surgery and evaluated for nutritional needs. What parameters will determine the type of nutrition this patient receives?
   A. If the patient has bowel sounds, he will require only intermittent boluses of enteral feedings.
   B. Because of the tissue damage that has occurred, the patient will require intermittent, hypertonic enteral feedings.
   C. If the patient has no bowel sounds, he will require only parenteral feedings.
   D. The patient requires an intake high in calories and protein, which usually is provided by total parenteral nutrition given through a central line.
10. A 20-year-old man presents with altered mental status, dehydration, and fever. His ABGs are: pH, 7.12; arterial carbon dioxide pressure ($Paco_2$), 7 mm Hg; bicarbonate (HCO_3), 8 mEq/L; base excess (BE), −12 mEq/L, and arterial oxygen pressure (Pao_2), 188 mm Hg. His blood sugar level is 580 mg/dL, and the lactate level is 30 mg/dL. Which statement explains why, once resuscitation has started, this patient's initial urinary output is 800 mL?
    A. He is showing signs of shock. The patient was thirsty and drank too much water.
    B. He is showing signs of DKA. The high level of glucose cannot be reabsorbed in the nephron, so the sugar spilled pulls water with it.
    C. ADH is secreted in DKA, causing removal of water from the renal system.
    D. He is showing signs of shock. The increasing lactate level causes renal failure and excess urine production.

CHAPTER 7

Multisystem Trauma

OBJECTIVES

1. Review the primary, secondary, and ongoing assessment and resuscitation techniques in trauma.
2. Describe the pathophysiology, clinical signs and symptoms, diagnostic procedures, and management techniques of system and organ trauma.
3. Apply the assessment findings, patient presentation observations, and selected management techniques to the critical care transport environment.

Scenario

The transport team has been called to a neighboring community hospital to transport a 22-year-old male patient who suffered multiple injuries in a motor vehicle crash approximately 1 hour ago. Your response time to this hospital will be 20 minutes, with an additional 60 minutes for transport to the level I trauma care facility.

On arrival, you find that the patient has been orally intubated with an 8-mm tracheal tube; he is being ventilated with a bag-valve system by the local respiratory therapist. The family medicine physician gives you a quick report and moves to the desk to complete the chart. The findings for this patient are as follows:

- Mechanism of injury: 70 mph one vehicle rollover crash in which the patient was ejected.
- Injuries found: Hemopneumothorax on the right, closed cranial trauma with altered mental status, open book pelvic fracture, multiple soft tissue injuries, and various other smaller fractures.
- Vital signs: Heart rate, 100-140 beats/min; temperature, 35.8° C (96.4° F). The patient has had several bouts of hypotension (82/60 and 78/50 mm Hg). The local hospital has been ventilating him at a rate of 12 breaths/min.
- Treatment: Oxygen with bag-valve system and intubation. A 32 Fr chest tube was inserted in the right axillary line. Two intravenous (IV) lines have been placed, and 2 L of normal saline (NS) have been infused. An orogastric tube and a Foley catheter have been placed. The patient has been removed from spinal immobilization. When asked about this, the physician stated, "I cleared his C-spine with a lateral x-ray."

As your partner applies your monitoring equipment, you note that the capnographer shows a good waveform, with an end-tidal carbon dioxide pressure ($PETCO_2$) of 28 mm Hg. Pulse oximetry is 100% with occasional loss of pleth. Lead II shows sinus tachycardia at a rate of 120 beats/min currently, and the blood pressure (BP) is 100/70 mm Hg.

You auscultate bilateral breath sounds, better on the left than on the right. You then apply your ventilator with these settings: rate, 10 breaths/min; oxygen, 100%; tidal volume (V_T), 10 mL/kg of ideal body weight; and positive end-expiratory pressure (PEEP), 5 cm H_2O. The right chest tube has been secured, and the pleural drainage system is operational, with tidal movement noted. The drainage container holds 400 mL of bright red blood. The current time is noted on the system with a line at the 400 mL mark.

Two 16-gauge IV lines are in place in the patient's left arm (the right arm was fractured). A total of 2 L of crystalloid have infused. The patient's skin is pale and cool to the touch. The Foley catheter shows 100 mL of blood-tinged urine. You apply a pelvic binder to reduce the open book pelvic fracture and control bleeding. You switch the IV fluid to lactated Ringer's solution (LR) and infuse 1 more liter. You place the patient back into full spinal immobilization.

The emergency department (ED) team reports that the patient's Glasgow Coma Scale (GCS) score was 10 upon arrival; this was a rapid drop from the GCS score of 14 obtained by the emergency medical services (EMS) crew at the scene. A computed tomography (CT) scan showed diffuse edema and no focal hemorrhage. The patient was sedated and chemically paralyzed with etomidate and succinylcholine for induction 30 minutes ago. He subsequently was given 2 mg of midazolam and 1.2 mg/kg of rocuronium.

Up to now, you have focused on a single body system at a time as you learn about the critical care environment in transport. Trauma affects the entire body. Attempts to describe the anatomy and physiology of the body are left to the individual system's descriptions in Chapters 3, 4, 5, and 6. Those chapters introduced you to the respiratory, cardiovascular, neurologic, and gastrointestinal (GI) systems, along with the renal anatomy, normal physiology, and pathophysiology. This chapter covers the old disease of trauma and the most common traumatic disorders of individual systems.

THE DISEASE OF TRAUMA

Worldwide, the disease process of trauma accounts for 12% of all deaths, and motor vehicle crashes are the leading cause. However, statistics cannot fully convey the physical, social, and economic effects of trauma on individuals, their families, culture, and government.

EMS and critical care transport teams manage trauma patients within the first hours after the event to days later, when complications arise and specialized care is necessary. Time is an enemy in the early phase of resuscitation, and the transport team must work with local trauma systems to streamline the movement of injured patients to the correct trauma care facility.

CLINICAL ASSESSMENT OF THE TRAUMA PATIENT

As a well-prepared critical care transport professional, you will have prepared yourself for this specialized world by gaining as much knowledge as possible in basic and advanced healthcare pathophysiology. In the world of trauma, this includes taking courses and maintaining certification in various trauma programs and remaining current in the science of trauma assessment and resuscitation. Whether you are caring for a patient with multisystem trauma during a 9-1-1 response or during the critical care transfer, the assessment follows a systematic approach taught in nearly every trauma program. This assessment begins with the primary or initial assessment: airway, breathing, circulation, and disability (ABCD).

Primary Assessment and Management

A better acronym for emergency care providers is A-(C)-B-C-D, because the airway evaluation includes assessing for and maintaining in-line stabilization of the cervical spine. Begin this assessment and resuscitation with basic maneuvers and reassess after each intervention.

A—Airway

- Is the airway open now?
- Are any threats to this airway present (e.g., facial fractures, dental injuries)?
- Will the patient require intubation in the next few minutes?
- What is the patient's projected clinical course? For instance, if the patient has serious burns, you know that swelling will put the patient at risk for airway compromise and respiratory failure. Early intubation protects the patient from that risk.
- If an airway was inserted before your transport team arrived, what type and size of tube was used?
- What is the position of the tube (i.e., the centimeter mark at the upper teeth)?
- Is the tube working?
- Attach monitors to confirm placement of the tube and monitor throughout transport.

Did You Know?

To quickly assess for adequate depth of insertion for a tracheal tube, multiply the size of the tube by 3; that centimeter marking should be at the lip, as long as bilateral breath sounds also are present.[1]

Insertion of an oral gastric tube (OGT) tube at this point helps secure the patient's airway and should be done before transfer. Placing the OGT tube before obtaining a chest radiograph also aids the diagnosis of diaphragmatic injuries and helps ensure proper placement of the OGT tube in the esophagus and stomach.

C—Cervical Spine

- Is the cervical spine immobilized properly?
- Are the head, neck, and torso in alignment and secured?
- If the local hospital has decided to remove the immobilization devices, what procedure was used to "clear" the spine of injuries (Figure 7-1)?

B—Breathing

- Is the patient breathing?
- What are the respiratory rate and rhythm?
- Is there evidence of an acidotic state? (**Quiet tachypnea** is a sign of shock.)
- Is there evidence of obstruction or trauma to the airway or chest?
- Does the chest move symmetrically?
- Are breath sounds equal?
- If a chest tube had been placed before you arrived, follow standard procedure for evaluating for proper function of the chest drainage system and secure the tube at the chest wall.

C—Circulation

Assess proximal and distal perfusion by evaluating the skin vital signs (color, temperature, and condition); include palpation of the pulses and capillary refill testing. Control obvious

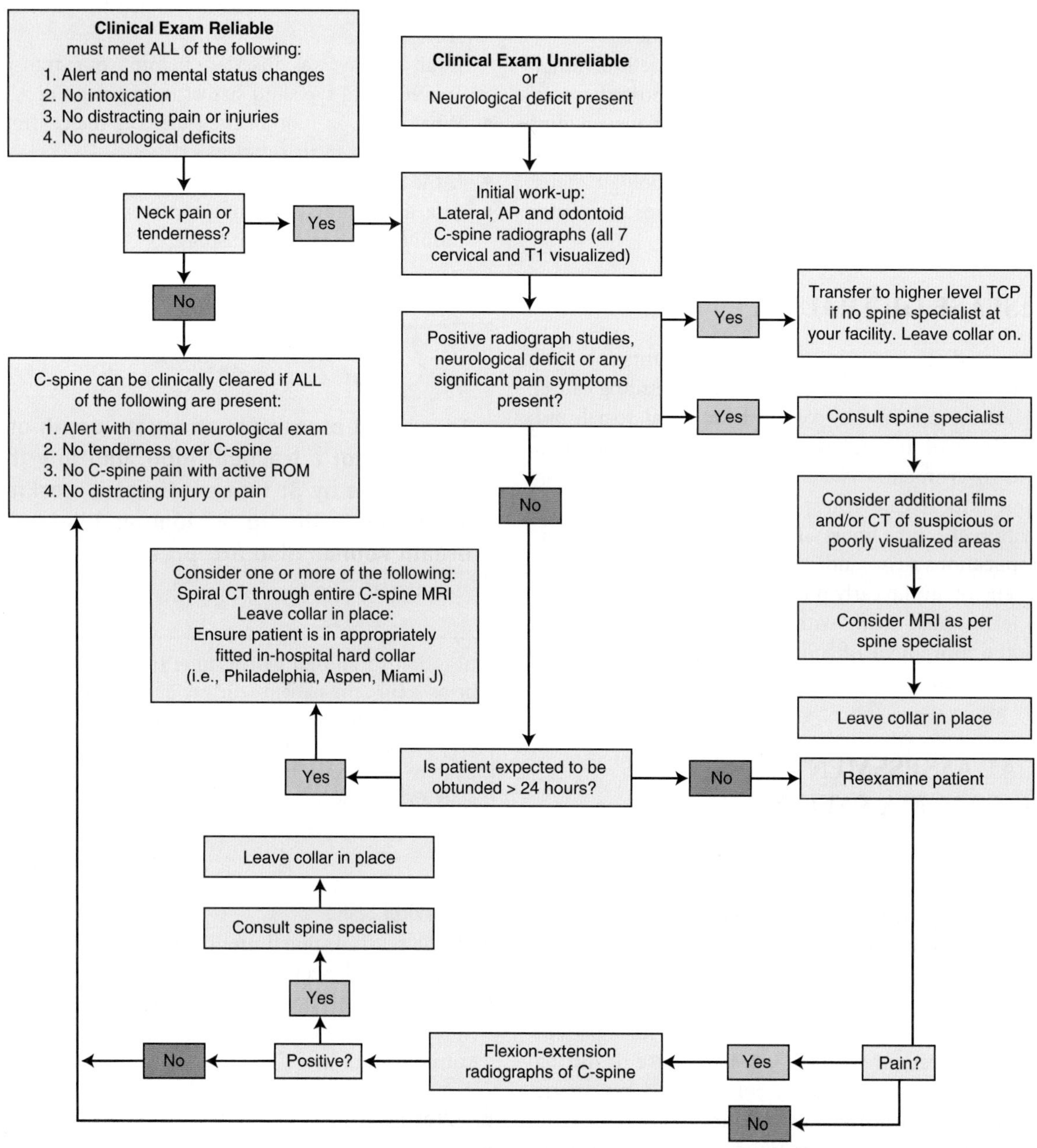

Figure 7-1

Protocol for cervical spine clearance.

external hemorrhage during this phase. The patient should have two large-bore (larger than 18 gauge) IV or intraosseous (IO) lines in place with crystalloid infusing. Do not place peripheral IV lines in extremities with major fractures, because often the vascular system is affected, and the infused fluids may end up in the soft tissues.

It is important to assess how much IV or IO fluid has been administered and the changes in vital signs that occurred with each bolus. Whether the patient responded to fluids completely or transiently helps the team determine the origin of the bleeding. Alert the receiving trauma center as early as possible if the patient is in hemorrhagic shock and specify the amount of crystalloid already infused. This information allows the receiving facility to order blood products early and helps prevent delays in the administration of blood products caused by blood bank logistics.

The urinary catheter, although usually considered a secondary tube, also should be inserted to aid assessment of the patient's perfusion status. Renal function can serve as a "window" that allows the critical care team to "see" shock and the effects of resuscitation. At minimum, urinary output should be 0.5 mL/kg/hour in adults, 1 mL/kg/hour in children, and 2 mL/kg/hour in infants.

Table 7-1 Identification and Management of Pelvic Fracture and Bleeding

Type of Fracture	Significance	Management
Pubic ramus fracture	Less blood loss	Volume replacement Possible use of blood products Avoid excessive manipulation
Open book fracture	Increase in pelvic size	Volume resuscitation Probable use of blood products Reduce pelvic size (binder) Internal hip rotation (binder) Use of a pneumatic antishock garment (PASG) Orthopedic surgery
Visceral organ injury	Potential for continuing blood loss	Volume replacement Possible use of blood products Surgical consultation

Modified from the American College of Surgeons, Committee on Trauma: *ATLS advanced trauma life support for doctors*, ed 7, St Louis, 2004, Mosby.

Splint long-bone fractures in the local facility before transport to help control bleeding sites. This might include stabilization of an **open book pelvic fracture** with a pelvic binder. If long-bone and pelvic fractures do not account for the amount of bleeding (Table 7-1), examine the abdomen for evidence of internal hemorrhage.

D—Disability

The critical care transport team should note previous neurologic examinations and their results but also should perform a personal baseline assessment using the Glasgow Coma Scale. Quickly assess for pupil shape and ability to react to light and then determine whether the patient has been using the extremities. Has the patient shown purposeful movement? Note any history or presence of seizure activity, keeping in mind that seizure activity can go undetected if **paralytic** agents have been administered.

Resuscitation in this phase of the assessment may include securing the airway and, if approved by the receiving neurosurgeon, administering medications and other therapy to reduce intracranial pressure (see the discussion of the neurologic system in Chapter 5).

Once the primary assessment is complete, the team should make transport decisions based on the patient's physiologic status. Time is an enemy when hemorrhagic shock continues. The complications awaiting the patient in the intensive care unit (ICU) will involve all eight systems and include acute respiratory distress syndrome (ARDS), renal failure, and multisystem organ dysfunction syndrome (MODS).

Secondary Assessment

The overall purposes of a secondary assessment are to reassess the patient, evaluate the effect of the resuscitation measures, and identify any additional injuries. Because time is a factor, this should be a quick examination that focuses on the prevention of further injury.

Packaging for Transport

A critically injured patient must be transported as soon as possible so that definitive treatment can be provided. The transport team's job is to prepare the patient for this trip by following the principles of good trauma patient care and safety. As stated previously, splinting of long-bone and pelvic fractures is part of the control of bleeding. This should be done as quickly as possible before transport. Pain control may be achieved by positioning the patient, splinting any fractures, and administering analgesics. The patient also may need to be packaged into in-line, neutral spinal immobilization.

DIAGNOSTIC PROCEDURES

Laboratory Values

Normal laboratory values are as follows:

Serum lactate: Venous, 0.9 to 1.7 mmol/L; arterial, less than 1.3 mmol/L

Arterial blood gases (ABGs): See Chapter 3.

Prothrombin time/international normalized ratio (PT/INR): The **international normalized ratio (INR)** is the PT corrected for the reagent used. For patients undergoing warfarin therapy, an INR of 2 to 3 usually is the goal.

Fibrinogen: 190 to 400 mg/dL

Platelets: 174,000 to 404,000/mcL

Hemoglobin
- Male: 13.5 to 17.5 g/dL
- Female: 12 to 16 g/dL

Hematocrit (proportion of red blood cells in whole blood)
- Male: 40% to 54%
- Female: 37% to 47%

Radiographs

Regardless of whether clinical interpretation skills are within the transport team's scope of practice, it is essential that all team members understand the basics of the following diagnostic radiographic techniques. These procedures are performed in the hospital, if possible, at the bedside of a trauma patient.

Radiographic Evidence of Diaphragmatic Injury

Anatomically, the diaphragm is described as having a left leaf and a right leaf. Placement of a gastric tube before a chest radiograph is taken may reveal the injury to the left leaf of the diaphragm described in the chest trauma section of this chapter. In Figure 7-2, note the radiographic image of the gastric tube as it courses down the esophagus and into the stomach. To aid the clinician, these tubes are manufactured with radiopaque lines so that they are visible on radiographs. Note the location of this particular gastric tube, in the left thorax.

Bedside Radiographic Evaluation of the Pelvis

To identify fractures that increase the volume of the pelvis (and thus result in massive bleeding), the clinician should evaluate the width of the symphysis pubis (greater than 1 cm indicates injury) and the sacroiliac (SI) joints; the symmetry of the internal ring; the integrity of the superior and inferior pubic rami on both sides; and the integrity of the acetabula, femurs, and ilium. In Figure 7-3, note the distance across the SI joint and pubic rami and the loss of symmetry in the ring.

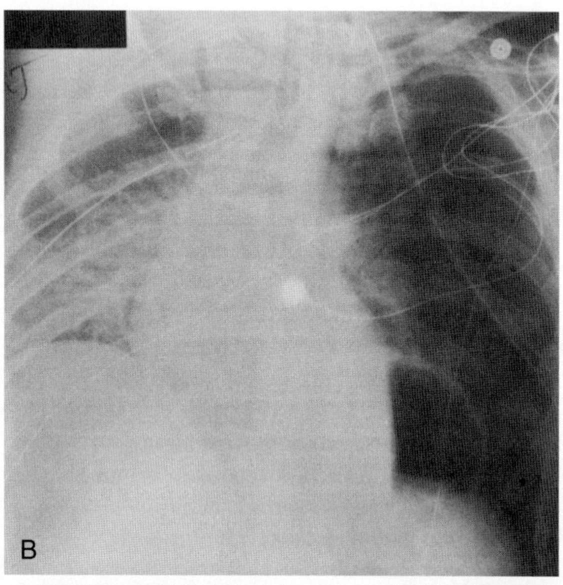

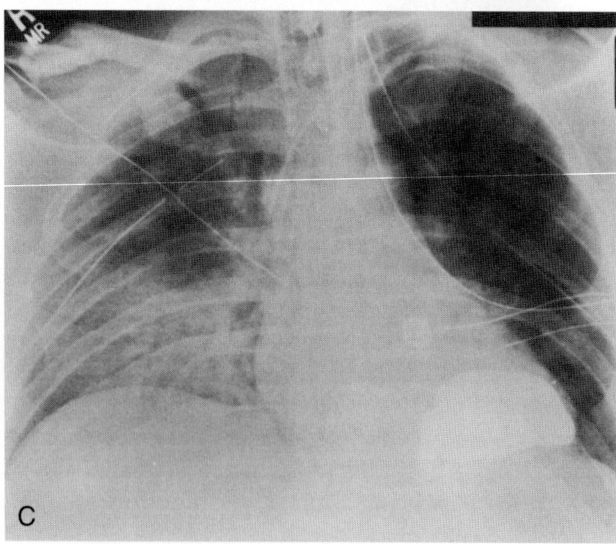

Figure 7-2

Left diaphragmatic rupture. A right-side-down decubitus radiograph demonstrates an air-fluid level in the left retrocardiac region. (From McLoud TC, Boiselle PM: *Thoracic radiology: the requisites*, ed 2, St Louis, 1998, Mosby.)

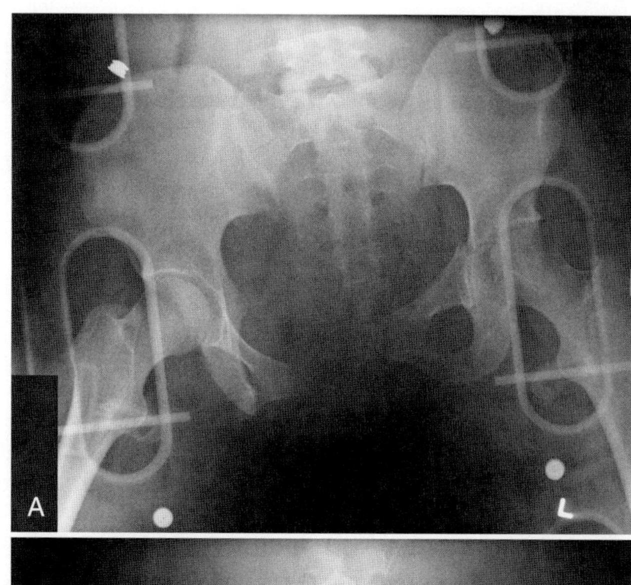

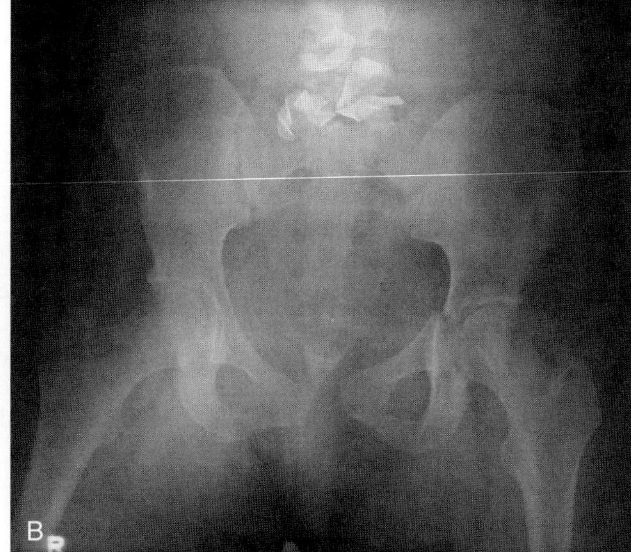

Figure 7-3

Open book pelvic fracture. **A,** Initial anteroposterior radiograph of an open book pelvic fracture. **B,** After application of pelvic binder. (From Canale ST, Beaty J: *Campbell's operative orthopaedics*, St Louis, 2008, Mosby.)

Bedside Ultrasound for the Trauma Patient

Focused Abdominal Sonography in Trauma

The focused abdominal sonography in trauma (FAST) examination (Figure 7-4) has become a standard of care for trauma resuscitation in larger trauma centers, because it is a noninvasive means of detecting the abnormal presence of fluid (blood) in the peritoneum, thorax, and pericardial sac. In addition, a variety of views can be obtained to diagnose a pneumothorax.

For the FAST examination, an ultrasound transducer transmits high-frequency sound waves into the target area. The sound waves are bounced back off the tissues to a receiver, which creates a live-action video or still pictures. The bounce-back shows fluid as dark. The following are some of the structures that may be visualized.

- Morrison's pouch can be visualized by placing the transducer in the midaxillary line over the seventh to eleventh ribs on the right side. This right upper quadrant view reveals the liver, kidney, and right leaf of the diaphragm. A black stripe may be seen between the liver and kidney if bleeding is occurring in this area. Injury around the diaphragm also may be viewed with subtle movements of the probe. Dark fluid above the diaphragm indicates a hemothorax on the right (Figure 7-5).
- The left upper quadrant parisplenic (splenorenal) view can be obtained by positioning the transducer over the fifth to eighth ribs in the postaxillary line on the left (Figure 7-6). Clockwise movement of the probe reveals the spleen and left leaf of the diaphragm. Blood (dark fluid) above the diaphragm indicates a hemothorax. Placing the patient in Trendelenburg's position aids visualization of areas of concern in both upper abdominal quadrants.

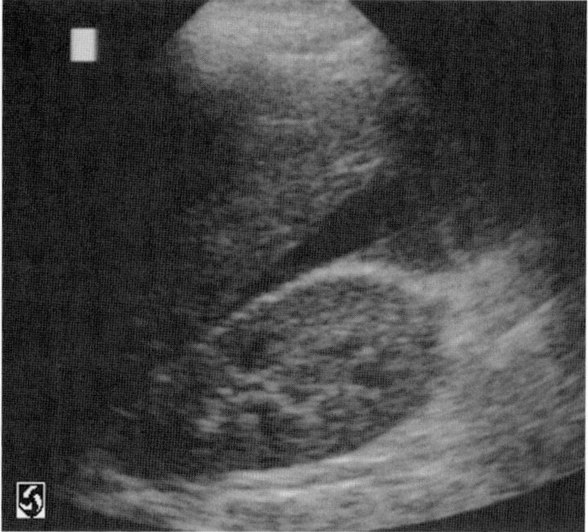

Figure 7-5

Positive findings on a focal abdominal sonography in trauma (FAST) study. A collection of fluid is seen as a black strip between the liver and kidney. The white area is fat around the kidney. These findings are consistent with the collection of fluid in Morrison's pouch. (From Goldman L, Ausiello D, editors: *Cecil medicine*, ed 23, Philadelphia, 2007, Saunders.)

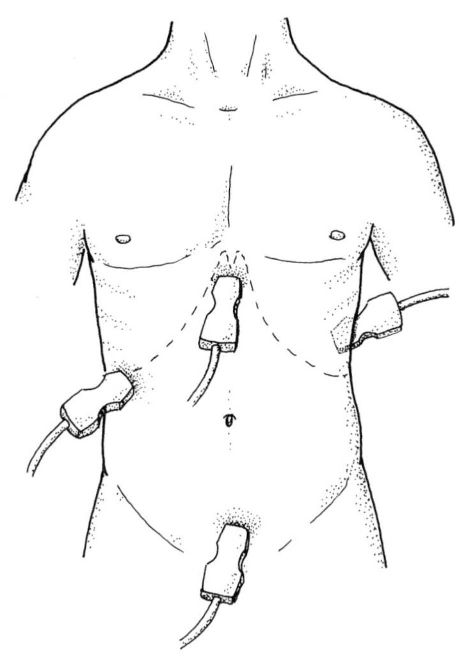

Figure 7-4

Schematic of a focused abdominal sonography for trauma (FAST) examination, with emphasis on views of the subxiphoid, right upper quadrant and Morrison's pouch, left upper quadrant and left paracolic region, and pelvic region and pouch of Douglas. (From O'Neill JA, Coran AG, Fonkalsrud E, et al: *Pediatric surgery*, ed 6, St Louis, 2006, Mosby.)

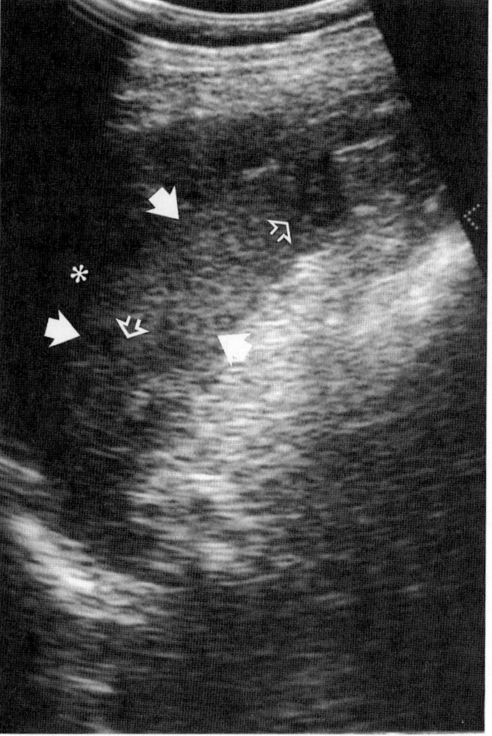

Figure 7-6

A longitudinal ultrasound shows splenic lacerations *(open arrows)* and perisplenic fluid/hematoma *(asterisk)* around the spleen *(arrows)*. (Courtesy Dr. JAW Webb.)

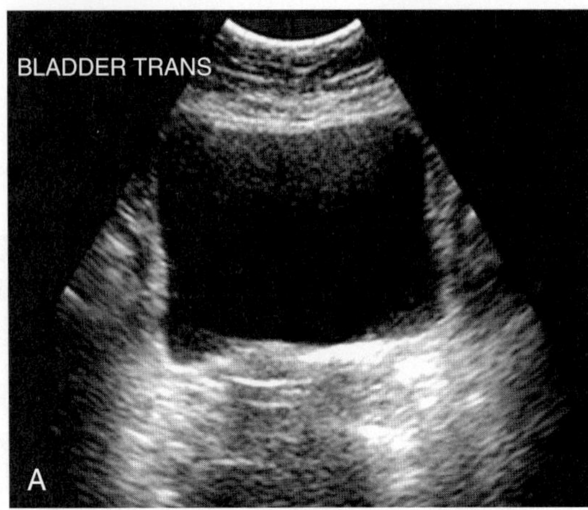

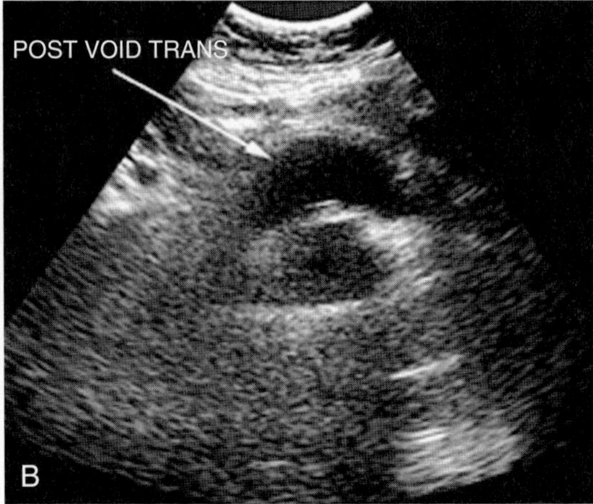

Figure 7-7

A, Suprapubic transverse view of a full urinary bladder. This "square" appearance of the bladder with a concave superior wall is typical of a moderately full bladder. An overdistended bladder has a large, globular shape (not shown). **B,** Suprapubic transverse view of an empty bladder. An empty bladder often is small and may be difficult to identify. (From Fink MP, Vincent JL, Kochanek PM: *Textbook of critical care,* ed 5, Philadelphia, 2005, Saunders.)

- A pelvic view is obtained by placing the probe just superior to the pubic rami. In females, this allows visualization of the bladder, uterus, and posterior cul de sac, along with the pouch of Douglas. In males, the bladder and retrovesicular space are observed. These views should be obtained with a full bladder; therefore, they should be done before a urinary catheter is placed, if possible. An alternative is to clamp the drainage tube from the urinary catheter to allow urine to collect in the bladder (Figure 7-7).
- A cardiac view is obtained by placing the probe transversely across the subxiphoid area. Some movement of the probe to just left of the sternum at the second to fourth ribs can aid viewing of the area. The tissues visualized include the liver, left atrium, mitral valve, ventricles, diaphragm, and aorta (Figure 7-8).

In this view, a pneumothorax may be seen first by viewing the normal side for the sliding lung sign (in a normal lung, the pleura can be seen sliding under the ribs); when air accumulates in this potential space, the sliding lung sign is absent.

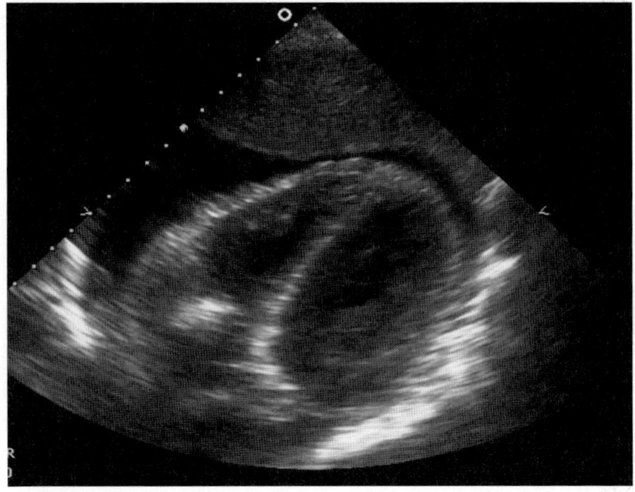

Figure 7-8

Subcostal view of a pericardial effusion. (From Marx JA, Hockberger RS: *Rosen's emergency medicine,* ed 7, St Louis, 2009, Mosby.)

REVIEW AND MANAGEMENT OF MAJOR TRAUMATIC INJURIES

Thoracic Injuries

Pneumothorax

The lower airways that are involved in the act of respiration are frequently injured. As described in Chapter 3, the two pleural layers work together to allow the smooth transition of lung tissue through the respiratory pattern. When an injury occurs, a potential space between the two layers becomes a real space.

A pneumothorax is the accumulation of either air or gas within the pleural space. If the defect is small and the accumulation of air is limited and under no pressure, the air can easily be reabsorbed by the body without intervention. This type of pneumothorax is called a *simple pneumothorax,* which may be well tolerated by the patient and not clinically evident to the critical care team. It can be diagnosed at the bedside using ultrasound, radiographic plain films of the chest, or CT scans. Clinical signs might include unilaterally diminished breath sounds with some increased work of breathing. Treatment might include insertion of a chest tube to restore the negative pressure in the thorax. Tube **thoracostomy** usually is not performed unless the patient will be transported at high altitudes or treated with positive pressure ventilation (PPV). However, the simple rule is, whenever even a small pneumothorax exists, PPV will create a tension pneumothorax.

Tension Pneumothorax

A tension pneumothorax is the result of air leaking from the lung into the pleural space; tension builds because the air does not escape, causing the affected lung to collapse. Venous return is compromised as a result of compression and shifting of the mediastinal structures to the contralateral side of the chest cavity, with collapse of the right side of the heart and lack of preload. This creates an obstructive shock state. Tension pneumothorax can result from **barotrauma** caused by mechanical ventilation; it also can be an adverse outcome of attempts to insert a central line or result from a parenchymal lung injury that fails to seal itself. It also can result from dressings applied to seal an open pneumothorax (sucking chest wound).

The diagnosis of tension pneumothorax is purely clinical, and treatment should never be delayed to confirm the diagnosis radiographically. The clinical signs include:

- Air hunger, increasing work of breathing (and, with the use of bag-valve devices, loss of chest wall compliance)
- Chest pain
- Acute respiratory distress
- Tachycardia
- Hypotension
- Decreased or absent breath sounds unilaterally
- Asymmetric chest wall motion.

Preterminal signs include neck vein distention, cyanosis, and tracheal deviation away from the affected side. Skill 7-1 reviews the steps for a needle thoracostomy (thoracentesis).

Skill 7-1

NEEDLE THORACOSTOMY (THORACENTESIS)

With a tension pneumothorax, the patient's condition often does not allow the time required to perform a tube thoracostomy. The accumulating air can be removed more quickly by inserting a long intravenous (IV) or spinal needle into the pleural space.

INDICATION

Tension pneumothorax

CONTRAINDICATION

Simple pneumothorax

PREPARATION

The critical care team should have needle decompression kits ready at all times; they should be included in the jump kits or easily accessible. Thoracentesis is indicated if the ongoing patient examination reveals increasing work of breathing and dyspnea with unilateral breath sounds.

EQUIPMENT

14- or 16-gauge, hollow catheter-over-needle device (needle must be at least 2 inches (or 5 cm) in length)
Skin cleansing agent
5-10 cc syringe with 2 cc of saline drawn up
One-way valve (Heimlich) (optional)

PROCEDURE

1. Observe standard precautions.
2. Identify the 2nd intercostal space in the midclavicular anatomic line on the side with no breath sounds. This can be done in two ways:
   a. Find the angle of Louis on the sternum and move your fingers laterally; this is rib no. 2.
   b. Palpate the clavicle on the affected side; remember that rib no. 1 is curved under it. Count down one more rib, to rib no. 2, and then to rib no. 3.
3. Confirm that you are performing the procedure on the correct side.
4. Cleanse the skin overlying the top of rib no. 3, in the midclavicular line on the affected side.
5. Remove the protective covering from a 2-inch needle. Using your nondominant hand, identify the top of rib no. 3, in the midclavicular line on the affected side. With your dominant hand, insert the needle over the top of rib no. 3 at a 90-degree angle. (The location of vessels and nerves under each rib precludes insertion of the needle under the rib; you must enter above the next rib inferiorly.)
6. Skin drag diminishes quickly as the needle tip enters the thoracic cage. Remove the hollow needle and discard it appropriately.
7. Confirm that air is being released.
   a. Saline that partially fills an attached syringe should bubble. (This technique can be quite helpful when fine-tuned listening is not possible.)
   b. Palpate for a rush of air from the open end of the catheter.
8. Reassess the patient for the most important clinical signs: The patient's condition has improved; the work of breathing has lessened; complaints of dyspnea have diminished; and signs of obstructive shock have been reduced.
9. The catheter may be kept in the insertion site until tube thoracostomy is performed. The catheter may serve as a reminder to the trauma resuscitation team that needle decompression was performed on that side. Report completion of the procedure during the hand-off to the nursing staff.
10. A one-way (Heimlich) valve may be attached; however, this is optional, because the opening of a 14- or 16-gauge catheter is not large enough to allow air to enter the thoracic cavity once pressures have nearly equalized.

11. Prepare for chest tube insertion (tube thoracostomy) by the clinician (see Figure 7-10).

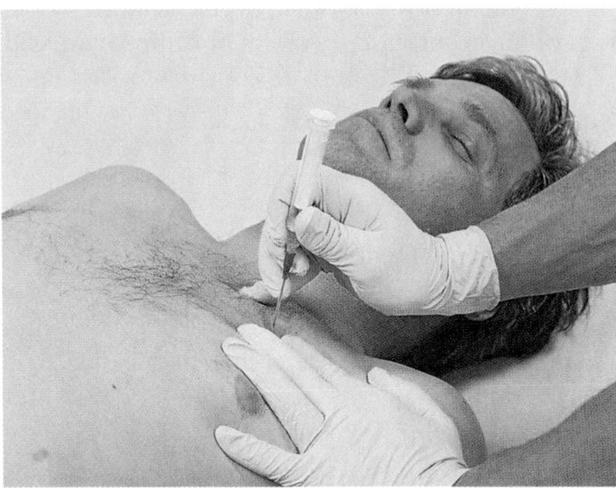

(From the National Association of Emergency Medical Technicians [NAEMT]: *PHTLS prehospital trauma life support: military version [NAEMT PHTLS, basic and advanced prehospital trauma support]*, ed 6, St Louis, 2007, Mosby.)

TROUBLESHOOTING

1. An alternative site for needle thoracentesis is the fourth or fifth intercostal space.
2. A standard $1\frac{1}{4}$-inch IV needle is not long enough to access the pleural space in most older children and adults.
3. If no air is obtained with thoracentesis, report completion of the procedure to the receiving healthcare professionals. Tube thoracostomy may still be required, because the patient may have just developed a pneumothorax with needle insertion.

The critical care team should have a working knowledge of the techniques for inserting a chest tube. Even if such procedures are not within the team's scope of practice, this knowledge enables the team to best facilitate the procedure and to anticipate the needs of the clinician. Skill 7-2 reviews the steps for a tube thoracostomy (chest tube insertion).

Skill 7-2

TUBE THORACOSTOMY (CHEST TUBE INSERTION)

Loss of negative pressure in the vacuum of the thorax can occur for a variety of reasons. In trauma cases, the accumulation of air or blood is the most common cause. Accumulation of air or fluid in the pleural space causes the affected lung to collapse. Insertion of a chest tube that is connected to a water-seal drainage system allows drainage of the air and/or fluid and subsequent reestablishment of the negative pressure and reinflation of the lung.

The chest tube is a sterile, flexible catheter with **nonthrombogenic** properties. It is approximately 20 inches long, and sizes range from 12 to 40 Fr. The tube has a **radiopaque** line that helps determine the location of the tube radiographically.

The size of chest tube chosen depends on the clinician's preference and the purpose of the tube. In general, drainage of blood or infectious material requires a larger tube. Some guidelines for tube size are:

- Pneumothorax or tension pneumothorax (air only): 12 to 26 Fr
- Pleural effusions (postoperative, **empyema, hydrothorax**): 26 to 36 Fr
- Hemothorax (blood): 36 to 40 Fr

INDICATION

Drainage of air or fluid from the pleural space

RELATIVE CONTRAINDICATIONS

Multiple **adhesions**, large **blebs**, or coagulopathies pose a risk for the patient; however, the need to reestablish negative pressure in the thorax usually outweighs relative contraindications.

PREPARATION

The patient is positioned supine with the arm on the affected side abducted and extended to at least 90 degrees, if possible.

EQUIPMENT

Sterile gloves (follow precautions)
Sterile towels or drapes
Skin cleansing agents
Small procedure instruments (three large Kelly clamps, scalpel, no. 11 blade, 4 × 4s, needle holder)
Local anesthetic, syringe, 18- and 25-gauge needles
Sterile chest tube (open onto sterile field and place a large Kelly clamp over the proximal end)
Pleural drainage system (assistants set up the system according to the manufacturer's recommendations and have the collection tubing ready for attachment to the chest tube)
Suction-connecting tubing and Y-connector
Securing tape (dove-tailed), Parham bands, or plastic straps for each connection
Dressings for skin (4 × 4s, split dressings, self-sealing wide tape, petroleum-impregnated gauze)

Chest Tube Position

1. Drainage of air: The distal tip of the tube is placed near the apex of the lung in a more anterior location.
2. Drainage of fluid: The distal tip of the tube should rest near the base of the lung posteriorly.
3. Postoperative cardiac procedure (mediastinum): The tube is placed with an open thorax in the operating room.

PROCEDURE

1. Put on a sterile gown and gloves. Wear facial protection with a mask.
2. Surgically prepare and drape the insertion site.
3. Inject a local anesthetic into the subcutaneous tissue, muscle, and then into the **periosteum**.
   a. Use a 25-gauge needle to inject the local anesthetic subcutaneously, creating a wheal at the insertion site.
   b. Continue administration of the local anesthetic by advancing a 1½-inch needle; aspirate as the needle is inserted into deeper tissue. Inject the local anesthetic into deeper tissues and continue as needle is withdrawn.
4. Make a 3 to 4 cm transverse incision directly over the inferior edge of the rib just below the insertion site and continue the incision into the subcutaneous tissue (see illustration).

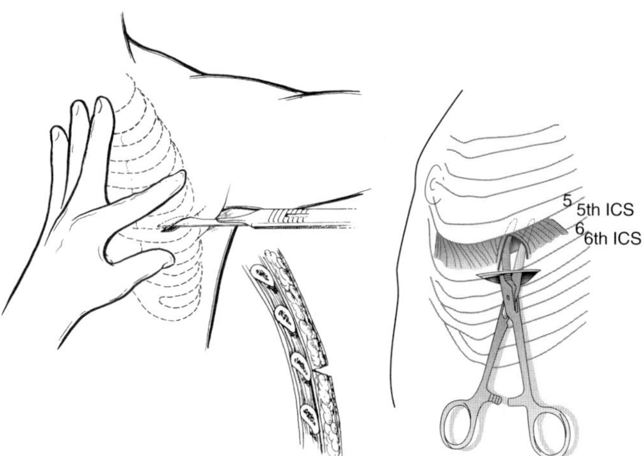

Left, A transverse skin incision is made directly over the inferior aspect of the anesthetized rib down to the subcutaneous tissue. *Right,* Blunt dissection is accomplished by forcing a closed clamp through the incision and by using an opening and spreading maneuver, creating a tunnel to the pleura. *ICS,* intercostal space. (*Left* figure from Dumire SM, Paris PM: *Atlas of emergency procedures,* Philadelphia, 1994, Saunders; *Right* figure from Wiegand D, Carlson K: *AACN procedure manual for critical care,* ed 5, Philadelphia, 2005, Saunders.)

5. Insert a closed Kelly clamp into the incision with the tips directed upward; then open the clamp. Repeat this technique with the clamp as you bluntly dissect the tissue. The goal is to create a pathway toward the superior portion of the rib and into the thorax. Some clinicians bluntly dissect with a gloved finger.

   NOTE: To prevent injury to the neurovascular bundle that lies beneath each rib, the Kelly clamp (and the chest tube pathway) must enter the thorax over the superior margin of the ribs.

6. When blunt dissection has created a pathway to the chest wall, stop and close the Kelly clamp. Place the forefinger of your dominant hand over the upper edge (tips) of the clamp and exert firm pressure until the clamp enters the pleural space. Open the clamp and create an entry pathway for subsequent insertion of a finger and then the chest tube (see illustration).

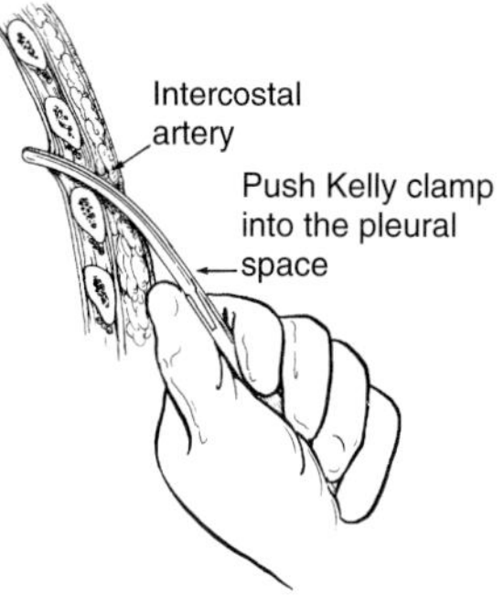

Left, Just over the superior portion of the rib, close the clamp and push with steady pressure into the pleura. *Right,* Grasp the tube with the curved clamp, with the tube tip protruding from the jaws of the clamp. (*Left* figure from Dumire SM, Paris PM: *Atlas of emergency procedures,* Philadelphia, 1994, Saunders; *Right* figure from Roberts JR, Hedges JR, editors: *Clinical procedures in emergency medicine,* ed 4, Philadelphia, 2004, Saunders.)

7. Remove the clamp as you slide your forefinger over and into the newly created pathway. Dilate the pleural hole with your finger and then sweep the curved finger around inside the hole to release any adhesions. Keep your finger in the pleural opening (see illustration).

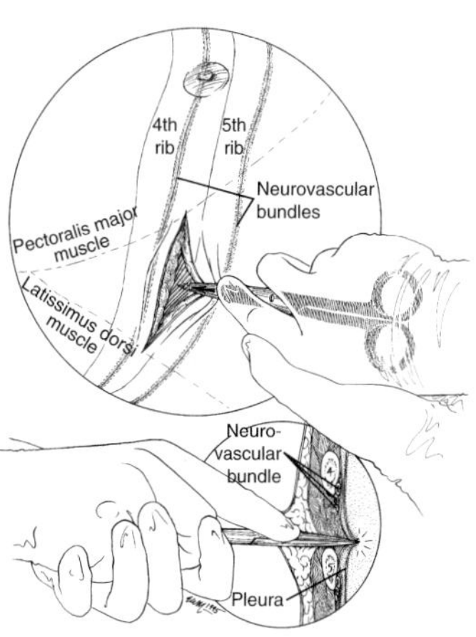

(From Proehl JA: *Emergency nursing procedures,* ed 4, Philadelphia, 2008, Saunders.)

8. Pick up the Kelly clamp attached to the proximal end of the chest tube. Direct this clamp into the pleural opening with the tips of the clamp (and the chest tube) under your finger (see illustration).

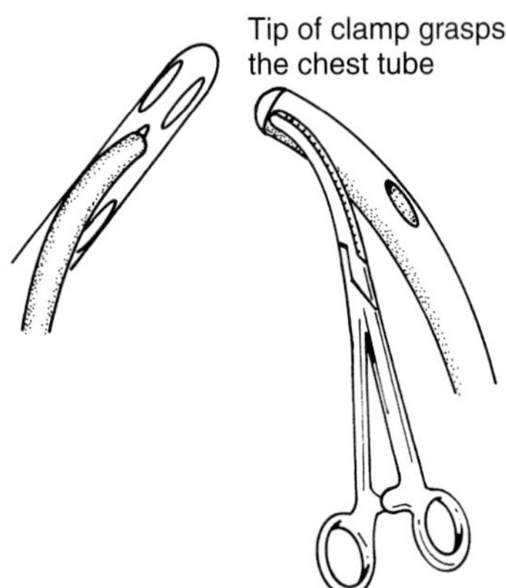

(From Wiegand D, Carlson K: *AACN procedure manual for critical care,* ed 5, Philadelphia, 2005, Saunders.)

9. As the proximal tip enters the chest, remove the clamp and your finger. With a rotating motion, direct the tip of the chest tube to the desired area of the thorax. When the last drainage hole is in the thorax, you may stop inserting the tube.
10. You should see condensation, air, or fluid entering the chest tube.
11. Quickly attach the chest tube to the connecting tubing of the assembled pleural drainage system.
12. Watch the pleural drainage system for fluctuation (tidaling).
13. Secure the chest tube to the chest wall. Place a purse-string or stay suture through the skin and around the chest tube twice; then pull up the suture, giving the incision a puckered appearance around the tube (see illustration).

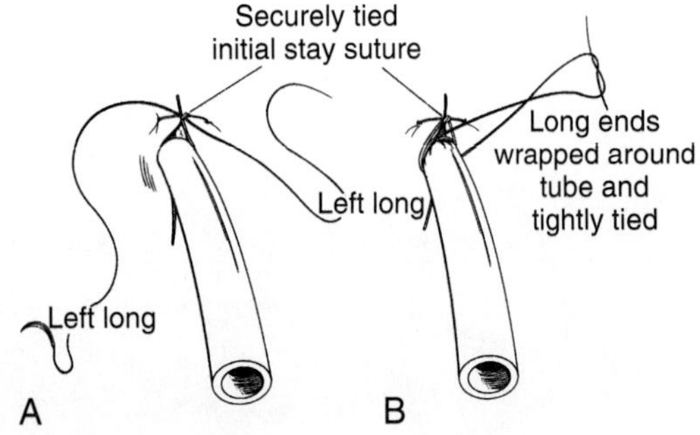

A stay suture is placed first, next to the tube, to close the skin incision. **A,** The knot is tied securely, and the ends are left long. **B,** The suture ends are wound twice around the chest tube, tightly enough to indent the tube slightly, and then tied securely. (From Roberts JR, Hedges JR, editors: *Clinical procedures in emergency medicine,* ed 4, Philadelphia, 2004, Saunders.)

14. Apply a petroleum-impregnated gauze dressing over the incision site and cover the dressing with split 4 × 4s. Tape the dressings in place.
15. Tape or place Parham bands or binding bands around all connections. If tape is used, dove-tail all ends (see illustration).

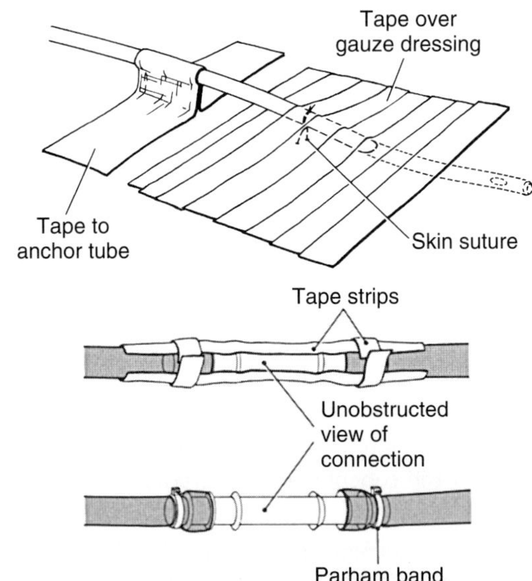

(From Proehl JA: *Emergency nursing procedures,* ed 4, Philadelphia, 2008, Saunders.)

16. Turn on the suction and turn the dial on the pleural drainage system to the desired level; the initial setting usually used is −20 cm H_2O.
17. Obtain a chest radiograph to confirm placement of the tube and expansion of the lung.
18. Document the procedure in the patient care record; include the size of the tube, its location, and the results of the chest radiograph, along with patient tolerance, vital signs, and the initial fluid output of the pleural drainage system.

TROUBLESHOOTING

1. Prevent kinking or clamping of the chest tube system by draping the tubing along the length of the patient. Do not position the patient on top of the tubing.
2. Check the output of the pleural drainage system at least every 2 hours. Notify a thoracic surgeon if bloody pleural drainage initially exceeds 1200 to 1500 mL or if it amounts to more than 200 mL/hour for several hours. Mark the time on the face of the collection chamber every 2 hours at the level of the drainage.
3. Monitor the chest tube, incision site, and pleural drainage system. The chest tube should show condensation (fog). The skin around the incision site should not have increasing subcutaneous air (subcutaneous emphysema). The tubing should be clear of clots and kinks.
4. Continuous bubbling without the suction on indicates an air leak. Follow the procedure outlined in Chapter 3 for maintaining a pleural drainage system and troubleshooting an air leak.

Open Pneumothorax

Large chest wall defects create equal pressures between the thorax and the atmosphere, and if the defect is larger than the trachea, air passes through the chest defect with each breath. The initial management of this type of wound involves covering it with an occlusive dressing (defibrillator pads, plastic wrap, petroleum gauze, a gloved hand); however, some controversy exists as to whether a three-sided dressing (which allows an exhalation port) or a four-sided dressing (which provides total coverage of the wound) should be used. Regardless of whether complete or partial coverage is used, you must be alert for the development of a tension pneumothorax. Initiate or assist with tube thoracostomy quickly, along with surgical exploration and closure of the wound.

Hemothorax

As is a pneumothorax, a hemothorax usually is resolved by insertion of a chest tube, which allows the lung to reexpand. Occasionally the patient must be taken to the operating room. You must monitor the amount of blood in the pleural drainage system initially and then hourly. Surgical intervention is indicated if initially more than 1200 to 1500 mL of blood accumulates in the drainage device, or if 200 mL/hour accumulates over several hours in a patient with shock who fails to respond to fluid resuscitation and has unaccounted-for blood loss. Some pleural drainage systems provide a separate chamber for thoracic blood accumulation and subsequent transfusion back to the patient (**autotransfusion**) (Figure 7-9). However, always make sure the drainage is from the thoracic cavity.

Flail Chest

Flail chest has many definitions. In essence, it is a free-floating island of the thoracic bony structure (ribs, sternum) that creates unstable thoracic wall movement. As with most fractures, soft tissue injury is a large part of the clinical picture. The underlying pulmonary contusion, increasing difficulty moving the chest wall, and associated pain result in hypoventilation and hypoxia.

Patients with some reserve may tolerate this injury for quite some time, and the clinical picture in these cases is very similar to that for a pneumothorax, with increased work of breathing and pleuritic pain. The increasing dyspnea often is confused with tension pneumothorax, and clinicians often perform a needle thoracentesis, with no results. Flail chest requires insertion of a chest tube. Be cautious in your examination and make sure to determine whether the patient has unilaterally or bilaterally diminished breath sounds.

Patients who have used up their pulmonary reserves and those who had little to start with (e.g., children and the elderly) may present with the classic flail or paradoxical motion of the chest wall (Figure 7-10). Ventilator support is imperative, and ventilating this patient can be quite a challenge. Analgesia must be included in the continuing care, along with close monitoring of **capnography** results. The lung-protective therapies described in Chapter 3 may need to be instituted, even in the early phase.

Injury of the Tracheobronchial Tree

Although rare, injury to the trachea or bronchus is a life-threatening event. Most injuries that occur within 1 inch of

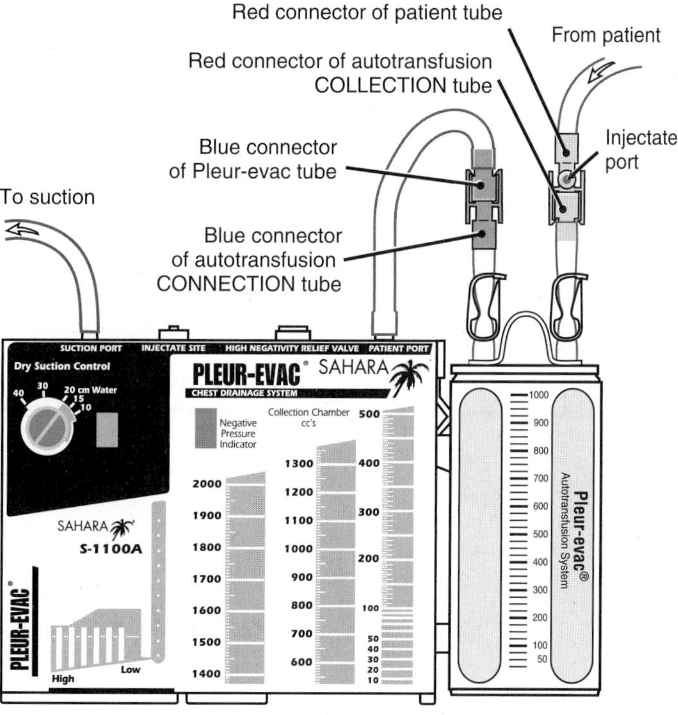

Figure 7-9

Standard pleural drainage system with autotransfusion attachment. (From Mims BC, Roberts MK, Tyner T et al: *Critical care skills: a clinical handbook*, Philadelphia, 2003, Saunders.)

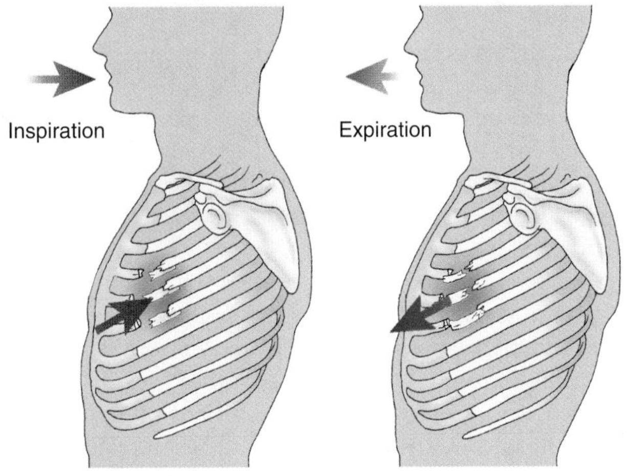

Figure 7-10

Paradoxical motion. Rib fractures in two or more places can disrupt the stability of the chest wall. In such cases, the intrathoracic pressure decreases during inspiration, and the external air pressure forces the chest wall inward. When the intrathoracic pressure increases during expiration, the chest wall is forced outward.

the carina are fatal at the scene. Even patients who survive the initial injury are critically ill with hemoptysis, subcutaneous emphysema (especially of the upper chest and neck), tension pneumothorax with mediastinal shift, and persistent pneumothorax with air leakage after chest tube insertion. Bronchoscopy confirms this injury.

Management of a tracheobronchial injury can be challenging. As stated, the patient requires a chest tube, and a persistent air leak warrants investigation for this defect and insertion of a second chest tube. Intubation can be difficult because of the anatomic distortions caused by the large amount of subcutaneous emphysema. Associated injuries to the maxillofacial and neck areas often are present as well. If possible, the endotracheal tube should be directed to the uninvolved bronchus. This is fairly easy if you are attempting to intubate the right mainstem bronchus; a bronchoscope usually is required to facilitate intubation of the left bronchus.

Cardiac Tamponade

With a traumatic defect of the heart (most commonly from penetrating injury), the fixed pericardial sac is unable to stretch and accommodate much blood within a short period. Sometimes removal of as little as 10 to 15 mL of blood from the pericardial sac through **pericardiocentesis** can relieve most of the classic signs of this injury. The clinical picture is described through **Beck's triad**: venous pressure elevation (seen as jugular venous distention [JVD]), low arterial pressure, and muffled heart tones. Despite its classic presentation, this injury sometimes is difficult to diagnose:

- JVD can be difficult to evaluate in a patient who is supine or in spinal immobilization or who has flat neck veins because of concomitant hypovolemia.
- Muffled heart tones are almost undetectable in loud environments (all heart tones are difficult to hear, let alone muffled tones).

Kussmaul's sign (elevated venous pressure with spontaneous inspiration) may be present with left-sided pneumothorax and pericardial tamponade. A patient with tamponade usually loses central pulses or presents with pulseless electrical activity without signs of hypovolemia *and* equal breath sounds.

An **echocardiogram** can be quite helpful in the diagnosis of tamponade. It also can aid pericardiocentesis by imaging the site while a needle is inserted. As mentioned, the FAST examination is becoming a standard in bedside ultrasound detection of several injuries, including tamponade. The pericardial sac is one of four areas examined by the clinician during this diagnostic test. Pericardiocentesis may be both diagnostic and therapeutic in pericardial tamponade. Skill 7-3 reviews the steps for pericardiocentesis.

Skill 7-3

PERICARDIOCENTESIS

Pericardial tamponade can occur through both medical and traumatic disease processes. The accumulation of serosanguineous fluid is called *pericardial effusion.* Whether blood or effusion, the rapid accumulation of fluid within the space creates a high-pressure environment outside the heart, resulting in collapse of the right side of the heart, loss of preload, and obstructive shock. When effusion accumulates at a slower rate, the heart is able to accommodate and remodels into a hypertrophic state marked by distention; as much as 1 to 2 L of fluid can accumulate before hemodynamic compromise occurs. Pericardiocentesis is geared toward emergency, life-saving removal of as little as 15 to 50 mL of blood after traumatic pericardial tamponade.

INDICATIONS

Pericardial tamponade with obstructive shock (emergency)

Removal of fluid (effusion) for laboratory analysis (elective)

CONTRAINDICATIONS

As an emergency procedure, no contraindications exist if tamponade has occurred. However, the risks of this procedure cannot be overstated, because it involves the insertion of a long, sharp needle into an area of crucial tissue. Possible complications include epicardial, myocardial, or pericardial laceration; coronary artery laceration; pneumothorax; and puncture of the great vessels, esophagus, or peritoneum.

EQUIPMENT

Sterile supplies (4 × 4s, gloves, alligator clip and cable, two three-way stopcocks)
Sterile drapes or towels
Skin cleansing agent
5-, 10-, and 20-mL syringes
16- or 18-gauge, 6-inch cardiac or spinal needle or catheter-over-needle device
12-lead electrocardiograph machine at bedside, prepared for procedure

Ultrasound machine and transducer gel at bedside (if available)

PREPARATION

The critical care team must have protocols in place, and the professional credentialing agency must have approved the procedure as falling within the team members' scope of practice. The employer should routinely reeducate and recertify each team member for this procedure in a skills laboratory. If the procedure is within the team's scope of practice, the agency should have an assembled pericardiocentesis kit ready at all times.

PROCEDURE

1. Put on sterile gloves and facial protection.
2. Cleanse the skin over the xiphoid and subxiphoid areas with an approved agent (a chlorhexidine-based solution usually is recommended).
3. Attach a sterile three-way stopcock to the 6-inch cardiac needle and then to a 20-mL syringe.
4. The sterile alligator clip may be connected to the distal aspect of the needle already attached to the syringe. An assistant connects the ECG machine end to lead V_1 or a bedside monitoring display. If the clinician chooses not to attach the alligator clamp, the monitor can be observed for cardiac irritability (premature ventricular contractions [PVCs], ventricular tachycardia [V tach]) while the needle is advanced.

   NOTE: An alternative is to use a bedside ultrasound device with the pericardial view as you observe the needle enter the space.
5. Note the anatomic landmarks for this procedure:
   a. Puncture the skin 1 to 2 cm just below and slightly to the left of the junction of the xiphoid process and the costal margin in the left anterior chest wall.
   b. Direct the angle of insertion at 45 degrees to the skin.
   c. Direct the tip of the needle toward the tip of the left scapula.
6. Monitor the ECG continuously. The V_1 lead, attached to your needle, may indicate improper positioning. If the needle is advanced too far, an ECG pattern known as a "current of injury" is seen. This finding appears as an extreme ST-T wave change or a widened and large QRS complex. Withdraw the needle until the baseline ECG rhythm reappears. If the injury pattern persists, withdraw the needle completely.
7. Apply negative pressure to the syringe as you insert the needle. Advance the needle until you aspirate blood, and then advance it about 2 mm farther. If you are using a catheter-over-needle device, withdraw the needle and leave the catheter attached to the stopcock and syringe.
8. Aspirate pericardial fluid until signs of shock subside.
9. The clinician may want to maintain the catheter within the pericardial sac (if positioning has been confirmed). In such cases, a guide wire is inserted into the catheter and directed around the heart. The guide wire then is removed, and the catheter is connected to a three-way stopcock and drainage bag for intermittent or continuous fluid removal. The catheter is secured to the chest wall with tape.

Ultrasound-Aided View

1. View the probable insertion site with the ultrasound wand as the procedure begins.
2. Check the position of the needle in the pericardial sac.
3. If the procedure is done in the cardiac catheterization laboratory, a small amount of contrast may be used to facilitate the view.

TROUBLESHOOTING

1. If pericardiocentesis is performed with a mediastinal shift occurring, the location of the needle insertion site will alter the angle of insertion (see illustrations).

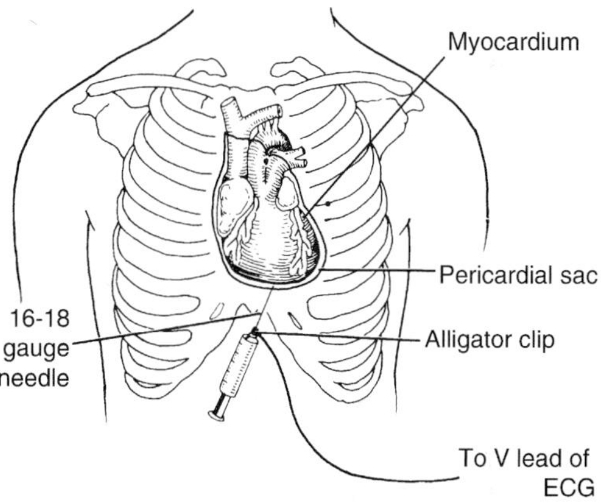

Pericardiocentesis. (From Sheehy SB: *Emergency nursing: principles and practice*, ed 3, St Louis, 1992, Mosby.)

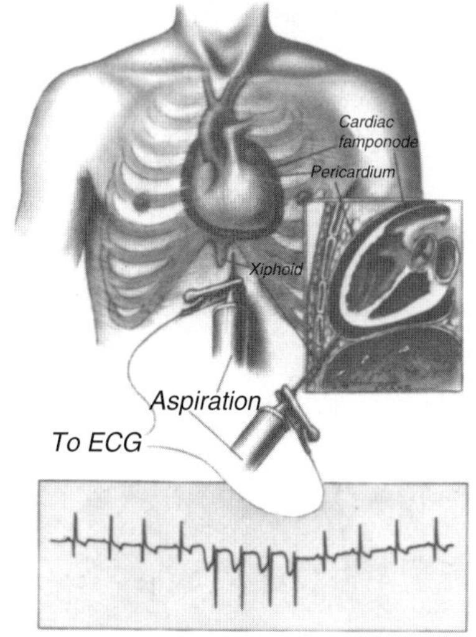

Subxiphoid pericardiocentesis with electrocardiographic monitoring. Note the negative QRS deflection, which indicates myocardial contact. (From Sellke F, Swanson S, del Nido PJ: *Sabiston and Spencer surgery of the chest*, ed 7, Philadelphia, 2004, Saunders.)

Aortic Disruption Caused by Trauma

In the first few seconds or minutes after blunt trauma caused by extreme forces, an aortic tear usually takes the person's life. With a partial tear near the **ligamentum arteriosum**, the patient may survive long enough for the condition to be identified and treated if you are suspicious, tenacious, and sometimes lucky. The trick is to identify a contained hematoma in the intimal layer of the aorta. Unexplained, intermittent hypotension may serve as a signal of such an injury, but most signs and symptoms are vague and usually missed. The chest radiograph may show some clues to aortic disruption, such as the following:

- Widened mediastinum
- Obliteration of the aortic knob
- Tracheal deviation to the right
- Left mainstem bronchus depression
- Right mainstem bronchus elevation
- Lack of an aortopulmonary window (i.e., the space between the pulmonary artery and aorta is missing)
- Esophageal deviation to the right (nasogastric [NG] tube moved to the right)
- Left hemothorax
- Presence of a pleural or an apical cap (thickened pleura at the apex)

In a small number of patients (10% to 20%), the chest radiograph may be normal despite aortic disruption.

If the chest radiograph shows a widened mediastinum, most primary physicians transfer the patient for further evaluation in a higher level trauma center with facilities for cardiothoracic surgery. CT scans, angiographic studies, and transesophageal echocardiography may help identify the defect; however, prolonged investigation is not recommended for a patient showing signs of shock.

Diaphragmatic Tears

The diaphragm often is torn in traumatic events, leading to herniation of gastric contents into the chest cavity. As mentioned previously, the diaphragm is described anatomically as having a left leaf and a right leaf. If the tear occurs in the left diaphragm, the stomach and bowel may enter the chest cavity. If it occurs in the right diaphragm, the liver tends to keep the GI contents where they belong, but the injury creates problems for the patient later on.

With a diaphragmatic tear, the patient may show signs of high intrathoracic pressure, including shortness of breath with unilaterally diminished breath sounds (usually on the left). After insertion of a gastric tube, radiographic identification of the tube's lines in the chest cavity is a clear indicator of this phenomenon. (This is yet another reason to insert a gastric tube fairly early in the resuscitation of a trauma patient.) This defect can confuse the assessment of whether the injury is a pneumothorax or a tear in the left leaf of the diaphragm. The appearance of GI contents in a chest drainage system is ominous. A chest radiograph that shows an elevated diaphragm on the left should dictate insertion of a gastric tube and a repeat chest radiograph.

Shock

Shock is the lack of perfusion and oxygen delivery to the cells (oxygen debt). In the cardiovascular system, three components ensure perfusion and oxygen delivery to each cell; in common terms, these can be summed up as pump, pipes, and volume. Any derangement in these components results in shock.

Obstructive Shock

Injuries to the chest that cause a change in pressures can affect cardiac output by reducing preload to the heart. This is obstructive shock, which can be caused by tension pneumothorax and pericardial tamponade, which already have been discussed. Obstructive shock also can be caused by a pulmonary embolus, which is less common in the resuscitation phase of trauma.

Distributive Shock

Distributive shock is caused by damage to sympathetic tracts in the spinal cord. **Neurogenic shock** is classified as a distributive shock because it causes vasodilation in the pump-pipes-volume circulatory system. This unusual presentation of hypotension in a trauma patient usually is accompanied by bradycardia, because loss of the sympathetic tracts allows dominance of the parasympathetic system. Initial fluid resuscitation followed by administration of vasopressors usually helps maintain perfusion.

Septic shock is another type of distributive shock, but it is not usually encountered in the resuscitation phase of trauma management. This type of shock manifests itself in the ICU, sometimes as part of systemic inflammatory response syndrome (SIRS), which occurs secondary to prolonged hypovolemic shock.

Hypovolemic Shock

Volume also can be a factor in the pathophysiology of a shock state. Many types of blunt and penetrating injuries can cause hemorrhagic shock, including thoracic, abdominal, and multiple long-bone fractures and major pelvic disruptions. A normal cardiovascular system has way too much "pipe" in relation to the volume available in a healthy patient; therefore, moving volume throughout the system by means of changes in vessel size and pressure is the key to maintaining a "normal" state. When a volume deficit occurs, the system must react to compensate. The ability to recognize the various shock states, the pathophysiology, and symptoms and a knowledge of how to resuscitate a patient in shock are the keys to good trauma management.

As you have learned, the classic signs and symptoms of shock are:

- Tachycardia
- Tachypnea
- Cool skin
- **Oliguria** (diminishing urinary output)

The release of natural vasoconstricting agents from the suprarenal and renal areas helps shunt blood appropriately (i.e., moves blood to priority tissues), and the quick

Table 7-2 Classification of Hemorrhagic Shock

	Class I	Class II	Class III	Class IV
Amount of blood loss (% total blood volume)	<750 mL (<15%)	750-1500 mL (15% to 30%)	1500-2000 mL (30% to 40%)	>2000 mL (>40%)
Heart rate (beats/min)	Normal or minimally increased	>100	>120	>140
Ventilator rate (breaths/min)	Normal	20-30	30-40	>35
Systolic blood pressure (mm Hg)	Normal	Normal	Decreased	Greatly decreased
Urine output (mL/hour)	Normal	20-30	5-15	Minimal

Modified from the American College of Surgeons, Committee on Trauma: *ATLS advanced trauma life support for doctors*, ed 7, St Louis, 2004, Mosby.

Table 7-3 Approximate Internal Blood Loss Associated with Fractures

Type of Fracture	Internal Blood Loss
Rib	125 mL
Radius or ulna	250-500 mL
Humerus	500-750 mL
Tibia or fibula	500-1000 mL
Femur	1000-2000 mL
Pelvis	1000 mL to massive

National Association of Emergency Medical Technicians (NAEMT): *NAEMT's PHTLS prehospital trauma (PHTLS basic and advanced prehospital trauma life support)*, ed 6, St Louis, 2007, Mosby.

development of anaerobic metabolism at the cellular level leads to the signs and symptoms of hemorrhagic shock. The other signs and symptoms are related to the stage of shock (Tables 7-2 and 7-3).

For effective management of hemorrhagic shock, a thorough but quick assessment must be done to estimate blood loss. The three major sites of blood loss are:

- Long-bone fractures
- Intraabdominal injuries
- Pelvic fractures

After this assessment, the patient's response to volume replacement may help determine whether the shock is due to fractures alone or whether other sites of hemorrhage may exist. For instance, you note humeral and femoral fractures. Administer a fluid bolus of 2000 mL, and the patient's vital signs normalize and are maintained; this should indicate to you that the long-bone fractures may be the only source of bleeding (Table 7-4).

Stopping External Bleeding in Shock

The definitive management of hemorrhagic shock is to *stop the bleeding*. Although this sounds simple, it may mean transporting a patient great distances to an operating room. As a critical care team member, you should perform the initial steps of bleeding identification and control: apply direct pressure to sites of external bleeding, splint long-bone fractures, and place a pelvic binder. Certain types of fracture stabilization, once considered secondary steps in resuscitation, now are considered part of the primary circulatory/perfusion management effort when shock is present.

Allowing blood loss from external wounds to continue is considered poor patient care, especially if you take the time to start an IV line while the wounds bleed. Renewed emphasis is being placed on aggressive management of external bleeding. If your initial management steps fail (pressure dressings, direct pressure), a tourniquet should be applied. No research actually supports the use of pressure points and extremity elevation to control bleeding. Controlling bleeding is extremely important, and although their use is controversial, tourniquets are the next logical step if direct pressure fails. The use of topical **hemostatic** agents has yet to be researched in nonmilitary settings and is secondary to direct pressure.

Stopping the Bleeding with an Open Book Pelvic Fracture

To assess for pelvic injury, first look for deformities of the legs and their positioning. Often these patients persistently keep their legs apart, and they complain of pain when the legs are abducted. When palpating, avoid excessive manipulation of the pelvis. The preferred assessment involves pushing gently on the iliac crests, toward the midline. Once a fracture has been identified, do not perform repeat examinations, which may cause more bleeding.

If an open book pelvic fracture is identified, leaking vessels posteriorly can cause massive loss of blood into a now open pelvis with little tamponade effect. Application of a pelvic binder can stabilize the pelvis, "closing" the open book, and help tamponade the bleeding. As an alternative to a manufactured binder, a thick sheet, such as a draw sheet, can be used. The sheet is placed under the patient and cinched, and surgical clamps are used to secure it. No matter which pelvic binding technique is used, before the procedure a Foley catheter should be inserted if there are no contraindications. Blood at the urethral meatus, one of the contraindications to insertion of a urinary catheter, may be a sign of a significant genitourinary system injury, which can occur with open book pelvic factures. Skill 7-4 presents the steps in the application of a pelvic binder.

Table 7-4 Responses to Initial Fluid Resuscitation*

Parameter	Rapid Response	Transient Response	No Response
Vital signs	Return to normal	Transient improvement, recurrence of decreased BP and increased HR	Remain abnormal
Estimated blood loss	Minimal (10% to 20%)	Moderate and ongoing (20% to 40%)	Severe (>40%)
Need for more crystalloid	Low	High	High
Need for blood	Low	Intermediate to high	Intermediate
Blood preparation	Type and cross-match	Type specific	Emergency blood release
Need for surgery	Possible	Likely	Highly likely
Need for early presence of surgeon	Yes	Yes	Yes

From the American College of Surgeons, Committee on Trauma: *ATLS advanced trauma life support for doctors,* ed 7, St Louis, 2004, Mosby.
BP, Blood pressure; *HR,* heart rate.
*In adults, give 2000 mL of Ringer's lactate solution (RLS); for children, give a bolus of 20 mL/kg RLS.

Skill 7-4

APPLICATION OF A PELVIC BINDER

PROCEDURE

1. Confirm radiographically that the patient has an open book pelvic fracture. Consult the receiving hospital or follow the trauma transfer arrangements made with the orthopedic surgeons at the level I trauma facility.
2. Adduct and internally rotate the patient's legs. Place the binder beneath the pelvis, including the trochanters within the garment. Use the pubis as the reference point for the middle of the garment anteriorly.
3. If the binder is too large, cut off the excess (following the manufacturer's recommendations). Then cinch the garment to "close the book" and secure it.

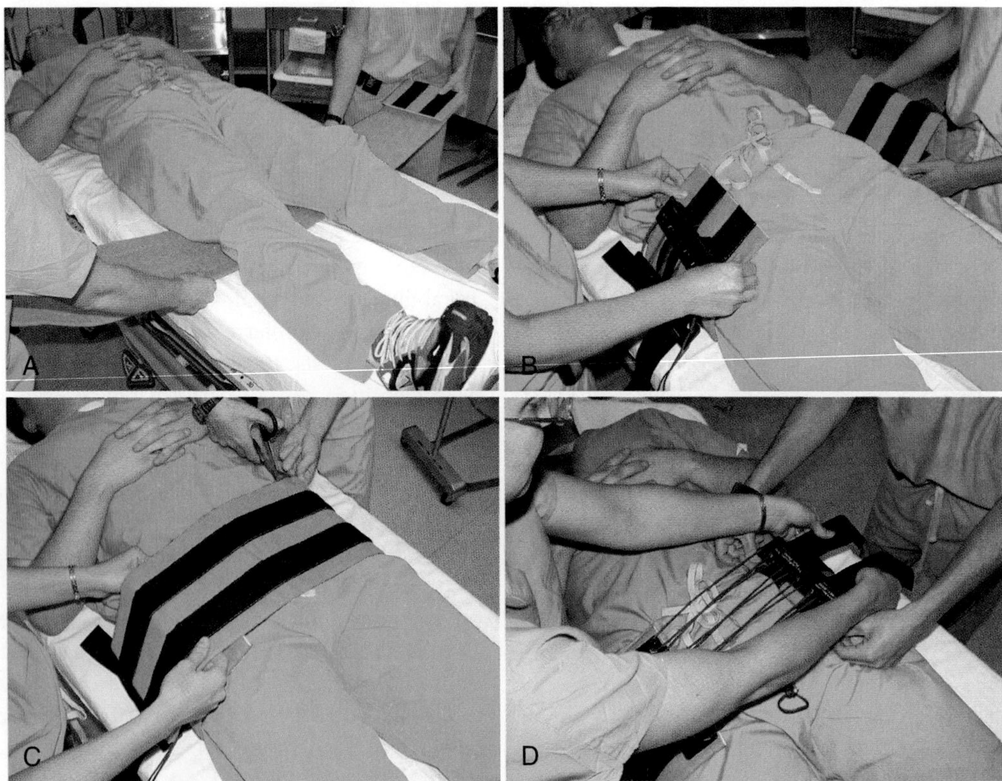

(Courtesy the University of Iowa Hospitals and Clinics, Iowa City, Iowa.)

Treatment of Hemorrhagic Shock

Resuscitation of hemorrhagic shock also includes the replacement of fluids. Resuscitation of blood loss by administration of blood products is best for the patient. Whenever possible, the critical care transport team should obtain the appropriate blood products from the transporting facility for transfusion during the trip. When blood products are not available, volume replacement with crystalloids can serve as a temporary measure. With an isotonic crystalloid solution, about one third of the product remains in the intravascular space for about 1 hour after infusion. Although NS can be used, LR has become the preferred solution for this type of volume replacement because it is buffered, and administration of large amounts of saline can cause hyperchloremic metabolic acidosis. In fact, a combination of LR with blood products has been shown to be better than blood alone.

Did You Know?

A patient who is in shock or who has a spinal cord injury should be packaged into a supine position. The Trendelenburg position, the old shock position, can inhibit good ventilations and increase intracranial pressure, and it does not improve blood flow.

Recent trauma research on the shock state and its current therapy has resulted in the introduction of new ideas about this age-old disease. It must be noted that controversy exists in hemorrhagic shock management regarding whether *any* fluids should be infused. Some studies show that if fluids are administered before bleeding is controlled surgically, the protective compensatory mechanisms of the body are disrupted, especially with penetrating injuries to the trunk. Some advocate fluid resuscitation only after surgery. Others contend that the best plan is to allow some fluid therapy, with strict controls, and to keep the patient hypotensive (permissive hypotension) throughout. Local protocol also may distinguish between penetrating trauma and blunt trauma in the decision on infusion of IV fluids.

Colloid solutions (albumin, dextran, Hespan) are an alternative to crystalloids in the resuscitation of hemorrhagic shock. However, the use of colloids poses the risk of an allergic reaction; also, they are expensive, and currently no end-outcome evidence shows them to have an advantage over other therapeutic methods.

Blood substitutes are another alternative to blood products. **Perfluorocarbons (PFCs)** carry 50 times more oxygen than blood. However, their role in resuscitation is undetermined because of technical and logistic problems in their manufacture. **Hemoglobin-based oxygen carriers (HBOCs)** may show promise in the future, but as yet they cannot be used by transport teams because most recent versions require refrigeration. **Recombinant Factor VIIa** has been used in patients with massive blood loss with limited success. Factor VIIa, a natural part of the clotting cascade, usually is used to treat patients with Alexander's disease. This product has shown potential for reducing blood loss, but further studies are needed.

Did You Know?

Because type O– blood is in short supply, blood banks now recommend the use of type O+ blood in males and other individuals who will never become pregnant. O– blood is used in females of childbearing age so that the Rh antigen (positive) is not introduced into a woman who may encounter the antigen again through pregnancy, which results in an immune response and fetal demise.

Ongoing Assessment and Management of Shock

The longer a patient in hemorrhagic shock is allowed to remain hypoperfused, the greater the oxygen debt. The tissues require oxygen, and a deficit builds; this is reflected in laboratory studies in the serum lactate and base deficit levels. Elevated lactate levels indicate continued hypoperfusion; a decreasing pH with metabolic acidosis indicates a base deficit and shock.

The body tries desperately to save itself when massive hemorrhage occurs. It makes and dissolves clots repeatedly in an attempt to stop the bleeding. **Coagulopathy** is a rare but devastating complication in a patient with multisystem trauma. Massive fluid resuscitation, along with transfusion of blood products, dilutes the clotting factors and platelets and increases the risk of this deadly complication. Be alert to the patient's PT/INR and partial thromboplastin time (PTT) and the platelet and fibrinogen levels, especially when a massive transfusion protocol has been implemented. The risk of coagulopathy is compounded if the patient takes medications that affect clotting, such as warfarin and aspirin.

In severely injured patients, the triad of hypothermia, acidosis, and coagulopathy indicates a poor prognosis and often leads to death in trauma patients. Therefore, measures should be taken to prevent these conditions:

- *Prevention of hypothermia:* Keep the patient warm. Take special care to ensure that the patient is packaged appropriately for transfer in the elements. Prevent heat loss by covering the head when feasible. Administer warmed IV fluids if possible.
- *Prevention of acidosis:* Stop what bleeding you can and resuscitate with blood products to transport oxygen to cells with oxygen deficit.
- *Prevention of coagulopathy:* Monitor and resuscitate the clotting factors with appropriate blood products, which may include cryoprecipitate, fresh frozen plasma, or both.

Ideally, through the coordinated efforts of healthcare providers, a trauma patient arrives at the ICU **euthermic,**

euvolemic, and with a normal pH and INR and minimal edema.

Head and Spinal Cord Injuries

Head Injury

The cranium essentially has three components: brain tissue, cerebrospinal fluid (CSF), and blood. The brain regulates its own pressure, and dilation or constriction of vessels and control of the amount of CSF are elements of this autoregulation. When injury results in an expanding mass (**focal brain injury**) or generalized edema (**diffuse brain injury**) or both, the brain attempts to shift blood or CSF by increasing the respiratory drive and raising the blood pressure. However, this process has limitations; blood is easily shifted, and CSF is allowed to expand around the brain and in the ventricles, but the brain itself has no room to give.

As noted in Chapter 5, perfusion of the brain is essential. Perfusion of the brain is reflected in the cerebral perfusion pressure (CPP). To perfuse the brain, the body must provide a minimum arterial blood pressure (mean arterial pressure [MAP]) and maintain pressure within the system (intracranial pressure [ICP]). The autoregulation of the brain is reflected in this formula: MAP – ICP = CPP. When the pressure within the brain increases, the blood pressure also must increase, or perfusion of the brain is altered.

Recognizing that an injury to the brain may affect autoregulation is important. Good patient care involves helping the brain regulate itself through resuscitation efforts as the patient is transported to a neurosurgeon for definitive treatment. Whether the patient has a focal or diffuse brain injury, a neurologic assessment must be performed at your first encounter and frequently throughout transport. Although it is not the only assessment performed, the Glasgow Coma Scale (Box 7-1) is the recognized standard for determining the level of consciousness. This three-section assessment helps provide a universal system for describing consciousness (instead of using terms such as "lethargic" or "semiconscious"). The patient's best eye opening and verbal and motor responses are assessed. If the patient has been intubated, a T is recorded to indicate that the patient, even if conscious, is unable to speak.

The size, shape, and reactivity of the pupils also should be assessed. A unilateral change in pupil size and reactivity usually indicates compression of cranial nerve III (the oculomotor nerve) as a result of impending **herniation** of the brain.

Some diffuse brain injuries, such as concussion and diffuse axonal injury, can cause secondary edema in the brain, leading to increased ICP. Focal injuries include epidural and subdural hematomas, cerebral contusion, and intracerebral hemorrhage. Because focal injuries may include expanding masses that shift the brain, lateralizing (one-sided) neurologic signs may be present.

Early signs of increasing ICP include:

- Headache
- Altered level of consciousness
- Amnesia about events surrounding the injury
- Nausea and vomiting

Box 7-1 Glasgow Coma Scale

Parameter	Score
Eye Opening	
Spontaneously	4
Open in response to voice	3
Open in response to pain	2
Do not open	1
Verbal Response	
Oriented to time, place, and person	5
Confused but speaks	4
Incomprehensive, inappropriate words	3
Incomprehensible sounds, no words	2
Does not speak	1
Motor Response	
Obeys commands	6
Localizes painful stimuli	5
Withdraws from painful stimuli	4
Posturing with flexion	3
Posturing with extension	2
No movement	1
Total Points	
Severe head injury	≤8
Moderate head injury	9-12
Minor head injury	13-15

Late signs of increased ICP include:

- Dilated, nonreactive pupils (unilateral presentation is a lateralizing sign)
- Lack of eye opening to voice and pain
- Abnormal posturing to stimuli (flexion or extension)
- Elevated blood pressure
- Changes in the respiratory pattern
- Bradycardia

Cushing's triad is a set of three signs and symptoms that indicate impending herniation of the brain:

- Elevated systolic BP (widening pulse pressure [systolic-diastolic BP])
- Bradycardia
- Irregular respirations

The development of Cushing's triad, which may be accompanied by unilateral pupil dilation, indicates that the brain's attempts to autoregulate (i.e., compensate through changes in vessel size and the movement of CSF) have failed; now the brain physically has to give. Once the brain begins to push its way into the foramen magnum, brain death is imminent.

Management of a Brain Injury

Observing for and appropriately treating increased ICP are important; however, aggressive resuscitation of hypovolemic shock to maintain the CPP is even more important. Hypovolemia by itself is harmful; in combination with head trauma, it is worse. Although you should take care not to overload an edematous brain with IV fluids, allowing a low MAP causes secondary brain injury. Say, for instance, that a patient has a BP of 100/70 mm Hg (and therefore an MAP of 80 mm Hg). This seems perfect, *except* when the patient has a head injury and the ICP is 20 mm Hg. This seemingly excellent BP actually indicates that the brain is being poorly perfused. According to the formula MAP – ICP = CPP (80 – 20 = 60), the CPP is only 60 mm Hg; a normal CPP is about 80 mm Hg. The ICP is rarely monitored in the early resuscitative phase of trauma. It can be estimated based on the patient's neurologic status (i.e., the GCS score). The point is, a combination of hypoperfusion and increased ICP is not good.

In trauma resuscitation, **normocarbia** (normal partial pressure of arterial carbon dioxide [$Paco_2$]) is the goal. During autoregulation, the brain attempts to increase the respiratory minute volume to drive down the level of carbon dioxide (CO_2), which results in less blood flow in the brain. Attempts by rescuers to do this, in their efforts to help the brain, usually cause harm. Rescuers should perform hyperventilation (a $Paco_2$ of 25 to 30 mm Hg) only when Cushing's syndrome is present *and* only after consultation with a neurosurgeon. Hyperventilation is accomplished during critical care transport by increasing the rate by 5 breaths/min until the patient's neurologic condition improves. It must be guided by continuous monitoring of the $PETco_2$, which should not be allowed to fall below 30 mm Hg.

Mannitol, occasionally in combination with furosemide, is used to help the brain regulate pressures. Barbiturates and anticonvulsants often are administered prophylactically, because onset of a seizure automatically causes secondary brain injury. The receiving neurosurgeon should be consulted before these drugs are administered.

Prevention, early recognition, and prompt treatment of hypoxia are the keys to preventing secondary brain injury (see Chapter 5).

Vertebral and Spinal Cord Injury

Remember that A(C)BCD was the stated plan for your initial assessment and management. If you have followed this plan, your patient should already be positioned flat and supine on a long board with the head and neck in line and with straps providing immobilization. This positioning and immobilization must be maintained until spinal injury has been ruled out (Box 7-2). If you are transporting the patient to another trauma care facility, the patient usually has distracting injuries that require the transfer. That fact alone should convince you to keep the patient immobilized.

Restless, confused, and agitated patients may require sedatives and paralytics, along with intubation, to help ensure safe immobilization—however, *remember that hypoxia and head injury also can cause these symptoms.*

Management of Spinal Cord Injury

Many facilities immediately remove the long board when the patient is brought into the resuscitation room. This helps prevent pressure sores on the skin, which can have grave consequences for a patient with multisystem trauma who must spend time in the ICU. The long board is considered a transport mechanism for trauma patients and is not generally used while the patient is in the ED or ICU. Therefore, if protocols dictate, place the patient back into complete immobilization before transport in the early phase of care.

Spinal injury is suspected with radiographic evidence of vertebral injuries and neurologic deficits of the spinal tract. Management of these patients generally includes keeping the patient warm, immobilization, pain control, aggressive airway management (with insertion of a gastric tube and attachment to intermittent suction), and prevention of pressure sores.

You should know the difference between **spinal shock**, a variable state of paralysis after spinal cord injury, and neurogenic shock, mentioned earlier, which is a distributive type of shock in which the sympathetic tracts are impaired. Anticipating the presence of neurogenic shock in patients with injuries of the cervical spine (C-spine) and with some injuries of the thoracic spine (T-spine) can aid early recognition and management. Signs of neurogenic shock in a patient with a spinal injury include warm skin, hypotension, and bradycardia (or failure to become tachycardic in hypovolemia).

Resuscitation with crystalloid fluids must be done cautiously in neurogenic shock. If hypovolemia is not present, overloading this patient with fluids may lead to overhydration and pulmonary edema. The massive vasodilation seen with this phenomenon warrants judicious infusion of a vasoconstricting medication, such as phenylephrine, epinephrine, norepinephrine, or dopamine.

Anticipation and early recognition of the ventilatory complications of high spinal cord injuries also are important. Paralysis of the intercostal muscles and impairment of innervation from the phrenic nerve (which causes movement of the diaphragm) forces the body to use other (i.e., the abdominal) muscles to pull the chest wall out to create negative pressure. This hypoventilation is not tolerated, and early intubation and ventilation are needed.

Another controversial management issue is the administration of high-dose steroids to a patient who suffered spinal cord injury from blunt trauma. When this therapy was first conceived, it was believed that steroids helped reduce inflammation and prevented secondary injury of the cord tissue. Years of practice and outcome studies are inconclusive, but some spinal cord specialists still use this therapy; consult the accepting clinician. For a nonpenetrating spinal cord injury, within the first 8 hours of the event, methylprednisolone is used as follows:

- An initial dose of 30 mg/kg is given within the first 15 minutes;

Box 7-2 Cervical Spine Radiographs

Many hospitals continue to use cervical spine (C-spine) radiographs as part of their routine trauma examination. However, most experts believe that computed tomography (CT) imaging is much more sensitive for pathologic conditions, especially for C1 and C2 fractures. Some trauma care facilities eliminate the time-consuming (and sometimes pointless) plain radiographs in favor of continued stabilization of the spine for transfer or CT and clinical examination.

Cervical Spine Diagnostics: Statistics to Consider

- Detection rates for C-spine fractures on plain radiographs may be as low as 40% to 47%.
- A cross-table lateral radiograph was read as positive in only 68% of 216 patients who proved to have a C-spine injury. Even in retrospect, only 85% were positive.
- 58% of fractures and 93% of subluxations were visible on radiographs. CT demonstrated 90% of the fractures but only 54% of the subluxations. The combination of radiographs and CT found 98% of fractures and 99% of subluxations.
- 3.2% to 16.7% of patients with one vertebral fracture have another. In one study, the mean delay in detection was 53 days.

Clinical Criteria for Ruling Out a Cervical Spine Fracture

- The patient does not complain of neck pain when asked *and*
- The patient does not have neck pain on palpation of the midline (spinous process) *and*
- The patient does not have any history of loss of consciousness *and*
- The patient does not have any mental status changes caused by trauma, alcohol, drugs, and so on, *and*
- The patient has no symptoms referable to a neck injury, such as paralysis or sensory changes (including transitory symptoms now resolved), *and*
- The patient has no other distracting painful injuries (e.g., fractured ankle, fractured ribs)

Also see the Canadian C-spine rules (CCR) or the National Emergency X-Radiography Utilization Study (NEXUS) Low Risk Criteria (NLC). In addition, a comparison study can be found in the *New England Journal of Medicine.*

The evaluation and clearance of suspected C-spine injuries are considerably different in pediatric trauma patients. For example, 67% of children with cord damage had no radiographic evidence of fracture. Spinal cord injury without radiographic abnormality (SCIWORA) is a well-documented syndrome that must be taken into account in pediatric patients, particularly those under 8 years of age.

The next question, then, is why the transport team would care whether a radiograph of the C-spine was obtained and what results might be seen. Some critical care practitioners prefer to have one cross-table lateral C-spine radiograph during the evaluation of risk when performing the pre–rapid sequence intubation (RSI) assessment to rule out any severe pathologic condition. Others theorize that the provider should just consider that a severe pathologic condition of the cervical spine is present with certain trauma presentations and proceed from there, maintaining in-line C-spine stabilization during intubation.

Another question frequently asked is whether it is acceptable to intubate patients with a cervical fracture. In a study by Scannell and colleagues, neurologic deficits were present before intubation in 20 of 58 patients with unstable fractures. The deficits improved after intubation in 4 of the 20 patients and were unchanged after intubation in the remaining 16 patients. The other 38 patients with unstable C-spine fractures, as well as the 23 patients with stable fractures, showed no neurologic deficits before or after orotracheal intubation. The answer, therefore, is: *Yes, it is OK to intubate!*

Table adapted by Mark A. Graber, MD, Department of Emergency Medicine, the University of Iowa Hospitals and Clinics, Iowa City, Iowa.

- 45 minutes later, 5.4 mg/kg/min is infused over at least 24 hours

In 2005, the recommendation was that the maintenance dose be continued for only 24 hours if it was started within 3 hours of the injury; continued for 48 hours if it was started after the first 3 hours. Current ATLS© (2008), recommendation is simple: there is no evidence that steroids are of benefit in spinal cord injury.

Abdominal Injuries

In the assessment of a patient who has suffered blunt trauma, a quiet abdomen is inconclusive. Early in resuscitation, the examination results may be negative despite vigorous bleeding going on inside.

Remember that in the discussion of hemorrhagic shock, reference was made to observing for the patient's response to volume resuscitation and finding the cause of the bleeding. If the patient is a transient responder or a nonresponder to fluid therapy, intraabdominal bleeding should be suspected.

Penetrating trauma to the abdomen should be evaluated by a surgeon, because most of these injuries involve significant peritoneal damage. With blunt abdominal trauma, diagnostic studies usually should be performed to help determine whether operative intervention is necessary. The FAST examination (mentioned previously in the diagnosis of pericardial injury) includes evaluation of the junction of the liver and kidney, the spleen and kidney, and the pelvis for bleeding. In patients in stable condition, it usually is followed by an abdominal CT scan.

Management focuses on maintaining oxygenation, ventilation, and perfusion and frequent reassessment of the abdomen. Evaluation by a surgeon is crucial. Gastric and urinary catheters are placed early, and the output is monitored.

Burns

Injury to the skin, the largest organ of the body, can be catastrophic and can have lifelong or life-ending' consequences. The healthcare profession has learned much about the treatment and expected complications of burns, and specialized burn centers have been developed to deal exclusively with these injuries.

Your job, as a member of the critical care transport team, is to understand the pathophysiology of a burn, the complications likely to ensue, and the emergency management of the burn patient. In most patients with burns, energy is transmitted into the skin by thermal means (fire or heat or both). Extreme cold, chemicals, electricity, and ionizing radiation also may be mechanisms of injury in burn patients.

A severe burn has local, regional, and systemic effects. The most seriously damaged cells are dead and are clotted off locally. The cells surrounding this area are ischemic and prone to biochemical changes and swelling. Through the cardiovascular system and immune response, the body attempts to increase blood flow to the injured sites wherever possible. If the burn affects more than 20% to 30% of the body surface area (BSA), all systems are affected.

The injury to the capillary beds and the subsequent release of chemicals allow large plasma proteins to move into the tissues. This leakage of plasma from the vessels creates a fluid imbalance between the tissues and the cardiovascular system. Fluid is pulled from the vascular space into the tissues.

Added to the plasma pull of water is the typical immune response that is supposed to occur in a healthy body with this type of crisis. Histamine, prostaglandins, cytokines, leukotrienes, bradykinins, and oxygen free radicals are released, resulting in dilated, leaking vessels and clotting. The combination of regional **hyperemia** around burned tissue, the inflammatory response, and leaking capillaries leads to the following:

- Elevated hematocrit as a result of hemoconcentration (loss of plasma into tissues)
- High blood viscosity (thick blood with high pressures in the tissues)
- Blood cell agitation and destruction with clotting
- Tissue edema
- Intravascular hypovolemia and shock
- Hypermetabolism

The distal tissues are heavy with fluid, which increases the **afterload** compared to the heart's pumping function. If the patient is elderly or has a history of heart disease, the increased afterload may overburden the heart, causing ischemic events and cardiac failure.

Inhalation Injury

The inhalation of toxic substances and heat is the first concern in the assessment and management of a burn patient. Heat from the burning environment usually travels as far as the glottis. The chemical byproducts from burning furnishings create a lethal gas mixture that is toxic to the body's cells. The final insult to the respiratory system occurs minutes to hours later, when significant swelling narrows airways, causes atelectasis, and sets up the patient for ARDS or acute lung injury (ALI). Signs of inhalation injury include:

- Facial and neck burns
- Singed facial and nose hair
- Carbon deposits in the oropharynx or nasopharynx (or both) and sputum
- Hoarseness
- History of the event that includes disorientation in an enclosed burning environment
- Explosion that causes burns to the head and torso

Airway and ventilation assessment and management must be diligent and aggressive in the resuscitative phase. In the airway assessment, patency is presumed if the patient can speak. However, if an inhalation injury is possible and because you do not know the patient's normal tone of voice, ask the patient and family members whether the patient is hoarse. Intubate early to prevent airway obstruction from the expected edema. Choose the largest tracheal tube you can insert without causing trauma to the mucous membranes, because the patient may have repeated bronchoscopic examinations in the ICU. Remember that the fluid resuscitation you must begin adds to the tissue edema, which affects all areas of the body, including all airways. A helpful technique is to use the tracheal tube to splint the upper airway open to 8 to 9 mm.

Cyanide exposure often occurs with carbon monoxide (CO) poisoning. Most fire-related deaths are caused by smoke inhalation. CO and hydrogen cyanide are among the byproducts of burning synthetic substances, and both should be considered in the assessment and management of a patient with a thermal injury. Hemoglobin's attraction for CO is 200 times that for oxygen, and cyanide creates a combined toxic effect in which cells are unable to use any oxygen available to the patient. This combination effect sometimes is difficult to differentiate; however, laboratory tests will show metabolic acidosis with high lactate and venous oxygen levels (see the discussion of hyperbaric treatment in Chapter 10 for CO categorization and treatment recommendations). A new approach to the treatment of cyanide toxicity involves the use of hydroxocobalamin, which must be administered very early in the resuscitation of the patient with inhalation injury.

Assessment of the Burn Patient

As with any trauma patient, follow the A(C)BCD plan for the primary resuscitation. When possible obtain a history quickly to learn the circumstances surrounding the burn injury, the patient's past medical history, medications the patient uses, and the patient's immunization status. Assess whether blunt or penetrating trauma has occurred with the thermal burn. Determine the BSA involved using the rule of nines or the Lund and Browder chart or compare the patient's palmar surface (fingers and hand, which constitute 1% of the BSA) to the involved skin.

The depth of the burn is assessed by evaluating the appearance and texture of the skin. A superficial (first degree) burn appears red and painful but does not have blisters. A partial-thickness (second degree) burn appears red or mottled and shows swelling and blisters. Ruptured blisters may appear weeping or wet and are painful, especially when exposed to air currents. A full-thickness (third degree) burn appears dark, translucent, mottled, or waxy white and has a leathery feel to the rescuer's gloved hand. The skin does not blanch with pressure. When palpating severely burned skin with a gloved hand, sweep across it to see whether body hair comes off on the glove; if so, the injury is a full-thickness burn.

The location of serious burns adds to the patient's risk for complications. Determine whether the hands, feet, face, or genitalia are involved. **Circumferential burns** to the extremity or torso significantly increase the risk of complications.

Management of Burn Injuries

The first principle of burn management is "put out the fire"; this is a reminder that all clothing and jewelry must be removed from the patient's entire body. In the often chaotic resuscitation effort in a local ED, clothing may be cut off, but it sometimes is pushed to the side and may remain smoldering beneath the patient. Fluid resuscitation creates massive peripheral edema, and any jewelry still on the patient may impede distal blood flow as this develops.

Vascular access is important, even if it must be achieved through burned tissue as the last resort. A gastric tube and Foley catheter must be placed before transport for the reasons explained in the discussion of shock. Perform a rapid assessment for the percentage of BSA involved, determine the patient's weight, and begin fluid resuscitation. BP monitoring devices may have to be applied creatively, following the standard principles of application and proper fit (the cuff must fit two thirds of the extremity section).

At least three formulas have been recognized for calculating fluid replacement in burn resuscitation; these are the Parkland, Brooke, and modified Brooke formulas. All of these formulas are an estimate if a thermal injury is more than 20% partial thickness or full thickness. The standard 2 to 4 mL/BSA/kg is calculated, and one half is given over the first 8 hours *starting at the time of the injury*. Adults usually receive the 4 mL/BSA/kg dose; children may receive 2 mL/BSA/kg. If no fluids have been started when you arrive for the transfer, you must calculate the time of injury into the adjusted 8-hour calculation. Do not administer this 8-hour dose faster than prescribed. It must be spread out evenly, depending on output and the patient's clinical condition. As mentioned earlier, a burn injury causes a tremendous increase in afterload, and rapid administration of a large fluid bolus can be dangerous, especially in patients with vascular or heart disease.

Ongoing evaluation of the patient for the response to the fluid dose is vital. Just as in hemorrhagic shock, monitoring of the heart rate, urinary output, and general condition guide the rate and volume of fluid administration.

Pain management also plays a major role in initial and ongoing treatment. The patient's **hyperdynamic** state (tachycardia, tachypnea, and elevated BP with restlessness) may occur as a result of the immune response, but pain also causes these symptoms. Monitor for hypercapnia, hypoxia, and respiratory effort as you decide which analgesic to give the patient.

Another pain management technique, which may also help prevent infection, is appropriate wound care. Dry, clean or sterile cloth or plastic wrap should be placed directly over the burns once all clothing and jewelry have been removed.

Partial-thickness and full-thickness burns that encircle an extremity or a body area develop into a thick, leathery tourniquet when swelling begins. Distal perfusion may be impaired, and if the entire thorax is involved, ventilation is impaired. If this type of injury is found with hypoventilation or poor distal blood flow, the clinician may need to perform an **escharotomy.** Escharotomies are rarely required within the first 6 hours of a burn, but the transport team must be diligent in watching for early signs of poor circulation and ventilation.

Electrical Burns

The body acts as a conductor of electricity, allowing the transfer of heat from the inside out. This makes electrical burns difficult to assess for BSA involvement even though deep tissue injury may be quite severe. What may look normal on the surface may contain necrotic muscle. To prevent renal failure as a result of **rhabdomyolysis**, the team should provide fluid resuscitation to maintain urinary output at a minimum of 0.5 mL/kg/hour in adults (1 mL/kg/hour in children and 2 mL/kg/hour in infants). If the urine retains the unusual dark red color of the hemochromogens (the byproduct of muscle destruction) despite adequate fluids, mannitol may be administered to help pull the fluids out of the tissues and through the kidney. The key is to "water down" the **myoglobin** in the urine with crystalloid IV fluids, which allows the kidney to filter the myoglobin out of the body without damage.

Chemical Burns

With chemical burns, meticulous care must be taken to remove all traces of the agent before the patient is placed in an enclosed environment of any kind. Remember, this includes removing all clothing and jewelry. Follow standard protocols for diluting or cleansing chemicals from the body.

Scenario Conclusion

The critically injured trauma patient has tolerated the transport to the level I trauma care facility fairly well so far. At 90 minutes after your first encounter, his temperature is 36.8° C (98° F), the BP is 100/60 mm Hg (the MAP is 73 mm Hg), the pulse is 100 beats/min, the respiratory rate is 10 breaths/min via ventilator, and you have normalized the $PETCO_2$ to 38 mm Hg. You have given a total of 5 L of crystalloid, and the urinary output is 250 mL. The pleural drainage system shows 500 mL of bloody output. The patient's pupils remain equal and reactive. Upon arrival at the trauma resource hospital, the patient's lactate level is 3.2 mmol/L, and blood gases show a base deficit continuing at –6. The patient is quickly evaluated, a focused abdominal sonography in trauma (FAST) examination and CT scans are completed, and the patient is taken to the interventional radiology department for management of the retroperitoneal vessels injured by the pelvic fracture.

SUMMARY

Your plan for the initial assessment and resuscitation of a trauma patient is A(C)BCD: airway, C-spine, breathing, circulation, and disability. Assessment and resuscitation are performed simultaneously, and airway assessment and management include evaluation of any devices in use.

The first C in the plan, the evaluation and management of possible C-spine (and all vertebral) injuries, requires thoughtful consideration of how to package the patient for safe transfer. The breathing assessment includes evaluation for injuries that affect ventilation and oxygenation (including the possibility of toxic gases from fires), the pericardial sac, and diaphragm, and evaluation of any pleural drainage systems.

Management of the circulation in the initial phase includes finding the cause of poor perfusion, if present, and initiating resuscitation. Shock may arise from pump, pipes, or volume failure. External bleeding must be controlled, and an ongoing assessment of the patient's response to resuscitation must be performed and the plan amended based on those findings. This phase also includes the insertion of tubes (gastric and urinary), splinting of fractures, and observing for the response to LRS and blood product resuscitation.

The disability component involves evaluation and resuscitation of the central nervous system, including recognizing and initiating management of injuries that may affect the cerebral perfusion pressure or spinal cord function.

KEY TERMS

adhesions Fibrous bands or structures that cause parts to adhere abnormally.

afterload In cardiac physiology, the force against which cardiac muscle shortens. In isolated muscle, it is the force resisting shortening after the muscle has been stimulated to contract. In the intact heart, it is the pressure against which the ventricle ejects blood, as measured by the stress acting on the ventricular wall after the onset of contraction; it is determined largely by peripheral vascular resistance and by the physical characteristics and blood volume of the arterial system.

autotransfusion Reinfusion of blood or blood products derived from the patient's own circulation; also called *autologous transfusion*. The collection, processing, and reinfusion of blood shed from the chest after traumatic hemothorax.

barotrauma An injury caused by pressure, especially to enclosed cavities of the body, such as the lung. Also, trauma to the lung as a result of pressure changes, an injury often seen in divers; it usually is characterized by peribronchial rupture and pneumomediastinum.

Beck's triad The three symptoms characteristic of cardiac compression caused by pericardial tamponade: jugular venous distention (JVD), hypotension, and muffled heart tones.

blebs Large blisters. An *emphysematous bleb* is any space in a distended area of an emphysematous lung; these blebs vary in size, from tiny (1 cm) to involvement of most of the hemithorax. Also called *bullae.*

capnography Monitoring of the concentration of exhaled carbon dioxide. Capnography is used to assess the physiologic status of patients with acute respiratory problems and those receiving mechanical ventilation and also to determine the adequacy of ventilation in anesthetized patients.

circumferential burns Burns that encircle an area.

coagulopathy Any disorder of blood coagulation. The term may refer to diffuse intravascular coagulation or disseminated intravascular coagulation; also referred to as a *bleeding disorder.*

colloid solutions Glutinous or resembling glue; Solutions composed of infinitesimal insoluble particles (usually 1 to 1000 nm in diameter) that are uniformly dispersed or suspended in a finely divided state throughout a continuous dispersion medium and that do not settle readily; .

Cushing's triad A set of three signs and symptoms of impending herniation of the brain; These symptoms include bradycardia, systolic hypertension, and widening pulse pressure.

diffuse brain injury Injury spread throughout the brain, such as diffuse axonal injury.

echocardiogram A graphic recording of the position and motion of the heart's walls or the internal structures of the heart and neighboring tissue that is produced by the echo obtained from beams of ultrasonic waves directed through the chest wall.

empyema A pleural effusion containing pus; also called *thoracic empyema, purulent* or *suppurative pleurisy,* and *pyothorax;* an abscess.

escharotomy. Surgical incision of the constricting eschar of the circumferentially burned limb in order to permit the cut edges to separate and restore blood flow to unburned tissue distal to the eschar. This can also be performed on the chest wall to allow for normal chest excursion.

euthermic Having a normal temperature; another term for normothermic.

euvolemic Having a normal water volume; another term form normovolemic.

focal brain injury A brain injury that occurs in a specific location, such as an epidural hematoma.

hemoglobin-based oxygen carriers (HBOCs) A blood substitute, made of human or bovine hemoglobin, that is manufactured without a cell membrane; removal of the antigen from HBOCs eliminates the need for a specific blood type. .

hemostatic A descriptive term for an agent that arrests the flow of blood.

herniation Abnormal protrusion of an organ or other body structure through a defect or natural opening in a covering membrane, muscle, or bone.

hydrothorax A pleural effusion containing serous fluid.

hyperdynamic A state in which the body shows signs of hyperactivity; it is marked by elevated vital signs.

hyperemia an increase of blood in a part; also called engorgement.

international normalized ratio (INR) A laboratory value developed by the World Health Organization in 1982 to standardize prothrombin time (PT) results among clinical laboratories. It is used to guide anticoagulation therapy with warfarin.

Kussmaul's sign Distention of the jugular veins during inhalation, as is seen in constrictive pericarditis and mediastinal tumor; also called *paradoxical pulse.*

ligamentum arteriosum A short, thick, strong, fibromuscular cord that extends from the pulmonary artery to the arch of the aorta; it is the remains of the ductus arteriosus. Also called the *ligament of Botallo.*

myoglobin The oxygen-transporting pigment of muscle. It is a type of hemoprotein that resembles a single subunit of hemoglobin, composed of one globin polypeptide chain and one heme group (containing one iron atom). It combines with oxygen released by erythrocytes, stores it, and transports it to the mitochondria of muscle cells, where it generates energy by combustion of glucose, producing carbon dioxide and water.

neurogenic shock A condition of profound hemodynamic and metabolic disturbance, the result of inadequate vasomotor tone, that is characterized by failure of the circulatory system to maintain adequate perfusion of vital organs.

nonthrombogenic A descriptive term indicating that an agent or item has properties that help prevent the formation of a thrombus, or blood clot.

normocarbia Normal partial pressure of arterial carbon dioxide ($Paco_2$).

oliguria The condition of diminishing urinary output.

open book pelvic fracture An anterior-posterior compression fracture that includes the pelvic ring and occurs in about 15% of pelvic injuries. It is called an "open book" fracture, because the symphysis is separated and the volume of the pelvis is greatly increased.

paralytic A pharmaceutical agent that produces paralysis, which often is induced to allow endotracheal intubation.

perfluorocarbons (PFCs) Synthetic compounds that have been proposed as a blood substitute; they have a high oxygen solubility compared with blood products and are free of biologic materials. These agents remain under study.

pericardiocentesis Surgical puncture of the pericardial cavity for the aspiration of fluid.

periosteum A specialized connective tissue that covers all bones of the body and has bone-forming capabilities. In adults, it consists of two layers that are not sharply defined; the external layer is a network of dense connective tissue containing blood vessels, and the deep layer is composed of more loosely arranged collagenous bundles with spindle-shaped connective tissue cells and a network of thin elastic fibers.

quiet tachypnea A rapid rate of breathing without the use of accessory muscles.

radiopaque Not penetrable by x-rays or other forms of radiant energy; radiopaque areas appear light or white on the exposed film.

recombinant factor VIIa A manufactured form of Factor VII produced by genetic recombination. Factor VII (proconvertin), which is heat and storage stable, participates in the extrinsic pathway of coagulation. It is activated by contact with calcium, and in concert with Factor III, it activates Factor X. Deficiency of Factor VII results in a hemorrhagic tendency.

rhabdomyolysis A condition marked by disintegration or dissolution of muscle; it is associated with the excretion of myoglobin in the urine.

septic shock See *neurogenic shock.*

spinal shock A variable state of paralysis after a spinal cord injury.

thoracostomy The surgical creation of an opening in the chest wall to allow drainage. In tube thoracostomy, a chest tube is inserted to remove fluid and air from the pleural space. Needle thoracostomy is performed to remove air from the pleural space.

REFERENCES

1. Orebaugh S: *Atlas of airway management: techniques and tools*, Philadelphia, 2006, Lippincott Williams & Wilkins.

Bibliography

American College of Surgeons, Committee on Trauma: *Advanced trauma life support for doctors, student course manual (ATLS)*, Chicago, 1996, American College of Surgeons.

American College of Surgeons, Committee on Trauma: *ATLS advanced trauma life support for doctors*, ed 7, St Louis, 2004, Mosby.

Argall J, Teece S: Factor VIIA for intractable blood loss in trauma. *Best BETs* (online), November 11, 2002. www.bestbets.org/bets/bet.php?id=371. Accessed May 5, 2010.

Dorland NW: *Dorland's illustrated medical dictionary*, ed 31, Philadelphia, 2007, Saunders.

Graber MA: *C-spine essentials*, Iowa City, 1998, The University of Iowa Hospitals and Clinics.

Hoffman JR, Schriger DL, Mower W, et al: Low-risk criteria for cervical spine radiography in blunt trauma: a prospective study, *Ann Emerg Med* 21:1454-1460, 1992.

Holcomb JB, Jenkins D, Rhee P, et al: Damage control resuscitation: directly addressing the early coagulopathy of trauma, *J Trauma* 62:307-310, 2007.

Howes DW, Stratford A, Stirling M, et al: Administration of recombinant Factor VIIa decreases blood loss after blunt trauma in noncoagulopathic pigs, *J Trauma* 62:311-315, 2007.

Keenen TL, Antony J, Benson DR: Noncontiguous spinal fractures, *J Trauma* 30:489-491 1990.

Kenet G, Walden R, Eldad A, et al: Treatment of traumatic bleeding with recombinant Factor VIIa, *Lancet* 354:1879, 1999.

Kirshenbaum KJ, Nadimpali SR, Fantus R, Cavallino, RP: Unsuspected upper cervical spine fractures associated with significant head trauma: role of CT, *J Emerg Med* 8:183-198, 1990.

National Association of Emergency Medical Technicians (NAEMT): *NAEMT's PHTLS prehospital trauma (PHTLS basic and advanced prehospital trauma life support)*, ed 6, St Louis, 2007, Mosby.

Pang D, Pollack IF: Spinal cord injury without radiographic abnormality in children: the SCIWORA syndrome, *J Trauma* 29:654-664, 1989.

Rotondo MF, McGonigal MD, Schwab CW, et al: Urgent paralysis and intubation of trauma patients: Is it safe? *J Trauma* 34:242-246, 1993.

Scannell G, Waxman K, Tominaga G, et al: Orotracheal intubation in trauma patients with cervical fractures, *Arch Surg* 128:903-905, 1993.

Woodring JH, Lee C: Limitations of cervical radiography in the evaluation of acute cervical trauma, *J Trauma* 34:32-39, 1993.

Woodring JH, Lee C: The role and limitations of computed tomographic scanning in the evaluation of cervical trauma, *J Trauma* 33:698-708, 1992.

REVIEW QUESTIONS

1. In the chapter scenario, the local physician said he "cleared the C-spine." The transport team placed the patient back into immobilization because:
   A. The safest practice is to immobilize the patient completely.
   B. The local trauma care should always be questioned.
   C. The patient has distracting injuries and cannot speak.
   D. The pelvic fracture can be immobilized only with a long board.
2. In the chapter scenario, the patient had identified arm and pelvic fractures. After 2 L of normal saline (NS) had been administered, why did the crew infuse 1 L of lactated Ringer's solution (LR)?
   A. The patient's blood pressure should be much higher.
   B. Three liters of fluid are always given.
   C. LR is a better resuscitation fluid in hemorrhagic shock.
   D. The patient needed warming.
3. In the chapter scenario, if hemorrhagic shock continues after you administer another liter of crystalloids, what treatment should be added?
   A. Administration of blood products: type O+ would be allowed.
   B. Administration of blood products: type O– must be given.
   C. Administration of more NS: probably 1 to 2 L.
   D. Administration of more LR: at least 2 L.
4. In the chapter scenario, what condition does the patient have?
   A. Respiratory acidosis as a result of overventilation
   B. Metabolic acidosis as a result of continued shock
   C. Overhydration as a result of administration of resuscitation fluids
   D. Metabolic acidosis as a result of the use of NS
5. What treatment is necessary for the condition in question 4?
   A. Reduce the rate on the ventilator
   B. Resuscitate the shock and transport the patient to a surgeon
   C. Stop all fluid resuscitation and give a diuretic
   D. Switch the fluids to a solution containing dextrose
6. Your trauma patient has a 20% pneumothorax, and the hospital is not going to place a chest tube. You are about to transport this patient a long distance by fixed-wing aircraft at approximately 32,000 feet. What complication may develop en route?
   A. Pericardial tamponade
   B. Diaphragmatic hernia
   C. Tension pneumothorax
   D. Distributive shock
7. A patient with multisystem trauma has both head and chest injuries and a unilateral reduction in breath sounds. You are ventilating the patient by the bag-valve method. What complication is likely to result?
   A. Tension pneumothorax
   B. Rising intracranial pressure with herniation
   C. Diaphragmatic hernia
   D. Distributive shock

8. Your patient is pale, and your assessment reveals these findings: pulse, 128 beats/min; respiratory rate, 40 breaths/min; BP, 110/88 mm Hg. The patient is restless and in obvious respiratory distress. He is fully immobilized and has decreased breath sounds bilaterally. What may be causing these symptoms?
   A. Bilateral flail segment with massive pulmonary contusion
   B. Pericardial tamponade
   C. Pneumothorax
   D. Anxiety
9. What treatment may be necessary for the patient in question 8?
   A. Sandbags to the chest wall and positive pressure ventilation
   B. Pericardiocentesis
   C. No treatment necessary
   D. Sedatives and anxiolytics
10. A patient with multisystem trauma who weighs 176 pounds (80 kg) is in full immobilization, is receiving oxygen, and has received 4 L of crystalloids. He is tachycardic and tachypneic and has an occasional drop in BP. His urinary drainage system, inserted 3 hours ago, shows 75 mL of reddish urine. On the pelvic radiograph, the sacroiliac (SI) joint is 5 cm across. What resuscitation is required before transport?
   A. Immobilization of the pelvis
   B. IV infusion of sodium bicarbonate to alkalinize the urine
   C. Urology consultation
   D. Changing of the Foley catheter to eliminate the hematuria
11. You are about to transport a patient burned in a house fire that occurred 2 hours ago. He weighs 220 pounds (100 kg) and has a 40% BSA burn. The IV fluids should run at how many milliliters per hour?
   A. 1000 mL/hour
   B. 1333 mL/hour
   C. 2000 mL/hour
   D. 3000 mL/hour
12. What laboratory tests should be added for the patient in question 11?
   A. Blood gases and carboxyhemoglobin
   B. Carboxyhemoglobin and a cyanide level
   C. Blood gases and a platelet count
   D. Drug and alcohol levels
13. With regard to question 11: After 2 hours of fluid resuscitation, the patient rates his pain at 1 when awakened. However, his heart rate remains tachycardic with quiet tachypnea at 26 beats/min. The urinary output is only 80 mL over 2 hours. What should be done?
   A. Increase the rate of IV fluid administration
   B. Administer meperidine
   C. Alkalinize the urine with mannitol
   D. Sedate the patient with haloperidol
14. You arrive at the side of a trauma patient 90 minutes after a motor vehicle crash. He has known femoral and humeral fractures. He has received 3 L of fluid; his vital signs have normalized, and urinary output is good. About 10 minutes later, he is tachycardic and tachypneic with occasional drops in BP. What type of response is this?
   A. Normal
   B. Transient response to fluid resuscitation
   C. Nonresponder to fluid resuscitation
   D. Terminal stage of shock
15. In the midst of a massive shock resuscitation for a patient with multisystem trauma, you note that all IV sites are bleeding, and bruises that once were small are becoming large hematomas. What complication has begun and what treatment is necessary?
   A. This is the terminal stage of shock; pronounce the patient expired.
   B. The patient is approaching the terminal stage of shock; administer sodium bicarbonate IV.
   C. This is a transfusion reaction; stop the blood administration.
   D. This is a coagulopathy; transfuse platelets, fresh frozen plasma, and Factor VIIa.
16. A patient has been resuscitated from cardiac arrest that occurred secondary to a high-voltage electrical injury. When you arrive, the emergency department (ED) nurse is inserting a urinary catheter, and the urine is reddish-brown. You know that:
   A. This is normal after an electrical injury, and only monitoring is required.
   B. This is normal after an electrical injury, and the urinary catheter should be removed.
   C. This is a sign of myoglobin in the urine. Vascular access should be obtained, and fluid rates should be at least 100 mL/hour to keep the urine yellow.
   D. This is a sign of myoglobin in the urine. Vascular access should be obtained, and fluid rates should be calculated by the modified Brooke formula.

17. A patient with unilaterally decreased breath sounds on the left is pale and tachycardic. When you arrive to transport this patient, the local clinician is inserting a chest tube in the 4-5 intercostal space (ICS), left axillary line. A yellowish fluid is appearing in the chest tube with flecks of brown. What may be happening?
    A. Diaphragmatic tear with entry of the chest tube into the stomach
    B. Hemopneumothorax with an acute infectious process
    C. Inadvertent insertion of the chest tube into the large bowel
    D. Bowel perforation with leakage into the chest
18. What change in the resuscitation plan could have helped prevent the situation described in question 17?
    A. Insertion of a gastric tube, followed by a chest radiograph
    B. Use of a special filter system on the chest tube and pleural drainage system
    C. Turning the patient onto the left side
    D. Use of diagnostic peritoneal lavage or a FAST examination before insertion of the chest tube
19. You have arrived at a midsize hospital to transport a patient who suffered thermal trauma about 12 hours ago to a burn center. He has a 50% partial-thickness and full-thickness burn on his neck, entire chest, abdomen, and upper arms. The patient, who weighs 154 pounds (70 kg), has received a total of 8000 mL of LR. He shows signs of respiratory distress but has no signs of smoke inhalation. His arterial blood gas (ABG) results are: pH, 7.30; partial pressure of arterial carbon dioxide ($Paco_2$), 65 mm Hg; partial pressure of arterial oxygen (Pao_2), 88 mm Hg (12 L on a nonrebreather mask); bicarbonate (HCO_3), 22 mEq/L; base excess (BE), 0. What may be the cause of this problem?
    A. Hypovolemia with continued metabolic acidosis and hyperkalemia
    B. Respiratory failure secondary to tissue swelling around the chest
    C. Respiratory acidosis from cyanide poisoning
    D. Fluid overload with a high afterload
20. What treatment may be necessary for the patient in question 19?
    A. Increase in fluid resuscitation to 20 mL/kg
    B. Escharotomy of the chest
    C. Administration of a cyanide antidote
    D. Decrease in fluid resuscitation and clamping of all IV lines.

CHAPTER 8

Multisystem Organ Dysfunction Syndrome and Systemic Inflammatory Response Syndrome

OBJECTIVES

1. Integrate the pathophysiologic principles and assessment findings to implement a treatment plan for the patient with multiple organ dysfunction.
2. Explain the process of the immune response.
3. Explain the pathophysiology, assessment, and treatment of sepsis.
4. Discuss the precipitating factors that can cause multiple organ dysfunction syndrome (MODS).
5. List assessment findings into the field care plan for a patient with MODS.

Scenario

After responding to a 9-1-1 call for a trauma patient, your ambulance service rapidly transports the patient, a 22-year-old male who has hemorrhagic shock related to pelvis, spleen, and head injuries, to the closest level II trauma center. During the first few hours, the patient is treated with intraabdominal surgery to control bleeding and is intubated to protect his airway. His prognosis for recovery is optimistic at the time he is placed in the surgical intensive care unit (ICU).

As the first 36 hours pass, the patient seems to be recovering. He then begins an unexpected and rapid deterioration. The respiratory therapist is having difficulty oxygenating the patient on the ventilator. The laboratory work indicates signs of renal failure, and the patient has diminishing urinary output.

At 48 hours after the original trauma, the hospital calls your ambulance company and requests a transfer of this patient to the level I trauma center because of respiratory and renal failure that is secondary to trauma and shock. During the bedside report, you ask whether the lungs and kidneys were injured during the primary trauma event. The nurse answers, "no," and you wonder what happened to cause the deterioration. The original event injured his head, spleen, and pelvis, which contributed to the co-existing shock. What caused the lungs and kidneys to fail?

The current healthcare industry has been successful in extending the lives of many patients and in saving the lives of those that formerly would have died from catastrophic surgical and medical conditions. This same industry has been less successful in preventing, recognizing, and managing the complicated immune response of the patient's body during these life-extending, life-saving endeavors. The nervous, immune, and endocrine systems initiate a series of interrelated responses during a crisis and subsequent resuscitation efforts. These responses are designed as a defense mechanism but can become quite offensive to the body when they create further tissue damage and destruction.

Sepsis is a major healthcare problem worldwide. Severe sepsis is the eleventh most common cause of death in the United States; mortality ranges from 28% to 60%. Sepsis affects all ages and occurs in the community, in long-term care facilities, and among patients admitted to hospital under the care of any, and every, medical specialty. Large epidemiologic studies of up to 6 million people have demonstrated the incidence of sepsis to be 3 per 1000 population per year or about 750,000 cases of sepsis a year in the United States. These figures result in approximately 2% of all hospitalizations, with hospital costs exceeding $16 billion for the care of these septic patients. The average hospital stay for patients with sepsis is 20 days and requires admission to the ICU in more than half of the cases. The annual mortality associated with sepsis is estimated to be between 30 and 50 deaths per 100,000 population. This corresponds to approximately 215,000 deaths or about 10% of all deaths in the United States, ranking sepsis as one of the top 10 causes of death. Therefore, sepsis has a significant impact on health care, and that will continue to be the case because by the year 2020, more than 1 million cases of sepsis per year are estimated to occur in the United States.

In this chapter, we describe the body's immune response (locally and systemically) and explain how the immune response leads to tissue destruction in the body, how it relates to sepsis and septic shock, and how these mechanisms can progress to multisystem organ dysfunction syndrome (MODS). Risk factors, clinical assessment, and management of this complicated syndrome are also discussed. We first reacquaint you with the immune system.

ANATOMY AND PHYSIOLOGY OF THE IMMUNE SYSTEM

When the human body is invaded or attacked by infectious materials, foreign tissue, or cancer cells, a defense system must be organized and implemented or the host will die. The **immune system** is made up of multiple organs and many specialized cells that move freely about the body, ready to attack and defend it as a whole. These highly specialized proteins, called antibodies and complement proteins, are unique to the system.

Antibodies and Complement Proteins

Antibodies have three major functions in the immune system. When an **antigen** (foreign protein or particulate) enters the system, antibodies seek out and attach themselves to the structure to create an **antigen-antibody complex**. This attachment is like a key in a lock; the complex has unique properties that neutralize the antigen. This unique attachment changes the shape of both the antigen and the antibody. The second function of the antibodies is stimulating production of phagocytes that engulf the target antigens. The last and most important function of the antibody is stimulation of a complement cascade.

A **complement** is a group of enzymes that are in the bloodstream in an inactive state at all times. They are activated when the antigen-antibody complex is formed. A cascade or series of events called the **complement cascade** are set in motion. Protein rings are formed by these sequential steps, which facilitate a rapid influx of sodium and water into the targeted cell, causing it to burst as a result of the high osmotic pressure.

The **complement system** is an important part of the immune response. There are 25 inactive proteins available within the circulatory system at all times. Complement activation can occur in three ways:

1. Classic pathway—set in motion by antibodies bound to their specific antigens
2. Lectin pathway—set in motion by particular bacterial carbohydrates
3. Alternative pathway—set in motion by gram-negative bacterial and fungal cell walled polysaccharides

Cells of the Immune System

The two primary cell types of the immune system are phagocytes and lymphocytes. Those identified as phagocytes are named neutrophils, monocytes, and macrophages. The lymphocytes are identified as B lymphocytes and T lymphocytes.

Phagocytes

Phagocytosis is the process of ingestion and digestion of targeted antigens. The phagocytes that perform phagocytosis are initially white blood cells that are recruited from the bloodstream when an infection begins. This recruitment triggers a conversion that activates their special immune system function. For instance, monocytes in the bloodstream are transformed into macrophages when they are drawn into the tissues at the site of the infection.

Lymphocytes

The major classes of **lymphocytes** are B cells and **T cells**. B cells arise from stem cells in the bone marrow and T cells arise from the thymus gland and circulate through the lymph nodes. The B cells identify and tag a previously unknown **antigen** by stimulating production of antigen-specific **immunoglobulins** and thereby are able to "remember" the invader when encountered in the future. Such encounters trigger a secondary immune response. These cells are called *memory B cells.*

T cells respond in three ways:

1. **Cytotoxic T cells** kill invading cells. Stimulated by **macrophages**, these cell killers gain assistance from the helper T cells to destroy marked antigens.
2. **Helper T cells** stimulate the immune system to create B cells, start antibody production, and activate cytotoxic cells and macrophages. Macrophages process the invader and mark it for destruction; then the "package" is presented to the helper T cells. Chemical mediators, called **interleukins**, are also released from the macrophages, and they assist the helper T cell in activating other immune system cells.
3. **Suppressor T cells** slow or control the immune system response once the foreign invader has been suppressed.

Inflammatory Cellular Response

Foreign proteins, local tissue injury, autoimmune reaction, and ischemia can trigger an inflammatory response. The degree of response depends upon the amount of injury to the tissues; an exaggerated response can overwhelm the patient's protective mechanisms. The biochemical response can be confined at a local level or be systemic.

Local Inflammatory Response

Let's say that you cut your arm while working on your dirty car in the garage. Bacteria enter this wound and trigger a response from your immune system. The local blood vessels become permeable and dilate to get a better blood supply to the area. A combination of plasma and cells (called *exudate*) is moved into the tissue. This slows movement of fluids around the site. Bradykinin, a mediator, creates spaces between cells so that leukocytes can emerge. Neutrophils (granulocytes) move to the inflamed area to phagocytose foreign debris. This is accomplished by three plasma protein systems initiated to engage the infection:

1. *Complement system* is initiated by the development of the antigen-antibody complex or sugar released from bacteria; lysis of the target is the goal.
2. *Kinin-kallikrein system* controls blood vessel size and permeability. Kinins are biochemicals controlled by the kinase enzymes. Production of bradykinin is the end result of this process.
3. *Coagulation system* traps the bacteria within the injured tissue to prevent its spread to other tissues and also helps control bleeding.

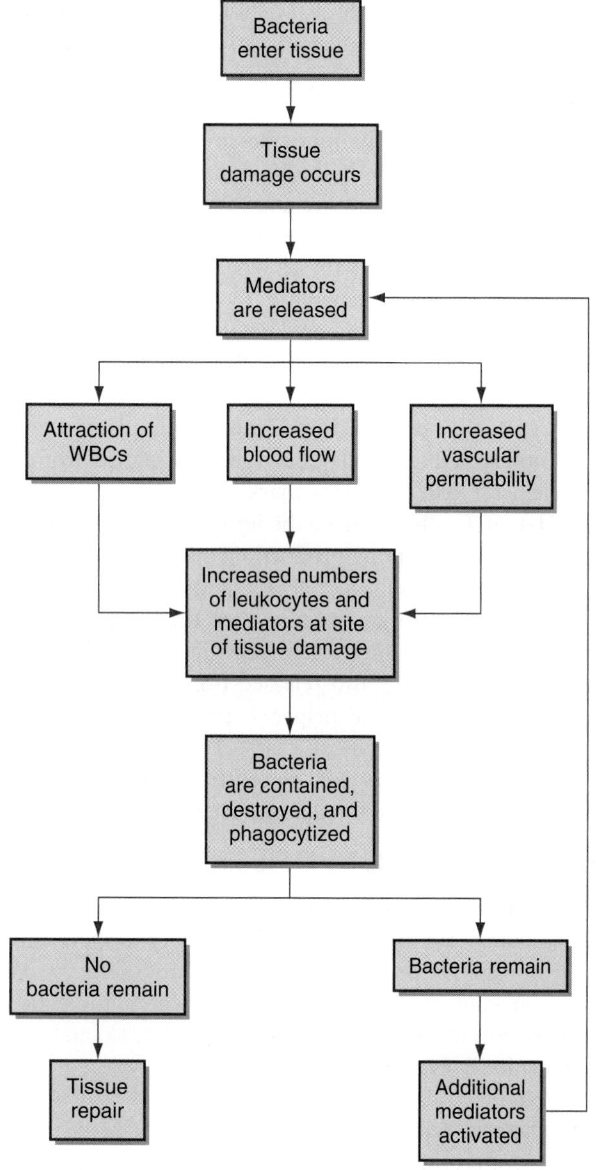

Figure 8-1

Inflammatory response. In this example, bacterial infection triggers a set of responses that tend to inhibit or destroy the bacteria. (From Thibodeau G, Patton K: *The human body in health & disease*, ed 4., St. Louis, 2010, Mosby.)

A delicate balance is at work in the coagulation cascade as thrombosis occurs alongside fibrinolysis. One process keeps bleeding under control and the other keeps the blood vessels patent. Platelets work with the coagulation system to stop bleeding.

Your arm injury has had a local inflammatory response. It's a good day and all the little foreign invaders are destroyed. This is called a **local inflammation.** Figure 8-1 demonstrates the local and systemic immune responses.

Systemic Inflammatory Response

If, on the other hand, it's a bad day, the bacteria are too many/too strong, your immune system is not up to par, or you have an unhealthy body, the bacteria will not be destroyed by merely a local response, and additional mediators from the immune system must then respond. This may become an overwhelming response that progresses into a **systemic inflammation**. In this instance, normal tissues may also become damaged. In fact, tissue destruction may result more from the systemic inflammatory response than from the original infection. If the suppressors of the immune system cannot slow the immune response (or stop the response), an overwhelming **positive feedback loop** of events occurs that causes tissue destruction. In other words, the inflammatory cascade must be slowed and stopped at some point or negative consequences will develop: first tissues, then organs may be destroyed.

Systemic inflammatory response syndrome, or **SIRS,** occurs when widespread biochemical reactions are occurring in tissues and organs remote from the original insult. Some clinical conditions can be predicted to lead to SIRS. (See Box 8-1.)

Box 8-1 Conditions That May Lead to SIRS

Vascular infections (heart and lungs)
Pancreatitis
Ischemia
Multisystem trauma with massive tissue injury
Hemorrhagic shock
Immune-mediated organ injury
Aspiration of gastric contents
Massive transfusion
Host defense abnormalities
Infectious processes like pneumonia, influenza
Exogenous administration of tumor necrosis factor or other cytokines

Modified from Urden S, et al: *Thelan's critical care nursing*, ed 5, St. Louis, 2006, Mosby.
SIRS, Systemic inflammatory response syndrome.

Immunity

Two different pathways are involved with the immune response to sepsis. These are the **innate immune system** and the **adaptive immune system.** The innate immune system activates and is responsible for protection during the first few hours of the infectious event. **Innate immunity** is also known as the *natural* or *native immunity* because this type of defense is always present in healthy individuals. Immunity is provided by epithelial barriers and by specialized cells and natural antibiotics present in epithelia, all of which function to block the entry of microbes. The innate immune system uses **toll-like receptors** to recognize different bacterial, fungal, and viral **pathogens**. The structures that the receptors bind to are present on a wide variety of organisms, and microbes have not been able to alter these binding structures. The toll-like receptors generate a response specific to that particular organism when activated. Signal pathways increase production of **pro-inflammatory cytokines**, such as **tumor necrosis**

factor-alpha (**TNF-α**), **interleukin-1-beta** (**IL-1-β**), and **nuclear factor-kappa-beta** (NF-κβ). They also activate IL-10, which is an **antiinflammatory cytokine.** Understanding and investigation of these receptors may lead to new strategies for treatment of sepsis.

The adaptive immune system, also called *specific* or *acquired immunity*, takes a more direct approach against the organisms. There are two types of adaptive immunity: humoral immunity and cell-mediated immunity. Several specific cell-mediated and **humoral** adaptive immune responses assist in this response. Both T cells and B cells are involved, and memory cells are developed during an infection that can lead to a faster response in a repeated exposure. Type 1 helper cells (Th1) secrete pro-inflammatory cytokines and type 2 helper T cells (Th2) form antiinflammatory cytokines during the immune response. B lymphocytes release **immunoglobulins** that bind to organism-specific antigens, which, in turn, lead to a greater recognition and destruction by other immune cells, such as natural killer cells and **neutrophils.**

Table 8-1 Laboratory Values Encountered in Sepsis

Lab Results Found	Reasons/Comments
High or low white count	Stress response with increased number of neutrophils
Thrombocytopenia	Watch for hemolysis DIC may appear
Hyper- or hypoglycemia	Stress response Inhibition of glucose release
High PT, aPTT	Coagulopathy with endotoxin release
Positive blood cultures	Sepsis can occur with AND without positive blood cultures
Elevated lactate (>2.2 mmol/L)	Anaerobic and hypermetabolism, hypoperfusion
Respiratory alkalosis	Found early in sepsis
Metabolic acidosis	Found late in sepsis

Modified from Dale D, Federman D: *ACP medicine,* ed 3, American College of Physicians, 2007, WebMD, Inc., Table 3, p. 1449.
aPTT, Activated partial thromboplastin time; *DIC,* disseminated intravascular coagulation; *PT,* prothrombin time.

DIAGNOSTICS

Laboratory Tests and Microbiology

Complete Blood Count (CBC) with Differential

Leukocytosis (elevated white blood cell count [WBC]) is the hallmark sign of infection and activation of the inflammatory cascade. Leukocytosis can also be misleading and nonspecific. Those who are being treated with steroids or who are suffering from stress may have signs of leukocytosis and yet do not have an infection. At the other end of the spectrum, there are cases of patients who are febrile and **neutropenic** and suffering from severe sepsis and yet do not have signs of leukocytosis.

Within the WBC differential, having **bands** at more than 10% represents release of immature cells from the bone marrow and is considered a sign of infection and/or **inflammation.** The CBC will also yield a hemoglobin and hematocrit level; these should be assessed to ensure adequate oxygen delivery. The hematocrit should be maintained at greater than 30% and hemoglobin at greater than 10 gm/dL. Platelets may be elevated in the case of an acute inflammation. On the other hand, a very low platelet count in a patient suffering from shock is a predictor of poor outcome.

Clotting Factors

Thrombocytopenia (low platelet count), elevated prothrombin time, elevated activated prothrombin time, decreased fibrinogen, and increased fibrin split products are associated with disseminated intravascular coagulation (DIC), one of the serious complications of shock and SIRS/MODS.

Chemistry

Identification of electrolyte disturbances and the subsequent correction of such is a high priority. A low bicarbonate level indicates acidosis and poor perfusion. When acidosis occurs in the setting of septic shock, lactic acidosis or diabetic ketoacidosis is usually the cause. Creatinine should be assessed for renal function. Elevated creatinine in the presence of sepsis may indicate early renal failure.

Evaluation of the lactate level and subsequent identification of an elevation indicates poor perfusion, shock, and a poor outcome if it is allowed to remain high (see further discussion of shock under the heading *Trauma* in Chapter 7). The lactate level also can be an indicator of sepsis. An arterial blood gas evaluation will help identify oxygenation level, ventilation perfusion, and overall acidosis and base deficits.

Liver function tests should be assessed to identify organ dysfunction or failure early. If a high total bilirubin level is identified early in a sepsis workup, along with an elevated aspirate aminotransferase/alanine aminotransferase (AST/ALT) ratio, "shock liver" may be present, indicating acute ischemia of the liver. Elevations in amylase and lipase may represent pancreatitis, a serious noninfectious cause of SIRS. Standard laboratory values encountered during sepsis are shown in Table 8-1.

Microbiology

Testing for and obtaining microbes in blood, urine, cerebrospinal fluid (CSF), and other tissue cultures is important. Specimens are placed in a nutrient-filled agar medium to facilitate growth of any microbes present. Within 1 to 2 days, the pathogens have multiplied sufficiently that they can be identified by their shape and growth pattern. Two other tests can be performed on collected specimens. The first is Gram's staining, which has been discussed previously. This can be done within a few hours of specimen acquisition to help identify the best antibiotic treatment for the patient. Another specimen test involves injecting certain types of antibiotics within the growing cluster of microbes to determine which agent is best suited to suppress or kill that particular organism. This is referred to as testing for the *sensitivity*.

Did You Know?

When the microbiology report states that a certain microbe is "resistant" to a group of antibiotics, it means the sensitivity examination conducted on the culture medium showed no suppression or lysis of the microbes—thus the involved antibiotic should not be used for this patient. For instance, vancomycin-resistant *Enterococcus* on a microbiology report would indicate that the microbes are growing on the culture plate as gram-positive cocci with no change in growth when vancomycin (a broad-range antibiotic) is injected into that area of the plate.

From Thibodeau G, Patton K: *The human body in health and disease*, ed 4, St. Louis, 2005, Mosby.

Blood Cultures

Obtaining blood cultures from patients with chills and fever is an important part of the septic workup. See Box 8-2 for predictive clinical signs of a positive blood culture (septicemia). All patients with suspected bacteremia should have blood drawn from two separate sites. These specimens are placed into culture medium; specimens from suspected sources of infection should be obtained and cultured as well.

Box 8-2 Predictions for a Positive Blood Culture

Fever >38.3° C
Presence of a rapidly fatal (<1 month) or ultimately fatal (<5 years) disease
Shaking chills
IV drug abuse
Acute abdominal findings or a major co-morbidity

From Marx, J et al: *Rosen's emergency medicine: Concepts & clinical practice*, ed 6, St. Louis, 2006, Mosby.

Other Laboratory Tests

A urinalysis identifies the number of white cells present and whether nitrites are positive or negative. Nitrites normally are not found in urine but do result when bacteria reduce urinary nitrates by converting them into nitrites. Many gram-negative and some gram-positive organisms are capable of this conversion. A subsequent specimen of urine should be cultured to determine potential urosepsis when nitrites are found. A lumbar puncture (LP) should be performed to obtain CSF to be used to identify leukocytosis and culture for foreign microbes if meningitis is suspected.

Radiographs

Each patient with suspected sepsis should have a chest x-ray (radiograph) completed to rule out a pulmonary infiltrate and to rule out the classic white, fluffy appearance of noncardiogenic pulmonary edema or acute respiratory distress syndrome (ARDS). The presence of free air under the diaphragm helps identify a perforated bowel. Pneumomediastinum helps differentiate an esophageal perforation. X-rays or other imaging studies should be completed on areas of the body thought to be involved in the infection.

DISEASE PROCESSES AND MANAGEMENT

Pathogens, cancer cells, tissue damage from trauma or ischemia are just a few examples of a trigger to an immune response that is identified as a disease process of the immune system. This section will review the pathogens, sepsis, and the positive feedback loop of SIRS and MODS.

Pathogens

Disease-producing organisms, called *pathogens*, initiate an immune response in a healthy body. There are many different types of pathogens or microbes including bacteria, fungi, protozoa, viruses, and prions.

Bacteria

Bacteria produce a variety of diseases and can gain access to the body through numerous sites. Bacteria secrete toxic substances that damage tissue as they are released. There are four major types of bacteria, identified by their shape and size.

1. Bacilli are large, rod-shaped cells found in singles or in groups.
2. Cocci are large, round cells that form in pairs (diplococci), in strings (streptococci), or in clusters (staphylococci).
3. Curved or spiral rods are arranged singly or in colonies.
4. Small bacteria are either round or oval in shape and are so small that many are just now being correctly identified. These are considered parasitic in nature because they must live inside another living cell to reproduce. Examples of this type of bacteria are *Rickettsia* and *Chlamydia*.

Some bacteria develop resistance to suppressive activity by producing spores. This action protects the bacteria by making them resistant to certain chemicals and temperature extremes. Examples of gram-positive and gram-negative bacteria are listed in Table 8-2.

Table 8-2 Pathogenic Bacteria

Structural Classification	Gram Stain	Name of Bacteria	Diseases Caused by Bacteria
Bacilli (rods)	Gram positive	*Bacillus*	Anthrax and gastroenteritis
	Gram positive	*Clostridium*	Botulism, tetanus
	Gram negative	*Enterobacteria*	Salmonella
	Gram negative	*Pseudomonas*	Otitis, endocarditis
Cocci (spheres)	Gram positive	*Staphylococcus*	Staph infections, food poisoning, UTI, toxic shock syndrome
	Gram positive	*Streptococcus*	Pharyngitis, pneumonia, sinusitis, otitis, rheumatic fever, dental caries
	Gram negative	*Neisseria*	Meningitis, gonorrhea, PID
Curved or spiral rod	Gram negative	*Vibrio*	Cholera, gastroenteritis, wound infections
	Gram negative	*Campylobacter*	Diarrhea
	Gram negative	Spirochetes	Syphilis and Lyme disease
Small bacterium	Gram negative	*Rickettsia*	Rocky Mountain spotted fever and Q fever
	Gram negative	Chlamydia	Genital infections, conjunctivitis

Modified from Thibodeau G, Patton K *The human body in health and disease*, ed 4, St. Louis, 2005, Mosby.
PID, Pelvic inflammatory disease; *UTI*, urinary tract infection.

Did You Know

The Gram's staining method is one tool the laboratory uses to identify which pathogen has entered a patient's tissues. A specimen from an infectious site is smeared on a slide and then stained. This stain colors only certain types of cells. The violet stain is quickly taken up by bacteria referred to as *gram positive.* If the Gram's staining result is negative, the suspect cells appeared, or rather did not become stained.

From Thibodeau G, Patton K: *The human body in health & disease*, ed 4, St. Louis, 2005, Mosby.

Bacterial Toxins

The human body is able to recognize and respond to molecules within bacterial microbes. The best studied is a special lipid (fat) on gram-negative bacteria. This **endotoxin** can either enter in its free form or be bound to the cell wall of bacteria, which then interact with toll-like receptors. The endotoxin causes a systemic inflammatory response while alerting the host of its presence. This systemic inflammatory response is more lethal to the host than the actual endotoxin itself.

Fungi and Protozoa

Both fungi and protozoa must live within a human host cell to survive. This parasitic relationship allows the pathogens to reproduce. Some examples of diseases produced by these pathogens include thrush and histoplasmosis caused by *Candida* and *Histoplasma* fungi. Examples of protozoan pathogens include amoebae and sporozoans, which cause dysentery and malaria, respectively.

Viruses

Viruses, although technically not living cells, can invade human cells, insert their own genetic code, and reproduce like a parasite. Microbiologists assist clinicians in the identification of viruses by determining their shape, DNA or RNA content, and their method of reproduction.

Prions

Prion is actually a shortened name for a microbe called a *proteinaceous infectious particle.* These pathogens convert proteins and alter cells. Being a recently discovered pathogen, not much is known yet about these microbes. We do know that they are the pathogen involved in mad cow disease (bovine spongiform encephalopathy or BSE) and its relative, Creutzfeldt-Jakob disease.

Treatment of Infections

The best way to treat disease caused by infection of pathogens is prevention. Immunity to some bacteria and viruses may be obtained through vaccines. The single most effective way to prevent the spread of these infections is good hand hygiene and use of standard precautions. Once an infection has begun, several mechanisms may be instituted to kill or slow the growth of the invading pathogen. Antibiotics are compounds produced to kill or inhibit pathogenic growth. Antiviral agents can inhibit the growth of certain viruses.

How does the clinician choose the correct antibiotic? The clinical presentation, the organ or system infected, and quick identification of whether the pathogen is a bacterial or viral infection can assist the clinician in determining the best antibiotic for the patient. Gram staining exudate or excretions

Table 8-3 Definitions of SIRS, Sepsis, Severe Sepsis, and Septic Shock by Consensus Conference

Syndrome	Definition by Consensus
Systemic inflammatory response syndrome (SIRS)	Two or more of the following: • Temperature > 38° C (100.4° F) or <36° C (96.8° F) • Pulse rate > 90 bpm • Respiratory rate >20 or $Paco_2$ < 32 mm Hg • WBC >12,000 mm^3 or <4000 m^3 or >10% immature forms (bands)
Sepsis	SIRS due to suspected or confirmed infection
Severe sepsis	Sepsis with organ dysfunction, hypoperfusion, or hypotension
Septic shock	Sepsis-induced hypotension despite adequate fluid resuscitation along with other signs of poor perfusion

Modified from Parillo J, Dellinger RP: *Critical care medicine: principles of diagnosis and management in the adult*, ed 3, St. Louis, 2007, Mosby.

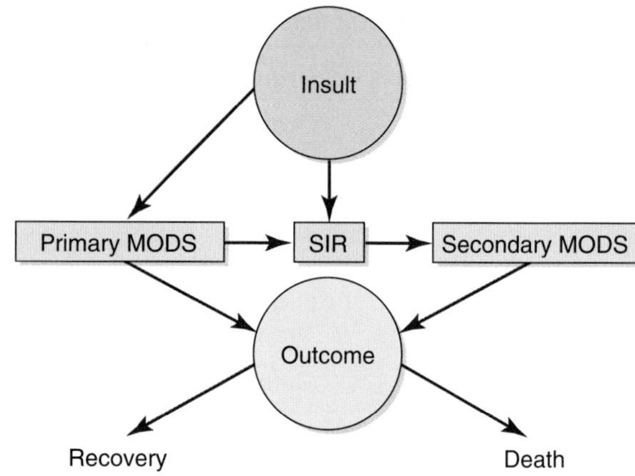

Figure 8-2

Different causes and results of primary and secondary multiple organ dysfunction syndrome (MODS). *SIR,* Systemic inflammatory response. (From American College of Chest Physicians/Society of Critical Care Medicine Consensus Conference Committee, *Crit Care Med* 20:868, 1992.)

from infected areas may aid in the quick identification if the pathogen is a type of bacteria. Once a course of treatment is determined, it is important that the critical care team follow through with antibiotic or antiviral administration. The treatment agent can be referenced in a pharmacology resource to determine correct administration techniques.

Sepsis

How does the immune response progress to sepsis? How does this cascade of events lead to a systemic immune response? What causes organs to fail as a result of this cascade? Some answers to these questions are emerging as researchers delve into this complex issue.

The complexity involves the very terminology within the healthcare language. In 2001, the International Sepsis Definitions Conference was undertaken. A product of that conference is a list of signs and symptoms that takes into account the complex nature of this disease process (Table 8-3).

Pathogenesis of Sepsis or Septicemia

Bacteremia (presence of bacteria in the blood) creates a systemic immune response in the body known as *septicemia.* **Septicemia,** or **sepsis,** is caused by a failure of the immune system to destroy a foreign invader, and the body then becomes ill as a result. In the recent past, the major organisms responsible for cases of sepsis were gram-negative bacilli. The trend has slowly shifted over time to gram-positive bacteria and opportunistic fungi being the causative agents. The definition of sepsis does not describe mechanisms of disease, but rather focuses on nonspecific clinical criteria. Before the 1990s, the definition of sepsis varied widely. In the early 1990s, a consensus conference defined sepsis as a systemic inflammatory response syndrome(SIRS) caused by presumed or confirmed infection (see Table 8-3). Severe sepsis is defined as sepsis plus sepsis-induced organ dysfunction or tissue hypoperfusion. The term *septic shock* is reserved for patients with sepsis-induced hypotension despite adequate fluid resuscitation in addition to the presence of perfusion abnormalities. Assessment of the severity of sepsis is important for clinical management, particularly in view of the new therapies for sepsis syndrome currently being evaluated in clinical trials. Increasing severity correlates with an increase in mortality, which rises from 25% to 30% for severe sepsis and up to 40% to 70% for septic shock.

Although the detailed mechanisms involved early in the cause of sepsis have not been clearly defined, a number of clinical risk factors for sepsis have been identified (Table 8-4). Bacteria are often considered the sole causative agents; however, any microorganism can cause sepsis, including fungi (fungemia), parasites (parasitemia), and viruses (viremia). Respiratory and intraabdominal infections are the most common associated sites of infection, with **gram-positive** organisms now outnumbering **gram-negative** organisms as causes of sepsis. Cases of fungal infections leading to sepsis are increasing rapidly, making up approximately 15% of the cases.

The human response to sepsis is complex and involves activation of both pro-inflammatory and antiinflammatory cascades, previously described. The **endothelium** is felt to be important in the cellular response to sepsis. Adhesion molecules act to enhance attachment of leukocytes to the endothelium and then enhance the passage of the leukocytes through the endothelium. Complex mechanisms exist that work to allow migration of neutrophils from the intravascular space into the interstitium. The activated neutrophils can then **degranulate,** which exposes the endothelial surfaces to species such as oxygen radicals and nitric oxide (Figure 8-2).

Death generally occurs as a result of complications of immunosuppression and multiple organ failure later in the

Table 8-4 Reported Association of Clinical Risk Factors with Sepsis and Severe Sepsis

Risk Factor	Description	Odds or Risk (95% CI)
Demographics		
Age	Greater than 65 years vs. ≤ 65 years	13.1 (12.6 to 13.6)*
Race	African American vs. Caucasian	1.9 (1.8 to 2.0)*
	Other non-Caucasian race vs. Caucasian	1.9 (1.8 to 2.0)*
Sex	Male vs. female	1.3 (1.2 to 1.3)*
Co-morbidities		
HIV	HIV vs. no HIV	5.1 (1.2 to 21.2)†
Cancer	Any cancer vs. no cancer	2.8 (2.8 to 2.8)*
	Solid tumor vs. no cancer	1.8 (1.8 to 18.2)*
	Hematologic cancer vs. no cancer	15.7 (15.6 to 15.9)*
Cirrhosis	Cirrhosis vs. no cirrhosis	2.6 (1.9 to 3.3)*
Alcohol dependence	Ongoing alcoholism or alcohol withdrawal vs. no alcohol dependence	1.5 (1.2 to 1.9)
Complications of Medical Care		
Venous access devices	Central venous catheter vs. peripheral venous catheter	64 (54 to 76)*
Transfusion	Packed red cell transfusion vs. no transfusion	6.0 (4.0 to 9.2)†

From O'Brien, JM Jr, Ali NA, Aberegg SK, et al: Sepsis, *Am J Med* 120:1012-1022, 2007.
95% CI, 95% confidence interval; *HIV*, human immunodeficiency virus.
*Relative risk; †Odds ratio.

disease process. The involvement of endothelium tissue (which is present throughout much of the body) would explain the high incidence of multiple organ dysfunction and failure. The inflammatory mediators that increase in sepsis create an increased demand for oxygen in the body. Oxygen extraction is altered during this process, and cardiac contractility is lessened, which alters the delivery of oxygen to tissues. The resulting cellular **dysoxia** leads to the release of more inflammatory mediators, which creates a repeating and worsening cycle of imbalance between oxygen supply and demand.

Fever is a natural response of the body that actually works to inhibit the progression of the infection. Bacteria do not tolerate high temperatures well, and fever in the body also works to increase phagocytosis. Some patients do not become febrile with sepsis, and this lack of an acute phase response has been linked to increased mortality.

Clinical Assessment of Sepsis

The early phase of sepsis generally is associated with fever; however, in some patients hypothermia may be present. Neurologic symptoms may be present and include confusion, altered sensorium, and disorientation. Physical examination findings are based on the causative organism and location of the infection. Patients may experience decreased urinary output, abdominal pain, hypotension, tachycardia, and shortness of breath. A variety of symptoms may occur in a wide range of organ systems (Figure 8-3).

It is imperative that early recognition and treatment of sepsis occur because this will determine final outcome in many cases. Microbiologic and radiologic evidence is not necessary; only clinical suspicion is needed to diagnose sepsis. Rapid assessment and treatment must occur as soon as the diagnosis is made. Septic shock can rapidly turn into multiple organ dysfunction syndrome (MODS). Multiple clinical and metabolic abnormalities occur with MODS (Table 8-5).

Some illnesses can mimic sepsis and should be included in the differential diagnosis. These include pulmonary embolism, acute pancreatitis, relative adrenal insufficiency, acute myocardial dysfunction, acute gastrointestinal (GI) bleed, diabetic ketoacidosis, and hypovolemia.

Did You Know?

Besides the immune response cascade, the coagulation cascade is also initiated when sepsis occurs.

From Naim R: *Immunology for medical students*, ed 2, St. Louis, 2006, Mosby.

Hemostatic Balance

The **coagulation cascade** is activated during sepsis via thrombin generation from **tissue factor** and **factor VII**. Tissue factor does not normally come into contact with blood; however, with the activation of **cytokines** in cases of sepsis, tissue factor is expressed on monocytes, neutrophils, and endothelial cells. The tissue factor activates factor VII, which then produces thrombin by way of the extrinsic pathway. Thrombin is also generated via the intrinsic pathway by the process of feedback. Disseminated intravascular coagulation (DIC) can develop, which can then consume coagulation factors leading to bleeding, although generally the bleeding is not severe.

In a healthy person, any increase in coagulation would be immediately stopped by antithrombin III, proteins C and S, and tissue factor pathway inhibitor. In a septic patient, reduced

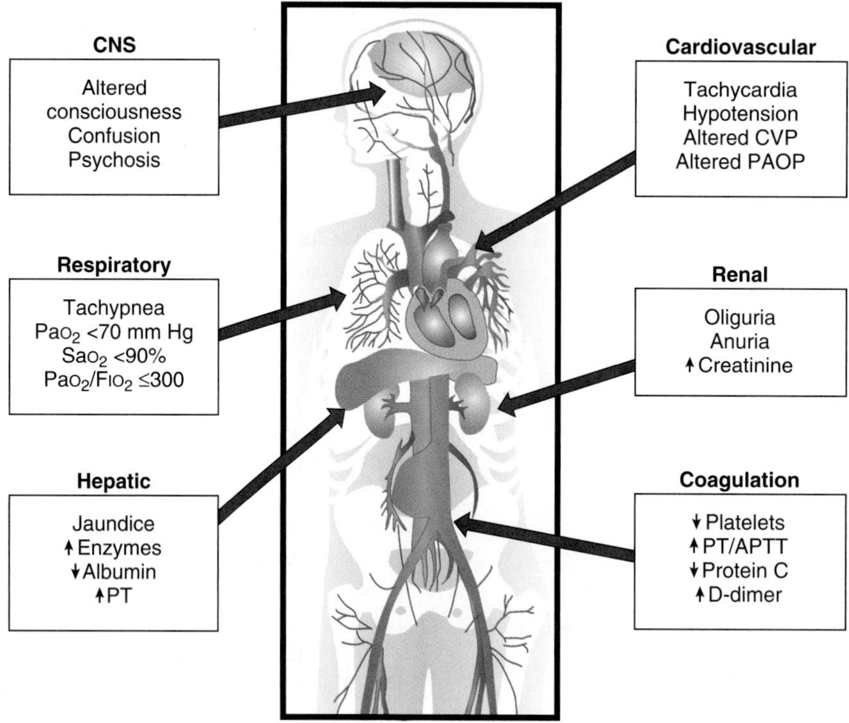

Figure 8-3

Identification of organ failure in severe sepsis. Clinical and laboratory criteria to identify organ failure are shown for each organ system. *APTT*, Activated partial thromboplastin time; *CNS*, central nervous system; *CVP*, central venous pressure; *PAOP*, pulmonary artery occlusion pressure; *PT*, prothrombin time. (Modified from Balk RA: Pathogenesis and management of multiple organ dysfunction or failure in severe sepsis and septic shock, *Crit Care Clin* 16:337-352, 2000.)

Table 8-5 Severe Sepsis with MODS

Clinical Presentation	Cellular Changes
Decreased level of consciousness	Cerebral edema, microthrombi
Decreased myocardial performance	Altered calcium influx, interstitial edema
ARDS/ALI	Fluid exudates into alveolar space, neutrophil plugging, hyaline membrane formation
Acute renal tubular necrosis	Low perfusion, focal ischemia, microthrombi
Adrenal insufficiency and hemorrhage	Focal or diffuse hemorrhage, necrosis
Jaundice, presence of clotting factors	Necrosis in liver and failure of gallbladder
Gut permeability and movement of bacteria	Interstitial edema, breaks in gut membrane, mucosal necrosis

Modified from Dale D, Federman D: *ACP medicine*, ed 3, American College of Physicians, 2007, WebMD, Inc., Table 5, p. 1450.
ALT, Alanine aminotransferase; *ARDS*, acute respiratory distress syndrome; *MODS*, multisystem organ dysfunction syndrome.

levels of protein C and antithrombin III are found due to consumption and reduced production of these factors. The hemostatic balance is altered and a shift toward a pro-coagulant state occurs. Protein C acts as both an anticoagulant and an antiinflammatory. Activated protein C has been shown to reduce cytokines, including TNF and IL-1. It also inhibits the macrophage response to lipopolysaccharide. The relationship of the inflammatory and coagulation systems in a septic response is illustrated in Figure 8-4.

Cardiac Dysfunction in Sepsis

Initial stages of sepsis are characterized by a distributive shock due to increased capillary leak that results in reduced venous return to the heart. The low intravascular volume that is coupled with sepsis-induced cardiac dysfunction leads to decreased stroke volume. Administration of fluids can improve blood pressure, reduce heart rate, and improve cardiac output. The presence of tissue hypoperfusion must also be assessed. Physical examination findings that increase suspicion include hypotension, decreased urine output, tachycardia, altered mentation, lactic acidosis, decreased mixed venous oxygen saturation, and delayed capillary refill.

Cardiac dysfunction, in the form of left ventricular impairment, affects up to 50% of those with severe sepsis. The mechanism is not completely understood; however, it is felt to be mediated by TNF-α and IL-1-β. When transporting patients with severe sepsis, it is important to understand that septic

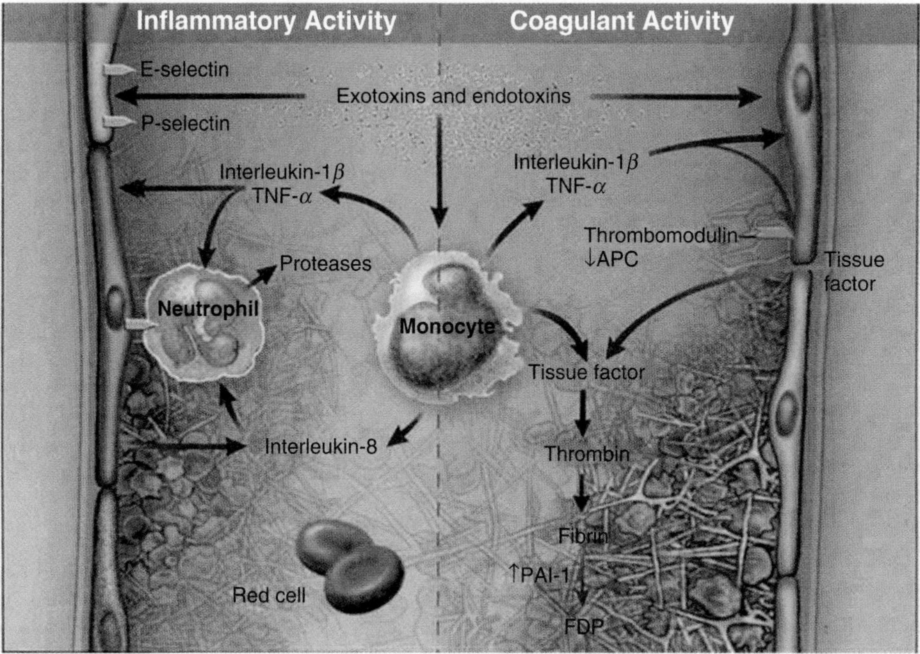

Figure 8-4

Relationship between inflammatory and coagulation systems in sepsis. Monocytes are activated by endotoxins and exotoxins from bacteria; they release tumor necrosis factor-alpha (TNF-α) and interleukin-1-β (IL-1-β). TNF-α and IL-1-β activate the inflammatory cascade via neutrophils and the production of other proinflammatory cytokines, and in combination with tissue factor, also activate the coagulation cascade, with production of fibrin and fibrin degradation products (FDP). *APC*, Activated protein C. (Modified from Matthay MA: Severe sepsis: a new treatment with both anticoagulant and antiinflammatory properties, *N Engl J Med* 344:759-762, 2001, figure 1A, p 761.)

shock is characterized by a **hypercirculatory** or **hyperdynamic** state. When pulmonary artery (PA) catheters or noninvasive cardiac output monitors are used, the majority of septic patients are found to have a decreased systemic vascular resistance and a significantly increased cardiac index. This may not be initially evident if the patient is significantly hypovolemic. At the same time, studies have demonstrated that patients suffer from decreased contractility of the left ventricle. It has also been demonstrated that stroke volume is maintained due to an increase in left ventricular end-diastolic and end-systolic volumes. Those patients that were unable to increase these volumes did not survive the episode of septic shock. Most patients had a recovery of left ventricular function within 10 days after the onset of sepsis.

Laboratory Findings

Laboratory abnormalities are common during episodes of sepsis but can be different based on patient characteristics and type of infection present. The more common abnormalities include **leukocytosis with left shift, thrombocytopenia,** and **hyperbilirubinemia**. Some patients, however, may actually develop **leukopenia.** As patients progress, they may develop a more severe thrombocytopenia coupled with a **coagulopathy**. This coagulopathy is characterized by prolongation of the prothrombin (PT) time, decreased fibrinogen, and positive D-dimer (fibrin degradation products), which is termed *disseminated intravascular coagulation (DIC)*. Many septic patients have **azotemia**, characterized by elevated blood urea nitrogen (BUN) and creatinine and may also have liver injury, characterized by hyperbilirubinemia and **aminotransferase** elevation. Many will become hyperglycemic and control of blood sugars has been shown to improve outcome.

Metabolic acidosis is one of the hallmark signs of severe sepsis and septic shock, most commonly caused by an increased lactate level. Hyperventilation may induce a respiratory alkalosis early in sepsis (due to hyperdynamic state), but this is quickly replaced by the more common metabolic acidosis. Most patients with sepsis are hypoxemic requiring supplemental oxygen. As the right-to-left shunt worsens, many require intubation and mechanical ventilation.

Management of Sepsis

Key objectives in the management of sepsis include initial resuscitation, source identification and control, appropriate antimicrobial therapy, ensuring adequate perfusion to tissues, and supportive therapy. Current guidelines emphasize early diagnosis and intervention as key factors in improved rate of survival in these patients.

Early goal-directed therapy (EGDT) has been shown to improve patient survival among patients with septic shock. Resuscitation in the first 6 hours after diagnosis aimed at achieving a mean arterial pressure (MAP) greater than 65 mm Hg, central venous pressure (CVP) of 8 to 12 mm Hg, urine output of greater than 0.5 mL/kg/hr, and central venous oxygen saturation ($Scvo_2$) of greater than 70% (or mixed venous oxygen saturation, or Svo_2, of greater than 65%) has been shown to significantly reduce 28-day mortality among patients with septic shock. In patients on mechanical ventilation, higher central venous pressure targets of 12 to 15 mm Hg are recommended. If despite achieving central venous pressure targets, the $ScvO_2$ remains less than 70% (or SvO_2 less than 65%), current recommendations suggest increasing oxygen delivery to tissues by either increasing the hematocrit to 30% or starting a dobutamine infusion, up to 20 mcg/kg/min.

Appropriate samples should be drawn and sent for gram staining and culture, including at least two blood cultures, at least one of which should be from a fresh skin puncture. A blood culture sample should also be acquired from each vascular access device that has been in place for more than 48 hours. Imaging studies may be necessary to confirm any other source of infection, and if such a source is present, it should be promptly sampled.

Although antibiotic therapy should be started after culture samples have been obtained, all efforts should be made to prevent delay in starting antibiotics. In a retrospective study of over 2000 septic shock patients in Canada, effective antimicrobial administration within the first hour of documented hypotension was associated with increased survival to hospital discharge in adult patients with septic shock. Antibiotics are subsequently stopped as soon as therapy is considered complete.

Did You Know?

Each hour delay in administering antibiotics in the septic patient is associated with a measurable increase in mortality.

From Urden LD, Stacy KM, Lough ME: *Thelan's critical care nursing: diagnosis and management*, ed 5, St. Louis, 2006, Mosby.

After initial resuscitation, it is common for patients with severe sepsis and septic shock to become hypotensive again. Patients should initially be resuscitated with a fluid bolus (crystalloids or colloids) with a target CVP of greater than 8 mm Hg (greater than 12 mm Hg if mechanically ventilated). The volume of the fluid bolus can depend on the patient's cardiac or renal status, that is, a patient with no cardiac or renal compromise should receive a fluid bolus of 10 to 20 mL/kg, whereas those with such organ dysfunction should receive a smaller fluid bolus of 5 to 10 mL/kg. It is prudent to monitor the patient's response to the fluid bolus, with regard to heart rate, blood pressure, urine output, and rise of central venous pressure. If the CVP increases without any hemodynamic improvement, it is likely that further fluid boluses will not benefit the patient.

The goal during treatment of septic shock is to maintain an MAP greater than 65 mm Hg. Once the patient stops responding to fluids, one can start a vasoactive agent to try and achieve this target. Norepinephrine and dopamine are the agents of choice for initial vasopressor therapy (see Table 8-1) because of the pathophysiology of septic shock, which involves peripheral vasodilation along with myocardial depression. Vasopressin infusion may also be added as an adjunct in some patients. Invasive blood pressure monitoring with an arterial line is common and recommended in all patients on vasopressor therapy. In patients with high cardiac filling pressures and low cardiac output, inotropic therapy is started to boost oxygen delivery to tissues.

In patients who continue to require vasopressor therapy and are judged to have relative adrenal insufficiency, steroid replacement is initiated, using dexamethasone, hydrocortisone, and fludrocortisone. The usual dose of hydrocortisone is 200 to 300 mg/day intravenously in two to three divided doses. Steroid therapy may be weaned once vasopressor therapy is no longer required. The efficacy of steroids in patients with sepsis is controversial; however, in patients with hypotension refractory to vasopressors and resuscitation, steroids appear to have a role in reducing dosages of vasopressors and a suggestion of mortality benefit is seen.

Did You Know?

Many agents have been evaluated for the treatment of severe sepsis without much success until the recent addition of recombinant human activated protein C. Protein C is a natural element within the body that, when activated, interrupts the coagulation cascade and increases fibrinolysis. It has been shown to reduce coagulopathy and inflammation.

From Urden LD, Stacy KM, Lough ME: *Thelan's critical care nursing: diagnosis and management*, ed 5, St. Louis, 2006, Mosby.

Administration of **recombinant human activated protein C (rhAPC)** has been shown to improve survival when initiated early in patients with septic shock. Protein C is a vitamin K–dependent protein that circulates in the blood as an inactive precursor. Once activated, it modulates endothelial cell function and has antithrombotic, profibrinolytic, and antiinflammatory properties. Available under the brand name Xigris (Eli Lilly) and generic name drotrecogin alfa, it is administered as a continuous infusion over 96 hours at a dose of 24 mcg/kg/hr intravenously. It is only beneficial in patients at a high risk of death, usually quantified as an **APACHE (Acute Physiology, Age, and Chronic Health Evaluation) score** of greater than 25, or sepsis-induced multiple organ failure. The major side effect with activated protein C is bleeding. It is hence contraindicated in patients with active internal bleeding, recent (less than 3 months) hemorrhagic stroke, head or spine surgery, or presence of an epidural catheter.

Did You Know?

Acute Physiology, Age, and Chronic Health Evaluation (APACHE) scoring is done in the first 32 hours after admission to the ICU and can predict outcomes.

Score	Mortality Rate
0-5	2.3%
6-10	4.3%
11-15	8.6%
16-20	16.4%
21-25	28.6%
26-30	56.4%
31+	70%

The APACHE scoring system evaluates 12 physiologic variables, age, and chronic health status to generate a total point score. The systems/parameters are allowed the following variables as the score is tallied: cardiovascular 7, respiratory 3, renal 3, GI 6, hematologic 4, septic 4, metabolic 6, and neurologic 1. A value of 0-4 is assigned, based on the patient's status. For instance, in the respiratory system, the three variables are nonventilated respiratory rate, po_2 with Fio_2 at 1.0, and pco_2.

(From McCance KL, Huether SE: *Pathophysiology: the biologic basis for disease in adults and children*, ed 5, St. Louis, 2005, Mosby.)

Once initial resuscitation is complete, red blood cells are transfused only if the hemoglobin decreases to 7.0 gm/dL to target a hemoglobin of 7 to 9 gm/dL. Unless the patient has myocardial ischemia, acute hemorrhage, lactic acidosis, or cyanotic heart disease, transfusing to a higher target hemoglobin has been shown to offer no additional advantage. Although platelet counts of 5000 to 30,000/mm^3 are acceptable in most patients, higher counts (greater than 50,000/mm^3) are required for surgery or invasive procedures.

Patients with sepsis-induced acute respiratory distress syndrome (ARDS) requiring mechanical ventilation should be ventilated with a tidal volume of 6 mL/kg (predicted body weight, see Table 8-2) and to a target maximum inspiratory plateau pressure of 30 cm H_2O. Sedating, and occasionally paralyzing, patients can help reduce airway pressures required to provide adequate mechanical ventilation. If necessary, $Paco_2$ can be allowed to increase above normal to minimize plateau pressures and tidal volumes. Noninvasive ventilation may be considered in patients with mild to moderate hypoxemic respiratory failure who are hemodynamically stable, comfortable, easily arousable, and able to protect/clear their airway.

Maintain mechanically ventilated patients in a semirecumbent position (head of the bed raised to between 30 degrees and 45 degrees) unless contraindicated. Patients in the ICU should be assessed daily for suitability for a spontaneous breathing trial, and if they pass the trial, considered for extubation. A conservative strategy of fluid management has been shown to improve lung function and shorten the duration of mechanical ventilation and intensive care in patients with acute lung injury, without increasing nonpulmonary organ failures.

Other supportive therapy includes managing sedative infusions. These should be titrated to a predetermined end point. Maintaining a blood glucose level of less than 150 mg/dL using an insulin protocol improves survival. Because keeping a tight control on the glucose level increases the risk of hypoglycemia, always provide a glucose calorie source and monitor blood glucose values every 1 to 2 hours (4 hours when stable) in patients receiving intravenous insulin. Bicarbonate therapy is not useful in improving hemodynamics or reducing vasopressor requirements in patients with lactic acidosis.

Providing nutritional support is essential to patient preservation, especially as the patient withstands the hyperdynamic state (hypermetabolism) with weight loss, **cachexia**, and loss of organ function. Nutritional support may not reverse organ dysfunction but can preserve gut function and provide essential calories to support tissue. As described in Chapter 6, there are several ways to administer this nutrition. **Enteral** is preferred (as long as there is bowel function) to **parenteral** routes. Besides the ability to meet the high-caloric demands of the body, the addition of glutamine, arginine, and omega-3 fatty acids may lessen the tissue damage of SIRS.

You may encounter ICU patients who are being treated prophylactically for DVT (deep vein thrombosis) (also called *VTE* [*venous thromboembolism*]) prophylaxis. All critically ill patients, and patients with septic shock in particular, should be given **DVT prophylaxis** with compression stockings or an intermittent compression device along with either unfractionated or low-molecular-weight heparin unless contraindicated. Stress-ulcer prophylaxis should be provided using an H_2 blocker or a proton-pump inhibitor.

Because the mortality associated with severe sepsis and septic shock can be more than 30% to 40% and increases as the number of organs involved increases, it is prudent to discuss advance care planning with the patient, family, or surrogate decision-maker. (See Tables 8-6 and 8-7 and Box 8-3.)

Disseminated Intravascular Coagulation

Disseminated intravascular coagulation (DIC) is a complex set of signs and symptoms that arise as a complication of another serious disease. Examples of conditions that have been known to trigger DIC include hemorrhagic shock and sepsis (especially gram-negative organisms). See Box 8-4 for common causes of DIC. Called also *consumptive coagulopathy*,

Table 8-6 Vasopressors and Inotropes

Medication	Dose	Contractility	Heart Rate	Vasoconstriction	Vasodilation
Dobutamine	2-20 mcg/kg/min	3-4+	1-2+	0	2+
Dopamine	1-4 mcg/kg/min	1+	1+	0	1+
	4-20 mcg/kg/min	2-3+	2+	2-3+	0
Epinephrine	1-20 mcg/min	4+	4+	4+	3+
Isoproterenol	1-5 mcg/min	4+	4+	0	4+
Milrinone	0.125-0.5 mcg/kg/min	4+	0	0	3+
Norepinephrine	2-40 mcg/min	2+	1+	4+	0
Phenylephrine	20-200 mcg/min	0	0	3+	0
Vasopressin	0.01-0.04 units/min	0	0	4+	0

Table 8-7 Estimating Predicted Body Weight

Height		Predicted Body Weight
Males	cm	50 + 0.91 (height in cm – 152.4)
	inches	50 + 2.3 (height in inches – 60)
Females	cm	45.5 + 0.91 (height in cm – 152.4)
	inches	45.5 + 2.3 (height in inches – 60)

Box 8-3 Ideal Body Weight Calculation

Females: 105 lb + 5 × (Height in inches – 60)
Males: 105 lb + 6 × (Height in inches – 60)
Example: Ideal body weight for a 6-foot male (72 inches)

105 lb + 6 × (72 – 60)
105 + (6 × 12)
105 + 72 = 177 lb (80.5 kg).

Box 8-4 Common Causes of DIC

Obstetric Complications

Toxemia
Abruptio placentae
Retained dead fetus
Septic abortion
Amniotic fluid embolism

Infections

Gram-negative sepsis
Meningococcemia
Rocky Mountain spotted fever
Histoplasmosis
Aspergillosis
Malaria

Massive Tissue Injury

Extensive surgery
Burns
Trauma

Neoplasms

Cancer of pancreas, prostate, lung, stomach
Acute promyelocytic leukemia

Others

Snakebite
Shock
Heat stroke
Aortic aneurysm

Modified from Urden L, Stacy KM, Lough ME: *Thelan's critical care nursing: diagnosis and management*, ed 5, St. Louis, 2006, Mosby.
DIC, Disseminated intravascular coagulation.

DIC can present in two unique ways: excessive bleeding or excessive clotting.

The coagulation cascade, which can be associated with an inflammatory response, was described earlier in this chapter.. Direct damage to endothelial layers with release of TNF activates the coagulation cascade. DIC develops when a secondary release of thrombin formation occurs and the delicate balance of hemostasis is tipped. Coagulation factors are rapidly consumed with depletion of proteins C and S and antithrombin. Clots will then form in the damaged endothelial walls, and distal tissue ischemia results with occlusion of the vessels. This secondary tissue damage stimulates another round of cascade release and subsequent worsening of the condition (**negative feedback loop**). This triggers both anticoagulant release and the fibrinolytic system to activate and break apart all the clots disseminated. This may then result in excessive bleeding.

With too much clotting or too much bleeding secondary to a serious illness, resuscitation will be needed. That is the presentation of DIC in a broad sense. Too much clotting will create cyanotic fingers, toes, ears, and nose. As this progresses, central cyanosis appears along with respiratory failure, acute tubular necrosis in the kidneys, bowel infarctions, and stroke. Too much bleeding commences as the fibrinolysis process begins. All IV and other puncture sites in the skin will bleed. Ecchymotic areas will appear on the skin wherever pressure is applied (e.g., blood pressure, body position). Blood may appear within the urinary and pleural drainage systems.

Management of this serious complication includes two goals: maintain organ perfusion and slow the consumption of the clotting factors. MODS frequently results from this complication. Use of IV fluids, inotropic agents, infusion of blood products (packed RBCs, platelets, plasma) can help maintain organ perfusion. Administration of cryoprecipitate and fresh frozen plasma may help replenish clotting factors. Inhibiting clot formation with use of heparin is controversial because use of this drug in patients who present with DIC is contraindicated (e.g., patients who have had surgery or experienced trauma). It may be helpful in the obstetric patient. Administration of aminocaproic acid (Amicar) may also benefit the patient who is clotting. Recombinant human protein C has been discussed in the treatment of SIRS but is contraindicated for patients with DIC who present with severe sepsis.

Multisystem Organ Dysfunction Syndrome

Multisystem organ dysfunction syndrome (MODS) is defined as the presence of altered organ function in an acutely ill patient that requires intervention to maintain homeostasis. Either a systemic infection or a systemic inflammation (shock) has triggered a series of events and two cascades that are overwhelming the body's tissues. Organ dysfunction will eventually lead to organ failure and subsequently death. MODS will occur during severe sepsis if not treated promptly.

MODS is a leading cause of mortality in surgical intensive care units. Mortality will increase in patients to 54% with two failing organ systems and to 100% mortality with five failing organ systems. Furthermore, mortality rates have not improved much over the past 15 to 20 years. There are primary and secondary mediators that cause activation of both the complement and coagulation cascades and produce prostaglandins and leukotrienes that create tissue and organ damage. MODS occurs when this catastrophe creates an indirect effect that is undesirable—something to be prevented, and if not possible, at least recognized early and aggressively managed. Although the term *organ failure* alludes to a terminal event, some organs may be salvaged if the patient survives. The paradox in this phenomenon is that the organs that show dysfunction were not damaged or infected in the original insult or injury. Figure 8-5 describes the pathogenesis of MODS.

Primary and Secondary MODS

1. **Primary MODS** is a relatively rare syndrome in which an organ is injured directly through an inflammatory process; this relates to a small percentage of MODS cases. Some examples include respiratory failure after a pulmonary contusion or aspiration events, burns, or acute tubular necrosis in the kidneys. Primary MODS cannot be detected clinically. Primary MODS has three possible outcomes: patients may recover without experiencing an inflammatory response or have a limited systemic inflammatory response (SIRS) and then recover or die.
2. **Secondary MODS** is the physiologic failure of two or more organs that were not initially affected by the original infectious or noninfectious insult that triggered SIRS. Exactly how secondary MODS progresses is still being questioned; one theory suggests the progression of this stage occurs in a cumulative pattern, starting with the lungs, which are considered to be the most commonly affected organs, followed by the liver, the abdominal region, and ending in the kidneys. As secondary MODS develops into a late stage, bone marrow dysfunction may develop and eventually cardiac arrest can occur. Some of the specific signs and symptoms are described in Box 8-5.

Scenario Conclusion

The patient with remote organ failure, secondary to severe shock and major surgery, is being readied for transport. The patient's chest radiograph shows the white, fluffy appearance of ARDS; ventilator settings are at 100% oxygen; positive end-expiratory pressure (PEEP), 10 cm H_2O; tidal volume of 10 mL/kg; and respiratory rate at 10. The patient is administered a sedative and long-acting paralytic for the short-term facilitation of ventilation during the trip. You dial in pressure support on your ventilator. The patient's perfusion is being supported by two vasoactive agents: dopamine and phenylephrine. Urinary output is diminished, despite aggressive fluid resuscitation, and the patient's creatinine is 3.1. Blood chemistries show elevated liver enzymes and a lactate at 3.5 mmol/L.

The patient is successfully transported to the resource hospital where alternative methods for ventilation in ARDS are implemented, and continuous dialysis is initiated. Despite intense therapy for the patient's MODS, he succumbs to his illness 5 days later.

SUMMARY

- A delicate balance exists in our body.
- There are certainly benefits to an active immune system and the local and systemic inflammation that can result when tissues have been damaged or a foreign invader enters. A controlled mild to moderate response is appropriate and beneficial. But there are detrimental effects of this same response when severe SIRS initiates a cascade of events that can create organ failure and kill the host.
- Bacterial and nonbacterial products initiate primary and secondary mediators that activate both the complement and coagulation cascades, along with production of prostaglandins and leukotrienes.
- When SIRS appears, an inflammation exists, not necessarily an infection. A lack of balance is the ultimate result—inflammation vs. antiinflammation; coagulation vs. fibrinolysis.
- As the healthcare industry continues to progress toward the improved and successful resuscitation of a tissue crisis (medical and surgical), early recognition and goal-directed therapy toward suppressing the imbalance created in the body during the resuscitation must also improve. Efforts are proving to be more effective, but ongoing research is needed to find the best approach to the crisis.

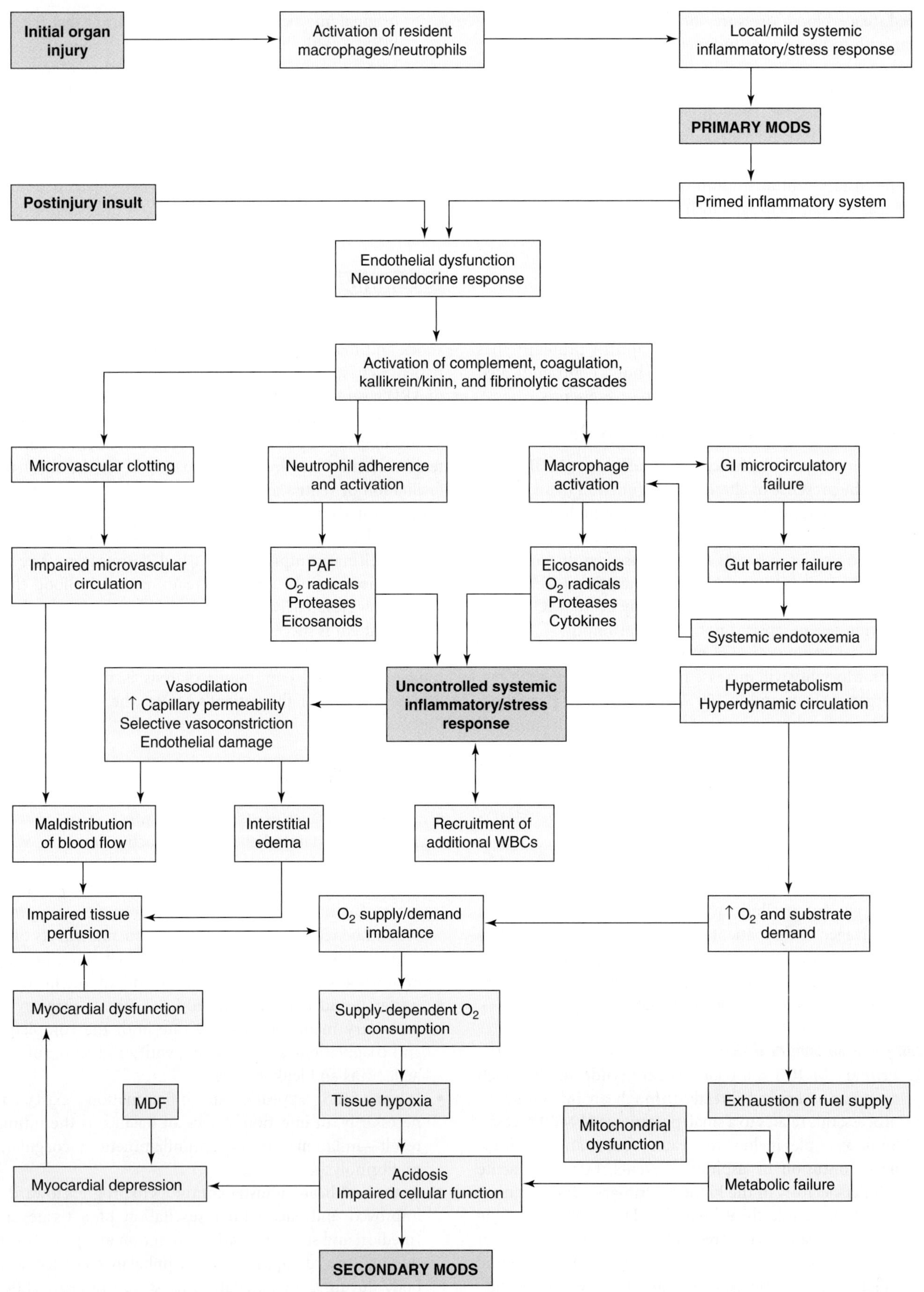

Figure 8-5

Pathogenesis of multiple organ dysfunction syndrome. *MODS*, Multiple organ dysfunction syndrome; *GI*, gastrointestinal; *PAF*, platelet activating factor; *WBCs*, white blood cells; *MDF*, myocardial depressant factor. (From McCance KL, Huether SE: *Pathophysiology*, ed 5, St. Louis, 2006, Mosby.)

Box 8-5 Clinical Manifestations of Organ Dysfunction

Gastrointestinal

Abdominal distention
Intolerance to enteral feedings
Paralytic ileus
Upper/lower GI bleeding
Diarrhea
Ischemic colitis
Mucosal ulceration
Decreased bowel sounds
Bacterial overgrowth in stool

Liver

Jaundice
Increased serum bilirubin (hyperbilirubinemia)
Increased serum ammonia
Decreased serum albumin
Decreased serum transferrin

Gallbladder

Right upper quadrant tenderness/pain
Abdominal distention
Unexplained fever
Decreased bowel sounds

Metabolic/Nutritional

Decreased lean body mass
Muscle wasting
Severe weight loss
Negative nitrogen balance
Hyperglycemia
Hypertriglyceridemia
Increased serum lactate
Decreased serum albumin, serum transferrin, prealbumin
Decreased retinol-binding protein

Immune

Infection
Decreased lymphocyte count
Anergy

Pulmonary

Tachypnea
ARDS pattern of respiratory failure (dyspnea, patchy infiltrates, refractory hypoxemia, respiratory acidosis, abnormal O_2 indexes)
Pulmonary hypertension

Renal

Increased serum creatinine, BUN levels
Oliguria, anuria, or polyuria consistent with prerenal azotemia or acute tubular necrosis
Urinary indexes consistent with prerenal azotemia or acute tubular necrosis

Cardiovascular

Hyperdynamic

Decreased pulmonary capillary occlusion pressure
Decreased systemic vascular resistance
Decreased right atrial pressure
Decreased left ventricular stroke work index
Increased oxygen consumption
Increased cardiac output, cardiac index, heart rate

Hypodynamic

Increased systemic vascular resistance
Increased right atrial pressure
Increased left ventricular stroke work index
Decreased oxygen delivery and consumption
Decreased cardiac output and cardiac index

Central Nervous System

Lethargy
Altered level of consciousness
Fever
Hepatic encephalopathy

Coagulation/Hematologic

Thrombocytopenia
DIC pattern

ARDS, Acute respiratory distress syndrome; *BUN*, blood urea nitrogen; *DIC*, disseminated intravascular coagulation; *GI*, gastrointestinal.
From Urden L, Stack KM, Lough ME: *Thelan's critical care nursing: diagnosis and management*, ed 5, St. Louis, 2006, Mosby.

KEY TERMS

adaptive immune system One of two pathways toward immunity, this system can stop or prevent challenges to the system and is initiated by the evolutionary innate system. Eventually, this system adapts the immune response through memory B and T cells.

adaptive immunity Passive immunity of the cell-mediated type conferred by the administration of sensitized lymphocytes from an immune donor.

aminotransferase (also called *transaminase*) A sub-subclass of enzymes of the transferase class that catalyze the transfer of an amino group from a donor to an acceptor.

antigen Any substance capable, under appropriate conditions, of inducing a specific immune response and of reacting with the products of that response, that is, with specific antibody or specifically sensitized T lymphocytes , or both. Antigens may be soluble substances, such as toxins and foreign proteins, or particulates, such as bacteria and tissue cells.

antigen-antibody complex The complex formed by the noncovalent binding of an antibody and an antigen; complexes of antibodies belonging to certain immunoglobulin classes may activate complement.

antiinflammatory cytokine A type of cytokine that counteracts or suppresses inflammation.

APACHE score Acute Physiology, Age, and Chronic Health Evaluation. This is a system for classifying patients in the intensive care unit. Patients are evaluated by physiologic scores in 8 classes (cardiovascular, respiratory, renal, GI, hematologic, septic, metabolic, and neurologic) with 34 variables. The evaluation is completed in the first 32 hours after admission to the ICU and is a reliable predictor of patient outcomes.

azotemia An excess of urea or other nitrogenous compounds in the blood; also called *uremia.*

band A late metamyelocyte in which the nucleus is in the form of a curved or coiled band, not having acquired the typical multilobar shape of the mature polymorphonuclear neutrophil. Called also *band form* or *neutrophil, rod neutrophil.*

cachexia A profound and marked state of constitutional disorder; general ill health and malnutrition.

coagulation cascade The series of steps that begins with activation of the intrinsic or extrinsic pathways of coagulation, or of one of the related alternative pathways, and proceeds through the common pathway of coagulation to the formation of the fibrin clot; each step is catalyzed by the activated zymogen.

coagulopathy Any disorder of blood coagulation; called also *bleeding disorder.*

complement A group of enzymes in the bloodstream; the term originally used to refer to the heat-labile factor in serum that causes immune cytolysis, the lysis of antibody-coated cells.

complement cascade Activation of a series of events in which activation can occur by two different sequences—classic and alternative pathways—with cell lysis being the goal.

complement system The functionally related system of complement, comprising at least 20 distinct serum proteins (C1 through C9 with fragments), their cellular receptors, and related regulatory proteins that is the effector not only of immune cytolysis but also of other biologic functions including anaphylaxis, phagocytosis, opsonization, and hemolysis.

cytokine A generic term for nonantibody proteins released by one cell population (primed T lymphocytes) upon contact with a specific antigen, which act as intercellular mediators, as in the generation of an immune response. Examples include lymphokines and monokines.

cytotoxic T-cell (CTL) Differentiated T lymphocyte that can recognize and lyse target cells bearing specific antigens recognized by their antigen receptors.

degranulate Release of the contents of secretory granules from the cell by fusion with the plasma membrane.

disseminated intravascular coagulation (DIC) (also known as *diffuse intravascular coagulation*). A bleeding disorder (coagulopathy) resulting from overstimulation of clotting and anticlotting processes in response to disease or injury such as septicemia; it is characterized by abnormal reduction of the elements involved in blood clotting.

DVT prophylaxis (deep vein thrombosis or deep venous thrombosis). A therapy intended to prevent clot formation; may include both pharmacologic and nonpharmacologic strategies.

dysoxia Difficulty in oxygenating cells, tissues, and organs.

endothelium The layer of epithelial cells that lines the cavities of the heart, the lumina of blood and lymph vessels, and the serous cavities of the body; it originates from the mesoderm.

endotoxins Heat-stable toxins associated with the outer membranes of certain gram-negative bacteria, including the brucellae, the enterobacteria, neisseriae, and vibrios. Endotoxins are not secreted but are released only when the cells are disrupted; they are less potent and less specific than the exotoxins; and they do not form toxoids. They are composed of complex lipopolysaccharide molecules, of which the polysaccharide unit (somatic O antigen) is responsible for antigenicity, occurring in hundreds of variations, and the phospholipid moiety (lipid A) is the source of toxicity. When injected in large quantities, the endotoxins produce hemorrhagic shock and severe diarrhea; smaller amounts cause fever, altered resistance to bacterial infection, leukopenia followed by leukocytosis, and numerous other biologic effects.

enteral Within the small intestine.

exotoxins Toxic substances formed by species of certain bacteria (e.g., *Bacillus, Bordetella, Clostridium, Corynebacterium, Escherichia, Pseudomonas, Salmonella, Shigella, Staphylococcus, Streptococcus, Vibrio, Yersinia)* that are found outside the bacterial cell or are freely present in the culture medium. Exotoxins are protein in nature and heat-labile; they are detoxified with retention of antigenicity by treatment with formaldehyde (formol toxoid), and are the most poisonous substances known to humans.

factor VII (coagulation factor VII or proconvertin). A heat- and storage-stable factor participating in the extrinsic pathway of coagulation. It is activated by contact with calcium, and, in concert with factor III (tissue thromboplastin), activates factor X. Deficiency of this factor, which may be hereditary (autosomal recessive) or acquired (associated with vitamin K deficiency), results in a hemorrhagic tendency. Called also *serum prothrombin conversion accelerator* (SPCA) and *stable f.* The activated form is also called *convertin.*

feedback loop To help maintain homeostasis, the body uses sensors and effectors to control systems in response to disturbances. Information from the body's sensors feeds information back to a control center where effectors make changes.

gram negative Describes a bacterium that loses stain or is decolorized by alcohol when subjected to the Gram method of staining; a primary characteristic of bacteria that have a cell wall composed of a thin layer of peptidoglycan covered by an outer membrane of lipoprotein and lipopolysaccharide.

gram positive Describes a bacterium that retains stain or resists decolorization by alcohol when subjected to the Gram method of staining; a primary characteristic of bacteria that have a cell wall composed of a thick layer of peptidoglycan with attached teichoic acids.

helper T-cells (helper T-1s, T-4 cells [CD4]) Major regulatory cells that secrete interleukin-2 (IL-2), which stimulates the activity of B cells and other T lymphocytes. These are the primary cells attacked by HIV in AIDS.

humoral (1) Pertaining to elements dissolved in the blood or body fluids (e.g., humoral immunity from antibodies in the blood as opposed to cellular immunity). (2) Pertaining to one of the humors of the body or to humoralism.

hyperbilirubinemia Excessive bilirubin in the blood, which may lead to jaundice; the hyperbilirubinemias are classified as either *conjugated* or *unconjugated*, according to the predominant form of bilirubin involved.

hypercirculatory Characterized by elevated rate, pressure, pumping functions of the circulatory system.

hyperdynamic Pertaining to or characterized by hyperdynamia; hyperactivity.

immune system A system designed to protect the body against infectious diseases by either specific or nonspecific mechanisms.

immunoglobulins Any of the structurally related glycoproteins that function as antibodies, divided into five classes (IgM, IgG, IgA, IgD, and IgE) on the basis of structure and biologic activity. The basic structural unit of the immunoglobulin molecule, referred to as a *monomer,* is a Y-shaped molecule composed of two heavy (H) chains and two light (L) chains. IgD, IgG, and IgE occur only as monomers; IgM and IgA may occur as monomers or polymers. The polymeric forms contain an additional polypeptide called the *component* (SC). Immunoglobulins (monomeric IgM and IgD) first appear on the surface of B cells as antigen receptors. When a cell is activated by contact with antigen and differentiates into a plasma cell, the cell continues to produce the same arrangements and chains but gene rearrangement may occur; thus the secreted immunoglobulin may be of any class but has the same antigenic specificity as the antigen receptors of the parent B cell. In addition to the effects produced solely by the binding of antigen by antibody, for example, viral neutralization or the inability of some bacteria to invade mucosal surfaces when coated by antibody, certain classes of antibodies can trigger other processes when bound to antigen: IgM and IgG activate the classic complement pathway; IgA and IgG3 act as opsonins, triggering phagocytosis of the bound antigens by macrophages and neutrophils. IgE has the unique function of mediating immediate hypersensitivity reactions; it binds to specific receptors on basophils and mast cells and triggers the release of mediators on contact with antigen. IgG is the only class transferred across the placenta, providing the fetus and neonate with protection against infection.

inflammation A localized protective response elicited by injury or destruction of tissues, which serves to destroy, dilute, or wall off (sequester) both the injurious agent and the injured tissue. It is characterized in the acute form by classic signs of pain, heat, redness, swelling, and loss of function. Histologically, it involves a complex series of events, including dilation of arterioles, capillaries, and venules, with increased permeability and blood flow; exudation of fluids, including plasma proteins; and leukocytic migration into the inflammatory focus.

innate immune system A generic and immediate response to pathogens that is derived through human evolution. Initiation of this immune response activates the complement cascade.

innate immunity Immunity based on the genetic constitution of the individual, (e.g., immunity of humans to canine distemper). Called also *familial i., genetic i., inherent i., inherited i.,* and *native i.*

interleukin-1-beta (IL-1-β) A lymphokine produced by antigen- or mitogen-activated T cells; its principal role is regulation of IgE- and eosinophil-mediated immune reactions. It stimulates switching of B cells, particularly TH_2 cells; is a growth factor for mast cells; and stimulates the expression of some adhesion molecules on endothelial cells. Formerly called *B lymphocyte stimulatory factor 1.*

interleukins A generic term for a group of multifunctional cytokines that are produced by a variety of lymphoid and nonlymphoid cells and have effects at least partly within the lymphopoietic system; originally believed to be produced chiefly by and to act chiefly upon leukocytes.

leukocytosis A transient increase in the number of leukocytes in the blood; seen normally with strenuous exercise and pathologically accompanying hemorrhage, fever, infection, or inflammation.

leukocytosis with left shift If the laboratory reports leukocytosis with greater than 10% *bands* (immature neutrophil cells), a left shift is demonstrated. This indicates that the bone marrow is generating many neutrophils in the setting of an acute infection.

leukopenia Reduction in the number of leukocytes in the blood below about 4000/mm^3. Types are named for the type of cell, such as *agranulocytosis* and *neutropenia;* may also be called *aleukia, aleukocytosis,* and *leukocytopenia.*

local inflammation Focal; an infection confined to a single spot or to a few limited spots.

lymphocyte Any of the mononuclear, nonphagocytic leukocytes found in the blood, lymph, and lymphoid tissues; these are the body's immunologically competent cells and their precursors. They are divided on the basis of ontogeny and function into two classes, B and T lymphocytes, responsible for humoral and cellular immunity; characteristically they have a round or slightly indented heterochromatic nucleus that almost fills the cell and a thin rim of basophilic cytoplasm that contains few granules. When activated by contact with antigen, small lymphocytes begin macromolecular synthesis, the cytoplasm enlarges until the cells are 10 to 30 μm in diameter, and the nucleus becomes less completely heterochromatic; they are then referred to as *large lymphocytes* or *lymphoblasts*. These cells then proliferate and differentiate into B and T memory cells and into the various effector cell types—B lymphocytes into plasma cells and T cells into helper, cytotoxic, and suppressor cells.

macrophages Any of the many forms of mononuclear phagocytes found in tissues. They arise from hematopoietic stem cells in the bone marrow, which develop according to the stages of the monocytic series until they are monocytes; these then enter the blood, circulate for about 30 hours, and subsequently enter tissues, where they increase in size, phagocytic activity, and lysosomal enzyme content to become macrophages. Two types, *fixed macrophages* and *free macrophages* are distinguished.

multiorgan dysfunction syndrome (MODS) Clinical syndrome of progressive physiologic dysfunction or failure (absolute or relative) of two or more separate organ systems; the presence of altered organ function in an acutely ill patient such that homeostasis cannot be maintained without medical support. Also known as *systemic inflammatory response syndrome (SIRS).*

negative feedback loop Those communication loops that oppose or negate a change in conditions, hopefully back to normal. Example: increased muscle activity creates a lack of oxygen, therefore creating an increase in the respiratory effort to increase oxygen.

nuclear factor-kappa-beta (NF-κ-β) A protein complex that is involved in cellular response to cytokines, antigens, free radicals, and stress.

neutropenic A decrease in the number of neutrophils in the blood.

neutrophil A mature granular leukocyte that is polymorphonuclear (the nucleus has three to five lobes connected by slender threads of chromatin and the cytoplasm contains fine granules); neutrophils have the properties of chemotaxis, adherence to immune complexes, and phagocytosis. Also called *neutrocyte* and *neutrophilic leukocyte.*

parenteral A route of injection that does not make use of the alimentary canal (GI tract); includes subcutaneous, intramuscular, intraorbital, intracapsular, intraspinal, intrasternal, or intravenous routes.

pathogen Any disease-producing agent or microorganism, such as a bacterium, fungus, protozoon, or virus.

positive feedback loop Those loops of communication that enhance a process or stimulate it. An ever-increasing rate of events occurs until something stops the process. Examples include the clotting process involving platelet aggregation and labor contractions while giving birth.

primary MODS Direct trauma to the organ system that causes progressive dysfunction (e.g., pulmonary contusion creating acute respiratory dysfunction syndrome [ARDS] or acute lung injury [ALI]).

pro-inflammatory cytokine A type of cytokine that is capable of stimulating inflammation.

recombinant human activated protein C (rhAPC) Recombinant refers to a new entity (e.g., gene, protein, cell) that results from genetic recombination. Activated protein C exerts an antithrombotic effect by inhibiting factors Va and VIIIa and may have indirect profibrinolytic activity through its ability to inhibit plasminogen activator inhibitor-1 and may exert an antiinflammatory effect by limiting the chemotactic response of leukocytes to inflammatory cytokines. This agent may also reduce interactions between leukocytes and the microvascular endothelium. Developed as drotrecogin alfa (activated) (brand name *Xigris; Eli Lilly*), this pharmaceutical is given via IV to ICU patients for the reduction of mortality in adult patients with severe sepsis with high risk of death (MODS, SIRS).

secondary MODS A latent development of organ dysfunction from a systemic inflammatory response (SIRS). The organs affected are not involved in the initial insult.

sepsis The presence in the blood or other tissues of pathogenic microorganisms or their toxins; *septicemia.*

septicemia Systemic disease associated with the presence and persistence of pathogenic microorganisms or their toxins in the blood. Called also *blood poisoning* and *sepsis.*

suppressor T cells (also called T-8 cells [CD8]) These cells stop a specific immune response after several days and create memory cells.

systemic inflammation Diffuse inflammation; an infection spread over a large area.

systemic inflammatory response syndrome (SIRS) Pertaining to or affecting the body as a whole; a cascade of immune response events that leads to tissue destruction.

T cells Primarily responsible for cell-mediated immunity; they originate from lymphoid stem cells that migrate from the bone marrow to the thymus and differentiate under the influence of the thymic hormones thymopoietin and thymosin.

thrombocytopenia Decrease in the number of platelets, such as in thrombocytopenic purpura.

tissue factor Tissue thromboplastin: a lipoprotein functioning in the extrinsic pathway of coagulation, activating factor X. Also known as *coagulation factor III* and *tissue f.*

toll-like receptors Protein receptors involved as part of the innate immune system that recognize microbes and initiate a response.

tumor necrosis factor-alpha (TNF-α) Produced primarily by macrophages in response to infection with gram-negative bacteria; this cytokine facilitates inflammation by causing the vascular endothelium to become stickier, which results in increased adherence of neutrophils from the vessels. TNF acts directly on the brain to induce fever, on the liver to produce plasma proteins; in high doses, creates MODS and death.

Bibliography

Abbas AK: *Basic immunology: functions and disorders of the immune system*, ed 3, St. Louis, 2008, Saunders.

Abbas AK, Murphy KM, Sher A: Functional diversity of helper T lymphocytes, *Nature* 383:787-793, 1996.

Abraham E, Laterre PF, Garg R, et al: Drotrecogin alfa (activated) for adults with severe sepsis and a low risk of death, *N Engl J Med* 353:1332-1341, 2005.

Acute Respiratory Distress Syndrome Network: Ventilation with lower tidal volumes as compared with traditional tidal volumes for acute lung injury and the acute respiratory distress syndrome, *N Engl J Med* 342:1301-1308, 2000.

Aird WC: Vascular bed-specific hemostasis: role of endothelium in sepsis pathogenesis, *Crit Care Med* 29(7 Suppl):S28-S34, 2001.

Angus DC, Linde-Zwirble WT, Lidicker J, et al: Epidemiology of severe sepsis in the United States: analysis of incidence, outcome, and associated costs of care, *Crit Care Med* 29:1303-1310, 2001.

Annane D, Sebille V, Charpentier C, et al: Effect of treatment with low doses of hydrocortisone and fludrocortisone on mortality in patients with septic shock, *JAMA* 288:862-871, 2002.

Bernard GR, Vincent JL, Laterre PF, et al: Efficacy and safety of recombinant human activated protein C for severe sepsis, *N Engl J Med* 344:699-709, 2001.

Blumen IJ, Abernathy MK, Dunne MJ: Flight physiology: clinical considerations, *Crit Care Clin* 8:597-618, 1992.

Bone RC, Balk RA, Cerra FB, et al: Definitions for sepsis and organ failure and guidelines for the use of innovative therapies in sepsis, The ACCP/SCCM Consensus Conference Committee, American College of Chest Physicians/Society of Critical Care Medicine, *Chest* 101:1644-1655, 1992.

Braman SS, Dunn SM, Amico CA, et al: Complications of intra hospital transport in critically ill patients, *Ann Intern Med* 107:469-473, 1987.

Cunha BA: Sepsis and its mimics, *Intern Med* 13:48-55, 1992.

Dellinger RP, Levy MM, Carlet JM, et al: Surviving Sepsis Campaign: international guidelines for management of severe sepsis and septic shock, *Intensive Care Med* 34:17-60, 2008.

Dorland's Illustrated Medical Dictionary, ed 31, Philadelphia, 2007, Saunders.

Drake TA, Cheng J, Chang A, et al: Expression of tissue factor, thrombomodulin, and E-selectin in baboons with lethal *Escherichia coli* sepsis, *Am J Pathol* 142:1458-1470, 1993.

Friedman G, Silva E, Vincent JL: Has the mortality of septic shock changed with time? *Crit Care Med* 26:2078, 1998.

Grinnell BW, Joyce D: Recombinant human activated protein C: a system modulator of vascular function for treatment of severe sepsis, *Crit Care Med* 29(7 Suppl):S53-S60, 2001.

Hébert PC, Wells G, Blajchman MA, et al. A multicenter, randomized, controlled clinical trial of transfusion requirements in critical care, *N Engl J Med* 340:409-417, 1993.

Kaiser ML, Wilson SE: Intra-abdominal surgical infections and their mimics in the critical care unit. In Cunha BA, editor: *Infectious disease in critical care medicine*, New York, 2007, Informa Healthcare, pp. 291-304.

Kumar A, Roberts D, Wood KE, et al: Duration of hypotension prior to initiation of effective antimicrobial therapy is the critical determinant of survival in human septic shock, *Crit Care Med* 34:1589-1596, 2006.

Kumar A, Thota V, Dee L, et al: Tumor necrosis factor-α and interleukin-1-β are responsible for depression of in vitro myocardial cell contractility induced by serum from humans with septic shock, *J Exp Med* 183:949-958, 1996.

Lever A, Mackenzie I: Sepsis: definition, epidemiology, and diagnosis, *BMJ* 335:879-883, 2007.

Luster AD: Chemokines: chemotactic cytokines that mediate inflammation, *N Engl J Med* 338:436, 1998.

Mallamaci F, Zocali C, Parlongo S, et al: Diagnostic value of troponin T for alterations in left ventricular mass and function in dialysis patients, *Kidney Int* 62:1884-1890, 2002.

McCance KL, Huether SE: *Pathophysiology: the biologic basis for disease in adults and children*, ed 5, St. Louis, 2005, Mosby.

Minimum standards for transport of critically ill patients, Australasian College for Emergency Medicine Policy Document, *Emerg Med* 15:197-201, 2003.

Martin GS, Mannino DM, Eaton S, et al: The epidemiology of sepsis in the United States from 1979 through 2000, *N Engl J Med* 348:1546-1554, 2003.

O'Brien JM Jr, Ali NA, Aberegg SK, et al: Sepsis. *Am J Med* 120:1012-1022, 2007.

Olson CM, Jastremski MS,Vilogi JP, et al: Stabilization of patients prior to inter hospital transport, *Am J Emerg Med* 5:33-39, 1987.

Osterud B, Flaegstad T: Increased tissue thromboplastin activity in monocytes of patients with meningococcal infection: related to an unfavourable prognosis, *Thromb Haemost* 49:5-7, 1983.

Parillo JE, Burch C, Shelhamer JH, et al: A circulating myocardial depressant substance in humans with septic shock: septic shock patients with a reduced ejection fraction have a circulating factor that depresses in vitro myocardial cell performance, *J Clin Invest* 76:1539-1553, 1985.

Parker MM, Shelhamer JH, Bacharach SL, et al: Profound but reversible myocardial depression in patients with septic shock, *Ann Intern Med* 100:483-490, 1984.

Pridmore AC, Wyllie DH, Abdillahi F, et al: A lipopolysaccharide-deficient mutant of *Neisseria meningitidis* elicits attenuated cytokine release by human macrophages and signals via toll-like receptor (TLR)2 but not via TLR4/MD2, *J Infect Dis* 183:89, 2001.

Recommendations on the transport of critically ill patient, SIAARTI Study Group for Safety in Anesthesia and Intensive Care, *Minerva Anestesiol* 72: XXXVII-LVII, 2006.

Rivers E, Nguyen B, Havstad S, et al: Early goal-directed therapy in the treatment of severe sepsis and septic shock, *N Engl J Med* 345:1368-1377, 2001.

Sands KE, Bates DW, Lanken PN, et al: Epidemiology of sepsis syndrome in eight academic medical centers, *JAMA* 278:234, 1997.

Smith I, Fleming S, Cerniana A: Mishaps during transport from the intensive care unit, *Crit Care Med* 18:278-281, 1990.

St. Andrá AC, Del Rossi A: Hemodynamic management of patients in the first 24 hours after cardiac surgery, *Crit Care Med* 33:2082-2093, 2005.

Thibodeau G, Patton K: *The human body in health & disease*, ed 4, St. Louis, 2010, Mosby.

Todoroki H, Nakamura S, Higure A, et al: Neutrophils express tissue factor in a monkey model of sepsis, *Surgery* 127:209-216, 2000.

Underhill DM, Ozinsky A: Toll-like receptors: key mediators of microbe detection, *Curr Opin Immunol* 14:103-110, 2002.

Urden L, Stacy K, Lough M: *Thelan's critical care nursing: diagnosis and management*, ed 5, St. Louis, 2006, Mosby.

Van den Berghe G, Wouters P, Weekers F, et al: Intensive insulin therapy in critically ill patients, *N Engl J Med* 345:1359-1367, 2001.

Warren J, Fromm ER, Orr RA, et al: American College of Critical Care Medicine guidelines for the inter- and intra-hospital transport of critically ill patients, *Crit Care Med* 32:256-262, 2004.

Wiedemann HP, Wheeler AP, Bernard GR, et al: Comparison of two fluid management strategies in acute lung injury, *N Engl J Med* 354:2564-2575, 2006.

REVIEW QUESTIONS

1. In the case study at the beginning of this chapter, the initial assessment, recognition, and resuscitation of shock seemed to generate a recovery in your trauma patient. What syndrome developed that prompted a transfer to a higher level ICU?
   A. Primary MODS
   B. Secondary MODS
   C. Local inflammatory response
   D. Cushing's disease
2. There is usually a paradox that occurs in MODS. Choose the best description of this paradox.
   A. Once the organ shows early signs of failure, nothing can save it.
   B. Even though signs of organ failure may be evident, all organs will recover.
   C. The organs that fail are remote from the original tissue damage.
   D. Those that are healthiest are at most risk for developing MODS.
3. The two cascades initiated by SIRS are:
   A. Complement and coagulation
   B. Complement and anticoagulation
   C. Coagulation and anticoagulation
   D. Coagulation and antigen-antibody
4. Sepsis is:
   A. A local inflammation
   B. The inflammatory response with clinical signs of infection
   C. A sign of MODS
   D. The presence of pathogens (or their toxins) in the blood
5. B cells are:
   A. Immunoglobulins that recognize antigens for the immune system
   B. Lymphocytes that stimulate production of immunoglobulins
   C. Monocytes that remember past antigens for quick lysis
   D. Lymphocytes that suppress the immune response
6. T cells are:
   A. Immunoglobulins that recognize the antigen-antibody complex and target it for lysis
   B. Lymphocytes that place tags on the foreign pathogen for future immune responses
   C. Lymphocytes that stimulate production of B cells, lyse the marked antigens, then slow the immune response
   D. Cytokines that function as messengers among the white cells and complement system
7. Cytokines are:
   A. T cells that either identify and kill the antigen or suppress the response
   B. Messengers that promote the inflammatory response (such as TNF-α).
   C. Messengers that can fight against an inflammatory response (such as IL-10)
   D. B and C are both examples of cytokines
8. An infection that creates a drop in blood pressure (hypoperfusion) despite fluid resuscitation is termed:
   A. Severe sepsis
   B. Systemic inflammatory response syndrome
   C. Multiple organ dysfunction syndrome
   D. Septic shock
9. After a latent recovery period and discharge from the ICU, a multisystem trauma patient develops quiet tachypnea, (with respiratory alkalosis), tachycardia, slightly elevated blood pressure with a temperature of 35° C (95° F). This patient may be suffering from:
   A. Acute coronary syndrome
   B. Pneumonia
   C. Systemic inflammatory response syndrome
   D. Septic shock
10. Certain patients are at risk for developing sepsis. They include:
    A. The very young, very old, and those non-Caucasians
    B. The elderly and those who have received blood transfusions
    C. The very young and those who have a central line placed
    D. Females, the very young, and those with peripheral IVs

11. A hemostatic imbalance may occur with SIRS. This may include:
    A. Tissue necrosis factor 1 (TNF-1) coming into contact with blood and activation of factor VII
    B. DIC, leading to consumption of coagulation factors that leads to bleeding
    C. A coagulation cascade that is activated by thrombin
    D. A, B, and C all describe this imbalance
12. The objective of early sepsis therapy is:
    A. Source identification and control
    B. Appropriate antimicrobial therapy
    C. Ensuring adequate perfusion
    D. A, B, and C are all goals in the treatment of sepsis
13. A goal in the treatment of septic shock is:
    A. Maintaining urinary output at greater than 2 mL/kg/hr
    B. Achieving a mean arterial pressure (MAP) of greater than 65 mm Hg
    C. Maintaining a mixed venous oxygen saturation (SvO_2) at greater than 100%
    D. A, B, and C are all goals in septic shock therapy
14. A treatment plan for septic shock might include:
    A. Fluid therapy only; boluses of 20 mL/kg should be considered
    B. Fluids and vasopressor therapy
    C. Vasopressor therapy only; epinephrine is the drug of choice
    D. Steroid therapy only; hydrocortisone at 200 to 300 mg/day is ideal and always effective
15. ARDS is a common organ failure associated with MODS. One strategy for ventilator therapy includes:
    A. Maintaining the tidal volume at 15 mL/kg of predicted weight; example: 5 foot, 100 kg, Pt might receive 1500 mL of tidal volume
    B. Maintaining the tidal volume at 6 mL/kg of predicted weight; example: 5 foot, 100 kg, Pt might receive 300 mL of tidal volume
    C. Maintaining the patient in a flat, supine position at all times
    D. Hyperventilation therapy to maintain the $paCO_2$ at less than 35
16. A previously healthy 68-year-old male has had emergency heart surgery to repair an aortic valve. His operating room course was troublesome, and he had to be given several units of blood, along with vasoactive agents, and other resuscitation. Three days later, he was discharged from the ICU and is now awaiting discharge to home in 2 more days. Today, the patient's laboratory work results are listed as follows: BUN 50 mg/dL; creatinine 2.8 mg/dL. This may indicate:
    A. Laboratory error
    B. Hemolytic reaction from the blood transfusion
    C. Early renal failure from SIRS
    D. Terminal signs of renal failure
17. Following what appears to be the successful resuscitation of a multisystem trauma patient, the post-op surgical floor is reporting that the patient's laboratory work today is as follows: lactate 5.1 mEq/L, WBC 21,000 with 15% bands. This may indicate:
    A. Leukopenia with right shift and alkalosis from shock
    B. Leukocytosis with left shift and acidosis from shock
    C. Leukocytosis with right shift and renal failure from early MODS
    D. Agranulocytosis with degradation of the cell wall in the renal system
18. Select the correct statement regarding cultures and the administration of antibiotics.
    A. Blood cultures should always be obtained prior to the administration of antibiotics.
    B. Blood cultures should be done approximately 8 hours after antibiotic administration.
    C. The laboratory will perform Gram staining (violet stain) on the culture to see whether the organism retains the stain (gram positive) or loses the stain (gram negative) to determine whether it is bacterial or viral in nature.
    D. Antibiotics should be given as soon as sepsis is identified clinically although cultures would be helpful.
19. A patient with identified MODS has both renal failure and ARDS, secondary to septic shock. On the third ICU day, his laboratory results are as follows: total bilirubin: 2.2 mg/dL, AST: 45 Units/L, LDH: 220 Units/L, CK: 310 U/L, albumin: 2.8 gm/dL, PT/INR: 18 seconds/2.7, with signs of jaundice in the palms of his hands and the sclera of his eyes. What complication has arisen?
    A. Liver failure
    B. Splenic failure
    C. Gallbladder failure
    D. Renal failure
20. A positive or negative feedback loop may occur in human physiology and pathophysiology. Which statement is true of these two phenomena.
    A. Platelets rapidly sticking together to create a plug that begins the clot formation is positive.
    B. Only positive loops help maintain homeostasis.
    C. Complement and coagulation cascade implementation during SIRS is a positive feedback loop.
    D. Anaphylaxis is a positive feedback loop.

CHAPTER 9

Special Patient Groups in Critical Care

OBJECTIVES

1. Discuss the physiologic changes in anatomy and physiology associated with pregnancy, infancy, childhood, and older age and apply this knowledge to the assessment and management of such patients requiring critical care.
2. Identify preexisting conditions, diseases, or complications of pregnancy and explain the monitoring and management of each condition.
3. Discuss common pathophysiologic conditions and their management in pediatric patients.
4. Analyze the special preparation necessary for the service, crew, and system to provide neonatal and pediatric critical care transport services.
5. Describe the challenges in communication, subtleties in assessment, and fragile nature of the elderly that accompany resuscitation.

The preceding chapters presented the different body systems and the ways they function. This chapter discusses special patient groups with unique anatomic or physiologic changes associated with age or pregnancy. These groups include obstetric (OB), neonatal, pediatric, and geriatric patients. Because of the unique characteristics of some of these groups, your transport service and crew may need to make special preparations to provide good care.

CRITICAL CARE OF THE OBSTETRIC PATIENT

Scenario

You are called to an outlying hospital to transport a 45-year-old female, gravida 1, para 0, who is at 34 weeks' gestation with twins. The patient has a history of gestational diabetes, pregnancy-induced hypertension (PIH), and asthma. Currently, she is insulin dependent, takes metoprolol for the PIH, and has a rescue inhaler with albuterol. The patient sought treatment at the local community hospital for symptoms of a urinary tract infection (UTI); however, the emergency department (ED) evaluation also revealed these findings: pulse, 96 beats/min; respirations, 24 breaths/min; BP, 200/110 mm Hg; blood sugar level, 128 mg/dL, and protein in the urine.

The patient was given a quick infusion of 5 gm of magnesium sulfate, and a maintenance infusion of magnesium sulfate, 10 gm/hour, was started approximately 1 hour ago.

On your arrival, the patient responds to you verbally but does not open her eyes. She shows some signs of respiratory failure and has fine crackles in the bases. Your findings are: pulse, 110 beats/min; respirations, 6 breaths/min with use of accessory muscles; and BP, 188/106 mm Hg.

1. What conditions does this patient have?
2. What diagnostics should be performed?
3. What treatment should be instituted?
4. What is the normal dose of magnesium sulfate? What are the complications of magnesium sulfate administration?
5. What are some special techniques for endotracheal intubation of a patient in the third trimester of pregnancy?

A pregnant patient presents challenges to critical care providers because of the dynamic changes that occur both in the mother's body and in the developing fetus. During pregnancy, practically every organ system undergoes change. Determining a baseline or a specific reaction to those physiologic changes will be a challenge in the pregnant patient. As the healthcare system develops specialized critical care areas for obstetric patients, the transport of these patients will also need some attention. When you consider the care for critical care obstetric patients, you have to remember the patients came into our care as result of either having preexisting diseases before becoming pregnant, or those who became pregnant and have developed some injury or a critical illness.

ANATOMY AND PHYSIOLOGY OF PREGNANCY

Intrauterine development begins with **gametogenesis** and progresses to the term fetus. Gestation occurs over about 40 weeks, including fetal membranes, umbilical cord, placenta, and amniotic fluid. Factors that affect this normal growth and development may be chromosomal, congenital, environmental, infectious, or toxicologic. From the first week of pregnancy to approximately six weeks after delivery, the woman's body (and nearly all systems) undergo changes.

Pulmonary System

The patient's increasing metabolic demands, along with a growing fetus, mandate some anatomic and physiologic changes within this system.

Did You Know?

The pulmonary system is affected only indirectly in pregnancy. Although airway changes are not dramatic, management can be. The patient's increased overall girth and thicker soft tissue in the face and neck create a sense of anatomic change, along with an increased risk of aspiration (see section on gastrointestinal and genitourinary systems).[1]

As the uterus enlarges, it encroaches on the upper abdomen, pushing the diaphragm upward about 4 cm. As this occurs, it compresses the lungs, flaring the lower ribs outward and enlarging the thoracic cage. As the need for oxygen increases by approximately 15% to 25% during the pregnancy, the tidal volume and respiratory rate increase to meet the need for the additional oxygen demand. These changes increase minute volume by as much as 50%. This, along with the stimulation of progesterone on the respiratory center, causes a chronic state of compensated respiratory alkalosis. As progesterone stimulates the respiratory center, a natural hyperventilation will occur. This results in a decrease in the $PaCO_2$ levels to approximately 28 to 32 mm Hg. Secondary to the alkalosis, there will be an increase in renal excretion of bicarbonate.

Respiratory Changes with Pregnancy

- Minute ventilation increases by 40% to 50%.
- Tidal volume increases by 40% to 50%.
- $Paco_2$ decreases to 28 to 32 mm Hg.
- Normal maternal Pao_2 is 101 to 108 mm Hg.
- Functional residual capacity decreases 20%.
- Oxygen reserve decreases.

Cardiovascular System

The rapidly changing needs of the pregnant body mandate adjustment of blood volume, structure, output, afterload, and rate to create a high flow, low resistance environment for the cardiovascular system. During pregnancy, blood volume increases 20% to 25% above normal by the end of the first trimester, and 30% to 50% near term. There is an increase in plasma volume versus red blood cells, creating a slight decrease in hematocrit to an average of about 32% to 34% by week 32 or 34.

Cardiac output increases by 30% to 40% from a normal average of 4.5 L/min to 6 to 7 L/min from week 10 until the end of pregnancy. This occurs, despite a decrease in the average central venous pressure from 9 mm Hg in nonpregnant women to about 4 mm Hg in the third trimester. The heart rate increases by 10 to 15 beats/min throughout pregnancy. During the pregnancy both the systolic and diastolic blood pressure decreases from an average of 110/70 mm Hg to about 102/50 mm Hg at the end of the second trimester. At term, the blood pressure often returns to normal.

The heart is displaced slightly upward and to the left with slight rotation to the front. This may create an axis deviation on the otherwise normal diagnostic electrocardiogram (ECG).

Some patients develop pulmonic, systolic, and apical systolic murmurs, resulting from decreased blood viscosity and increased blood flow. S-1 heart tones tend to exhibit a pronounced splitting and each component tends to be louder. An occasional S-3 sound may occur after 20 weeks of gestation.

Supine hypotension results from obstructed blood flow caused by the weight of the growing fetus and uterus pressing the vena cava against the vertebrae as the patient lies in a supine position. This creates a decrease in blood return to the heart, and the patient experiences an immediate decrease in cardiac output with marked hypotension.

The placenta is extremely reactive to hypovolemia or sympathetic stimulation. Even a relatively mild decrease in maternal blood flow can cause a severe decrease in placental perfusion. Hemodynamic monitoring may need to occur; the normal variations are shown in Table 9-1.

Cardiovascular Changes with Pregnancy

- Plasma volume increases 40% to 50%.
- Hematocrit decreases from a mean of 40% to 32%.
- Cardiac output increases by 30% to 40%.
- Heart rate increases by 10 to 15 beats/min.
- Systolic blood pressure decreases slightly (10 to 15 mm Hg).
- Peripheral vascular resistance decreases.
- Central venous pressure falls from a mean of 9 to 4 mm Hg.
- Electrocardiogram shows left axis deviation (10% to 15%).

Did You Know?

Looking for shock in the pregnant patient takes on a whole new perspective because of the tachycardia, slightly lower blood pressure, resting tachypnea, decrease in hematocrit, and anemias commonly present. Assessing lactate levels, base deficit, and other assessment for poor perfusion is imperative.[2]

Table 9-1 Hemodynamic Monitoring in a Pregnant Patient

Hemodynamic Parameter	Pregnancy	
	Normal	Variation
Mean arterial pressure (MAP)	90 ± 6	No difference
Central venous pressure (CVP)	8 ± 2	No difference
Pulmonary artery wedge pressure (PCWP)	4 ± 3	No difference
Cardiac output (L/min)	6.2 ± 1.0	43% Increase
Systemic vascular resistance (dynes/sec/cm^{-5})	1210 ± 266	21% Decrease
Pulmonary vascular resistance (dynes/sec/cm^{-5})	78 ± 22	14% Decrease

Modified from Urden L, Stacy K, Lough M: *Thelan's critical care nursing: diagnosis and management*, ed 5, St. Louis, 2005, Mosby.

Endocrinologic System

Progesterone and estrogen at high levels are crucial to maintaining the pregnancy but also affect the entire body. The most prominent change in the endocrine system is the hyperglycemia due to the anti-insulin effects from lipid breakdown. The thyroid enlarges and has increased stimulation throughout pregnancy.

The pituitary gland gets 30% to 100% heavier during pregnancy. As a consequence, shock may cause necrosis of the anterior pituitary, resulting in postpartum pituitary insufficiency (Sheehan's syndrome).

Endocrinologic Changes with Pregnancy

- Increased progesterone and estrogen
- Hyperglycemia
- Increased thyroid stimulation
- Heavier pituitary gland

Hematologic System

During pregnancy, a relative leukocytosis occurs, increasing the white blood cell count from a previous rate of 7200/mm^3 to about 9800/mm^3 in the third trimester. Blood also becomes "hypercoagulable" with increases in factors VII, VIII, IX, X, and XII. Plasma fibrinogen levels may also double, and the plasma levels of plasminogen activator tend to decrease. Normal concentrations of coagulation factors in a critically ill pregnant woman should make you suspicious for the presence of disseminating intravascular coagulation (DIC), which is discussed later in this chapter.

Hematologic Changes with Pregnancy

- Hematocrit decreases to about 32%.
- A white blood cell count of 12,000 per mm^3 may be normal.
- Fibrinogen increases to 400 mg/dL.
- Coagulation factors VII, VIII, IX, X, and XII all increase.
- Coagulation times decrease.

Gastrointestinal and Genitourinary Systems

Pregnant women are especially susceptible to aspiration of gastric contents because of the decrease in gastrointestinal motility that accompanies pregnancy. Compression by the gravid uterus and overall reduction in smooth-muscle tone cause delays in gastric emptying and prolonged intestinal transit lines. Hormonal influence causes the lower esophageal sphincter of the stomach to remain open. Increased progesterone during pregnancy tends to cause ureteral dilation, which can be increased by compression by ovarian vessels and the uterus. There is also delayed urinary bladder emptying that can lead to bacteremia and pyelonephritis.

Gastrointestinal and Genitourinary Changes with Pregnancy

- Reduced motility creating heartburn, constipation, and risk of aspiration
- Displaced lower esophageal sphincter with open conduit from stomach to esophagus
- Decreased gallbladder emptying
- Renal blood flow increased by 25%-50%
- Increased size of kidney with genitourinary (GU) dilation
- Bladder displaced upward and forward
- Enhanced filtration creates a normal pregnant creatinine level of 0.46 mg/dL and BUN of 8.2 mg/dL.
- Glycosuria and proteinuria may occur due to decreased reabsorption of both (but must be investigated)

BUN, Blood urea nitrogen.

Reproductive System

The uterus grows, from a 7-cm long, 70-gm organ in the adult nonpregnant state, to a 36-cm long, 1000 gm organ at term. The combined weight of the uterus, fetus, placenta, and amniotic fluid at term is about 4500 gm. Blood flow to the uterus increases from 60 mL/min to 600 mL/min at term. This predisposes a pregnant woman to massive blood loss if the uterine vasculature is disrupted. During the first trimester the uterus is a thick-walled organ confined within the safety of the bony pelvis. In the second trimester, the uterus leaves its protected intrapelvic location, but the small fetus is still relatively well protected because it is cushioned by a large amount of amniotic fluid. By the third trimester, the uterus is large and thin-walled. During the last 4 weeks of gestation, the fetus slowly descends as the fetal head engages in the pelvis. The placental vasculature exists in a state of maximal vasodilation throughout gestation, but is sensitive to catecholamine stimulation so that mild to moderate maternal hypovolemia can cause severe placental vasoconstriction and hypoperfusion. The uterus may fill with as much as 2000 mL of blood with little evidence of bleeding.

ASSESSMENT OF THE OBSTETRIC PATIENT

During resuscitation of a critically ill or injured pregnant patient, airway, breathing, circulation, and disability(ABCDs) are approached in the same manner as for a nonpregnant individual. As you apply the physiologic changes of pregnancy discussed above, you can then relate your assessment to the "normals" of this condition. There are some unique assessment techniques that should be discussed here. During the primary survey, all pregnant patients in their third trimester should be in a left side-lying position. Additionally, special assessment techniques for gestational age and fetal heart tones should be added to the secondary exam.

Position

Positioning is very important. Before examining the patient, pay particular attention to the pregnant patient's position to facilitate perfusion. If the fundal height is at or above the umbilicus, it is reasonable to position your patient into a left side-lying position to prevent supine hypotensive syndrome. If side lying is not possible, adaptation of the patient's position to allow for the uterus to be tipped to the side is recommended.

Obstetric History

Most due dates are estimated, based on a regular menstrual period of 28 days. Many women have irregular cycles and the range may be 22 to 35 days between periods. Further confounding this true estimate is the occurrence of small amounts of vaginal bleeding during implantation of pregnancy in the endometrial wall, which can confuse the patient and cause her to think that a period has occurred when it has not.

Nearly 12% of women who answer, "No way could I be pregnant," when asked, actually have a positive pregnancy test. Nagele's rule for estimating due date is based on regular cycles and the last "normal" menstrual period:

(Last Menstrual Period First day + 7 days) − 3 months

Assessment of Gestational Age

The critically ill or injured patient may be unable to relate to you her due date for delivery. It is important that, during your secondary assessment, you evaluate the patient for approximate gestational age. The following information will help you make that approximation:

- Determine normal physiology for current gestation
- Determine fetal age in case emergency delivery occurs

A full-term gestation is now considered to be at 37 to 40 weeks. The occurrence of a preterm delivery (between 22 and 37 weeks) presents a second patient who is also critically ill and requires specialized resuscitation.

Table 9-2 Relationship of Gestational Age to Fundal Height

Gestational Age	Fundal Height
12 weeks	Uterus just palpable over the top of the pubis
16 weeks	Halfway between pubis and umbilicus
20-22 weeks	Umbilicus level
24 weeks	1-2 finger breadths above umbilicus
32 weeks	3-4 finger breadths above umbilicus
36-38 weeks	1 finger breadth below xiphoid process
40 weeks	2-3 finger breadths below xiphoid (post lightening)

Modified from Gruenberg B: *Essentials of prehospital maternity care*, 2006, Brady.

By measuring from pubic bone to fundus, the provider can compare the fundal height to charts to predict the gestational age. After 22 to 24 weeks of pregnancy, if using centimeter (cm) markings on a measuring tape, the number of centimeters measured should approximately equal the weeks of gestation (Table 9-2).

Fetal and Uterine Monitoring

There are two ways to monitor both the fetal heart rate and the patient's uterine contractions: (1) Intermittent, simple diagnostics or (2) continuous, external or internal devices.

Intermittent Fetal and Uterine Monitoring

Fetal heart rate (FHR) monitoring may be done via intermittent auscultation. With an amplified stethoscope (or Doppler), fetal heart tones may be auscultated at approximately 10 to 12 weeks, but are best heard after week 20. They are heard best through the fetus' back. To determine the best location, palpate the patient's abdomen for the firmest part of the uterus. Place the bell of the device over this location. With the fetus in a cephalad presentation (head down), heart tones are usually auscultated in the lower quadrants of the mother's abdomen. Palpate for the fetal buttocks and follow the fetus down that side of the abdomen to determine which side will present the back of the fetus. Figure 9-1 demonstrates suggested locations for FHR auscultation.

Once you auscultate this fairly rapid heart rate, compare it to the mother's radial pulse to rule out unintended auscultation of her heart rate. Normal fetal heart rate is 120 to 160 beats per minute. The rate has significant beat-to-beat variability, especially with an active fetus. Consistent bradycardia is an ominous sign. Decelerations (drop in heart rate) can be due to a compressed fetal head during labor, umbilical cord compression, or a low perfusion state to the fetus.

Monitoring for uterine contractions may also be done in a simple, intermittent fashion. Palpate the fundus of the uterus for a rise within the abdominal wall as the muscle

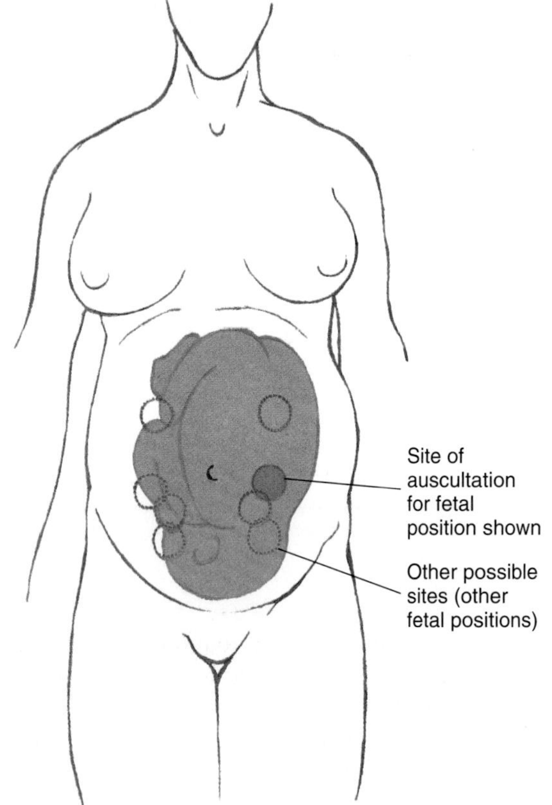

Figure 9-1

Sites for auscultation of fetal heart tones.

contracts or tightens. You may note both duration (length of contraction) and frequency (timed from beginning of one contraction to the beginning of the next).

Continuous Fetal and Uterine Monitoring

Continuous monitoring of fetal heart rate may be done with an external Doppler or internal fetal scalp electrode. External monitoring includes application of two belts that hold sensors into position on the mother's abdomen. One sensor is placed in the lower quadrants for fetal heart and one is placed over the fundus for contractions. Movement (of both mother and fetus) causes many problems with the sensors.

Electronic monitoring of FHR and the patient's contractions (tocometer) with internal monitoring is deemed better than external monitoring. A skin-penetrating spiral electrode is placed directly on the fetal presenting part via an introducer placed within the mother's vagina after the amniotic sac has been ruptured. Fetal scalp pH and oximetry may also be evaluated through a specialized internal electrode.

Many well-controlled studies have shown that intermittent evaluation (every 15 minutes in active, every 5 minutes in second stage labor) via external auscultation is just as reliable at identification of fetal distress.

Some patients may be transported with tocometer and fetal monitoring devices in place. The monitor that displays the FHR and uterine contractions also records these measures onto paper very similar to ECG displays. The graph paper shows the FHR on the top and the contractions on the bottom with notation of time. Special initial and ongoing training are required to accurately interpret these recordings; and such training is considered outside the scope of knowledge for standard critical care transport personnel. Specialized, high-risk obstetric healthcare professionals should accompany any patient who requires continuous fetal and tocometer monitoring.

Table 9-3 Unexpected Laboratory Results in a Pregnant Patient

Laboratory Results	Rationale/Management
Complete Blood Count (CBC)	
WBCs > 18,000/mm^3	
RBCs <6,500,000/mm^3	
Hgb <12 gm/dL	Hgb and Hct values are below normal; at risk for hypoxia
Hct <32%	
Platelets <200,000/mm^3	
Fibrinogen >400 mg/dL	
Chemistries	
BUN <9 mg/dL	
Creatinine >0.5 mg/dL	
Sodium, slightly elevated	
Glucose, slightly decreased	
Kleihauer-Betke	If positive, indicates a break in the fetal/maternal circulation because fetal cells are present
Special Tests	
12-lead ECG	Left axis deviation is a normal variant
Lecithin/sphingomyelin (L/S) and phosphatidylglycerol (PG)	Tests for fetal lung maturity/amniocentesis

BUN, Blood urea nitrogen; *ECG*, electrocardiogram; *Hgb*, hemoglobin; *Hct*, hematocrit; *RBCs*, red blood cells; *WBCs*, white blood cells.

DIAGNOSTICS FOR AN OBSTETRIC PATIENT

Laboratory Testing

The full array of laboratory testing should be evaluated for an obstetric patient, just as it is for any critically ill patient. This patient is at risk for hematologic complications, and clotting factors should be evaluated carefully. See Table 9-3 for variables in laboratory analysis for the pregnant patient.

Ultrasound Testing

Sonography or ultrasound testing of the pregnant patient has become routine at approximately 15 to 16 weeks' gestation. The usual approach is transabdominal. Occasionally, this technique may be nondiagnostic, especially if early in the pregnancy. An alternative approach is transvaginal.

Radiography

Although x-rays are a known **teratogen,** the clinician must weigh this risk versus the risk of an undiagnosed problem in the critically ill patient. Exposure of the fetus to ionizing radiation is of concern when the dose exceeds 5 to 15 rads (cGy). For example, a standard chest radiograph of the pregnant patient exposes the fetus to 8 rads, a thoracic spine radiograph exposes the fetus to 402 rads. Radiation from computed tomography (CT) scanning is a concern, but with appropriate shielding and technique, fetal exposure can be kept at acceptable levels. Spiral CT scans further reduce radiation dosage by as much as one third.

Magnetic Resonance Imaging

The effect of a strong magnetic field on fetal development is unknown, therefore, magnetic resonance imaging (MRI) is not recommended.

CONDITIONS THAT AFFECT THE HEALTHY OBSTETRIC PATIENT

As mentioned earlier, generally one of two pathways is followed based on the patient's condition when an obstetric patient enters the arena of critical care: (1) a preexisting disease that worsens, or (2) a normal pregnancy that becomes complicated by an illness or injury. Below you will find some conditions that may affect the healthy obstetric patient. As you proceed through these conditions, remember the presentation and management learned from the preceding chapters.

Preexisting Conditions

Heart Disease

Although the healthcare system is doing better at managing commonly encountered cardiac disease, the physiologic changes of pregnancy can create unusual stress upon the cardiovascular system. Congenital heart defects are described in the pediatric section of this chapter. Chapter 5 describes all other heart diseases.

Septal Defects

The left-to-right shunt within the heart is a result of atrial septal defect, (ASD), ventricular septal defect (VSD), or patent ductus arteriosus (PDA), any of which may affect this structural defect, with varying degrees of tolerance by the patient. ASD is the most common congenital irregularity seen during pregnancy. Women with ASD endure pregnancy, labor, and delivery without difficulty. The most common complication is dysrhythmias. Occasionally, heart failure and embolism formation are present.

Patent Ductus Arteriosus

Usually well tolerated by the pregnant patient, PDA, a congenital defect, should elicit precautions against the increased risk of infection and embolism formation, along with monitoring for pulmonary hypertension.

Valvular Disease

Right-sided valvular disease is well tolerated because of the high-flow, low-resistant state of the pregnant patient's cardiovascular system. Left-sided valvular disease may restrict cardiac output and create an increased chance of clot formation, infections, and dysrhythmias. Tachycardias treated with the use of beta blockade should be avoided (especially during delivery). Any treatment that may decrease preload should be avoided (epidural anesthesia, diuresis). Hemodynamic monitoring may be necessary. The most vulnerable time for this patient is the immediate postpartum period during which major fluid shifts and increases in cardiac output occur.

NOTE: All patients with prosthetic valves in place must maintain anticoagulation therapy (Lovenox, heparin).

History of Acute Myocardial Infarction

The obstetric patient's cardiovascular pumping function is key to a successful pregnancy. Our role is usually supportive, and outcome depends on early recognition of pump failure and keeping preload within reasonable limits.

Marfan Syndrome

In a patient with **Marfan syndrome,** the classic thinning and weakness of the aorta, along with mitral valve prolapse, warrants cautious monitoring of this patient. Prognosis is usually based on the diameter of the aortic root. An aortic root diameter greater than 4 cm is associated with significantly increased mortality. Treatment should include the prevention of tachydysrhythmias and hypertension. Beta blockade therapy is common to optimize cardiac output while minimizing pressures.

Chronic Hypertension

Known hypertension in the patient who becomes pregnant warrants high-risk obstetric monitoring and care. The diagnosis of hypertension in the first 20 weeks of pregnancy may be lumped into this group and can be confused with pregnancy-induced hypertension (PIH) and the toxemias of pregnancy (discussed later in this chapter).

Elimination of vasospasm and reduction of diastolic pressure to less than 90 mm Hg are the goals of therapy in the obstetric patient with preexisting hypertension. Specific interventions are discussed later in the chapter.

Asthma

The severity of a patient's asthma before pregnancy will dictate the outcome for both mother and passenger. The one-third rule applies to this disease during pregnancy: one third have no change in condition, one third improve, and one third get worse. Peak period for exacerbation is from 24 to 36 weeks of gestation. Judicious monitoring of peak flow rates helps the clinician with early detection of problems and quick adjustments of therapy.

Seizure Disorders

The most common reason for problems in the patient with known seizure disorder who becomes pregnant is a combination of factors that lead to decreased therapeutic levels of antiseizure medications: (1) increased clearance from the body and (2) failure to adjust doses according to pregnancy changes.

The overriding goal of managing the obstetric patient with a seizure disorder is to maintain a minimal drug dosing to prevent seizures but keep risks down for the fetus. Supplementing the mother with folic acid throughout pregnancy and adding vitamin K in the ninth month will help counter the effects of the antiseizure medications.

Substance Abuse

A patient's substance abuse may include the misuse or overuse of substances including alcohol, prescription, over-the-counter, and illicit drugs. Substance abuse during pregnancy can cause fetal harm, is most detrimental during the first trimester, and may be compounded by malnutrition, sexually transmitted diseases, and a poor self-image. Complications from substance abuse include an increased risk for infection, cellulitis, septic phlebitis, superficial abscesses, acute pulmonary edema, and delivery of a drug-addicted neonate.

Sexually Transmitted Diseases

Sexually transmitted diseases (STDs) can place a woman at greater risk for problems because of their potential effect on the pregnancy, fetus, or neonate. The most common STDs are **trichomoniasis,** bacterial vaginosis, chlamydia, syphilis, genital herpes, gonorrhea, **condyloma acuminata,** and group B streptococci infection. Negative side effects of STDs are preterm labor, premature rupture of membranes, neonatal conjunctivitis or pneumonia, neonatal congenital herpes, **ophthalmia neonatorum,** and respiratory distress syndrome.

Human Immunodeficiency Virus Infection

Human immunodeficiency virus (HIV) is the causative organism for acquired immunodeficiency syndrome (AIDS). HIV can have serious implications for the pregnant woman and fetus. It integrates itself into the cell's genetic makeup, ultimately causing cellular dysfunction, and may be transmitted through vertical communication across the placenta to the fetus during pregnancy, labor, and delivery or by breast milk to the neonate. Signs and symptoms of HIV infection are lymphadenopathy, bacterial pneumonia, fevers, night sweats, and weight loss. Tests to be performed are enzyme-linked immunosorbent assay, western blot test, and CD4+ T lymphocyte count.

Diabetes

Diabetes, a metabolic disorder characterized by hyperglycemia, affects the body's use of carbohydrates, protein, and fat metabolism. The three general classifications of diabetes are type 1—absolute insulin insufficiency, type 2—insulin resistance of varying degrees of insulin secretory defects, and gestational diabetes, which emerges during pregnancy. Hyperglycemia lends itself to an increased incidence of **candidal infection, hydramnios,** and macrovascular and microvascular changes. Management of diabetes includes monitoring blood glucose with a target of less than 100 mg/dl fasting glucose level and less than 120 mg/dl **postprandial.** Diet, exercise, adjusted insulin administration, and routine evaluation of glycosylated hemoglobin (hemoglobin A1c) are also part of the plan. Negative effects of diabetes include an increase of congenital anomalies, hydramnios, **macrosomia,** pregnancy-induced hypertension, spontaneous abortion, and fetal death.

Sickle Cell Anemia

Sickle cell anemia, a recessive, autosomal disorder, causes the red blood cells (RBCs) to become sickle-shaped and occurs primarily in those of African and Mediterranean descent. Pregnant women with the sickle cell trait experience an increased incidence of asymptomatic urosepsis, resulting in increased incidence of pyelonephritis.

A sickle cell crisis is triggered by illness, exposure to cold, stress, acidotic states, and any pathophysiologic processes that cause water to move out of the sickle cells. Some key findings are anemia, fatigue, burning and pain on urination, pooling of blood in lower extremities, and severe pain. Key tests for sickle cell anemia include hemoglobin electrophoresis and may reveal hemoglobin S, sickled cells on stained blood smear, hemoglobin level of 6 mg/dL or less, decreased RBC count and erythrocyte sedimentation rate, and increased indirect bilirubin level (during a crisis). Management includes evaluation of blood studies, avoidance of contributing factors, prevention of thrombophlebitis, folic acid supplementation, blood transfusion therapy, oxygen therapy and fluids during labor, and analgesics during crisis.

Illness and Injury in a Healthy Obstetric Patient

Cardiac Disorders

Peripartum Cardiomyopathy

Those obstetric patients with no prior evidence of cardiac disease who present with heart failure in a timeframe that includes the ninth month of gestation through 6 months postpartum are given the diagnosis of peripartum cardiomyopathy. Although rare, mortality may be as high as 50%. The cause of this unusual disease is yet to be determined but symptoms mimic classic congestive heart failure (CHF).

Treatment should include rest, fluid and sodium restrictions, inotropes, diuretics, and afterload reduction. Anticoagulation therapy is used to prevent thromboembolism.

Acute Myocardial Infarction

Acute myocardial infarction (AMI) is another rare event during pregnancy. The mortality from this dramatic event is related to the timing of the event, that is, the closer it occurs to time of delivery, the higher the mortality. Treatment is fairly standard but considerations for measures to ease the delivery as much as possible should be planned.

Treatment of AMI during pregnancy is focused on balancing myocardial oxygen supply and demand. Management may include nitrate and/or beta-blockade therapy, cardiac monitoring, oxygen therapy, management of pain and anxiety, and afterload reduction. Special consideration is given to the maternal physiologic demands required during the labor and delivery processes. Operative delivery interventions, such as forceps or cesarean section, may be necessary.

Shock

As stated earlier, the normal physiologic changes of pregnancy include a high-flow, low-resistant state with high oxygen demands and changes in the vital signs that may make recognition of shock, when it is occurring, rather tricky.

Obtaining a history that would include the possibility of shock is important (placenta previa, abruption, ectopic pregnancy, and post-partum hemorrhage). Evaluating both the fetus and the obstetric patient may also give clues to the presence of shock.

Management is aggressive; many important decisions are made that focus on salvage of the fetus versus emptying the contents of the uterus (to save the mother's life). Adaptations to the obstetric patient's position (left-side lying) during all resuscitation phases may help. The old saying has always been, "To save the baby, one must save the mother."

Pregnancy-Induced Hypertension

Remember that some patients come into the pregnancy with preexisting hypertension (previously discussed). The classification of hypertension in the obstetric patient (Table 9-4) helps with terminology and management controversy. The presence of hypertension in the pregnant patient adds a significant risk for complications (Table 9-5).

Preeclampsia

Pregnancy-induced hypertension (PIH) is a fairly common and sometimes fatal complication, whose cause is not well understood by the medical community. Preeclampsia and PIH are terms used interchangeably in many references. Many of those same references continue to call this complication toxemia of pregnancy. No matter the term, this complication of pregnancy is more common in African Americans, those with multiple gestation, teenagers, diabetics, and women over 35.

This complication usually presents as the triad of hypertension, proteinuria (albuminuria), and generalized edema that develops in the second or third trimester with widely variable development and severity in the individual patient.

There are three major effects of this disease process: arterial vasospasm with subsequent endothelial damage, platelet aggregation, and decreased vascular volume. The pregnant patient progresses from a high-flow, low-resistance cardiovascular state to a low-output, high-resistance disease with hypertension as the leading symptom. As with the earlier discussion regarding therapy for hypertension, the goal is to reduce the vasospasm and keep the diastolic pressure at less than 90 mm Hg.

Management includes facilitating a quiet environment, left side-lying position, and careful monitoring. Methyldopa may be used by some clinicians for treating hypertension during pregnancy because it decreases vascular resistance with little or no change in cardiac output or heart rate. It has less fetal effect, as well. Use of nifedipine or labetalol has few fetal side effects. Other beta blockers may cause fetal growth retardation and newborn distress at birth. Avoid diuretics unless pulmonary edema or oliguria is present. Angiotensin-converting enzyme (ACE) inhibitors should be avoided during pregnancy.

The physician may prescribe IV corticosteroids to the patient with PIH if delivery is to be induced within 24 to 48 hours to help mature the fetal lungs.

Table 9-4 Classification of Hypertension in a Pregnant Patient

Class	Description
I	Chronic hypertension: Hypertension before conception or diagnosed before 20 weeks' gestation
II	Preeclampsia-eclampsia: Systemic syndrome of hypertensive disease with proteinuria diagnosed after 20 weeks' gestation
III	Preeclampsia superimposed on chronic hypertension: May be before 20 weeks' gestation or have sudden onset
IV	Gestation hypertension: Hypertension without proteinuria

Table 9-5 Complications from Hypertension in a Pregnant Patient

System	Complication
Pulmonary	Pulmonary edema, acute airway obstruction
Cardiovascular	Dysrhythmias, congestive heart failure, severe hypertension
Neurologic	Cerebral edema, eclampsia, stroke, coma
Renal	Acute tubular necrosis, acute renal failure, oliguria
Hepatic	Necrosis, rupture, portal bleeding
Hematologic	Disseminated intravascular coagulation, hemolysis, thrombocytopenia

Eclampsia

When PIH and preeclampsia progress to a severely diminished level of consciousness, the condition is termed *eclampsia*. This convulsive presentation occurs between 24 weeks' gestation and the end of the first postpartum week. The incidence increases among women who are pregnant for the first time, have multiple fetuses, and have a history of vascular disease. Findings include blood pressure over 140/90 or increase of 30 mm Hg systolic and 15 mm Hg diastolic over the base line blood pressure. You can have an increase in generalized edema associated with a sudden weight gain of more than 5 lb per week and **proteinuria.**

Remember to differentiate those obstetric patients with preexisting seizure disorders with subtherapeutic medication levels vs. eclampsia once the resuscitation from the seizure is concluded. The PIH patient may decompensate rapidly into a convulsive state, especially when albumen levels are 2+ or more and mean arterial pressure (MAP) remains high. This condition may exist for as long as 2 weeks after delivery.

Control of the seizures is accomplished through administration of magnesium sulfate, 4 to 6 gm IV over 10 to 30 minutes (4-5 gm in 250 mL D_5W). This is followed by an IV infusion of 2 to 3 gm/hr. Magnesium sulfate may be used to treat any seizure because it has a depressant effect on the central nervous system and prevents or controls seizures by blocking peripheral neuromuscular transmission. When administered for seizures in PIH, the drug crosses the placenta and achieves nearly the same blood levels in the fetus as in the mother. This causes decreased reflexes, muscle tone, blood pressure, and respiratory depression in both patients.

Caution must be taken by healthcare providers who are monitoring these high-risk obstetric patients receiving magnesium sulfate because toxic levels may occur. Signs of toxicity include hypotension, respiratory depression, heart block, and depressed neuronal reflexes (decreasing deep tendon reflexes). Treatment of hypermagnesemia includes ventilation support and administration of calcium.

Many protocols add the use of benzodiazepines to stop an active seizure in the eclamptic phase of this disease. You must be cautious during this period because the seizures themselves can cause placental disruption, end-organ failure, and death. Diligent assessment and management of the ABCs while transitioning the patient to the care of a high-risk obstetrician and probably cesarean section delivery are a priority.

Hemolysis, Elevated Liver Enzymes, Low Platelet Count Syndrome

Hemolysis, elevated liver enzymes, low platelet count (HELLP) syndrome is a complication of pregnancy that occurs when pregnancy-induced hypertension (PIH) or preeclampsia is occurring. This additional problem involves changes in blood components and liver functions. As many as 12% of women with PIH are at risk for HELLP syndrome, and there is a high maternal and infant mortality rate. The exact cause of HELLP is unknown. It is diagnosed through laboratory studies in the patient with PIH.

This syndrome may present clinically as pain in the right upper quadrant of the abdomen, along with epigastric and lower chest discomfort. Symptoms such as nausea and vomiting, general malaise, severe edema, and signs of preeclampsia are included. Laboratory abnormalities include hemolysis of the RBCs, thrombocytopenia, and elevated liver enzymes.

Management of HELLP syndrome includes frequent assessment of maternal vital signs and fetal heart rate, along with hemodynamic monitoring. Treatment for PIH (as discussed) must also be continued.

The goals of management include prevention of seizures, decrease of vasospasms, and facilitation of prompt delivery of the fetus. Administration of magnesium sulfate is standard, with serum levels of 4 to 7 mEq/L considered therapeutic. Avoid use of phenytoin, diazepam, or phenobarbital because of their mechanism of action on neurologic dysfunction (vs. vasospasm in PIH). Complications of HELLP syndrome are fetal or maternal death, hemorrhage, hypoglycemia, hyponatremia, subcapsular liver hematoma, and renal failure.

Respiratory Failure

Maternal hypoxia has significant consequences in the fetal/maternal unit and is usually the result of an infectious process, asthma, trauma, ARDS, or pulmonary embolus.

Did You Know?

Maternal hypoxia is indicated by the following[2]:
$Pao_2 < 100$
$Spo_2 < 95\%$
$Svo_2 < 60\%$

Remember that the pregnant patient many times presents with some signs of dyspnea and hyperventilation. A thorough physical examination must be completed to differentiate maternal complaints of pregnancy versus serious underlying pathology.

Acute Respiratory Distress Syndrome

Noncardiogenic pulmonary edema is a result of many low perfusion states (sepsis), but can also occur from **tocolytic** administration and amniotic fluid embolism (AFE). Management of acute respiratory distress syndrome (ARDS) in the obstetric patient can be quite a challenge because of the physiologic differences and the consequences to both mother and fetus. Hemodynamic monitoring may assist the clinician in assessing the balance between fluid resuscitation and overload.

Management of ARDS during pregnancy has two main goals: airway maintenance and ventilation:

1. Airway maintenance: A complacent approach to advanced airway management and noninvasive ventilation management is usually avoided because of the risk of aspiration.

Placement of a gastric tube and vacuuming out stomach contents prior to advanced airway management may be helpful, along with proper positioning of the patient's body to facilitate viewing the cords in a patient who has a major change in the center of gravity.

2. Ventilation: When setting mechanical ventilators, tidal volume should be set slightly higher than for the nonpregnant patient in order to mimic the resting hyperventilation of the obstetric patient. Administer oxygen at a high flow rate to achieve an optimal PaO_2 greater than 100 mm Hg and an SpO_2 greater than 95%.

Did You Know?

Considerations for all obstetric patients being mechanically ventilated: Capnography should be implemented and $ETCO_2$ levels maintained at normal levels with frequent reassessment for compliance. Considerations for maintaining the $ETCO_2$ at 30 to 32 mm Hg to mimic the chronic hyperventilation of pregnancy may be done. The most important consideration should be that lung protective strategies (permissive hypercapnia) discussed in Chapter 3 should NOT be done because the fetus does not tolerate hypercapnic states.[2]

Pulmonary Embolism

There are many reasons for the obstetric patient to develop a pulmonary embolism (PE), especially in those high-risk obstetric patients already on bed rest for a complication of pregnancy. Women have a greater risk of developing a PE in the immediate postpartum period.

Heparin (unfractionated or low-molecular weight) is the drug of choice for anticoagulation therapy because warfarin is considered too risky; it is a known fetal teratogen and easily crosses the placenta. Suprarenal placement of a vena caval filter is usually considered in these patients.

Anaphylactoid Syndrome of Pregnancy

Anaphylactoid syndrome of pregnancy, formerly called an *amniotic fluid embolism* (AFE), was renamed because of the pathology and presentation, that is, the patient presents with anaphylactic versus PE symptoms. Those patients at risk are those with a large fetus or multiparous placenta previa, difficult labor, placental abruption, and intrauterine fetal distress. The sudden onset of symptoms (usually immediately post partum) includes respiratory distress, shock, chills, fever with chills, and cardiovascular collapse (similar to standard anaphylaxis). Some present initially with a generalized seizure alone. Morbidity and mortality is quite high (as much as 60%-70%) with this dramatic ailment. If fetal tissue (**lanugo, vernix caseosa,** meconium, fetal **squamous cells**) is aspirated from the pulmonary artery via invasive therapy or monitoring, diagnosis is confirmed. The chest x-ray will show an enlarged cardiac silhouette with pulmonary edema and effusions.

Management includes support of oxygenation and cardiovascular function with inotropes, fluids, and blood products.

Trauma

Trauma is the leading cause of death in pregnant women and accounts for twice as many deaths in women as do all other cases of maternal mortality combined. Among the mothers who survived their injuries, placental abruption was the most common cause of fetal loss. Abruptio placentae from direct trauma are caused by maldistribution of shearing forces between the elastic and flexible uterine wall and the inelastic placenta. Disruption of 25% or less of the placenta from the uterus is compatible with fetal survival but often causes intrauterine bleeding and premature labor. Disruption of 50% or more of the placenta is almost always fatal to the fetus. High pressure injuries can be generated during deceleration forces and may cause relatively little extrauterine damage, but may create marked uterine distortion and a shearing effect on the placental insertion site.

Consequently, abruption and fetal injury can occur with little or no external sign of trauma to the abdominal wall. Vaginal bleeding is likewise often absent, and fetal distress is frequently the initial sign. This combination of factors mandates that healthcare personnel monitor the obstetric patient judiciously, even after relatively minor traumatic forces. Penetrating wounds to the midabdomen during the late second and all of the third trimester are very likely to involve the uterus and its contents with resulting very high fetal mortality.

Gunshot wounds to the gravid uterus involve the fetus 60% of the time and have a fetal mortality approaching 80% if wounding is sustained preterm, versus 40% if the fetus is near term.

Of the pregnant women who die as a result of trauma, head injury and hemorrhage are the most common causes of death. Splenic injuries and retroperitoneal hemorrhage caused by blunt trauma are also major causes. Burns exceeding one third of the total body surface area usually result in termination of the pregnancy within 1 week. Even if the fetus survives the first week of such a burn, eventual fetal loss from sepsis can be expected.

A third trimester major burn may allow some fetuses to be saved by cesarean section within the first 5 days.

Hypotension from compression of the inferior vena cava by the gravid uterus in the third trimester can be corrected rapidly by turning the patient about 10 to 15 degrees to the left. For spinal precautions, the patient's backboard can be turned or one can displace and try to hold the uterus manually to the left. An alternative is to position the pregnant patient on her side on the backboard with padding and straps. Vena cava compression by the uterus also can increase venous pressure in the lower part of the body and increase bleeding from injuries to the pelvis and lower extremities.

Obstetric Disseminated Intravascular Coagulation

Placental abruption, preeclampsia-eclampsia, dead fetus syndrome, septic abortion, and AFE are all causes of the potentially fatal onset of DIC. Finding and removing the cause of this terminal spiral, along with administering volume, blood products, and anticoagulation therapy if the disease is the clot-making form are all measures to be taken. DIC is described in Chapter 8.

Placenta Previa

Placenta previa occurs when the placenta implants in the lower uterine segment, where it encroaches on the internal cervical opening; this is one of the most common causes of bleeding during the second half of pregnancy. The location of the placenta in relation to the cervix will determine the degree of placenta previa. There are three degrees of placenta previa:

- **Marginal**—where the placenta is 2 to 3 cm from the cervical opening
- **Partial**—where the placenta partially covers the cervical opening
- **Total**—where the placenta totally covers the cervical opening

Signs of placenta previa include painless, bright red bleeding after the twentieth week of gestation that starts without warning and stops spontaneously. Bleeding increases with each successive incident, a soft nontender uterus is present, and **Leopold's maneuver** (uterine fundal palpation for fetal position) reveals various malpresentations.

Managing placenta previa is usually accomplished through conservative measures, including limiting activity, monitoring vital signs, and restraint of healthcare personnel from performing rectal and vaginal examinations.

Abruptio Placentae

Abruptio placentae is the premature separation of the normally implanted placenta from the uterine wall, usually occurring after 20 to 24 weeks of gestation. It is most common in the multigravid patient, and fetal prognosis depends on the gestational age and amount of blood loss. The presence of pain is an important symptom that will determine placenta previa vs. abruptio placentae. Painful bleeding will be dark red and will occur when the blood leaks past the edges of the placenta. The uterus will be tender and will be firm or "boardlike" secondary to blood leaking into the muscle fibers. The woman will have frequent uterine irritability, which is described as cramp-like contractions.

Maternal prognosis is good if hemorrhage can be controlled, and it is classified according to the degree of the placental separation. Factors that can contribute are multiple gestations, hydramnios, cocaine use, decreased blood flow to the placenta, trauma to the abdomen, low serum folic acid levels, vascular or renal disease, and pregnancy-induced hypertension. Abruptio placentae is classified as one of three severities:

- *Mild*—gradual onset, mild to moderate bleeding, minimal lower abdominal discomfort and uterine irritability, but strong and regular fetal heart tones
- *Moderate*—gradual or abrupt onset; moderate, dark red vaginal bleeding; continuous abdominal pain with a tender uterus that remains firm between contractions; barely audible or irregular and bradycardic fetal heart tones
- *Severe*—abrupt onset of agonizing, unremitting uterine pain; boardlike, tender uterus; moderate vaginal bleeding; rapidly progressive shock; and absence of fetal heart tones

Management of abruptio placentae includes monitoring maternal vital signs, fetal heart rate, uterine contractions, and vaginal bleeding while transporting the patient for vaginal delivery for mild and cesarean delivery for moderate to severe placental separation. Vascular access, fluid and electrolyte replacement therapy, along with infusion of blood products are usually necessary. Cesarean section may need to be performed secondary to the risk of shock, clotting disorders, and fetal death.

Dead Fetus Syndrome

The pathology of dead fetus syndrome is caused by a gradual onset of DIC (over 2-4 weeks) that causes fetal demise. This is a chronic DIC condition; 80% of the women who experience fetal demise will have a spontaneous onset of labor, and treatment for the stable patient is allowing this vaginal delivery to occur. Heparin may be considered for patients with associated coagulopathy, along with support of the ABCs if unstable.

Septic Abortion

Any loss of the products of conception is called an *abortion* by the medical community, whether surgically related or spontaneous. Bacterial infection after this event creates sepsis with a real possibility of DIC. The sepsis pathology is described in Chapter 8. Management usually includes surgical tissue debridement, aggressive antibiotic therapy, and perfusion support along with treatment of the coagulopathy.

Ectopic Pregnancy

Ectopic pregnancy refers to the implantation of the fertilized ovum outside the uterine cavity. Most ectopic pregnancies occur in a fallopian tube, but other sites include the cervix, ovary, or abdominal cavity (Figure 9-2). This is a significant cause of maternal death due to hemorrhage. Indications of an ectopic pregnancy include mild abdominal pain, amenorrhea or abnormal menses, slight vaginal bleeding and unilateral pelvic pain over the mass, an abnormally low **beta hCG titer,** sudden severe abdominal pain radiating to the shoulder, **boggy** and tender uterus, syncope, nausea and vomiting, and shock.

As described in introductory emergency medicine references, this illness is like a medical gunshot wound to the abdomen and should be treated as such because intraabdominal bleeding can be life-threatening. Surgical management includes laparoscopic removal of the ruptured tube. Transport management includes treatment of hemorrhagic shock.

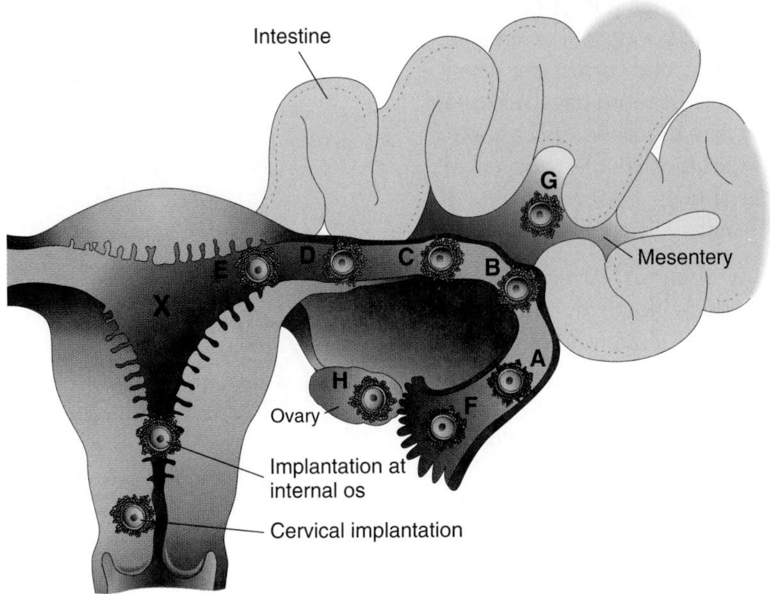

Figure 9-2

Sites of abnormal implantation in the uterus and fallopian tubes. **A** to **F,** Tubal pregnancies, the most common type of abnormal implantation. **G,** Abdominal pregnancy (the x indicates the wall of the uterus where implantation normally occurs). (From Leifer G: *Introduction to maternity and pediatric nursing,* ed 5, Philadelphia, 2006, Saunders.)

Isoimmunization

Isoimmunization is also known as *Rh sensitivity,* and it refers to a condition in which the pregnant woman is Rh negative but her fetus is Rh positive (or AB/O type incompatibility). A mixing of these blood types between the fetal-maternal unit sets up antigens for subsequent immune response. If left untreated, it can lead to hemolytic disease in neonates. Findings of isoimmunization include an increased concentration of bilirubin and RBC breakdown products in amniotic fluid, anti-D antibody titer 1:16 or greater, and edema revealed in radiologic studies. Management includes monitoring of the indirect Coombs test, delta optical density analysis of amniotic fluid at 26 weeks, and intrauterine transfusion.

Scenario Conclusion

This patient is a high-risk obstetric patient for many reasons: age, preexisting diabetes, and now PIH with signs of preeclampsia. Treatment before your arrival involved aggressive administration of magnesium sulfate. The patient now appears to be in respiratory failure and may have pulmonary edema.

You administer beta blockers to lower the MAP. You also discontinue the magnesium infusion and administer calcium to reduce the toxic magnesium levels. The patient's condition does not improve rapidly, so you prepare her for intubation. A gastric tube is inserted, and you put the patient in reverse Trendelenburg position, placing a blanket under her right hip to facilitate left uterine tilt. You place the patient on a ventilator with these settings: positive end-expiratory pressure (PEEP), 5 cm H_2O; tidal volume, 8 mL/kg (ideal); rate, 10 breaths/min (because of her stage of gestation). You then administer benzodiazepines to reduce her seizure threshold further. As a result of this care, she tolerates transport well and the fetal heart tones are normal throughout the trip.

CRITICAL CARE TRANSPORT OF NEONATAL AND PEDIATRIC PATIENTS

Scenario

You have been notified by your hospital's ED that a very sick infant needs rapid transport to a high-level pediatric ICU (PICU). The 6-month-old patient, who weighs 17.6 pounds (8 kg), originally presented with status epilepticus and had to be intubated by the local physician. The patient has been difficult to ventilate and requires high airway pressures. The cause of the seizures is unknown. So far, diagnostics are all negative.

Because you work for a hospital-based, adult critical care transport program, you are not sure that this patient should be transported by your service. The local physician is making arrangements for a specialized pediatric transport crew from a competing agency to manage the care of this child. You notice some unrest among your fellow crew members, who are wondering why they cannot transport the child.

The pediatric transport crew arrives 30 minutes later. This crew is staffed by personnel who have been credentialed by the receiving PICU, and they carry sophisticated equipment specially designed for neonatal and pediatric patients. One nurse gets on the phone to the PICU physician, and another evaluates the patient's airway, breathing, and circulation (ABCs) and obtains the history.

The IV bags are replaced with syringe pumps and medications calculated for the patient's weight. The endotracheal tube is checked for air leaks and correct placement. A capnographic device and monitors are attached to the patient. The ventilator settings are as follows: assist-control (A/C); inspiratory to expiratory (I:E) ratio, 1:1; inspiratory/expiratory time (T_I/T_E), 1 second; rate, 30 breaths/min; oxygen, 100%; PEEP, 3 cm H_2O.

A capillary blood sample is obtained 10 minutes later from the infant's heel, and bedside blood gas and glucose tests are done. The results are: pH, 7.36; partial pressure of arterial oxygen (PaO_2), 78 mm Hg; partial pressure of arterial carbon dioxide ($PaCO_2$), 42 mm Hg; base excess (BE), −1; bicarbonate (HCO_3), 23 mEq/L; glucose, 120 mg/dL. The current ventilator settings are maintained with the patient sedated.

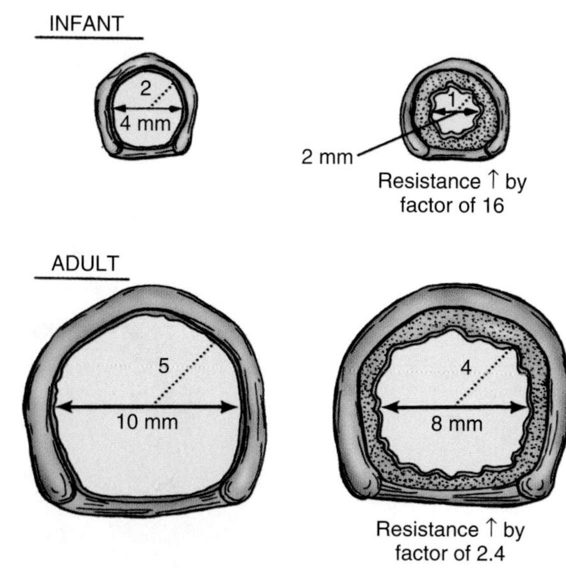

Figure 9-3

Effects of edema on airway resistance in infants. In infants, 1 mm of circumferential edema produces a substantial increase in airway resistance compared with the effect in adults. (From Zander J, Hazinski MF: Pulmonary disorders. In Hazinski MF, editor: *Nursing care of the critically ill child,* ed 2, St Louis, 1992, Mosby.)

The care of infants and children in a medical crisis is a challenge to any healthcare system. You can prepare for the special transport needs of this population by taking focused classes and learning some new skills. The education, resources, and equipment necessary to provide high-quality care to children will require more of your transport company and of yourself.

ANATOMY AND PHYSIOLOGY OF THE NEONATAL AND PEDIATRIC PATIENT

It seems from time to time you hear the old adage that pediatric patients are just little adults. Nothing could be further from the truth. This special population needs to be cared for with the knowledge and understanding of their anatomic and physiologic differences. In the section below we examine the differences in the pediatric patient via the ABCs.

Airway Differences

Your first patient priority is always airway management. The pediatric airway is different from that of the adult. This makes children more vulnerable to insults and can quickly lead to a compromised airway or suboptimal ventilation. These differences include the following:

- A child's airway is much smaller.
- These smaller airways are much more likely to be obstructed by mucus and edema. The cross-sectional area of a circle (such as an airway) is derived from the formula Πr^2, where r represents the radius. So a small change in the radius can make a huge difference in the area through which a child needs to breathe. Even 1 to 2 mm of edema can substantially increase the resistance to airflow and increase the work of breathing (Figure 9-3).
- The tonsils and adenoids are larger and the mucosa more delicate. Equipment such as a nasogastric tube passed through the nose is more likely to cause bleeding and mucosal edema. Special care needs to be taken to avoid irritation of these tissues.
- The tongue is larger in relation to the size of the mouth. The tongue can easily fill the back of the pharynx and cause obstruction when the child is on the back. Oral airways should be inserted with the use of a tongue blade to bring the tongue forward while the airway is inserted, with the curved portion following the natural curve of the tongue and palate, in other words, the right side down. This helps prevent pushing the relatively larger tongue backwards and then pinning it at the back of the pharynx—potentially worsening or even creating an obstruction. Delicate mucosal tissues are also less likely to be traumatized with this technique.
- The larynx is more anterior. The pediatric larynx is at about the level of the first or second cervical vertebrae whereas an adult's is at the fourth or fifth vertebrae. This may make visualization of the cords more difficult in a child. Gentle cricoid pressure may be helpful during intubation.
- The epiglottis is larger. The larger size and striking oblong or U-shape of a child's epiglottis makes it preferable to use a straight (Miller) laryngoscope blade during intubation. This blade is designed to directly elevate the epiglottis to allow vocal cord visualization. It provides better control of the epiglottis as well. The curved (McIntosh) blade fits into the vallecula and is designed to indirectly lift the epiglottis to reveal the glottic opening. The use of such a blade in a child usually results in the large epiglottis flopping down and causing visual obstruction of the cords. The larger size

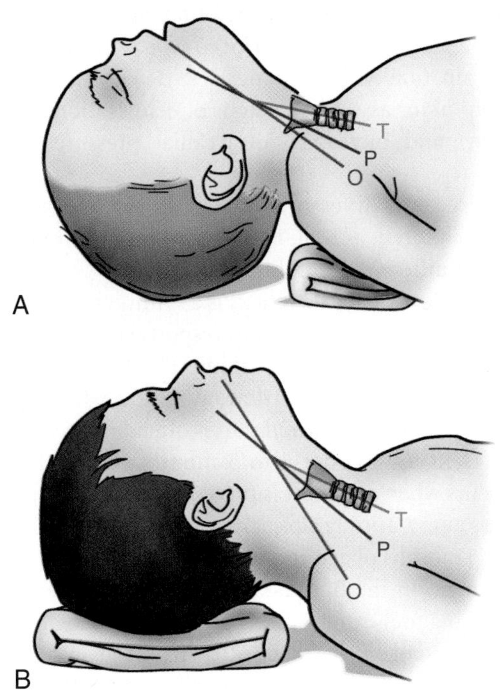

Figure 9-4

Correct airway positioning for ventilation of an infant **(A)** and a child **(B)**. Better airflow is provided with straight alignment of the oropharynx *(O)*, pharynx *(P)*, and trachea *(T)*. (From Urden LD, Stacy KM, Lough ME: *Thelan's critical care nursing: diagnosis and management*, ed 5, St Louis, 2005, Mosby.)

of the epiglottis can also make it more susceptible to injury and swelling.

- The larynx is smaller and more collapsible. The immaturity of the supportive structures of the voice box allows it to collapse—especially when higher negative pressures are created in the chest. This can be seen, for example, when an infant is in respiratory distress.
- The tracheal rings have less cartilaginous support. The immature trachea is more pliable and vulnerable to collapse as well. Hyperextension or hyperflexion of the neck may lead to a partial or complete occlusion of the airway. Foreign bodies trapped in the cervical esophagus are more likely to bulge into the trachea and block the airway.
- The narrowest part of the pediatric airway is the cricoid ring. This allows younger children to be intubated with an uncuffed endotracheal tube and still maintain a good seal.
- The combination of a more anterior larynx, a relatively larger head size, and a smaller body can make head/neck positioning for infants and toddlers a challenge during resuscitation. See Figure 9-4 for best practice suggestions on positioning for ventilation in this age group.

Differences in Breathing

Children's breathing is greatly impacted by their physiologic differences from adults. The basal metabolic rate is much higher in infants and young children. In fact, oxygen consumption can be about 50% higher per unit of body weight in early childhood. This causes infants and young children to breathe at a much higher rate at rest than that of adults. As children get bigger, their respiratory rate drops.

Normal respirations in the first months of life can be irregular and include cessation of breathing for up to 20 seconds. This may require you to count respirations for at least 30 seconds, ideally 60 seconds, to establish a rate. Any apnea greater than 20 seconds, however, is abnormal and requires intervention.

Structural differences in children as compared to adults also affect their breathing. Infants have much fewer and more primitive alveoli. This increases their risk for atelectasis. Grunting is a compensatory mechanism of infants in respiratory distress to create some positive end-expiratory pressure to keep their alveoli sacs inflated. Infants less than 6 months are primarily nose breathers. So, infants in respiratory distress often have nasal flaring to help decrease the resistance of air movement through the nose.

The pediatric chest wall has ribs that are more horizontal, a softer sternum, and weaker accessory muscles than adults. Their bones are not completely calcified, which makes them more pliable. The more horizontal and less rounded nature of ribs in pediatric patients provides them less leverage to increase the anterior-posterior diameter of the chest. All of these factors cause children to be predominantly "belly breathers" until about 3 years of age.

Normal respiratory tidal volumes in children are about 8 to 10 mL/kg. Adults can often increase their tidal volume by increasing their depth of breathing when they are in respiratory distress. Children, on the other hand, usually rely on increasing their respiratory rate to compensate for respiratory problems. This is mostly because they have less ability to increase their tidal volume. Part of this is also due to their hearts being relatively larger, which leaves the lungs less space in the chest cavity.

Another factor is that a child's abdomen is small with a relatively larger liver and spleen compressed within it. This makes it difficult to increase the depth of breathing due to the abdomen's resistance to the diaphragm in moving further down. Thus infants and young children find great difficulty in generating negative pressures inside their chest in order to increase their tidal volumes when they are in distress.

All of these structural differences give younger children, particularly infants, much less pulmonary reserve than adults. This can lead to big problems if ventilation becomes compromised.

Differences in Circulation

There are a number of differences between the pediatric and adult cardiovascular systems. For one, pulses in children can be nearly impossible to feel over areas that are usually easily palpated in adults. A child's smaller cardiac output creates a lower palpable volume of blood through the vessels, which can make it difficult to feel the pulse. This difficulty is magnified by the overall smaller anatomy of the child.

Table 9-6 Normal Pediatric Cardiac Output and Stroke Volume

Age	Cardiac Output (L/min)	Heart Rate	Normal Stroke Volume
Newborn	0.8-1.0	145	5 mL
6 mo	1.0-1.3	120	10 mL
1 yr	1.3-1.5	115	13 mL
2 yr	1.5-2.0	115	18 mL
4 yr	2.3-2.75	105	27 mL
5 yr	2.5-3.0	95	31 mL
8 yr	3.4-3.6	83	42 mL
10 yr	3.8-4.0	75	50 mL
15 yr	6.0	70	85 mL

From Urden L, Stacy K, Lough M: *Thelan's critical care nursing: diagnosis and management*, ed 5, St. Louis, 2005, Mosby.

So it is recommended to check peripheral pulses in children over the brachial artery at the inside of the upper arm and central pulses over the femoral or carotid arteries. If you have problems palpating peripheral pulses you can always auscultate the apex of the heart. The heart tones are created by the opening and closing of the heart valves due to blood flow. If heart tones can be heard, there is blood flow and a pulse is likely present. However, remember that the presence of a pulse does not equal adequate perfusion.

Left atrial pressure (LAP), central venous pressure (CVP), and pulmonary artery pressure (PAP) in children are essentially the same as in adults. The differences lie in cardiac output and stroke volume (Table 9-6).

Cardiac index is higher in children because that measurement is derived in part from body surface area, which is higher in children. The normal cardiac index is 3.5 to 5.5 L/min/m^2.

Children primarily increase their cardiac output by increasing their heart rate. Unlike adults, they cannot increase their stroke volume much due to the pediatric heart's low compliance as it relates to volume. Therefore, the heart rate can be considered a significant clinical marker of the cardiac output of a child.

One can assume that the cardiac output has been drastically reduced when bradycardia develops. Most commonly this is due to hypoxemia. Bradycardia is an early sign of hypoxemia for the neonate, but can be an ominous sign of severe hypoxia in the infant and child. Fortunately, this bradycardia can usually be quickly reversed in the young child with treatment of the hypoxia and improved ventilation.

Differences in the Central Nervous System

One of the most striking differences between children and adults is that the head size in children is relatively larger, particularly the occiput. The skull is also more flexible due to unfused cranial bones and the increased plasticity of the bones themselves. There are two spaces between these unfused bones, called **fontanelles.** The posterior fontanelle closes at about 3 months of age and the anterior one closes at around 20 months. Palpation of the fontanelles to determine the contour can be helpful for assessing of signs of dehydration (described as sunken) and increased intracranial pressure (tense or bulging).

There are some differences in neurologic reflexes between adults and children, as well. Babies have infantile reflexes that disappear at different times during the first few months of life. The **Moro reflex** (or startle reflex) is a symmetric opening and closing of the arms that occurs in response to a loud noise or when infants feel as if they are falling. The Moro reflex is seen normally in infants up to 3 to 4 months of age. It is also called the *embrace reflex* or *startle reflex*. It is often followed by crying and is present until about 4 to 5 months of age. The **grasp reflex** occurs when an object is placed in the infant's palm and the fingers automatically close around it. This reflex is present until 5 to 6 months of age and may be confused with purposeful movement. In the **Babinski's reflex,** the toes fan out and the hallux (big toe) extends in response to stroking the side of the foot. Remember that a positive Babinski in an adult is *abnormal* and a sign of upper motor neuron pathology. This response in young children is caused by a lack of myelination in the corticospinal tract and is normally seen until about 2 years of age.

Differences in Temperature and Environment Regulation

Temperature regulation is very important in pediatric patients. Infants and children have a large body surface area compared to their volume. In fact, this ratio is 4 times greater than that of an adult whereas their heat production is only 1½ times as high. In addition, the very young cannot effectively induce muscular shivering to help boost core body heat. And generally, younger children have less adipose tissue to provide insulation to maintain their temperature. All of these factors make children particularly vulnerable to hypothermia. Hypothermia causes increased oxygen consumption, which can be extremely detrimental for the already ill or traumatized child. Your vehicle should be equipped with items to help prevent heat loss. This may include caps, foil blankets, heating pads, and commercial warmers.

Critically ill newborns are quite vulnerable to hypothermia. Their low fat stores make it extremely difficult for them to maintain their temperature. This is especially true of very low birth weight infants who often require neonatal transport. Such patients are susceptible to massive insensible losses due to their remarkably immature skin.

Hypoglycemia

Hypoglycemia is also a greater risk for infants and young children. Their immature liver will usually have decreased glycogen stores. This coupled with their high metabolic rate makes them particularly vulnerable. Stress from illness or injury may be all that it takes to overcome their glucose reserve. Regardless of the diagnosis, a glucose level should be checked on all infants.

Differences in Hepatic and Renal Physiology (Pharmacologic Applications)

Neonates are pharmacologically unique. Their immaturity frequently affects their ability to metabolize and eliminate many drugs. This can make them more vulnerable to adverse medication effects and warrant alterations in drug dosing or dosing interval.

Many enzymatic pathways may be reduced or even absent in the neonate. This is especially true for the liver. The more premature the infant, the less developed complex enzymatic processes will be in the liver. This means, for example, a drug that is typically metabolized in adults by an enzymatic pathway called **glucuronidation** may be metabolized by **sulfation** in the neonate—a completely different pathway. Sometimes this can result in unpredictable metabolism of a drug.

Neonates also have a decreased **glomerular filtration rate (GFR)** initially in their kidneys. This is especially true for critically ill and premature newborns. A general decrease in renal function in neonates means drugs that are eliminated through the kidney must be used with caution. Serum drug levels are often needed to monitor these medications. Prolonged dosing intervals for drugs with renal excretion may be required.

ASSESSMENT OF THE NEONATAL AND PEDIATRIC PATIENT

The key to any transport assessment is to identify any immediate life-threatening problems and treat them. In this section, we address the assessment of several selected areas of pediatric care.

Pediatric Assessment Triangle

The best approach to forming an immediate general impression of the severity of illness or injury in a child is the Pediatric Assessment Triangle (Figure 9-5). This tool was developed by the American Academy of Pediatrics and is based on the fact that you can usually determine whether a child is sick by just looking at the child.

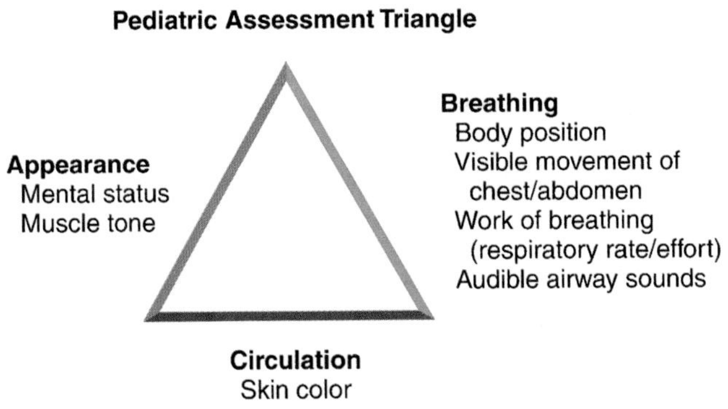

Figure 9-5

Pediatric Assessment Triangle. (From Aehlert BJ: *PALS pediatric advanced life support study guide*, ed 2, St Louis, 2006, Mosby.)

This assessment can be performed before any physical contact is made with the patient and used even when the local hospital has provided some resuscitation to the patient.

The triangle is composed of assessments of the following:

1. *Appearance*: The child's overall mental status, body position, and muscle tone
2. *Breathing:* The visual effort or audible sounds associated with the work of breathing
3. *Circulation:* The determination of the skin color and general perfusion status

By applying this assessment one can quickly determine the patient's problem category and whether he or she will require your immediate intervention. These categories include normal, respiratory distress/failure, shock, cardiopulmonary failure/arrest, and neurologic/metabolic. This assessment can become the basis from which further management can follow.

Subsequent evaluation includes the ABCs and vital signs. Of course, normal vital signs are a relative term and will vary in children depending on their age. The normal value range reflects the physiologic needs of children as they grow. There are many reference guides available to remind you of the normal values. Vital signs are beneficial but their greatest clinical value lies in trending changes in the patient's status over time.

Assessing for Shock

Children have a tremendous ability to compensate for significant volume losses in their circulatory system. They are able to vasoconstrict peripherally and maintain their normal blood pressure even with severe volume losses of 35% to 40% for prolonged periods.

Unrecognized bleeding is a common cause of preventable death in children with trauma. It is critical to identify when a child has poor perfusion while still in compensated shock and then treat the child. Once the blood pressure drops and the child has uncompensated shock, you know that both the patient and you are in trouble. It is going to take aggressive therapy to be able to successfully treat the child.

Because hypotension is an especially late finding in children, you must be able to recognize more subtle signs of shock in children. Tachycardia is an early sign of shock but can be elevated in children by other commonly seen problems such as fever, anxiety, and pain. The range of normal heart rates in children is also quite wide. It is probably most important to follow the heart rate over time. If you see it increasing, there may be worsening shock.

Patients in shock may be tachypneic, sometimes even with significant accessory muscle use, as the patient develops metabolic acidosis. This acidosis is due to an increased production of lactic acid as a result of inadequate perfusion of the intestine and muscle. The increased respiratory effort creates a respiratory alkalosis to help compensate for the metabolic acidosis. Sometimes this respiratory compensation is dramatic and fools providers into thinking there is a primary ventilation problem when the real problem is poor perfusion, for example, from septic shock.

Shock and the Skin

The skin is important in the evaluation of poor perfusion in children. You should be looking to see whether it is pale, mottled, cyanotic, cool, or diaphoretic. Altered mental status with agitation, restlessness, confusion, listlessness, and stupor may develop because there is worsening perfusion to the brain. Other signs of shock include delayed capillary refill and narrowed pulse pressure. Internal bleeding should be suspected in the trauma patient with shock when there is no significant external bleeding. Clues to hydration status include the tenseness of the anterior fontanelle, skin **turgor,** the moistness of mucous membranes, the presence or absence of tears, and urine output.

Assessing Neurologic Status

Assessing for and treating the patient with a rising intracranial pressure is integral to outcome, whether the pathology is medical or traumatic in nature. The child's cerebral perfusion pressure (CPP) must be maintained to ensure adequate blood flow to the brain.

As in adults, the AVPU (alert, verbal, painful, unresponsive) scale is used to delineate the level of consciousness in children. A tool to help assess neurologic appearance of the nonverbal child is the mnemonic TICLS (pronounced "tickles") (Box 9-1). The pediatric Glasgow Coma Scale (Table 9-7) is another evaluation used to determine the degree of mentation. As with the standard Glasgow Coma Scale, it is most clinically useful in following the improvement or deterioration of mental status over time.

DIAGNOSTICS

Laboratory Values

Common laboratory values in infants and children are listed in Table 9-8. For less common laboratory tests, the critical care team should use standard references.

Box 9-1 Appearance Mnemonic: TICLS

Tone: Is there vigorous movement with good muscle tone? Or, is the child limp?
Interactivity: Is the child alert and attentive to surroundings or apathetic? Will the child reach for a toy? Does the child respond to people, objects, and sounds?
Consolability: Does comforting the child alleviate the agitation and crying?
Look/Gaze: Do the child's eyes follow your movement, or is there a vacant gaze?
Speech/Cry: Are vocalizations strong, or are they weak, muffled, or hoarse?

From Urden L, Stacy K, Lough M: *Thelan's critical care nursing: diagnosis and management*, ed 5, St. Louis, 2005, Mosby.

Table 9-7 Modified Glasgow Coma Scale for Infants and Children

	Child	Infant	Score
Eye opening	Spontaneous	Spontaneous	4
	To verbal stimuli	To verbal stimuli	3
	To pain only	To pain only	2
	No response	No response	1
Verbal response	Oriented, appropriate	Coos and babbles	5
	Confused	Irritable cries	4
	Inappropriate words	Cries to pain	3
	Incomprehensible words or non-specific sounds	Moans to pain	2
	No response	No response	1
Motor response	Obeys command	Moves spontaneously and purposefully	6
	Localizes painful stimulus	Withdraws to touch	5
	Withdraws in response to pain	Withdraws in response to pain	4
	Flexion in response to pain	Decorticate posturing (abnormal flexion) in response to pain	3
	Extension in response to pain	Decerebrate posturing (abnormal extension) in response to pain	2
	No response	No response	1

Modified from Davis RJ et al: Head and spinal cord injury. In Rogers MC, editors: *Textbook of pediatric intensive care,* Baltimore, 1987, Williams & Wilkins; James H, Anas N, Perkin RM: *Brain insults in infants and children,* New York, 1985, Grune & Stratton; and Morray JP et al: *Crit Care Med* 12:1018, 1984.

Table 9-8 Common Laboratory Values for Various Age Groups

Parameter	Age	Normal Value	Parameter	Age	Normal Value
Red blood cell count (RBC)	1 week	3.9-6.3 millions of cells/mm^3	Alanine aminotransferase (ALT)	Infant	<48 U/L
	2 weeks	3.6-6.2		Child	<37 U/L
	3-6 months	3.1-4.5	Creatinine kinase	Newborn	40-474 IU/L
	2-6 years	3.9-5.3	Aspartate aminotransferse (AST)	Newborn	<50 U/L
Hematocrit (Hct)	3 days	44%-72% of packed cells		Child	<34 U/L
	2 months	28%-42%	Alkaline phosphatase (ALP)	Newborn	<310 U/L
	6-12 years	35%-45%		Infant	<360 U/L
Hemoglobin (Hgb)	1-3 days	14.5-22.5 gm/dL		1-10 years	<290 U/L
	2 months	9.0-14.0	Ammonia	Infant	50-84 μmol/L
	6-12 years	11.5-15.5		Child	12-38 μmol/L
Total white blood cell count (WBC)	Birth	9000-30,000 mm^3	Direct bilirubin	Child	0.1-0.4 mg/dL
	1 month	5000-19,500 mm^3	Total bilirubin	Infant	1-12 mg/dL
	1-3 years	6000-17,500 mm^3		Child	0.2-1.3 mg/dL
	4-7 years	5500-15,500 mm^3	Blood urea nitrogen (BUN)	1-3 years	5-17 mg/dL
Sedimentation rate (ESR)		0-10 mm/hr		4-13 years	7-17 mg/dL
Reticulocyte count	Infants	2%-5% of total RBCs	Creatinine	Newborns	7-10 mg/kg/24 hr
	Children	0.5-4.0% of total RBCs		Children	20-30 mg/kg/24 hr
Platelet count		150,000-400,000 mm^3	Albumin	Infant	3.9-4.6 gm/dL
Prothrombin time		11-15 seconds		Child	6.5-8.6 gm/dL
Partial thromboplastin time (PTT)		30-45 seconds	Base excess	Newborn	−10 to −2 mmol/L
				Infant	−7 to −1 mmol/L
Potassium	Premature	4.5-7.2 mmol/L		Child	−4 to +2 mmol/L
	Infant	3.7-5.2 mmol/L	Bicarbonate	Newborn	17.2-23.6 mmol/L
	Child	3.5-5.8 mmol//L		2 months-2 years	19-24 mmol/L
Sodium (Na^+)	Newborn	133-146 mmol/L		Child	18-25 mmol/L
	Child	135-148 mmol/L			
Calcium (Ca^+)	Premature	3.5-4.5 mEq/L	Carbon dioxide (pco_2)	Newborn	27-40 mm Hg
	Infant	4.0-5.0 mEq/L		Infant	27-41 mm Hg
	Child	4.4-5.3 mEq/L		Child	32-48 mm Hg
Chloride	<1 year	96-111 mmol/L	Oxygen (po_2)	Birth	8-24 mm Hg
	1-17 years	102-112 mmol/L		>1 hour	55-80 mm Hg
Glucose	Premature	20-80 mg/dL		>1 day	83-108 mm Hg
	Infant	30-100 mg/dL			
	Child	60-105 mg/dL			

Table 9-9 Comparison of Sample Sources for Normal Blood Gas Values

ABG Parameter	Arterial	Venous	Capillary
pH	7.35-7.45	7.31-7.41	7.35-7.45
O_2 saturation	95%-97%	60%-80%	Decreased arterial
po_2	80-100 mm Hg	36-42 mm Hg	Decreased arterial
pco_2	35-45 mm Hg	40-50 mm Hg	Same as arterial
HCO_3	22-26 mEq/L	Same as arterial	Same as arterial
Base excess/deficit	−2 to +2	Same as arterial	Same as arterial

Modified from Curley M, et al: *Critical care nursing of infants and children*, Philadelphia, 2001, Saunders.

Blood Gas Analysis

An arterial blood source is not always necessary to obtain valuable information from blood gas analysis. However, it is important to know the normal differences between various blood sources. Table 9-9 provides comparison between venous, capillary, and arterial blood gas values.

Lumbar Puncture

A lumbar puncture (LP) has become a standard diagnostic workup for certain types of pediatric presentations (sepsis). Although transport teams are not always involved in the emergency or critical care workup, it is reasonable that you understand the basics of the LP, especially the complications associated with positioning the patient.

A spinal needle is inserted into the subarachnoid space at either the L-3/L-4 or L-4/L-5 intervertebral space under local anesthetic for the purpose of obtaining cerebral spinal fluid for laboratory analysis. During the procedure, the patient is held with hips and neck flexed in order to "open" the lumbar intervertebral spaces. Because of this position, there is a risk of respiratory distress and/or respiratory failure. The patient must be monitored continuously via cardiac and respiratory monitors.

The clinician may evaluate the pressures within the space during the procedure. Fluid obtained will have cell counts and chemistries (glucose, protein) determined, and the presence of bacteria will be identified by microscopic examination under Gram's stain and by culture. Relative contraindications to lumbar puncture include those patients with coagulopathies and high intracranial pressure.

Imaging and Radiographs

The type of imaging examinations for diagnostic purposes is no different for the pediatric population than for the adult population. What is different is that younger pediatric patients cannot or will not hold still long enough to obtain a good image for many radiographic examinations such as CT or MRI screening. Procedural sedation often needs to be instituted, and the critical care team will need to follow institution protocols on assisting with this procedure.

Chest Radiographs

The seriously ill pediatric patient, like an adult, requires chest radiographs to determine multiple diagnostic parameters. Some of the important information gained from this examination includes heart size, chamber enlargement, and pulmonary blood flow. The presence of the normally large **thymus** gland in infants can obscure the upper portion of the heart and can often appear to be a chest mass as large as the heart. The thymus gland is located in the anterior mediastinum so a lateral view of the chest can be helpful if there is any question as to the origin of the silhouette seen.

Ultrasound Scans

Cranial Ultrasound Scans in Infants

In children young enough to have open cranial fontanelles, the clinician may use ultrasound to evaluate densities of the brain, especially intracranial hemorrhage.

Echocardiography

The most complete noninvasive diagnostic examination of the heart is obtained through using the echocardiograph. Transthoracic two-dimensional echocardiography, transesophageal echocardiography (TEE), and Doppler echocardiography have become important tools in evaluating the child with CHD.

Invasive Hemodynamic Monitoring

Arterial blood pressure measurement is always more accurate in children than cuff pressures because pulsatile blood flow distally is harder to measure. Size of catheters, potential for fluid overload, and blood loss concerns are the main issues when managing invasive hemodynamic monitoring in the pediatric patient. Careful consideration of heparin dosing in the lines, small blood sampling for laboratory testing, and measuring flush volumes judiciously are just a few considerations that make this different from adult hemodynamic procedures.

SPECIAL EQUIPMENT AND PROCEDURES

Cardiovascular Mechanical Support

Pediatric patients with persistently low cardiac output despite optimal intravascular volume replacement and pharmacologic management may require cardiovascular mechanical support. This support may include ventricular assist devices (VADs), intraaortic balloon pump (IABP), or extracorporeal membrane oxygenation. The choice largely depends on the size and condition of the child, the resources available, and institutional preferences. The descriptions and parameters for IABP and VAD use are described in Chapter 4.

Extracorporeal Membrane Oxygenation

Similar to a heart-lung or bypass unit, **extracorporeal membrane oxygenation (ECMO)** is initiated by placing catheters into large vessels and pumping blood from the patient to the device to provide gas exchange for those with lung and/or heart diseases. ECMO is preferred when both pulmonary and cardiac support is required and is gaining popularity among all intensivists, whether neonatal, pediatric, or adult.

There are two routes available for ECMO: (1) Venoarterial (VA), in which blood is drained through a catheter from the right atrium, is oxygenated through the system, and then is returned to the patient near the aortic arch. This method bypasses the pulmonary system. (2) Venovenous (VV), which is routed similarly for oxygenation as is VA but is taken back to the patient through a femoral vein and continues to perfuse the lungs.

Providing transport of a patient on ECMO is a logistical challenge and is usually reserved for specialty teams that must be credentialed for this highly technical treatment. There are three major concerns regarding transport of this patient:

1. If the originating hospital placed the patient on ECMO, why are they transporting the patient on to another facility? If they are sophisticated enough to initiate ECMO, what failure has created the need for another specialized facility?
2. If you are developing a specialized team to go out and initiate ECMO in the originating hospital, what specialized crew are you including? You need a clinician who can cannulate central vessels, possibly perfusionists to manage the special pump, and other crew members with special knowledge and skills.
3. What equipment have you included in your ground or air transport program to secure the heavy and cumbersome equipment needed on this transport? How will you lift/load all of the equipment and tubing in a safe way?

Detailed explanations of this very specialized treatment is beyond the scope of this book. Figure 9-6 demonstrates the amount of equipment necessary and explains why this therapy is a transport issue.

DISEASE PROCESSES AND MANAGEMENT OF THE NEONATAL AND PEDIATRIC PATIENT

Airway Compromise

It is crucial during any pediatric transport to control the airway. As discussed earlier, correct positioning, taking into account the larger head of the child, is an important step in maintaining an open airway. If the child is struggling to breathe but is conscious, you should allow the child to position himself as he feels most comfortable. Children will almost always assume the position that best keeps their partially obstructed airway open.

Opening the Airway

A chin lift or jaw-thrust maneuver can be used on less responsive patients to open the airway. You should manually remove any foreign material that is visible. Maneuver attempts to clear an airway of a foreign body should be considered if:

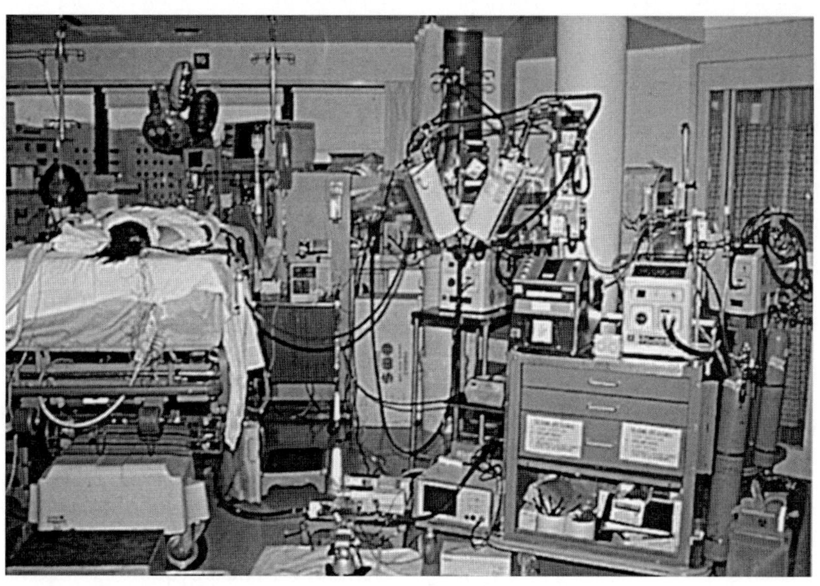

Figure 9-6

ECMO circuit. Blood drains from the right atrium by gravity to a blood reservoir. It then is pumped to the membrane oxygenator, heated, and returned to the patient. *ECMO,* Extracorporeal membrane oxygenation. (From Curley MA, Moloney-Harmon PA: *Critical care nursing of infants and children,* Philadelphia, 2001, Saunders.)

- A witnessed or strongly suspected aspiration has occurred
- A choking child is aphonic and/or the cough becomes ineffective
- An unconscious, nonbreathing child has significant resistance to positive pressure ventilation

Suctioning

Suctioning to remove secretions may be essential to maintain airway patency in some children. However, children can have vagal responses to suctioning causing significant bradycardia. So suctioning should be performed carefully with oxygenation before and afterward. Limiting catheter insertion time to about 5 to 10 seconds is also a good practice.

The opening of the catheter can also become stuck to the surfaces of the airway. Just remove your finger from the port to interrupt the vacuum seal, and the catheter will become free. The suction catheter needs to be at least 6 to 8 French in order to have a large enough internal diameter to remove secretions. A bulb syringe can be used in suctioning infants.

Intubation

Intubation may be important for some pediatric patients for resuscitation or to maintain an airway during transport. An uncuffed tracheal tube is generally recommended for children under 8 years of age in emergency settings. An audible air leak may be heard with an appropriately sized tube when the peak inflation pressure exceeds 20 to 30 cm H_2O.

A cuffed tube may be required if a child has a disease process that creates high airway resistance or stiff lungs, for example, from status asthmaticus or near drowning. In addition, when transporting intubated children from an operating room or from another hospital, recognize that a cuffed tracheal tube might have been used to help lessen air leak while providing the patient positive pressure ventilation.

The transport team should evaluate the tracheal tube cuff prior to transport and monitor the cuff throughout the transport. Maintain the cuff pressure to where there is a slight air leak, at less than 20 cm H_2O on the manometer. Back-up airway devices that are approved for pediatrics, including infraglottic airways, should be available for failed intubations that cannot be adequately ventilated by bag-valve mask. Box 9-2 presents the pediatric formulas for tracheal tube size and depth of insertion.

Box 9-2 Calculation of Tracheal Tube Size and Depth of Insertion for Pediatric Patients

Uncuffed tracheal tube: (Age in years/4) + 4 = mm (internal diameter (ID)

Cuffed tracheal tube: (Age in years/4) + 3 = mm ID

Depth of insertion: 2 yrs of age = (age in years/2) + 12 = cm

OR

Tube internal diameter (mm) × 3

From Urden L, Stacy K, Lough M: Thelan's *Critical care nursing: diagnosis and management*, ed 5, St. Louis, 2005, Mosby.

It is crucial to first listen over the stomach once a tracheal tube has been placed. It is so easy to be fooled by referred breath sounds from the child's stomach when there is an improperly placed tracheal tube in the esophagus. Transmitted breath sounds are much more of a problem in children because of their thinner chest walls and smaller size. In addition, one can often see the child's chest wall rise symmetrically as air is bagged into the stomach due to the compliancy of the pediatric chest.

Debating whether there are adequate breath sounds while you listen over the lung first will allow the stomach to be distended with more and more air. The ballooned stomach will push up on the diaphragm and make ventilation more difficult, even after the tracheal tube is properly placed and until a gastric tube can be inserted. If there are no breath sounds in the stomach, then you should listen over the upper lung fields. This is best done in the mid-axillary region just below the armpits.

Of the numerous methods of confirming correct placement of the endotracheal tube (described in Chapter 3), capnography has become a standard of care for any intubated patient and has been found to be superior to auscultation because of the issues described above. (Capnography is described also in Chapter 3.)

One of the most important aspects of intubation is ensuring adequate analgesia, sedation, and paralyzation both before and after the airway is secured. After intubation, this is usually best achieved with benzodiazepines and a long-acting nondepolarizing paralytic. Close monitoring of the sedation level is a must so that one can administer additional medications before there is significant patient movement and an accidental extubation.

Studies have shown that children are at much greater risk for accidental endotracheal tube dislodgement in the prehospital setting than adults. In fact, one study found it occurs between 16% and 25% of the time. Children's sensitivity to hypoxia may make it a little easier for you to identify a dislodged tube, but it still can be difficult.

Use of continuous waveform capnography is required to provide better monitoring, in large part due to this high frequency of accidental extubation. One should always be prepared for this possibility enroute with equipment and medications at the ready in order to reestablish the airway.

A chest x-ray is one of eight ways to confirm an endotracheal tube (ETT) placement. Figure 9-7 demonstrates proper and improper positions, especially as they relate to minor adjustments of the ETT. One note of caution: determining tracheal versus esophageal placement of an ETT can be difficult, but the x-ray can definitively determine depth of placement.

Respiratory Failure

Ventilation and adequate gas exchange is the next challenge for evaluation and treatment after airway management. Most pediatric medical emergencies are primarily respiratory rather than cardiac. It is important to recognize the early signs of respiratory distress and intervene before a child develops

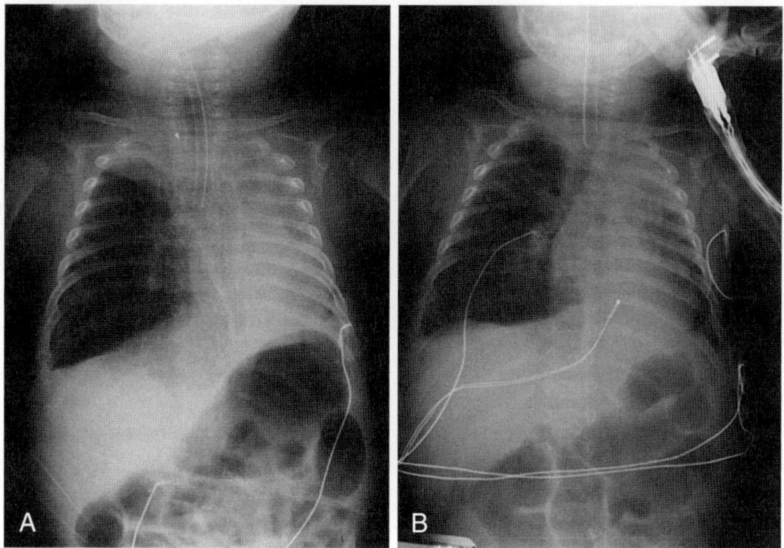

Figure 9-7

A, The right mainstem bronchus has been intubated, and the left lung has collapsed. **B,** After the endotracheal tube (ETT) is withdrawn just 1 cm, the left lung is partly reinflated. (From Curley MA, Moloney-Harmon PA: *Critical care nursing of infants and children,* Philadelphia, 2001, Saunders.)

respiratory failure if possible. Pulse oximetry can be very helpful in trending the patient's condition. A normal child should be able to easily maintain their oxygen saturation by pulse oximetry above 94%. Anything less is a clue that ventilation is probably impaired. Two common diseases are seen in the pediatric age group that may cause respiratory failure: viral infections and asthma.

Viral Respiratory Infections

Seasonal viral infections may cause respiratory failure in children. Influenza is one such infection and can be a problem in all age groups. Another is respiratory syncytial virus (RSV), which may cause severe bronchiolitis and pneumonia, particularly in those less than 1 year of age. These patients can have wheezing and significant air trapping that is not as responsive to bronchodilators or corticosteroids as that caused by asthma. However, it is reasonable to initiate bronchodilators for patients with bronchiolitis and then discontinue them if there is no significant improvement with the therapy. Other treatment is supportive including IV fluids and oxygen. Apnea is sometimes seen with RSV bronchiolitis, most commonly in young infants and those with underlying medical problems. These patients require ventilatory support.

Critical transport teams need to be cognizant of safety issues at all times. Patients with infectious diseases pose a risk to the team and to subsequent patients you care for if members become ill. One needs to use standard and special precautions such as respiratory/contact isolation when caring for patients with RSV. Consult epidemiology standards for other specific diseases and isolation precautions.

Asthma

Asthma is defined as recurrent episodes of reversible airway obstruction. These attacks are most commonly caused by viral respiratory infections but may have other triggers including allergens, cold, exercise, and anxiety. Physiologically, patients with asthma have bronchoconstriction, airway inflammation and increased secretions. Clinically, they present with wheezing and air trapping.

Most children with asthma have only intermittent problems and are well between episodes. These acute exacerbations require treatment with bronchodilators and sometimes short courses of systemic corticosteroids, usually oral. Moderate and persistent asthma is less common and is treated with a regular long-acting bronchodilator and inhaled steroids. Those with status asthmaticus are treated with oxygen, continuously nebulized β-2 agonists and IV corticosteroids. Those patients with more severe and resistant status may be considered for IV beta-agonists such as terbutaline, magnesium sulfate, and/or general anesthesia.

Oxygen Delivery

Oxygen delivery is important and should be provided to children in the most nonthreatening manner possible. Sometimes a care provider that the child trusts may be able to provide the oxygen by a mask more successfully. Other alternative methods include a "blow-by" stream via cupping the hand around the end of the oxygen tubing and holding it close to the patient or just directing the end of the tubing toward the patient's nose and mouth. Some providers have used a paper cup and fitted the oxygen tubing through the bottom of the cup. Children are usually familiar with paper cups and are more likely to accept such an item held over their face than they would an unfamiliar mask.

Supplemental oxygen is required for patients who cannot keep their saturations above 94% on room air. Those who remain less than 90% despite oxygen via a non-rebreather mask need assisted ventilations. However, many children in respiratory distress or otherwise sick may be able to maintain normal oxygen levels as measured by pulse oximetry. These patients still need supplemental oxygen and may even require positive pressure ventilation.

Bag-Mask Device

The ability to safely and effectively intubate children is a critical emergency skill. However, you should be aware that in the majority of cases, children do not require prehospital intubation and tend to do well by bag-valve mask (BVM) ventilation alone. This was found in a prospective, randomized controlled study comparing BVM ventilation with tracheal intubation of children in the prehospital setting.[4] In fact, in a subgroup of children with respiratory failure in the trial, bag-mask ventilation was associated with improved survival rate.

This study was performed in an urban setting where transport times were short. Therefore, the results may not apply to rural or other emergency medical services (EMS) settings where transport times may be much longer or to multitiered EMS systems where second tier providers have more training and experience in intubating pediatric patients. Still, it should be a comfort to know that pediatric patients may be effectively ventilated with a bag-valve mask in most situations. The more recent availability of infraglottic airways approved for pediatric patients adds key resources if endotracheal intubation is not possible or available and can be a nice backup with manual ventilation via bag-valve device.

You must be knowledgeable and skilled in using a bag-valve mask that is age and size appropriate. Bag-valve mask ventilation should be done via techniques taught in all basic pediatric courses, using the E-C clamp technique over the mask, with a lift of the patient's face toward the ventilation bag. Ventilation should be performed with only enough air to make the chest rise and at a rate appropriate to the age of the child. The breaths should be delivered slowly to provide adequate ventilation volume at the lowest possible pressure. This will help decrease the amount of air entering the esophagus, thereby preventing distention of the stomach. Remember though that gastric tubes should be inserted early in the secondary phase of resuscitation because gastric distention hampers good ventilation.

Mechanical Ventilation

Invasive Support for Ventilation

There are many ways to provide mechanical ventilation to intubated children. Inverse inspiratory/expiratory (I:E) ratio, high-frequency, and volume or pressure-controlled ventilation may be used, depending on the child's size, compliance, and ventilation requirements. Using adult ventilators for older children may be acceptable, but small children and infants will require special equipment.

Intermittent mandatory ventilation (IMV) or synchronized intermittent mandatory ventilation (SIMV) is commonly used with smaller children and infants. This age group is often unable to generate the negative pressure necessary to trigger the sensitivity of adult ventilators, so using continuous flow (positive end-expiratory pressure) will assist the patient.

Be cautious with synchronizing the patient's spontaneous ventilatory effort with positive pressure breaths from the ventilator. Several key differences between pediatric and adult ventilators are smaller tidal volumes and the ability to sense changes in pressure and alarm limits.

When placing the pediatric patient on your transport ventilator, there are several factors that may help you choose the best management method. Box 9-3 may aid you in the transition of the patient from the referring hospital's ventilator to yours.

You can evaluate the patient during bag-valve device ventilation to gain a "sense" of the patient's ventilatory needs prior to mechanical ventilation, especially if a manometer is used to gauge the compliance and resistance. An alternative strategy to determine initial ventilatory settings is based on the pathology present and the lung's compliance through time constraints (Table 9-10). For instance, some pathology creates decreased compliance, which causes the lung to fill and empty more slowly (longer time constraints). For other problems,

Box 9-3 Transport Checklist: Invasive Mechanical Ventilation Assessment Factors

1. Baseline breath sounds (quality, adequate expiratory time)
2. Work of breathing (rate, retractions, etc.)
3. Chest excursion and symmetry
4. Chest x-ray (ETT position, lung volume, pathology)
5. Pulmonary mechanics (resistance, compliance, auto-PEEP)
6. Blood gases (capillary, venous, arterial)
7. Non-invasive monitors on? Capnography on: good waveform?
8. Does patient require sedation? Paralyzing agents?
9. Is pulmonary hygiene required?
10. Need for aerosolized or systemic bronchodilator Rx?

Modified from Curley M, et al: *Critical care of infants and children*, Philadelphia, 2001, Saunders.
ETT, Endotracheal tube; *PEEP*, positive end-expiratory pressure.

Table 9-10 Ventilator Settings Based on Compliance/Time Constraints

Setting	Long Fill Time	Short Fill Time	Normal
Tidal volume (Vt)	8-10 mL/kg	6-8 mL/kg	6-10 mL/kg
Breaths/min (rate)	8-15	15-30	10-20
I:E ratio	>1:4	1:1	1:2
PEEP	0-5 cm H_2O	>5 cm H_2O	3-5 cm H_2O

Modified from Curley M, et al: *Critical care nursing of infants and children*, Philadelphia, 2001, Saunders.
I:E, Inspiratory/expiratory; *PEEP*, positive end-expiratory pressure.

such as neuromuscular diseases, compliance may be greater and time constraints shorter.

Noninvasive Positive Pressure Ventilation (NPPV)

NPPV is an option to provide ventilatory support for patients with a clear airway and spontaneous breathing. It may be used via mask (older children) or nasopharyngeal catheter (infants). More detailed instructions on use of NPPV are given in Chapter 3.

In general, NPPV is used in the following situations:

1. Early in the stabilization of patients with acute respiratory failure
2. As a bridge from the ventilator to unassisted breathing after extubation
3. Temporarily in those with end-stage disease

Cardiovascular Failure

Shock

Hypovolemic, cardiogenic, obstructive, and distributive shock have been described pathophysiologically in previous chapters. These types of shock are seen in children as well as in adults. However, how children act clinically may be much different, as described earlier in the physiology section.

Hypovolemic Shock

Hypovolemic shock is a common malady in children and can be caused by decreased intake, gastrointestinal (GI) loss, or traumatic blood loss. The treatment is aggressive fluid resuscitation and treating the cause.

Cardiogenic Shock

Cardiogenic shock is less common in children but can be seen in children with pump failure due to myocarditis or congenital heart disease (CHD). Tachycardia is the best way for children to increase cardiac output because their hearts are fairly stiff with smaller stroke volumes. Clinical presentation may include oliguria, weight gain, and pulmonary crackles similar to adults, but children can often present in cardiogenic shock without these classic symptoms. CHD is discussed in detail later in this section.

Obstructive Shock

Obstruction of blood flow through the major vessels of the chest occurs through pulmonary embolus (rare in children), tension pneumothorax, and pericardial tamponade, usually through traumatic causes. Medically, with any mechanical ventilation (BVM or ventilator), pneumothorax is a possibility. With continued positive pressure ventilation, tension pneumothorax occurs. Chapters 3 and 7 describe the identification and management of this serious complication.

Distributive Shock

Neurogenic and septic shock create a dysfunctional vascular system with either an unresponsive, flaccid vessel or a leaky one. Afterload is affected and cardiac output decreases. Treatment is aimed toward eliminating the cause and managing the vessels, usually through fluids and vasoactive agents.

Vascular Access in the Treatment of Shock

Vascular access can be a very difficult task to accomplish in children, especially when they are ill. Being able to place an intraosseous (IO) needle is a vital skill that should be moved to quickly and confidently when peripheral IV access is not able to be achieved. Technology-assisted IO devices are now available and many transport systems are using them. These devices have needles that are 15 gauge in diameter and are available in three lengths: 15 mm for patients weighing 3 to 39 kg, 25 mm for patients weighing more than 39 kg, and 45 mm for those greater than 40 kg and having excessive tissue over the insertion site. Just be certain to have a manually inserted IO device available in case of equipment malfunction.

Intraosseous access is not only for cardiopulmonary arrest. Its use may be critical for other medical situations when vascular access is difficult and needed, such as in status epilepticus or severe dehydration. Once you stop the seizure with an anticonvulsant or treat the dehydration with fluid boluses through the IO line, it will often be much easier to place an IV.

Initial treatment for shock in children is fluid boluses of 20 mL/kg of normal saline or lactated Ringer's. Use 10 mL/kg in neonates. Pressure infusion devices and blood warmers are welcome adjuncts.

It is easy to overinfuse pediatric patients, which can lead to fluid overload and electrolyte imbalances. A few ways to minimize this risk include the following:

- Use an IV pump and enter the desired rate and volume to be infused
- Use micro-drip tubing for IV
- Hang a smaller bag of fluid

One should monitor the clinical response to your treatment including improvement of tachycardia and other signs of perfusion. If there is inadequate response, arrangement for blood transfusion, surgical intervention, or transport to a tertiary facility needs to be considered. (See Box 9-4 for guidelines regarding pediatric fluid resuscitation.)

Box 9-4 Guidelines for Pediatric Fluid Resuscitation

Hemorrhagic Shock

20 mL/kg warmed crystalloid over 10 minutes × 2-3 boluses then 10 mL/kg of blood

Hypovolemic (Medical) Shock

20 mL/kg warmed crystalloid over 10 minutes, repeat as necessary

Maintenance Fluid

Weight	Fluid Requirements/Hour
<10 kg	4 mL/kg
10-20 kg	2 mL/kg for each kg above 10
> 20 kg	1 mL/kg for each kg above 20

From Curley M, et al: *Critical care of infants and children*, Philadelphia, 2001, Saunders.

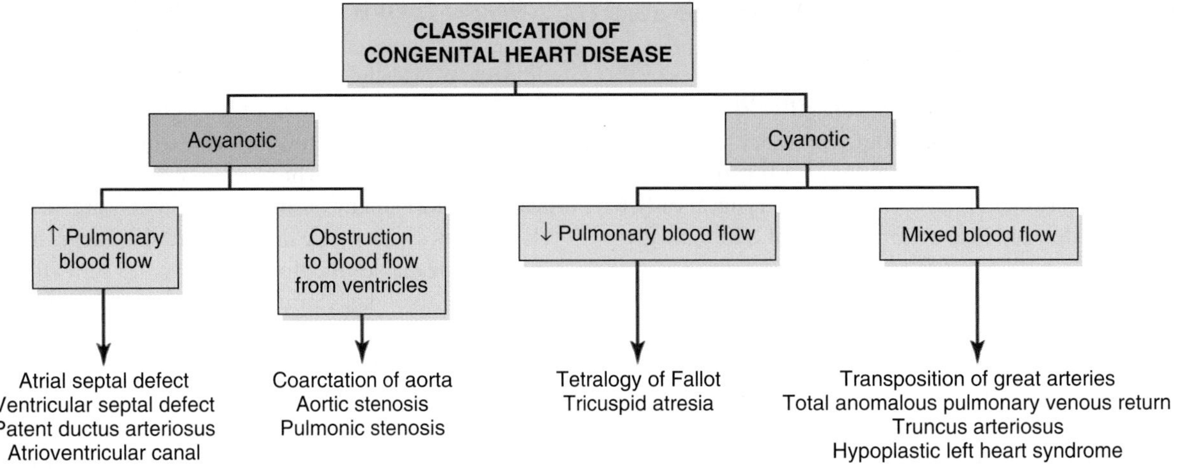

Figure 9-8

Comparison of acyanotic-cyanotic and hemodynamic classification systems of congenital heart disease. (From Wong DL, Hockenberry MJ, Wilson D, Winkelstein ML: *Whaley and Wong's nursing care of infants and children,* ed 6, St Louis, 1999, Mosby.)

Congenital Heart Defects

Encountering a young child with a CHD is not exclusive to the neonatal population. Some heart anomalies may not present until the child is older, or the child may need to grow before operative intervention can occur. It is important for you to have an understanding of the major CHDs.

There are two ways to categorize CHDs: cyanotic vs. acyanotic OR by defining them by their abnormal blood flow. Those that favor categorization by blood flow argue that even acyanotic heart defects may cause cyanosis. Abnormal blood flow can be defined by four basic routes as shown in Figure 9-8.

One of the major complications of CHDs is heart failure. This condition sometimes appears even after surgical repair of the defect. Both right- and left-sided failure may be present. Children do not always present with the classic signs of heart failure seen in adults. The work of the young child is eating, so infants in heart failure often present with a history of poor feeding during which they fatigue easily and become sweaty. This is the equivalent of dyspnea on exertion seen in adults. In fact, intake may be poor enough that the child may be dehydrated. Thus some of the signs of pump failure seen in adults such as rales in the lungs and lower extremity edema may not be evident.

Ductal Patency in the Neonate

Conversion from fetal to neonatal circulation includes closure of the ductus arteriosus, which may take several days. Some neonates with CHDs depend on the ductus to remain patent for pulmonary and/or systemic blood flow.

Administration of Prostaglandin

For some CHD patients, you may need to administer prostaglandin (PGE_1) therapy to prevent closure or reopen the patent ductus arteriosus (PDA) pathway. PGE_1 has a vasodilating effect on the ductus and can create a rapid improvement within 30 minutes of its IV administration. Side effects include respiratory depression, and many transport teams intubate the patient prior to PGE_1 administration. Table 9-11 lists the CHD lesions that might benefit from PGE_1 administration.

Table 9-11 Congenital Heart Defects That Would Benefit from PGE_1 Administration

Improve Pulmonary Blood Flow or Promote A-V Mixing of Blood	Maintain Systemic Perfusion
Pulmonary atresia	Interrupted aortic arch
Critical pulmonary stenosis	Critical coarctation of the aorta
Triscuspid atresia	Hypoplastic left heart syndrome
Transposition of great vessels (with intact septum)	Critical aortic stenosis
Tetralogy of Fallot (with pulmonary atresia or pulmonary artery hypoplasia)	

Modified from Curley M, et al: *Critical care nursing of infants and children,* Philadelphia, 2001, Saunders.
A-V, Atrioventricular.

Hypoxemia in Congenital Heart Defects

Cyanosis from hypoxemia is present in children with certain congenital heart defects (CHDs). This skin sign usually appears when arterial oxygen saturation drops to less than 75% to 85%.

Did You Know?

Cyanosis that decreases with crying is usually respiratory in nature, whereas cyanosis that increases with crying usually is cardiac in nature.[2]

A very dangerous and dramatic presentation called a **tet spell** may occur in some CHD patients. This is classically seen in children with tetralogy of Fallot, a four-lesion CHD. During these spells, there is a sudden increase in right to left shunting causing an acute increase in deoxygenated blood systemically. The child may lose consciousness, have a seizure, or become very cyanotic with tachypnea during the episode. Treatment includes placing the child's knees against the abdomen (or knee-chest position) and administering oxygen. This positioning increases systemic vascular resistance while the supplemental oxygen decreases pulmonary vascular resistance via vasodilation in the lungs. Both of these maneuvers cause a decrease in right to left shunting and improved oxygenation of the blood. If the episode is severe, resuscitation with intubation, ventilation, and fluids may be needed.

Dysrhythmias

The same dysrhythmias encountered in the adult population are also seen in the pediatric age group. In those with CHD, dysrhythmias may be more complicated and problematic. Supraventricular tachycardia (SVT) is the most common dysrhythmia seen in children. Treatment of dysrhythmias is also similar to that in adults, but dosing needs to be weight-based. For SVT, adenosine at 0.05 to 0.1 mg/kg for patients weighing less than 50 kg is standard dosing. The dose may be increased by 0.05 to 0.1 mg/kg, with a maximum total dose of 0.3 mg/kg. Cardioversion for pediatric patients with SVT is performed at 0.5 to 1.0 J/kg.

Nervous System Disease

The nervous system develops very rapidly in children and the central nervous system (CNS) cells and tissues have a high metabolic demand. The critically ill infant or child with illness or injury to the nervous system warrants very specialized care.

Seizures

Seizures are a fairly frequent pediatric emergency. Febrile seizures, or seizures due to fever, are commonly seen in preschool children over 6 months of age and affect about 4% of all children. Other seizures may be related to brain injury including child abuse, congenital abnormalities, CNS infections, or metabolic disorders. Children are more likely to develop hypoglycemia, which is an easily treatable cause of seizure.

Seizures in infants may be quite subtle and present in various ways. These include diverted eye gaze with or without nystagmus, repetitive eye blinking or fluttering, drooling, sucking, tongue thrusting, or lip smacking, and swimming or bicycle pedaling–like movements of the extremities. A postictal state must always be considered as the cause in any child in an unexplained, unconscious condition.

Management of Seizures

Seizures are treated with short-term anticonvulsants such as benzodiazepines, airway maintenance, and general support of the patient's vital signs. One should try to find the cause of the seizure, especially evaluating the blood sugar. Antipyretics are administered to children with febrile seizures.

You should remember that infants and children who have a combination of altered mental status with fever may have meningitis. Compliance with standard and respiratory precautions while caring for such patients is important. NOTE: Those patients with a history of looking well prior to the seizure and who are returning to normal neurologic status after the seizure are unlikely to have bacterial meningitis whether they have a fever or not.

Central Nervous System Infections

The brain and spinal column can be infected through abscess, encephalitis, or meningitis. Brain abscesses and severe encephalitis are rare in pediatric patients and will not be covered in this section. Fortunately, bacterial meningitis is becoming much less common as well outside the neonatal period thanks to childhood immunization programs.

Meningitis

Inflammation of the meninges may be caused by viral, bacterial, or fungal pathogens. Clinically, meningitis presents with fever and signs of meningeal irritation including headache and positive **Kernig's sign** and **Brudzinski's sign.** Fluid is obtained by lumbar puncture to confirm the diagnosis. For bacterial meningitis, cerebrospinal fluid (CSF) analysis will show leukocytosis, increased protein, and decreased glucose.

Meningitis due to viruses, or aseptic meningitis, is typically more benign and treated supportively. Bacterial infections are much more serious. One such infection is meningococcal meningitis, which classically presents with a purpuric rash. Purpura are nonblanching spots on the skin that are usually dark red or purple and caused by bleeding into the skin. Any patient with a suspected bacterial meningitis needs to remain in respiratory/contact isolation until appropriate antibiotics have been administered for at least 24 hours. Close contacts may need preventive antibiotics as well.

Trauma

Trauma is the leading cause of death in children over a year of age and a very common reason for critical care transport. The process for assessment of the child involved in trauma is the same as that for all other patients, keeping in mind the likelihood of physical injuries. How we treat the trauma is based on the physiologic changes already described. Treatment for hemorrhagic shock has been detailed. A very special set of circumstances exists, however, when you provide spinal immobilization in infants and children.

Pediatric Cervical Spine Immobilization

Cervical spine injury in children is uncommon. However, all children suspected of having a cervical spine injury or with a mechanism of injury putting them at risk for such injuries should be immobilized. This immobilization should be continued until an injury is ruled out clinically and radiographically.

Providers must be aware of a relatively common cervical spine injury that is most commonly seen in children less than 8 years of age called **spinal cord injury without radiographic abnormality (SCIWORA).** This syndrome usually presents with normal x-rays, and many have only transient neurologic symptoms that improve. Some patients have severe injuries, especially younger patients. The neurologic deficits that are initially present may subsequently worsen. Some signs are delayed, usually developing within 24 hours. Young children are predisposed to SCIWORA because they have a more tenuous spinal cord blood supply and greater elasticity in the vertebral column than in the spinal cord. The most common mechanism is a flexion/extension injury but can occur with other neck injury mechanisms. MRI is an important tool for evaluating these injuries.

Children have relatively larger heads, weaker neck muscles, and shorter necks than adults. These developmental differences will influence your method of cervical spine immobilization. This can be best accomplished by an appropriately sized and rigid cervical collar. Cervical collars that will fit the array of neck sizes seen in children are commercially available. These collars are more desirable for immobilization than more makeshift methods such as towels around the neck. Contraindications to cervical collar placement include fixed neck angulation, massive cervical swelling, or the need to perform cricothyrotomy.

Children, like all patients, will need to be adequately secured to a backboard to fully immobilize the spine. This can be accomplished with a full or half-sized rigid spine board depending on the size of the child. Infants requiring cervical spine stabilization should be immobilized ideally on a half-sized board; this has been found to be more effective than immobilization in an infant seat. Any gaps between the child and the edges of the board should be filled with blankets or towels to prevent shifting from side to side.

It is critical to maintain a neutral position when placing a patient on a backboard—in other words, without rotating or bending the spinal column. For children, this has been defined as a positioning of the head and torso to create a gaze preference perpendicular to the horizontal plane of the backboard. Unlike adults who require occipital elevation to maintain a neutral position, children will often require elevation of their back to achieve proper positioning due to their larger heads. Without this elevation, the larger occiput of the younger child will force the head into flexion when the child is placed supine.

Some pediatric backboards have a built-in depressed area for the head placement to maintain a neutral position. Regular backboards used for children may be modified to accomplish this as well. Figure 9-9 demonstrates this technique. Otherwise, you can elevate the back by placing some sort of padding under the shoulders and extending it to the buttocks.

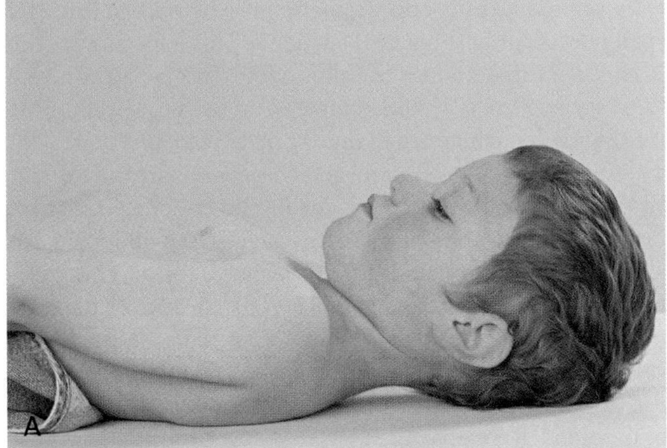

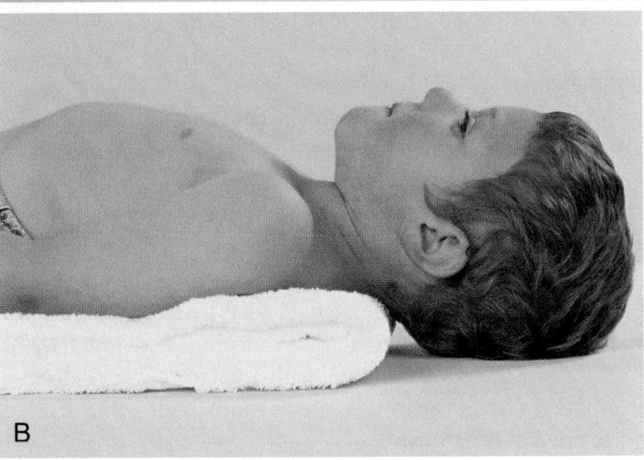

Figure 9-9

A, Because of the large size of a child's head, relative to body size, and the incomplete development of the posterior thoracic muscles, hyperflexion of the head occurs when a child is placed on a backboard. **B,** Padding beneath the shoulders and torso prevents hyperflexion. (From NAEMT: *PHTLS prehospital trauma life support*, ed 6, St Louis, 2007, Mosby.)

Hypoglycemia

Hypoglycemia is likely to develop in the stressed critical pediatric patient because of the lack of glycogen stores and the high demand of the pediatric body for ready sugars. Therefore, assessment of glucose is critical as part of your immediate post-resuscitation evaluation. Normal glucose levels are variable in the preterm, neonate, infant, and child age groups. In general, any blood sugar less than 30 mg/dL should be treated. Manage acute hypoglycemia by administering 10% dextrose in water at 5 to 10 mL/kg IV for young children or 25% dextrose in water at 2 to 4 mL/kg IV for older children. Using dextrose concentrations greater than this will be very harsh on the child's veins because of the hyperosmolality of the solutions.

Child Abuse

Child abuse is a leading cause of death in young children, especially in children between 1 and 12 months of age.

Transport team members play a very important role in identifying child abuse and in helping to break the cycle of violence. It may be one of your best ways to save a child's life.

For those transport teams that have both 9-1-1 and critical care transfer resources, one should closely assess the surroundings and mentally note the environment when responding to any emergency call. This may be critical when attending to pediatric patients who may be the victim of child abuse. Because you are being called into the homes of these children, you have a unique opportunity to identify and document vital information that could provide evidence of child abuse. Child abuse injuries may involve life-threatening problems that require involved medical interventions and necessitate immediate transport to an emergency department.

You need to particularly pay attention to and record the mechanism of injury. Note the area where the caregiver states the fall or impact took place. Estimate heights of couches or beds from which the child reportedly fell. What surface did the child fall onto? Document statements of any bystanders. Are the provided histories consistent? What is the affect of the caregiver and what emotions does the person display? You should keep in mind that children with special needs may be at increased risk for abuse or neglect.

Your initial scene contact may reveal important details that later on crime investigators may not see. This information needs to be preserved in writing. Clear, objective language should be used in your documentation. No matter how horrible the abuse, you must not use judgmental statements.

Child abuse and neglect cases can be very emotionally challenging. Your main role is still efficiently treating, stabilizing, and safely transporting the child. You should not confront the caregiver with your suspicions. This may lead to a confrontation that will interfere with your treatment of the patient or even be dangerous.

Your team members are mandatory reporters, just like other medical care providers. Suspected child abuse or neglect needs to be reported to the child protective services agency in the county in which the event occurred. Most state statutes call for reporting if there is merely a "reasonable cause to believe" or a "reasonable suspicion." Some require the reporter to "know or suspect," which is a slightly higher degree of knowledge. Regardless, you do not have to be certain that abuse or neglect occurred to make a report.

In most states, persons who report suspected child abuse or neglect in "good faith" are absolutely immune from criminal and civil liability. However, failure to report can result in criminal liability (typically a misdemeanor punishable by a fine) and, perhaps more importantly, can result in civil liability. Your suspicions should be shared with hospital personnel to whom you deliver the patient as well. You can have a great impact on identifying abused and neglected kids whose families need help and intervention to prevent further harm to their children.

Cardiopulmonary Arrest in Children

Unlike cardiac arrest in adults, children spiral toward death through two pathways: respiratory failure and/or shock. Thus the best way to manage critically ill children is to quickly identify and aggressively manage those in respiratory failure and shock to prevent the downward spiral toward cardiopulmonary arrest. It is much more difficult to have a satisfactory patient outcome once an arrest occurs. Even if the patient is resuscitated and death initially averted, multisystem organ failure and severe increased intracranial pressure with brain injury or death is a common post-arrest scenario.

Many intensive care units are managing cardiac arrest in children with therapeutic hypothermia during the resuscitation. For those with open fontanelles and sutures not yet fused, ice (or iced helmet) to the head is one method of preventing secondary reperfusion brain injury.

Cardiac arrest management in the newly born involves the steps taught in the neonatal resuscitation courses; 120 events per minute are organized around 90 compressions (encirclement technique) and 30 ventilations at a 3:1 ratio. Access to the umbilical vein for fluid and drug administration is also advised. For all other children in the healthcare setting, a 15:2 ratio is encouraged at this time. The sequence of cardiac arrest management is the same as that for adults. You must have current credentials in cardiopulmonary resuscitation (CPR) and ALS courses for pediatric care through your employer.

Termination of Pediatric Resuscitation Efforts

It is difficult to determine when to stop resuscitative efforts during a pediatric arrest. Transport services will usually have guidelines or protocols you will need to follow with regard to this issue. Previously, a child that failed to have a return of spontaneous circulation with two or more doses of epinephrine was considered unlikely to survive. However, with arrest in the in-hospital setting, prolonged resuscitation with intact patient survival has been more recently documented. The decision regarding when to stop resuscitation may be influenced by the cause of the arrest, available resources, where the arrest occurred, and the likelihood of reversible problems. Generally, resuscitative efforts may be discontinued if there is no return of spontaneous circulation despite ALS interventions. This often requires not more than 30 minutes. More prolonged resuscitation should be performed in children with the following: recurring or refractory ventricular fibrillation (VF) or ventricular tachycardia (VT), a history of a toxic drug exposure, or a primary hypothermic insult.

CARE AND TRANSPORT OF NEONATAL AND PEDIATRIC PATIENTS

Special Considerations

The pediatric and legislative community noticed a gap in the emergency care of infants and children in the 1980s. Several organizations joined forces to demonstrate need and seek standards. In 1984, the federal government of the United States passed legislation allocating funds to create the Emergency Medicine Services for Children (EMS-C) Program for the purpose of improving EMS care for children. EMS-C is a collaborative program between the Maternal and Child Health Bureau and the National Highway Traffic Safety Administration. It provides funding to all 50 states and United States territories.

All states have legislation that provides the basis for their statewide EMS systems. However, state agencies establish local regulations regarding the extent of services that can be provided by prehospital personnel and the procedures that they may perform on children. To improve outcomes for critically ill and injured infants, children, and young adults, all EMS-C components must be integrated into existing EMS systems.

The above initiatives, however, do not address the transport of the critically ill infant or child from one institution to another, usually a tertiary care center. *Guidelines for Air and Ground Transportation of Pediatric Patients*, published in 1986 by the American Academy of Pediatrics (AAP), and *Guidelines for Air and Ground Transport of Neonatal and Pediatric Patients*, published in 1993, provide some interfacility transport guidelines. In addition, the Emergency Medical Treatment and Active Labor Act (EMTALA) rules for transfer do address certain issues related to stabilization, equipment, and personnel (see Chapter 1).

There is general agreement that pediatric transport requires special preparation and skills. However, even the experts have different expectations and may disagree with regard to the systems that should be in place for child transport beyond the neonatal age. Transport of the newly born (within a few hours of delivery) and the newborn (1-31 days of age) is a well-respected system with accepted transport criteria. Hospital systems with obstetric capabilities have defined neonatal transport team arrangements and transfer agreements and will wait for that specialized team while stabilizing the baby. They do not ask the local EMS system to transport a neonate. They stabilize and wait for the specialized neonatal transport team.

What happens at 32 days of age? This well-established and standardized system of transporting neonates does not extend into the world of pediatric transport in many areas of the country. Critical Care Transport programs, knowledgeable and skilled in taking care of adult pathophysiology, are sometimes called upon to provide the same level of care for very ill children—often with a crew having very little experience in pediatric care. The AAP has pediatric transport recommendations, but these are not always followed by hospitals and providers. *Guidelines for Air Medical Crew Education*, jointly published by the Association of Air Medical Services (AAMS), Air Medical Physician Association (AMPA), the Air & Surface Transport Nurses Association (ASTNA), the International Association of Flight Paramedics (IAFP), the National Association of Air Medical Communication Specialists (NAAMCS), and the National EMS Pilots Association also provides standards and guidance to transport services who wish to provide care to ill or injured neonates and children.

Should your critical care transport system include neonate and pediatric patients? That answer depends again on the team you have, how they are prepared, and what equipment and resources you can promise to the hospitals and patients you serve. One of the basic tenets of pediatric critical care transport is that the program must develop multiple resources, particularly a critical mass of skilled healthcare professionals. In addition, there should be an adequate volume of transported pediatric patients to maintain appropriate skills and staff levels.

Let's begin by looking at our youngest special population, the neonate. And, to begin this discussion, you must look at the special process of neonatal transport.

Neonatal Transport

Neonates that require transport are an extremely high-risk population. These fragile babies often need emergent transfer for specialized neonatal care due to complicated medical and surgical problems. This includes prematurity, perinatal infections, and congenital abnormalities. Most healthcare providers do not have the skills and training necessary to adequately care for the smallest and most critically ill neonates. Transport of these babies is best provided by personnel skilled in critical neonatal care with specialized equipment.

The establishment of neonatal transport teams at tertiary care centers developed from this medical care necessity. These specialized teams are most commonly a component of a larger, sometimes regional, perinatal care system. Such systems usually include the perinatal care unit, the neonatal intensive care unit (NICU), a neonatal outreach program, and numerous medical and surgical pediatric subspecialists. Neonatal transport team members often fulfill other functions within the perinatal care system including on-site and outreach educational roles, and public relations.

Neonatal transport systems have played an important part in helping reduce the United States neonatal mortality rate. Despite this, the outcome of neonates with serious medical or surgical problems born outside a tertiary care center remains poorer than those born in-house. This underscores the importance of prenatal diagnosis and in identifying those at risk for perinatal problems. Mothers still make the best transport incubators!

Initiating Neonatal Transport

Good communication is vital for any transport. Upon receiving a neonatal transfer request, the medical control physician must be able to be contacted immediately to initiate the transport process. Usually this is a physician who is a subspecialist in neonatal/perinatal medicine or in pediatric intensive care. Discussion with the referring physician is imperative for the medical control physician to determine whether transfer is appropriate and what mode of transport to use. Some of the reasons for transport include the following:

- When a medically indicated procedure or service cannot be provided at a level I or II nursery or when a patient's best interest would be better served at another facility with appropriate capabilities, transport is undertaken.
- When there is no longer a need for tertiary care, an infant is transported to a level/II facility.

- In rare situations (because of lack of bed space and/or personnel) an infant may be transported to another facility capable of providing the same appropriate level of care.
- At request of parent(s) or legal guardian, transport is provided after explanation is given of the potential risks of transport.

Communication of vital signs, laboratory values, radiographic studies, and treatment already provided is essential. This allows for adequate preparation of the accepting hospital and transport team. In addition, the case details allow medical control to provide advice for stabilization and management by the referring hospital until the transport team arrives.

Predeparture Stabilization

The neonatal transport team usually assumes control of patient management under direction of medical control when they arrive at the transferring facility. Often, they will work under protocols that serve as standing orders and care guidelines. This allows the team to perform immediate actions to care for a critical neonate in the absence of direct physician input. The transport team needs to become familiar with the contents of the patient's chart prior to transport and obtain clarification as required.

The time the neonatal transport team spends at the transferring hospital depends greatly on the configuration of the team, the mode of transport, and the patient's medical status. The team always performs a careful assessment of the neonate. This includes vital signs, the ABCs, and a rapid blood glucose. Particular attention needs to be given to the airway and the adequacy of ventilation and oxygenation because they are such a frequent problem in this age group.

A method of quickly stabilizing and rapidly loading neonates for transport is sometimes employed. This practice is somewhat similar to the method often used for trauma calls. Much shorter out-of-hospital times are seen with this approach. It is more commonly used by teams of less experienced personnel, in helicopter transfers, and for neonates with rapidly progressing disease processes.

Frequently, neonates are maximally stabilized at the referring facility prior to departure. This can lead to extremely long stabilization times because high level critical care interventions are performed. But it minimizes the need for such interventions during the less controlled environment of a transport. This method is more commonly used when physicians or other highly skilled providers are members of the transport team. It is also more likely to be done if the transport will be a longer ground or fixed-wing transport.

Neonatal Care During Transport

Initial Patient Stabilization

Initial stabilization and assessment always starts with ensuring the airway is patent. Positioning of the infant should allow appropriate suctioning. Take note of the patient's color, breathing pattern, and effort. Attach needed monitoring devices such as cardiac, blood pressure, capnography.. Make certain vital signs are taken initially and as frequently as the condition indicates. Assess the need to empty the infant's stomach. Consider the use of an orogastric tube to perform gravity drainage if needed. Temperature should be stabilized and maintained between 96.8° to 98.6° F.[5] Review current blood gases for evidence of ventilation problems. Critical results of laboratory values would include a pH of less than 7.25 or greater than 7.5; a P_{CO_2} less than 30 or greater than 55; a P_{O_2} less than 60 or greater than 100 (if infant is less than 1500 gm). Once the decision is made to move the infant for transport, take the most direct route as quickly and safely as practical.

Airway and Ventilation Management

BVM ventilation is the first intervention to turn to for neonates who require positive pressure ventilation. Extremely small masks may be required to perform this skill. However, prolonged airway management during neonatal transport should not be attempted by BVM. Intubation is required. This should always be accomplished in the neonate with an uncuffed endotracheal tube of the appropriate internal diameter. The ETT size will vary from 2.5 to 4.0 mm.

Although hand bagging through an ETT may be acceptable for short transports, ventilators are generally used for most neonatal transports. Transport ventilators are different from models usually seen in the NICU and are technologically limited. Typically, they are not capable of patient synchronization, heated ventilation circuits, and patient triggered or high-frequency ventilation modes. Team members must be proficient in the setup and use of the transport ventilators they have available.

Temperature Control

Specially designed neonatal incubators are used during transport to help decrease heat and fluid losses (Figure 9-10). Thermal control can still be very difficult because of the less controlled transport environment. Cold weather, long transports, and less efficient equipment than what is available in

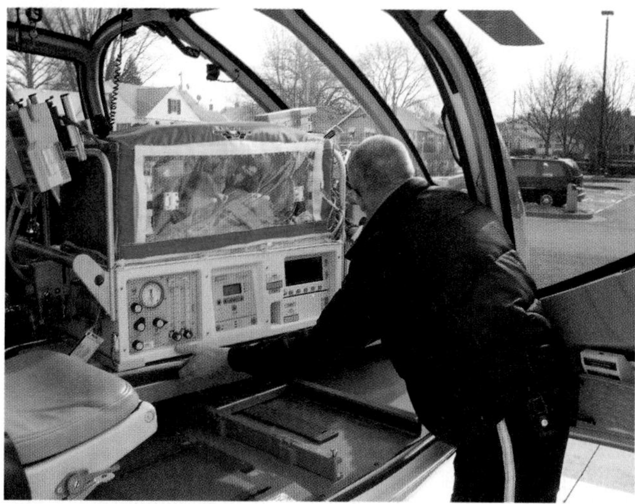

Figure 9-10

Neonatal incubator. (Courtesy the University of Iowa Hospitals and Clinics, Iowa City, Iowa.)

the NICU can all be contributory factors. An unusual technique to address this problem is used in extremely premature infants—polyethylene sheets or bags are placed over the neonate to help maintain body temperature.

If a newborn becomes hypothermic, he or she should be warmed in a carefully controlled manner. This should occur at approximately 1° C per hour. During transport, this can be a challenging but important task. Hypothermic neonates who are rapidly warmed have been found to have increased morbidity and mortality.

TRAINING FOR NEONATAL AND PEDIATRIC TRANSPORT

Only about 2% of pediatric EMS calls are for children with life-threatening problems. The good news is that children are usually well and don't get that sick. The bad news is that because we see so few sick kids, we are not very skilled in taking care of them.

Pediatric-focused training is an important component of all emergency healthcare professional development. You will need to achieve and maintain a competency (if not expertise) in the assessment and stabilization of children. Adequate initial training and ongoing experience with pediatric advanced life support (ALS) skills is essential. Most EMS systems require their professionals to have at least 10% of their training in pediatrics. But that is just the "basics" of pediatric care.

The Neonatal Resuscitation Program (NRP), Pediatric Advanced Life Support (PALS), Pediatric Education for Prehospital Professionals (PEPP), and Emergency Pediatric Care (EPC) courses are all programs available to both basic and advanced prehospital providers. For nurses, PALS and the Emergency Nursing Pediatric Course (ENPC) set the stage for basic pediatric resuscitation education. Respiratory therapists may gain knowledge from NRP and PALS. The Advanced Pediatric Life Support (APLS): The Pediatric Emergency Medicine Course is available to all potential transport team members.

The courses mentioned above are excellent for care providers involved in the emergency care of ill or injured pediatric patients. However, these courses may not provide care providers with enough critical care knowledge or with sufficient opportunities to develop the necessary skills with the special equipment required to provide bedside stabilization of a critically ill neonate or pediatric patient. This high level care demands a special educational approach by the programs and the personnel dedicated to these specialized services.

Transport Team

Neonatal Team

Neonatal transport teams are configured in a number of ways. Usually the team is composed of a highly skilled and experienced registered nurse (RN) combined with one of the following: another nurse, a paramedic, a respiratory therapist, or a physician. The most common configuration is that of an RN and EMT-P; the second most common being a two-RN crew. Because many critically ill neonates have existing or impending respiratory failure, a respiratory therapist is a popular choice for the second team member in some programs because of the ventilation management expertise such a member can provide.

Any particular system's team configuration is largely determined by tradition, the local availability of various personnel, and by the characteristics of patients that are transported. Members are often selected by the special skills, experiences, and abilities they bring to the transport team. Continuing education to obtain and retain competence is a necessity for team members. This often includes practical skill sessions with animals, models, or cadavers, or in clinical settings such as the delivery room, operating suite, or NICU.

Pediatric Team

At least one member of a specialized pediatric team must have experience in pediatric intensive bedside care. As the team leader on each mission, this person primarily operates via guidance of the Medical Director's protocols, but must be able to make critical decisions independently.

The Medical Director of the transport program is in charge of all aspects of care during transport. However, if a program commits to providing pediatric services, there should be a medical command from the referral center's neonatal and/or pediatric ICU. All team members, whether they have an EMS, nursing, or respiratory therapy background, must follow a detailed plan of initial training, credentialing, and ongoing education in the care of this special population.

Educational Programs for Neonatal and Pediatric Transport

Services should establish an initial orientation program for those assigned to neonatal and/or pediatric transports, including didactic sessions, case review, specialized skill credentialing, and then a program of ongoing experiential and continuing education maintenance and minimums. Supervised management of critically ill patients in the neonatal and pediatric ICU or high-level pediatric emergency department, as well as pediatric airway and ventilation management experience in the operating room are keys to success. In addition, preceptor supervision of new personnel during their initial patient contacts is necessary.

Airway and Ventilation

Pediatric airway and ventilation management, including intubation proficiency, may be accomplished with time spent in the operating room. This is best done on a regular basis. A minimum number of skills performed by the crew is established by the medical director of the program and should be monitored routinely. Manikins and animal models can also be helpful in skill establishment and retention, but they do have their limitations.

Needle and tube thoracostomy, tracheostomy care, emergency surgical airway skills, ventilator management, use of nitric oxide, interpretation of blood gases, and respiratory monitoring must all be included in crew preparation for critical care transport.

Perfusion, Vascular Access, Hemodynamic Monitoring, and Circulatory Support

Obtaining vascular access in a 2-kg patient can be quite challenging. Such demands will require transport personnel to obtain didactic and practical knowledge in circulatory access via intraosseous, umbilical venous and arterial, peripheral, arterial, and central lines as well as in the monitoring of hemodynamic parameters in the pediatric population. Medications and equipment used to support circulation are similar in all patients. But the unique dosing and size of young pediatric patients present challenges to all healthcare providers, especially those that more often care for adult patients.

Extracorporeal Membrane Oxygenation

ECMO is a sophisticated procedure in which blood is oxygenated and cardiac functions are performed by a mechanical pump outside the body. Similar to heart-lung bypass, this therapy is used for critically ill patients with ARDS, diaphragmatic hernia, meconium aspiration, pulmonary hypertension, and cardiorespiratory failure/arrest, and postoperative cardiac surgery support. Used in all patient populations, this bridge process is performed much more in pediatric age groups. Some European transport services establish ECMO at the referring hospital and transport the patient with the process ongoing.

Neonatal Considerations in Education and Preparation

The neonatal team takes control of the neonate's care in hospitals with lesser resources. They must communicate well and feel comfortable operating in the high-risk neonatal transport environment. Protocols need to be established and crew personnel need to have expertise in high-risk neonatal problems. These include the care of respiratory distress syndrome (RDS), transient tachypnea of the newborn (TTN), meconium aspiration syndrome (MAS), congenital heart disease (CHD), cardiac arrhythmias, persistent pulmonary hypertension in the newborn, seizures, intraventricular hemorrhage, hydrocephalus, neural tube defects, hypoglycemia, acid-base derangements, electrolyte disturbances, sepsis and surgical emergencies of the newborn including omphalocele, gastroschisis, malrotation, necrotizing enterocolitis (NEC), tracheoesophagel fistula (TEF), and diaphragmatic hernia. Skills in all aspects of neonatal airway management and vascular access (intraosseous (IO) and intravenous (IV), umbilical venous catheter [UVC], umbilical artery catheter [UAC]) are necessary for personnel. High-level skills in ventilator support, including use of high-frequency ventilation, nitric oxide and ECMO, and knowledge of the special fluid and electrolyte requirements of neonates are needed. Stabilization of the patient should be as complete as possible prior to transport so that, hopefully, only maintenance is required during the transport phase.

Suggested equipment, supplies, and medications for neonatal transport are included in Box 9-5.

Pediatric Considerations in Education and Preparation

The pediatric critical care team, usually based out of the referral center's ICU or specialized ER, must be knowledgeable in normal growth and development of children, as well as in pediatric medical and trauma assessment and management. Expertise in airway conditions, such as foreign body airway obstruction, croup, epiglottitis, tracheitis, retropharyngeal abscesses, asthma, pneumonia, and bronchiolitis due to respiratory syncytial virus (RSV), are required. High-level knowledge in cardiovascular emergencies in children, such as CHD (cyanotic and acyanotic), cardiomyopathies and dysrhythmia management, along with traumatic injuries that involve airway, breathing, and circulation, are mandatory. Specialized knowledge and skills in recognition and management of medical emergencies such as fluid and electrolyte abnormalities, toxic exposures, seizures, shock, child abuse, and complications in children with special healthcare needs are also required.

Skills necessary for initial and ongoing credentialing include all aspects of pediatric airway care, vascular access (IV, IO, peripheral intravenous central catheter [PICC], UVC, central venous catheter [CVC], central and hemodynamic lines), ventilator set-up and maintenance, and management of the unique fluid and electrolyte needs in this age group.

Suggested equipment, supplies, and medications for pediatric ALS care are presented in Box 9-6.

Continuing Education

A particularly important development in healthcare education is the availability of high-fidelity patient simulators in a pediatric size. These high-tech simulators provide learners with the opportunity to repetitively practice their pediatric critical care skills during a multitude of medical and trauma scenarios. The simulators model respiratory patterns, eye movements and responses, heart sounds, and even exchange of gases in simulated technology. They are realistic in appearance as well as in their ability to react to the treatment provided by the learner. This is usually based on preprogrammed scenarios. Providers can get hands-on experience in a near real-life setting without causing potential harm.

Emergency and critical care systems use simulation resources to improve their teamwork. The simulation experience allows them to condition themselves in improving communication, role assignments and in identifying potential problems in their treatments before they experience them in reality. Studies have shown that simulator laboratory participants feel better prepared and are more relaxed when dealing with common and uncommon emergency situations.

Most laboratories are able to teach critical thinking skills by working through a problem, which is the simulation, and then reviewing it. This is called the *debriefing*. The debriefing is important to help identify what was done right and what might need to be corrected or repeated. It allows both students and teams to recognize their strengths and weaknesses. Some laboratories use videotaping to help learners identify for themselves their strong and weak areas.

Box 9-5 Suggested Equipment, Supplies, and Medication for Neonatal Care

This list is not comprehensive and is intended to be an adjunct to equipment already used by the air medical team. The program mission, scope of practice and medical direction will determine the specific equipment and medications required.

The size of equipment and supplies is critical to the provision of appropriate neonatal care. Any air medical program that may be called to respond to a neonatal patient or potential delivery of a neonate should have size and age-appropriate neonatal transport equipment. Inventories can be organized according to the familiar A-B-C approach, or may be categorized by color as part of a larger pediatric response kit. Equipment must be maintained in a ready and operational state. All equipment must be secured in the transport environment to provide for both infant and air medical crew safety. Electronic equipment must have dependable power sources (inverter access and/or batteries).

Airway Support

- Bulb syringe
- Suction catheters (5, 6.5, 8, 10 Fr)
- Oral airways (0, 1)
- Respiratory saline irrigant
- Meconium aspirator
- Mucus suction trap
- Mechanical suction (wall and portable) with regulator, canister and tubing

Breathing Support

- Neonatal flow-inflating (anesthesia) bag
- Neonatal self-inflating bag
- Face masks (preemie, newborn, infant)
- Pressure manometer
- Feeding tube (5, 8 Fr)
- Replogle tube (10 Fr)
- Laryngoscope handle with Miller blades (0, 1)
- Spare batteries and bulbs
- Neonatal stylette
- Endotracheal tubes (2.0, 2.5, 3.0, 3.5, 4.0)
- ET tube holder, tape
- Heat/moisture exchanges (artificial nose)
- Pedi-cap
- Nasal CPAP prong set-up (sizes XS, S, L)
- Oxygen hood
- Thoracentesis kit
  - 21-gm butterfly
  - 3-way stopcock
  - 60-mL syringe
  - Betadine, alcohol preps
- Thoracotomy kit (umbilical cath kit used for surgical drapes, betadine swabs, instruments, and sutures)
  - Chest tubes (10, 12 Fr)
  - Heimlich valves
  - Neonatal transport ventilator with 50+ psi O_2 source
  - Ventilator monitor with alarms, oxygen analyzer
  - Oxygen source (with system back-up)
  - Air source (tank or compressor)
  - Blender capability
  - Flow meter, O_2 nipple adapter
  - O_2 tank key

Circulation Support

- IV catheters (22, 24 gm)
- Scalp vein needles (23, 25 gm)
- T-connectors
- Stopcocks
- Bio-occlusive dressing
- Extension tubing
- Syringes (assorted 1-60 mL)
- Assorted needles
- Tape
- Infusion pump with appropriate tubing (2-5 line capability)
- Rubber bands, cotton, safety pins
- Arm boards (preemie, newborn)
- Alcohol preps
- Umbilical catheter tray (sterile tray with drapes, iris forceps, curved forceps, scissors, needle holder, 2 × 2s, umbilical tape, 4.0 silk suture with curved needle, scalpel and blade, tape measure)
- Umbilical catheters (3.5, 5.0)
- Cloth limb restraints
- Surgical masks, cap, gloves
- Intraosseous needles

Monitoring/Miscellaneous

- Cardiac, respiratory, temperature monitor with appropriate supplies (neonatal electrodes, lead wires, tape, recorder paper)
- Invasive and noninvasive BP monitor with supplies (pressure transducer, BP cuffs: 2.5, 3, 4, 5)
- Pulse oximeter with disposable probes
- Blood glucose monitoring strips, lancets, cotton, Band-Aids
- Neonatal stethoscope
- Portable transilluminator
- Personal protection supplies (gloves, antimicrobial wipes, waterless hand wash, gowns, masks, eye shields, trash bag, sharps containers)

Environment

- Transport incubator with installed safety straps
- Infant blankets (warmed and sufficient enough to provide for nesting rolls)
- Disposable diapers
- Chemical heat mattress
- Infant hat
- Thermometer
- ViDrape© (useful for protection of open defects)
- Face mask, ear protection for sensitive neonates
- Infant safety seat or infant restraint device for term infants who do not need thermal support

Family Support, Facilitation of Continuity of Care

- Instant camera, film
- Parent information
- Facility phone numbers, maps/directions
- Transport consent forms
- Documentation supplies (chart forms)

Box 9-5 Suggested Equipment, Supplies, and Medications for Neonatal Care—cont'd

Medications for Neonatal Care

Resuscitation Medications

- Epinephrine 1:10,000 (0.1 mg/mL)
- Normal saline or Ringer's lactate-volume
- Sodium bicarbonate 4.2% (5 mEq/10 mL)
- Naloxone hydrochloride 0.4 mg/mL or 1.0 mg/mL
- Normal saline (without preservatives) vials—IV flush
- Dextrose 10% ($D_{10}W$)

Additional Neonatal Medications

- Dopamine
- Dobutamine
- 5% Albumin
- Furosemide
- Digoxin
- Adenosine
- Calcium chloride 10% or calcium gluconate
- Ampicillin
- Gentamicin
- Cefotaxime
- Sterile water (without preservative)—diluent
- Erythromycin ointment (eye prophylaxis)
- Phytonadione (vitamin K)
- Heparin (100 μ/mL)
- Albuterol
- Dextrose 5% (D_5W)
- Dextrose 25% or 50% (D_{25}, D_{50})
- Morphine sulfate
- Phenobarbital
- Diazepam
- Versed
- Midazolam
- Fentanyl
- Vecuronium or pancuronium
- Prostaglandin E_1
- Exogenous surfactant
- Xylocaine 1%

Miscellaneous Medication Supplies

- Neonatal code card references
- Calculator
- Medication labels
- Filter needles

From Association of Air Medical Services (AAMS): *Guidelines for air medical crew education*, Kendal/Hunt Publishing, 2004, Dubuque, Iowa, pp. 30-29 through 30-32.
BP, Blood pressure; *CPAP,* continuous positive airway pressure; *ET,* endotracheal.

The use of high-fidelity simulators with knowledgeable facilitators and well-thought-out scenarios and formalized debriefing will most certainly become an increasingly important element of healthcare provider curricula. Pediatric critical skill and emergency care learning and retention will undoubtedly rely heavily on this developing technology.

Ongoing experience and maintenance of skills is a must in providing high quality neonatal and pediatric critical care transport. A quality assurance/improvement program for the transport company should include a system by which the medical director evaluates the number of procedures performed and the types of patients encountered.

The medical director and transport company may need to focus the ongoing education program on maintenance of pediatric critical care knowledge and skills if the team is not completing the minimum number of procedures or patient encounters. This may include experiential-based training with supervised education in the neonatal and/or pediatric ICUs, or through classroom and laboratory sessions that focus on cognitive or skills gaps. If the predetermined numbers are being met through in-house or transport experience, the medical director may look at patient medical records to review quality of decisions made and successes as a way of determining the ongoing educational needs of crew members.

Routine team development education should be centered around case conferences and continuous quality improvement initiatives. The team should also be involved in community education and research and attend neonatal and pediatric critical care transport conferences.

Transport Safety for Pediatric Patients

The safety of a child in your transport vehicle is an important consideration. Children who are properly restrained in a motor vehicle have a greatly reduced likelihood of being seriously injured or dying in a crash. Pediatric patients transported in our ambulances and fixed or rotor-wing aircraft deserve at least the same level of protection that we advocate in private vehicles.

Crashes involving ambulances and aircraft are far too common. In the United States, they account for nearly one fatality each week and many more injuries. Of those involving occupants in an ambulance, most were positioned in the rear compartment and either improperly restrained or not restrained at all.

Safe and appropriate transport of children by ambulance never includes having the child being held by another person. All occupants need to be restrained, and all equipment needs to be safely secured including monitoring devices.

Car Seats

What about transporting children in their own car seat? Well, child car safety seats are not considered medical devices, nor are they designed to withstand more than one crash. Such wisdom would suggest that all children should be removed from their car seat and placed in an approved medical device or into a new car safety seat for transport. Although such action is reasonable, it is not necessarily a given.

If there is no concern of spinal damage, it may be necessary to temporarily violate the best practice of not using a car seat

Box 9-6 Suggested Equipment and Supplies for Pediatric ALS Care

0.9% normal saline or lactated Ringer's for intravenous infusion
Sodium chloride—bacteriostatic for injection
Water—bacteriostatic for injection
Activated charcoal
Adenosine
Atropine sulfate
Sodium bicarbonate—8.4% (1.0 mEq/mL)
Benzodiazepine (of choice)
Epinephrine—1:1000 (1 mg/mL)
Epinephrine—1:10,000 (.1 mg/kg)
Racemic epinephrine
Lidocaine—(10 mg/mL)
Naloxone—(1.0 mg/mL)
Flumazenil
Lorazepam
Diazepam
Midazolam
Phenytoin
Phosphenytoin
Paraldehyde
Pain medication per medical control
50% dextrose in water
25% dextrose in water
Inhalant beta–adrenergic agent of choice
Nebulizer

From Association of Air Medical Services (AAMS): Suggested equipment and supplies for pediatric ALS care. In AAMS: *Guidelines for air medical crew education*, Dubuque, Iowa, 2004, Kendal/Hunt Publishing, pp. 31-22 and 23.
ALS, Advanced life support.

that has already been in a crash under the circumstances of no other safety restraint device being available. The child's own restraint device, if intact, will be far superior to a stretcher alternative. A typical gurney's belt system provides poor restraint for a child in both the flat and back elevated positions. This is true even when the shoulder straps are used. Because the straps route over the back edge of the gurney and do not fit snugly against the back of the shoulders of the child, backward movement is possible. This has allowed children to slide off a gurney head first in actual crashes.

Infants and small children may be transported in their own safety seat as long as you can secure it to your vehicle and have adequate access to the patient. You may elect to use some additional padding. Use of a child safety seat integrated into the rear-facing captain's chair in the front of the ambulance patient compartment is another option. This seat can be used to transport uninjured children older than 1 year and weighing between 20 and 50 pounds.

Ambulance Cart Restraints

A great innovation for proper restraint of children during transport has been the recent development of ambulance-specific child safety seats. Initially, these were available for children up to only 40 pounds. Now there are models designed for the emergency transport of children weighing 22 to 100 pounds. This cot-mounted ambulance restraint device can be used at angles from flat to 70 degrees.

You should discuss with your medical director and legal staff what is the most reasonable and safe approach regarding restraint of pediatric patients for your service. Regardless of how you secure a child in your ambulance, continuous monitoring and reassessment must be done throughout the duration of your care to ensure the safety of your patient.

Family-Centered Care and Family Presence during Treatment

The care approach used with pediatric patients will vary depending on the patient's age and the severity of the injury or illness. You must be cognizant of both the medical and emotional needs of the child throughout the care you provide. Children's response to what is happening will vary greatly depending on their level of development. All team members should develop a comprehensive understanding of normal growth and psychosocial development. This will make it much easier to anticipate the effects of injury and illness on children and to meet their physiologic needs.

Any reasonable action that decreases a child's fear or anxiety during transport should be considered. Allowing a parent or guardian to accompany the child is usually one of the best ways to allay the child's fears. You should do this whenever possible. Sometimes the child's condition or other factors may make it prudent to not have the parent present. An extremely upset or distraught parent is not likely to be helpful and could create a disaster. Decisions need to be based on a case-by-case basis with the child's best interest in mind.

Making use of the family's knowledge of their child's condition and maintaining open communication with the family during your assessment and management is a must. Meeting the needs of the child and the child's family members are equally important. The concept of fulfilling these needs and actively involving the whole family in the medical care process is called *family-centered care*. Providing good family-centered care can be challenging, but it is especially so in the out-of-hospital setting. In this stressful environment, families are often upset and seeking answers to questions you may not be able to supply or are contrary to what they expected.

According to surveys, most family members want to be present during the attempted resuscitation of a loved one. Family presence during resuscitation is a practice being used in emergency rooms and ICUs in greater numbers all the time. Most families have very positive experiences with this practice, even when their loved ones die. One study found parents were more accepting of the death of their child if they were present during their child's attempted resuscitation. Parents or family members often fail to ask if they can be present, but all healthcare providers should offer the opportunity.

You should try to keep family-centered care in mind while treating children. This may mean having to break old habits and doing things in new ways. For some, this can be very difficult. Having a parent present in the ambulance or helicopter while you are providing acute care can be very stressful. The feelings and attitudes of the transport crew will need to be taken into consideration when making a decision to allow a parent to accompany a child.

Injury Prevention for Pediatric Patients

The outcome of pediatric cardiopulmonary arrest is dismal. Prevention saves many more lives than resuscitation attempts. Many of the major causes of fatal injuries in children can be prevented by simple strategies. Your involvement in efforts to promote these prevention methods and help pass state child safety legislation is greatly needed. Such efforts can be extremely satisfying both professionally and personally. Most people become healthcare providers because they want to make a difference and save lives. For kids, our prevention efforts are really our best opportunity to do just that.

Scenario Conclusion

The pediatric transport crew has just left with the very ill 6-month-old patient. You take a moment to investigate the unrest among your crew members. They express frustration and a little anger that they could not transport the infant. You discuss the fact that your service has chosen not to become credentialed to provide pediatric transport. The crew decides to form a committee to study the possibility of developing an educational program for pediatric transport and acquiring the equipment and medical oversight needed to include this service. You tell them to include the projected costs of each part of the plan (e.g., special ventilator, pumps, education), along with the potential revenue from the area served by your adult transport program.

Six weeks later, the committee has lost its steam. They report that the costs involved in starting up a pediatric program would be difficult for the service to recoup. The number of transports would be small, and the crew would need to spend a considerable amount of time keeping up-to-date on skills and knowledge.

CRITICAL CARE OF THE GERIATRIC PATIENT

Scenario

You are called to a small outlying hospital to transport a 72-year-old male to another acute care facility. The patient has a history of non-insulin-dependent diabetes, hypertension, a previous stroke, coronary artery disease, and glaucoma. His family brought him to the local ED earlier today because he had fallen several times the night before. He has a contusion on his forehead and has vomited once. The family states that the patient "just isn't acting normal." They use the word "delirious" to describe his actions this morning. The patient takes numerous medications, including warfarin, nifedipine, captopril, glimepiride, and Xalatan eye drops.

At the hospital, the patient's electrolyte and complete blood count (CBC) results were normal. A 12-lead ECG showed atrial fibrillation with a prolonged QT segment and left bundle branch block (LBBB). The CT scanner is not working at this facility, so the physician requests transfer of the patient for further workup.

The patient's vital signs are as follows: pulse, 60 beats/min, strong and irregular; respiratory rate, 16 breaths/min; BP, 170/100 mm Hg (MAP, 123 mm Hg); pulse oximetry (SpO_2), 95%; end-tidal partial pressure of carbon dioxide ($PETCO_2$), 38 mm Hg. The patient is on room air, in no obvious respiratory distress, and he has clear and equal breath sounds. His skin is warm and dry, and his temperature is 98.6° F (37° C). He shows a sinus rhythm on lead II.

He has one peripheral IV line with normal saline (NS) infusing at 60 mL/hr. The most significant finding in this patient is the decline in his Glasgow Coma Scale (GCS), which has dropped from 14 on admission 2 hours ago to 10. He shows no lateralizing signs, and the pupils are slow to react but equal. Because of the rapid decline in his GCS score and the 90-minute transport required, you prepare to perform rapid sequence intubation (RSI) to protect the airway.

When it comes to the EMS transport of older patients, it seems every transfer has many implications, including social, pharmacologic, and multisystem medical. **Senescence** is characterized by many cell, tissue, and organ changes. These changes, in combination with chronic health conditions, present a challenge to critical care providers. In this section we discuss some of the anatomic and physiologic changes expected in the geriatric patients and how those changes might impact the approach and treatment. You should begin this review by realizing the impact our older population has on the healthcare system and critical care.

Older Patients and Critical Care

An increasing amount of our population is occupied by our older citizens. As of 2002, the United States population older than 65 years of age accounted for 12.3%, with females at approximately 84 years and men at approximately 81 years in life expectancy.

Within the healthcare system, and especially the intensive care units, the older patient accounts for 40% to 50% of patient hospital days. The most common disease processes seen in this population are hypertension (49.2%), arthritis (36.1%), heart disease (31.1%), cancer (20%), and diabetes (15%).

On average, the 65 years and older population spends an average of 11% of their median income on healthcare costs, more than twice that spent by the rest of the population. People over 65 account for about 13% of the population, but consume more than 30% of all prescription medications and outpatient resources and account for 20% of all emergency department visits.

As people age, the rate of disability increases, but several factors determine the rate of this "disability." The speed with which a person ages depends on heredity, lifelong dietary patterns, the amount of habitual exercise, past illnesses, the presence of one or more chronic illnesses, and the stresses experienced throughout life. For instance, only 9% of those 65 to 69 years of age need help with daily activities. For those 85 years and older, 45% need similar assistance.

This is not all bad news. You have a tendency to read about the anatomic and physiologic changes of senescence and dread the aging of your body. The physical decline of the aging body occurs independent of diseases. Although senescence creates less reserve, the body has the ability to live to 115 years.

ANATOMY AND PHYSIOLOGY OF THE GERIATRIC PATIENT

Just as growth and development in children is predictable and expected, so are the changes of aging. These changes are described here through the organization of the primary assessment.

Airway

Most airway alterations are related to the musculoskeletal and dental changes listed in Box 9-7.

Breathing

The changes seen in the pulmonary system with senescence are presented in Figure 9-11 and Box 9-8.

Did You Know?

Senescent changes in the pulmonary system make the older patient more vulnerable to the hypoventilation side effects of narcotic analgesics.[2]

Circulation

Anatomic and physiologic changes in the circulatory system are rather extensive. They are listed in Box 9-9.

Did You Know?

Of individuals over 60 years of age, 70% to 80% have asymptomatic premature ventricular contractions (PVCs). Because of the side effects and possible toxicity, antidysrhythmics are not generally recommended for this asymptomatic group.[2]

Box 9-7 Changes with Aging: Effect on Airway

Alterations	Implications
Upper airway weakens	Mechanical airway obstruction
Facial shape changes	Mask positioning for ventilation
Dentures, partials	Obstructions
↓ ability to clear secretions	Aspiration, obstructions

Box 9-8 Breathing Changes with Aging

Alterations	Implications
Respiratory muscles weaken	↓ Reserve, easily fatigued
Kyphosis, barrel chest	↓ vital capacity
↓ recoil, ↑ compliance	↑ residual volume
↑ alveolar duct size, ↓ elasticity	↓alveolar surface area
↓ diffusion of gases by 8%/year	Average $PaO_2 = 74$; $PaCO_2 = 40$
↓ sensitivity of chemoreceptors	Sluggish response to changes

Box 9-9 Circulatory System Changes with Aging

Alterations	Implications
↑ **Collagen** in myocardium	↓ Compliance and diastolic filling = ↑ LV pressure (S4 sound)
Atherosclerotic build-up	Risk for ischemia/infarction
↓ or altered pain sensation	Absence of typical chest pain with AMI
(Males) LV wall thickening	LV hypertrophy
↑ Afterload and slow contraction	Prolonged systole
↓ Supine heart rate	Exercise intolerance
Aging electrical system	Dysrhythmias common: PVCs, V Tach, sinus node dysfunction (AF); AV node dysfunction (blocks); aberrant conduction defects
Baroreceptor altered	Slow changes in rate and vasomotor tone
Vessels become stiff	↑ Afterload; ↑ BP

AF, Atrial fibrillation; *AMI,* acute myocardial infarction; *AV,* atrioventricular node; *BP,* blood pressure; *LV,* left ventricle; *PVC,* premature ventricular contractions; *V tach,* ventricular tachycardia.

Central Nervous System

Changes in the brain and spinal column and cord are listed in Box 9-10, along with the implications to the patient and the healthcare provider.

Renal System

Because of blood flow and cellular changes, kidney function deteriorates with age. The implications of this are listed in Box 9-11; particular emphasis is placed on the effects of drug excretion, along with fluid and electrolyte balance.

Gastrointestinal System

The rigorous changes that occur in this system create difficulties with both digestion and absorption of nutrients. Liver changes add to the difficulty with pharmacokinetics. These changes are listed in Box 9-12.

Did You Know?

Even a small dose of alcohol on a routine basis in the elderly patient can contribute to an acute episode of hypoglycemia because stores of glucose in the liver are very low as we age.[2]

Box 9-10 Central Nervous System Changes with Aging

Alterations	Implications
Thinking and processing slowed	No cognitive impairment; timing slowed
↓ Brain size (20%)	Larger subdural masses before signs appear; more pull on bridging vessels with increased risk of SDH
Senile plaque formation	Risk of Alzheimer's disease
Neurofibrillary tangles	Reduced neuronal signaling
↓ Neurotransmitter functions	Certain drugs cause delirium with ease and low serotonin, dopamine levels; degeneration of blood-brain barrier
Arthritic spine	Central cord syndrome risk in trauma Difficult to diagnose fractures because of chronic changes
Pharmacokinetic changes	Diuretic Rx for increased ICP altered
Hardened pupil sphincter and rigid iris	Slow and limited pupil response to light
Subdural hematoma	

ICP, Intracranial pressure; *SDH*, subdural hematoma.

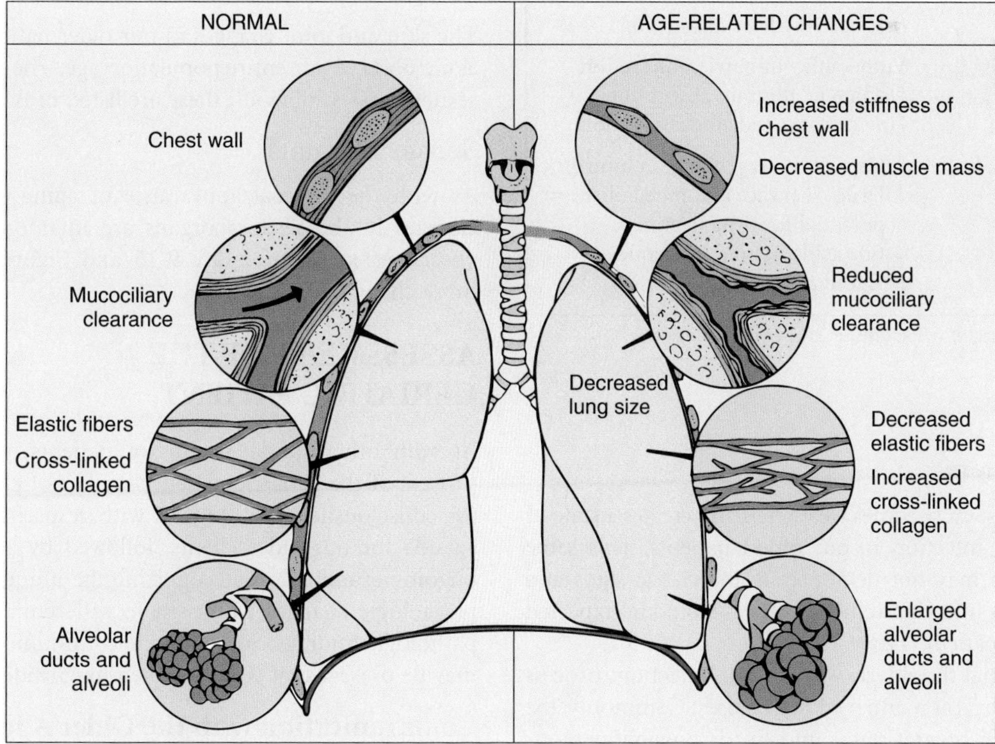

Figure 9-11

Age-related changes in the respiratory system. With advancing age, chest wall and lung tissue compliance diminishes. Also, clearance of mucus by the cilia lining the pulmonary tree decreases, and the alveolar ducts and alveoli enlarge. (From Urden LD, Stacy KM, Lough ME: *Thelan's critical care nursing: diagnosis and management*, ed 5, St Louis, 2005, Mosby.)

Box 9-11 Changes with Aging: Renal/Urinary

Alterations	Implications
↓Blood flow = ↓ number of nephrons	Small kidney size and weight Loss of renal reserve = vulnerable to injury in shock
↓ Glomerular filtration rate (GFR)	↓ Ability to regulate Na^+ and H_2O, and to excrete drugs.
↓ Tubular function	↓ Ability to regulate Na^+ and H_2O Inability to conserve H_2O High BUN, creatinine
↓ Response to sympathetic nervous system and **renin-angiotensin-aldosterone system (RAAS)**	Orthostatic hypotension Poor fluid homeostasis
Poor urinary bladder emptying	Susceptible to urinary tract infection

BUN, Blood urea nitrogen; *Na^+*, sodium.

Box 9-12 Changes with Aging: GI System

Alterations	Implications
↓ **Mastication,** swallowing motility, absorption	Potential obstructions, aspiration, **presbyesophagus,** GERD Less carbohydrate absorption
↓ Mucin, pepsin, and HCl secretion	Vulnerable gut barrier, ulceration Decline in albumin absorption Low calcium and zinc absorption
↓ **Hepatocytes,** liver blood flow (by 50%)	↓ Capacity to regenerate in injury ↓ Drug clearance and metabolism = ↓ potential for drug overdose ↓ Bile acids, steroid hormones Reduced carbohydrate storage

GERD, Gastroesophageal reflux disease; *HCl,* hydrogen chloride.

Immune System

The immune system becomes weathered and creates a state of vulnerability to infection in our oldest patients. This same immune system may not demonstrate the classic signs and symptoms of an infection (chills, fever) as would be expected in the younger patient (Box 9-13.)

Please note that the elderly who have an infectious process present in an atypical manner in many cases. Commonly, the first change is in mental status and this is possibly demonstrated by the occurrence of frequent falls. They many times do not present with chills and fever, as might be seen in other patients. There may be incontinence, poor appetite, or complaints of weakness. Just as in newborns, this special group of patients may present with subtle changes that, if unrecognized, may lead to serious consequences.

Box 9-13 Immune Changes with Aging

Alterations	Implications
↓ Cell-mediated immunity; shrunken lymphoid tissue	More susceptible to infections
Multiple concurrent chronic illness	System stressors to immunity

Box 9-14 Skin and Orthopedic Changes with Aging

Alterations	Implications
Loss of elastin and connective tissue	Wrinkled, sagging skin; loss of turgor; **capillary fragility**
Thinner cartilage	Lean body mass; narrower vertebral spaces
Less synovial fluid	Less joint mobility
Bone **demineralization** and **menopause**	**Osteoporosis,** especially women (loss of estrogen promotes osteoporosis)

Integumentary and Musculoskeletal Systems

The skin and joint changes in our older patients are obvious as we observe our entire population age. The implications are sometimes less obvious; these are listed in Box 9-14.

Sensory Organs

As with the external appearance of aging skin and joints, changes in the sensory organs are infamous among those observing senescence. Box 9-15 and Figure 9-12 illustrate those changes.

ASSESSMENT OF THE GERIATRIC PATIENT

As with other special groups of patients, your assessment process of the geriatric patient should not change. Assessing for consciousness and ABCDs with resuscitation is still the agenda for our older clients, followed by a secondary and ongoing examination. Recognizing the unique anatomic and physiologic changes will assist in differentiating normal vs. pathologic findings. Some unique communication challenges may be present that you may need to consider.

Communication with the Older Adult

Communicating with the elderly is essential while assessing and providing management. The patient, if aware, will note your verbal and nonverbal communication. If you display a positive attitude toward the older population, it will result in

Box 9-15 Sensory Changes with Aging

Alterations	Implications
Hardened pupil sphincter and rigid iris	Slow and limited pupil response to light Loss of visual acuity in dim light
↓ Opacity of the lens; ↓ ciliary movement	Slow and limited pupil response to light↓ Near and peripheral vision
↓ **Melanocyte** production, **arcus senilis**	Pale iris with fatty deposits
Loss of subcutaneous tissue	Shrunken/recessed eye appearance
↓ **Lacrimal** activity	Dry and itchy eyes
↓ Sense of smell, **polypharmacy**	Change in sense of taste/ appetite
Atrophy of auditory nerve	**Presbycusis;** inability to discern high vs. low pitch sounds
↓ Peripheral nerve sensation	↓ Sense of hot, cold, pain

a higher interest level, improved communication and assessment, and more effective care and management of older patients.

Communication tips:

1. Communicate openly and respectfully.
2. Provide information about your assessment and proposed plan of action.
3. Respect the patient's autonomy, and honor competent choices.
4. Allow some control over when, how, or if minor procedures occur.
5. Give prior explanation for assessments and treatment.
6. Allow for elimination prior to transport.
7. Remember to ask about hearing aids, dentures, and other personal needs.
8. Provide for comfort and warmth with extra blankets or padding.

Communication skills consist of gathering and providing information, listening and observing. The oldest and most vulnerable patients deserve nothing but the best.

Scene Size-Up in Assessment

The location of your assessment of the older adult may be an important factor. If you are part of a 9-1-1 response called to the patient's home, assessing for the patient's personal safety is part of your scene size-up. Awareness of environmental factors that may play a role in the client's health is also key. In most cases, however, the critical care team will be evaluating this patient in an emergency or ICU setting. Interviewing the patient's family about living arrangements may help if environmental factors are involved in the differential diagnoses.

Box 9-16 Changes in Laboratory Values with Aging

Decreased erythrocyte sedimentation rate
Increased blood glucose
Decreased serum albumin
> 60 years of age = PO_2 average of 74, PCO_2 average at 40

Modified from Urden L, Stacy K, Lough M: *Thelan's critical care nursing: diagnosis and management*, ed 5, St. Louis, 2005, Mosby.

Level of Consciousness

Assessing for level of consciousness (LOC) can be tricky in the senescent patient. It is important to note any alteration in LOC along with the complete neurologic examination. If multiple findings in your neurologic examination suggest a CNS disease, then alteration in consciousness may be part of that pathology. Also, sudden changes in orientation or LOC are not a normal part of aging.

Remember, the pathology of senility is a slow process. Any acute change in mental status in the older client should be considered to be acute pathology.

Airway and Breathing

Musculoskeletal and dental changes make airway management a challenge at times for the older patient. Assessment, however, remains unchanged. Because of a lack of pulmonary reserves, assessment of the patient's respiratory status is more of a challenge. Even application of spinal immobilization straps or devices can cause respiratory failure in this age group. Be judicious about conducting a thorough pulmonary examination in those with quiet tachypnea.

Circulation

The influence of medications, the common presentation of arrhythmias, and changes in skin parameters may create a challenge for assessing normal versus pathology. Be aware of symmetry in all aspects of your patient: pulse, skin parameters, and lateralizing neurologic signs. Evaluating urine output may help you determine end-organ perfusion.

DIAGNOSTICS

Most laboratory values are the same as in any other group of patients. However, some laboratory values, ECG readings, and pulmonary function test results do change with age and have clinical significance. They are listed in Box 9-16, Table 9-12, and Table 9-13.

DISEASE PROCESSES AND MANAGEMENT UNIQUE TO GERIATRIC PATIENTS

The older client presents with the same disease processes described in Chapters 3, 4, 5, 6, 7, and 8. There are two main considerations when managing the older patient in the critical care setting: The fragile balance in the older body during resuscitation and the changes made with medication use.

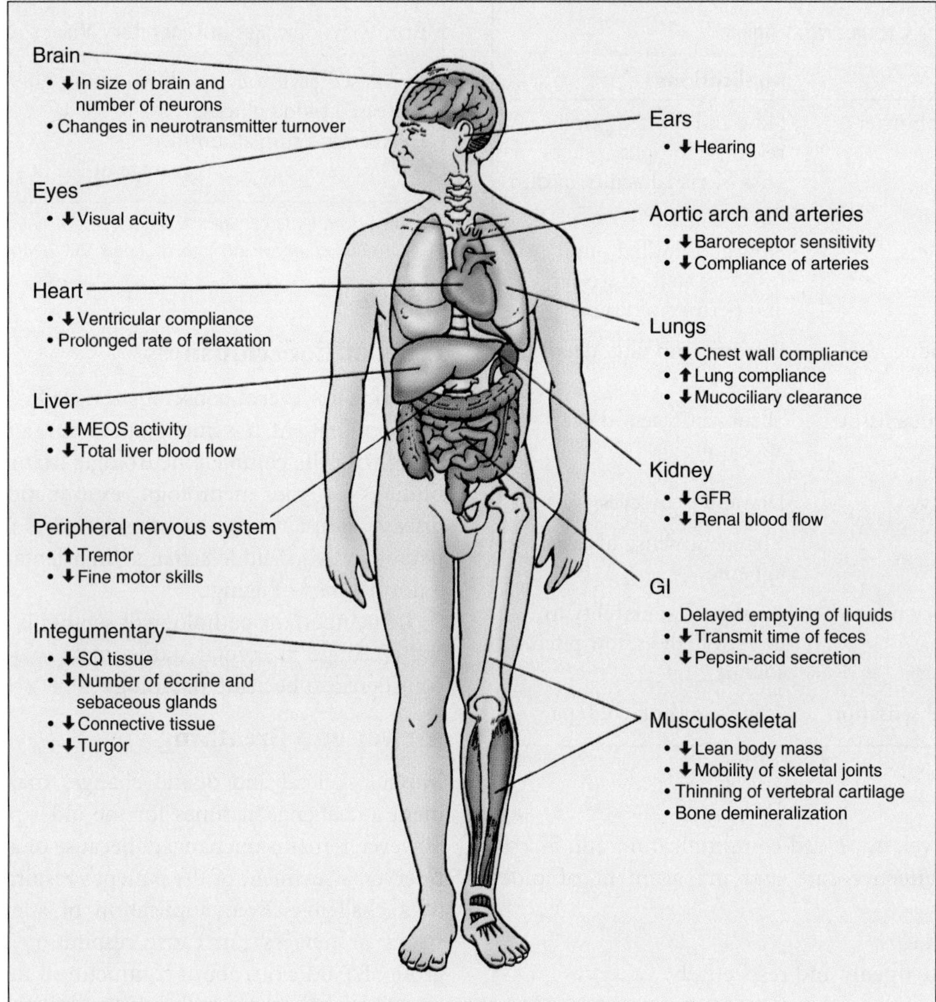

Figure 9-12

Physiologic changes that may be seen in elderly critical care patients. *MEOS,* Microsomal enzyme oxidation system; *GFR,* glomerular filtration rate; *GI,* gastrointestinal; *SQ,* subcutaneous. (Modified from Urden LD, Stacy KM, Lough ME: *Thelan's critical care nursing: diagnosis and management,* ed 5, St Louis, 2005, Mosby.)

Table 9-12 Age-Related Changes in Electrocardiographic Variables

	Age (in years)			
ECG Variable	**Younger Than 30**	**30-39**	**40-49**	**Older Than 49**
R wave amplitude (mm)	10.43	10.53	9.01	9.25
S wave amplitude (mm)	15.21	14.21	12.22	12.42
Frontal plane axis (degrees)	48.93	48.13	36.50	38.83
PR duration (ms)	15.89	16.23	16.04	16.25
QRS duration (ms)	7.64	7.51	7.36	8.00
QT duration (ms)	37.83	37.50	37.99	39.58
T wave amplitude (ms)	5.21	4.57	4.31	4.42

From Urden L, Stacy K, Lough M: *Thelan's critical care nursing: diagnosis and management, 5th Edition*, St. Louis, 2005, Mosby. Data from Bachman S, Sparrow D, Smith LK: Effect of aging on the electrocardiogram, *Am J Cardiol* 48:513, 1981.
ECG, Electrocardiogram.

Table 9-13 Age-Related Changes in Commonly Performed Pulmonary Function Tests

Pulmonary Function Test	Description	Standard Lung Volume and Capacity (mL)	Age-Related Change (mL)
Total lung capacity	Vital capacity plus residual volume	6000	No change
Vital capacity	Amount of air exhaled after a maximal inspiration	5000	3750
Tidal volume (V_T)	Amount of air inhaled or exhaled with each breath	500	No change
Residual volume (RV)	Amount of air left in lungs after forced exhalation	1200	↓ 1800
Inspiratory reserve volume (IRV)	Amount of air that can be forcefully inhaled after inspiring a normal V_T	3100	↓ 2800
Expiratory reserve volume (ERV)	Amount of air that can be forcefully exhaled after expiring a normal V_T	1200	↓ 1000
Forced expiratory volume in 1 sec (FEV_1)	Volume exhaled in the first second of a single forced expiratory volume; expressed as a percent of the forced vital capacity	80%	↓ 75%

From Urden L, Stacy K, Lough M: *Thelan's critical care nursing: diagnosis and management*, ed 5, St. Louis, 2005, Mosby.

Resuscitation of the Older Patient

You may find that certain trauma and medical disease processes will progress rapidly in the elderly because of a lack of reserve. The elderly may also present clinically in an altered fashion because of changes in the cardiovascular system. The best example is the presentation of shock in the elderly. Because the patient's normal blood pressure may be 180/90, a decompensated BP of 100/40, along with the lack of tachycardia, can be misunderstood. Additionally, dementia should always be considered pathology in this special population.

When considering the management approach in the primary phase of care, a quicker decision on providing airway and ventilation adjuncts, especially positioning, suctioning, positive-pressure ventilation, and tracheal intubation, should be completed. Whether to administer fluid resuscitation should be guided by hemodynamic monitoring because the struggle with preexisting afterload and slow changes in baroreceptor response can be difficult.

Medication Absorption, Distribution, Metabolism, and Elimination

Pharmacokinetics and **pharmacodynamics** are both processes in medication delivery that may be altered in the older patient. Medications are prescribed for their positive effects, but when combined with multiple other medications, and possibly with chronic diseases, in patients whose body tissues and organs do not function as they used to, the side effects are enhanced and adverse reactions may occur. This problem is so pronounced that some studies show that as many as 40% of all hospital admissions for this age group involve medication adverse reactions.

Absorption of drugs may be altered by the changes in the GI tract (oral medications) or body mass and water distribution (water and fat-soluble drugs). Distribution may be unbalanced because of decreased protein intake or liver disease (warfarin, phenytoin).

As noted above, both the liver and kidney undergo senescent changes; and these same organs are primarily responsible for drug elimination from the body. Those medications that are eliminated through the kidney must be evaluated for possible decreased dosing frequency to prevent toxicity (digitalis, **aminoglycosides**).

Another common adverse event precipitated by renal aging is the electrolyte imbalances created by diuretics. If a potassium-sparing diuretic is prescribed (e.g., spironolactone), hyperkalemia may result. Loop diuretics (e.g., furosemide) and thiazide diuretics (e.g., hydrochlorothiazide) may cause hyponatremia (Figure 9-13).

Did You Know?

Phenytoin administration for those older than 65 years of age should be 5 to 10 mg/minute, up to a maximum of 25 mg/minute. This rate is slower than the standard dose.[2]

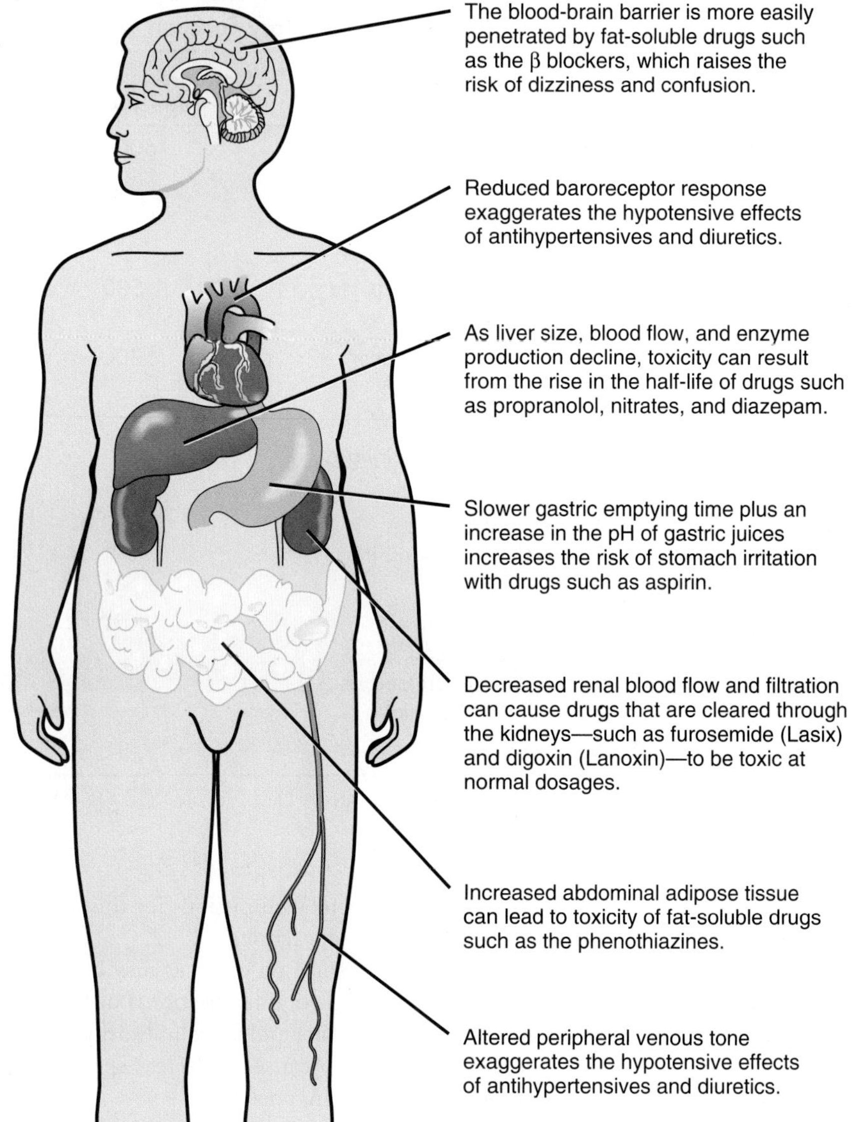

Figure 9-13

How physiologic changes of aging increase sensitivity to drugs and drug-inducted disease. (From McKenry LM, Tesser E, Hogan MA: *Mosby's pharmacology in nursing*, ed 22, St. Louis, 2006, Mosby.

Other drugs associated with critical care include digoxin, angiotensin II-converting enzyme (ACE) inhibitors and angiotensin II receptor blockers (ARBs) and show delayed excretion with longer duration of action and potential for excess concentrations. Additionally, the chronotropic and inotropic effects of beta agonists (isoproterenol, beta-dose dopamine) are decreased in the elderly.

Another caution regarding **delirium** in this special population: the presentation of delirium is commonly treated in the critical care setting with use of diphenhydramine or benzodiazepines, which may actually make agitation worse in older patients.

Pain Management in the Older Adult

Within the geriatric population living in their own homes, 50% report pain. Of those living in nursing homes, 80%

Did You Know?

Soft, disposable restraints are many times applied to wrists and ankles in the ICU to prevent flexion of hip/knee (femoral lines) and/ or to prevent accidental removal of essential equipment from the patient (such as tracheal tubes). Because of skin and vascular changes, it is imperative that you evaluate the patient's skin routinely for signs of irritation or diminished blood flow. This evaluation is charted routinely within a special documentation tool for the restrained patient. You should refer to the institution's policies on the use of restraints prior to obtaining an order.[2]

report pain. This is a factor when evaluating the patient's pain and how you manage it. As described above, the choice and dose of the drug may need to be adjusted because of the senescent changes in the body.

The patient's report of pain is different in this specialized population because of physiologic, psychologic, and cultural differences. In many cases, the older patient will not want to "bother" you because, "it's just pain," something they may have become accustomed to. If confusion or dementia is present, it adds to the challenge of eliciting an accurate assessment.

Lowering the doses of medication is not always the answer. Frequency of drug administration should be considered as well. It may be that too frequent administration accounts for the elimination problems explained.

Did You Know?

Because of senescent changes in the body, the following drugs are considered inappropriate for use in older patients[3]:
Propoxyphene (Darvon)
Indomethacin (Indocin)
Pentazocine (Talwin)
Meperidine (Demerol)

Nonsteroidal antiinflammatory drugs (NSAIDs) must be used with extreme caution because of potential GI, renal, and cardiovascular toxicity.

End of Life Issues

Dying is the final part of the life process. The healthcare system occasionally confuses issues surrounding resuscitation when a crisis occurs in our older patient's health. When asked, most of our oldest patients report that they do not want CPR performed when their heart stops. Commonly entitled "DNR" (do not resuscitate), this consent to do nothing is pretty well understood.

What happens though when the older patient suddenly suffers from a traumatic event or major illness? Does that mean that the patient's DNR status keeps them from being resuscitated *from* death or occupying a critical care bed in a hospital? There is a difference between DNR and the concept of do not attempt resuscitation (DNAR). Many critical care transports include the oldest of our population. Their wishes are to be resuscitated and saved FROM death.

Advance Directives

The patient should receive the amount of care desired and should be able to communicate those wishes throughout the healthcare process. Culturally, discussion of death is difficult and not well done in the United States. By the time the issue of potential death comes up, the patient may be deemed incompetent because of critical illness. Did they communicate their wishes to their family members prior to this illness? Hospitals generally ask the patient's family if there is an advanced directive (Living Will, Healthcare Power of Attorney) that expresses the patient's wishes or provides a decision-maker for healthcare issues. If the hospital then makes a decision to transfer the patient to a tertiary or specialized healthcare center, those directives should be communicated to your team. Those loved ones who have a legally designated power of attorney have the right to be involved in the discussion of healthcare decisions on behalf of the patient without fear of Health Insurance Portability and Accountability Act (HIPAA) violations (see Chapter 1).

Scenario Conclusion

This older male patient has multiple chronic diseases and is taking many medications that have significant side effects. Family members noted a sudden change in mental status with falls. He now has a rapidly deteriorating level of consciousness from a presumed subdural hematoma.

The intubation with RSI goes well. The patient is placed on your ventilator, and transport is essentially uneventful. On arrival at the tertiary care hospital, the warfarin is reversed with factor VIIa and vitamin K. With this therapy, his international normalized ratio (INR) drops from 3.2 (measured 1 week ago) to 1.6. The neurosurgeon evacuates a subdural hematoma, and the geriatrician determines that the patient had a urinary tract infection, which created the subtle changes in mental status that started the event. After treatment, arrangements are made to transfer the patient to a rehabilitation hospital in your area.

SUMMARY

- Each special population reacts differently in medical or traumatic crises.
- Your knowledge of the unique anatomic and physiologic changes in each of these three populations will assist in differentiating normal versus pathology during your assessment.
- Because of the special differences, especially in the youngest patient, special preparation is necessary in order to provide good care during critical care transports.

KEY TERMS

aminoglycosides A group of antibiotics derived from various species of *Streptomyces* or produced synthetically (e.g., amikacin, gentamicin, streptomycin). Aminoglycosides are bactericidal; they inhibit bacterial protein synthesis by binding with the 30S ribosomal subunit.

arcus senilis Fatty deposits that appear in the irides of the eyes in older adults.

Babinski's reflex Dorsiflexion of the big toe when the side of the foot is stimulated; it is normal in infants but in others is a sign of a lesion in the central nervous system, particularly in the pyramidal tract.

beta hCG titer Human chorionic gonadotropin titer; commonly known as a pregnancy test.

boggy Soft and watery; a term used to describe a uterus that is without tone.

Brudzinski's sign In meningitis, flexion of the hip and knee caused by flexion of the neck; called also the *neck sign.* Also, passive flexion of the lower limb on one side that causes a similar movement in the opposite limb; called also the *contralateral sign.*

candidal infection An infection caused by *Candida* organisms, often *C. albicans. Candida* is a genus of fungi that produces yeast cells. Although some species are part of the normal flora of human skin and mucous membranes, they also can cause infection.

capillary fragility An unusual capillary susceptibility to disruption under stress marked by extravasation, which usually is visible on the skin (e.g., ecchymoses, petechiae, or telangiectasias).

collagen A family of extracellular, closely related proteins that are a major component of connective tissue, giving it strength and flexibility.

condyloma acuminata Warty growths caused by the human papillomavirus that usually are found on the mucous membranes or skin of the external genitals or in the perianal region. Lesions may aggregate to form large, cauliflower-like masses. The disorder is infectious and autoinoculable. Also called *genital warts* or *venereal warts.*

delirium An acute, transient disturbance of consciousness, accompanied by a change in cognition, that follows a fluctuating course. Characteristics include reduced ability to maintain attention to external stimuli and disorganized thinking, manifested by rambling, irrelevant, or incoherent speech. A reduced level of consciousness; sensory misperceptions; disturbance of the sleep-wake cycle and level of psychomotor activity; disorientation to time, place, or person; and memory impairment also are possible. Delirium may be caused by a number of conditions that result in derangement of cerebral metabolism, including systemic infection, cerebral tumor, poisoning, drug intoxication or withdrawal, seizure or head trauma, and metabolic disturbances, such as fluid, electrolyte, or acid-base imbalance; hypoxia; hypoglycemia; and hepatic or renal failure.

demineralization Excessive elimination of mineral or inorganic salts, as occurs in pulmonary tuberculosis, cancer, and osteomalacia (i.e., inadequate mineralization of osteoid into mature bone).

extracorporeal membrane oxygenation (ECMO) A process in which the blood is passed through a mechanical pump that oxygenates it and returns it to the body.

fontanelles The membrane-covered spaces remaining in the incompletely ossified skull of a fetus or an infant.

gametogenesis Development of the male and female sex cells (gametes).

glomerular filtration rate (GFR) A calculated laboratory value that is determined by a patient's serum creatinine level, age, race, and gender. The GFR is the best overall index of kidney function. The normal range is 120 to 130 mL/min/1.73 m^2. A low GFR precedes the onset of kidney failure.

glucuronidation The process by which glucuronate forms conjugates with drugs and toxins during their biotransformation. Glucuronate is a salt, ester, or anionic form of glucuronic acid, which is derived from glucose.

grasp reflex A grasping motion of the fingers or toes that occurs in response to stimulation; it is normal in infancy but in later life is a sign of a pathologic condition.

hepatocytes Hepatic cells are diamond-shaped epithelial cells that constitute the substance of a liver's functional unit.

hydramnios An excess of amniotic fluid, usually more than 2000 mL; also called **polyhydramnios.**

Kernig's sign The ability to extend the lower limb easily and completely when in the dorsal decubitus position but not when sitting or lying with the thigh flexed on the abdomen. The presence of Kernig's sign is an indicator meningitis.

kyphosis An abnormally increased convexity in the curvature of the thoracic spinal column when viewed from the side.

lacrimal A term referring to tears.

lanugo Fine hair seen on the body of the fetus; called also *down, downy hair,* and *primary hair.*

Leopold's maneuver Four distinct actions used to palpate the abdomen of a pregnant woman to determine the position and presentation of the fetus; it may include manipulation of a malpositioned fetus.

macrosomia Abnormally large size; also called *macrosomatia.*

Marfan syndrome A autosomal dominant, congenital disorder of connective tissue characterized by abnormal length of the extremities, especially the fingers and toes; subluxation of the lens; cardiovascular abnormalities (commonly dilation of the ascending aorta); and other deformities.

mastication The process of biting and grinding food in preparation for swallowing and digestion; chewing.

melanocyte A type of dendritic clear cell found in the stratum basale of the epidermis; it synthesizes tyrosinase and contains melanosomes that produce melanin and can be transferred from melanocytes to nearby keratinocytes.

menopause The cessation of menstruation in the human female; it usually occurs around 50 years of age.

Moro reflex In infants, flexion of the thighs and knees and fanning and then clenching of the fingers, with the arms first thrown outward then brought together as if in an embrace. This reflex is produced by a sudden stimulus (e.g., striking the table next to the child); or by sudden extension of the neck when the head is allowed to fall backward; or by pulling the child up by both hands from a lying position and then letting go. The Moro reflex is seen normally in infants up to 4 to 5 months of age. Also called the *embrace reflex* or *startle reflex.*

ophthalmia neonatorum Severe inflammation of the eye or of the conjunctiva or deeper structures of the eye; any hyperacute, purulent conjunctivitis that occurs during the first 10 days of life. It usually is contracted during birth from infected vaginal discharge from the mother. The term formerly referred only to gonorrheal infections; however, an iatrogenic form sometimes occurs after administration of silver nitrate. Also called *neonatal conjunctivitis.*

osteoporosis A condition marked by a reduction in bone mineral density; it can result in fractures from minimal trauma.

pharmacodynamics The study of the biochemical and physiologic effects of drugs and their mechanisms of action, including the correlation of actions and effects of drugs with their chemical structure; also, such effects on the actions of a particular drug or drugs.

pharmacokinetics The processing of drugs by the body over a specific time, including absorption, distribution, location in tissues, biotransformation, and excretion.

polypharmacy The administration of many drugs together; the term also has come to mean the administration of excessive medication.

postprandial A term referring to the period immediately after a meal.

presbycusis Progressive, bilaterally symmetric sensorineural hearing loss that occurs with age.

presbyesophagus Impairment of the motor function of the esophagus as a result of degenerative changes that occur with advancing age.

proteinuria The presence of excessive serum proteins in the urine, as may occur with renal disease, after strenuous exercise, and with dehydration. Also called *albuminuria.*

renin-angiotensin-aldosterone system (RAAS) The regulation of sodium balance, fluid volume, and blood pressure by renal secretions. In response to reduced perfusion, renin is secreted, which hydrolyzes a plasma globulin to release angiotensin I. Angiotensin I is rapidly hydrolyzed to angiotensin II; this stimulates aldosterone secretion, which brings about sodium retention, an increase in blood pressure, and restoration of renal perfusion, which shuts off the signal for renin release.

spinal cord injury without radiographic abnormality (SCIWORA) An injury of the spinal cord syndrome in which the bony vertebrae show no evidence of fracture or trauma. The condition usually is seen in children under 8 years of age.

senescence The process or condition of growing old, especially the condition resulting from the transitions and accumulations of the deleterious aging processes; aging.

squamous cells Flat, scalelike epithelial cells that line the surface of the body.

sulfation The addition of a sulfate group to a molecule.

teratogen Any agent or factor that induces or increases the incidence of abnormal prenatal development.

tet spell An acute onset of symptoms when cardiac output falls and hypoxia occurs in a child with the congenital heart defect tetralogy of Fallot.

thymus The site of production of T lymphocytes. Precursor cells migrate into the outer cortex, where they actively proliferate. As they mature and acquire T-cell surface markers, they move to the inner cortex, where approximately 90% die (possibly as part of the acquisition of self-tolerance). The remainder move on to the medulla, become mature T cells, and enter the circulation. T cell maturation is regulated by hormones, including thymopoietin and thymosin, produced by thymic epithelial cells. Congenital athymia or neonatal thymectomy results in the complete lack of functional T cells. The thymus reaches maximum development at about puberty and then undergoes a gradual process of involution (replacement of parenchyma by fat and fibrous tissue), resulting in a slow decline of immune function throughout adulthood.

tocolytic A descriptive term indicating inhibition of uterine contractions (tocolysis).

trichomoniasis An infection of the vagina caused by *Trichomonas* protozoa.

turgor A reflection of the skin's elasticity as measured by the time required for the skin of the forearm to return to position after being lightly pinched between the thumb and forefinger. With normal turgor, this occurs within 3 seconds; skin that remains elevated (tented) longer than 3 seconds is a sign of decreased turgor.

vernix caseosa An unctuous substance composed of sebum and desquamated epithelial cells that covers the skin of the fetus.

REFERENCES

1. Walls RM, Murphy MF, editors: *Manual of emergency airway management*, Philadelphia, 2000, Lippincott Williams & Wilkins.
2. Urden LD, Stacy KM, Lough ME: *Thelan's critical care nursing: diagnosis and management*, ed 5, St Louis, 2005, Mosby.
3. McKenry LM, Tessier E, Hogan MA: *Mosby's pharmacology in nursing*, ed 22, St Louis, 2005, Mosby.
4. Gausche M et al: Effect of out-of-hospital pediatric endotracheal intubation on survival and neurologic outcome: a controlled clinical trial, *JAMA* 283:783-790, 2000.
5. Kenner C: *Neonatal nursing handbook,* Philadelphia, 2004, Saunders.

Bibliography

American College of Obstetricians and Gynecologists (ACOG): *Invasive hemodynamic monitoring in obstetrics and gynecology, Tech Bull 121*, Washington, DC, 1988, ACOG.

American College of Obstetricians and Gynecologists (ACOG): *Cardiac disease in pregnancy, Tech Bull 168*, Washington, DC, 1992, ACOG.

American College of Obstetricians and Gynecologists (ACOG): *Obstetric aspects of trauma management, Educ Bull 251*, Washington, DC, September 1998, ACOG.

American College of Obstetricians and Gynecologists (ACOG): *Hypertension in pregnancy, Pract Bull 29*, Washington, DC, 2001, ACOG.

Andres RL, Miles A: Venous thromboembolism and pregnancy, *Obstet Gynecol Clin North Am* 28:613-630, 2001.

Association of Air Medical Services: *Guidelines for air medical crew education*, Dubuque, Iowa, 2004, Kendall-Hunt.

Bayley EW, Turcke SA: *A comprehensive curriculum for trauma nursing*, Boston, 1992, Jones & Bartlett.

Boie ET, Moore GP, Brummett C et al: Do parents want to be present during invasive procedures performed on their children in the emergency room? A survey of 400 parents, *Ann Emerg Med* 34:70-74, 1999.

Boudreaux ED, Francis JL, Loyacano T: Family presence during invasive procedures and resuscitations in the emergency department: a critical review and suggestions for future research, *Ann Emerg Med* 40:193-205, 2002.

Centers for Disease Control and Prevention (CDC): Ambulance crash-related injuries among emergency medical services workers: United States, 1991-2002, *MMWR Morb Mortal Wkly Rep* 52:154-156, 2003.

Clark S: Central hemodynamic observations in normal third trimester pregnancy, *Am J Obstet Gynecol* 161:1439-1442, 1989.

Clark S: *Handbook of critical care obstetrics*, Boston, 1993, Blackwell Scientific.

Curley M, Moloney-Harmon PA: *Critical care nursing of infants and children*, ed 2, Philadelphia, 2001, Saunders.

Davies S: Amniotic fluid embolus: a review of the literature, *Can J Anaesth* 48:88-98, 2001.

DeJong JF, Fausett MB: Anaphylactoid syndrome of pregnancy: a devastating complication requiring intensive care, *Crit Care Nurse* 23:42-48, 2003.

Dildy G, Belfort MA, Saade GR et al, editors: *Critical care obstetrics*, ed 4, Boston, 2004, Blackwell Scientific.

Degutis LC, Greve M: Injury prevention, *Emerg Med Clin North Am* 24:871-888, 2006.

Snyder DR, Christmas C, editors: *Geriatric education for emergency medical services*, Boston, 2003, Jones & Bartlett.

Fleisher GR, Ludwig S, Henretig FM et al: *Textbook of pediatric emergency medicine*, ed 5, Philadelphia, 2006, Lippincott Williams & Wilkins.

Gausche-Hill M, Lewis RJ, Stratton SJ et al: Effect of out-of-hospital pediatric endotracheal intubation on survival and neurological outcome: a controlled clinical trial, *JAMA* 283:783-790, 2000.

Graves CR: Acute pulmonary complications during pregnancy, *Clin Obstet Gynecol* 45:369-376, 2002.

Harvey MG: Physiologic changes of pregnancy. In Harvey CJ, editor: *Critical care obstetrical nursing*, Gaithersburg, Md, 1991, Aspen.

Horton MA, Beamer C: Powered intraosseous insertion provides safe and effective vascular access for pediatric patients, *Pediatr Emerg Care* 24:347-350, 2008.

Hsu HE, Shutt KA, Moore MR et al: Effect of pneumococcal conjugate vaccine on pneumococcal meningitis, *N Engl J Med* 360:244-256, 2009.

Kahn CA, Pirrallo RG, Kuhn EM: Characteristics of fatal ambulance crashes in the United States: an 11-year retrospective analysis, *Prehosp Emerg Care* 5:261-269, 2001.

Lavery P: Asthma. In Queenan J, editor: *Management of high-risk pregnancies,* ed 4, Cambridge, 1996, Blackwell Science.

Lopez-Herce J, Garcia C, Rodriguez-Nunez A et al: Long-term outcome of paediatric cardiorespiratory arrest in Spain, *Resuscitation* 64:79-85, 2005.

Lough ME, Stacy KM, Urden LD: High risk and critical care obstetric issues. In Urden LD, Stacy KM, Lough ME: *Thelan's critical care nursing: diagnosis and management*, ed 5, St Louis, 2006, Mosby.

Mangurten J, Scott SH, Guzzetta CE et al: Effects of family presence during resuscitation and invasive procedures in a pediatric emergency department, *J Emerg Nurs* 32:225-233, 2006.

May K, Mahlmeister L: *Maternal and neonatal nursing: family centered care*, ed 3, Philadelphia, 1994, Lippincott Williams & Wilkins.

Meyers TA, Eichhorn DJ, Guzzetta CE: Do families want to be present during CPR? A retrospective survey, *J Emerg Nurs* 24:400-405, 1998.

NAEMT: *PHTLS prehospital trauma life support*, ed 6, St Louis, 2007, Mosby.

National High Blood Pressure in Pregnancy Education Program Working Group: *Working group report on high blood pressure in pregnancy*, 2000 (NHBPEP) Publication.

Naylor DF, Olson MM: Critical care obstetrics and gynecology, *Crit Care Clin* 19:127-149, 2003.

Parra DA, Totapally BR, Zahn E et al: Outcome of cardiopulmonary resuscitation in a pediatric cardiac intensive care unit, *Crit Care Med* 28:3296-3300, 2000.

Peters RM, Flack JM: Hypertensive disorders of pregnancy, *J Obstet Gynecol Neonatal Nurs* 33:209-214, 2004.

Pschirrer ER, Monga M: Seizure disorders in pregnancy, *Obstet Gynecol Clin North Am* 29:601-611, 2001.

Ralston M, Hazinski MF, Zaritsky AL et al: *Pediatric advanced life support course guide and PALS provider manual: provider manual*, Dallas, 2007, American Heart Association.

Reis AG, Nadkarni V, Perondi MB et al: A prospective investigation into the epidemiology of in-hospital pediatric cardiopulmonary resuscitation using the international Utstein reporting style, *Pediatrics* 109:200-209, 2002.

Richard J, Stiell IG, Osmond M et al: Management and outcomes of pediatric patients transported by emergency medical services in a Canadian prehospital system, *CJEM* 8:6-12, 2006.

Rutherford JD, Hands M: Pregnancy with preexisting heart disease. In Douglas PS, editor: *Cardiovascular health and disease in women*, Philadelphia, 1993, Saunders.

Shinnar S, Glauser TA: Febrile seizures, *J Child Neurol* 17(suppl 1):S44-S52, 2002.

Sole ML, Klein D, Moseley M: *Introduction to critical care nursing*, ed 4, Philadelphia, 2005, Saunders.

Springhouse: *Straight A's in maternal-neonatal nursing*, Philadelphia, 2003, Lippincott Williams & Wilkins.

Stone I: Trauma in the obstetric patient, *Obstet Gynecol Clin North Am* 3:459-785, 1999.

Taskforce on Interhospital Transport, American Academy of Pediatrics: *Guidelines for air and ground transport of neonatal and pediatric patients*, Elk Grove, Ill, 1993, American Academy of Pediatrics.

Vestergaard M, Christensen J: Register-based studies on febrile seizures in Denmark, *Brain Dev* 31:372-377, 2009.

Wendel PJ: Asthma in pregnancy, *Obstet Gynecol Clin North Am* 28:537-551, 2001.

Wilson RF: *Handbook of trauma: pitfalls and pearls*, Philadelphia, 1999, Lippincott Williams & Wilkins.

Young KD, Seidel JS: Pediatric cardiopulmonary resuscitation: a collective review, *Ann Emerg Med* 33:195-205, 1993.

REVIEW QUESTIONS

1. The scenario in the Obstetrics section described a middle-aged patient at 34 weeks' gestation with a complicated medical and obstetric history. What treatment should be instituted immediately in this patient?
   A. Nifedipine IV, reduce the magnesium sulfate infusion to 2 gm/hr, and prepare to intubate and ventilate with PEEP.
   B. Use Esmolol IV, maintain the magnesium sulfate infusion, and apply CPAP for noninvasive ventilation.
   C. Administer diltiazem IV, stop the magnesium sulfate immediately, and prepare to intubate and ventilate the patient.
   D. Administer metoprolol, reduce the magnesium sulfate infusion to 3 gm/hr, and prepare to apply CPAP.

2. Patients in the third trimester of pregnancy are considered high risk for endotracheal intubation. Choose the most important reason for this.
   A. Supine positioning is contraindicated.
   B. Change in body's center of gravity is altered and soft tissue in face has increased.
   C. Hormonal changes occur in the cardiac sphincter with reflux and aspiration.
   D. Bradycardia occurs during anoxic events.

3. CPAP is considered to be a common, viable option for ventilation in the third-trimester pregnant patient in respiratory failure.
   A. True
   B. False

4. A 35-week pregnant patient was positioned in the front passenger side during a 35-mile-per-hour rear-end collision. She was fully belted. She denies loss of consciousness and feels as though she's "just fine." BP 100/62, pulse 100, resp. rate 28, SaO_2 97% on room air, side-stream CO_2 assessment 32. She is sitting on the curb next to the vehicle and appears slightly short of breath. She contends that this is normal. Which course of action would be appropriate?
   A. Initiate prompt and aggressive resuscitation efforts as warranted by the patient's appearance and vital signs.
   B. Acknowledge that she's right. Send her home.
   C. Re-evaluate the patient's BP and pulse with her lying in a flat, supine position.
   D. Conclude that the vital signs, hypocapnia, and tachypnea may be normal for her pregnant state.

5. You have completed the primary examination and resuscitation of an obviously pregnant trauma patient who has a GCS of 9. Your partner has measured from her pubis to the top of the fundus and 35 cm is the result. What does this mean?
   A. She has a rapidly expanding abdomen, probably from hemorrhage.
   B. She should be quickly auscultated for fetal heart tones to determine whether the fetus is viable.
   C. This patient is approximately 35 weeks' pregnant.
   D. Fetal heart tones will be heard only at the top of the uterus.

6. You sensed that your adult critical care transport program should not assume care for the child in the case scenario. Your decision is:
   A. Correct because an adult program would not have the required knowledge, skills, or equipment necessary to properly care for this child
   B. Correct because the local physician agreed
   C. Incorrect in this case because the treatment given was straightforward and could have been done with the resources you currently have
   D. Incorrect because it will cause irrevocable harm to your crew's morale
7. The child's Po_2 was 78 in our case scenario. The transport crew should have:
   A. Increased the PEEP to 8
   B. Increased the I time to 1.5; E time decreased to 0.8
   C. Suctioned the tracheal tube
   D. Maintained current therapy because this is a normal result for a capillary gas
8. If the child in our scenario were placed on pediatric maintenance fluids, the pump should have been set to:
   A. 20 mL/hr
   B. 32 mL/hr
   C. 60 mL/hr
   D. 100 mL/hr
9. The proper size of a cuffed pediatric tracheal tube is determined by:
   A. (Age in years/4) + 4
   B. (Age in years/4) + 3
   C. The internal diameter of the patient's thumb
   D. Viewing the cords first and then choosing the right size
10. The appropriate depth of the tracheal tube is:
    A. Determined in children only by auscultating over the lateral chest wall for adequate breath sounds
    B. Determined in children only by palpating for symmetric chest rise
    C. Approximately 3 times the tube size AND verified by presence of bilateral breath sounds
    D. Calculated by (age in years/4) + 4, in children older than 2 years of age
11. You are evaluating a 6-year-old child with head trauma. He shows a positive Babinski's reflex.
    A. This is normal in this age group.
    B. This may indicate pyramidal tract, upper motor neuron damage.
    C. This is an unreliable test.
    D. When paired with a low Glasgow Coma Score, this may indicate impending uncal herniation.
12. A local hospital has preapproved an area transport team to care for all ages of patients transferred from their facility. In doing so, they used the PALS course as the standard for educational preparation for the pediatric population.
    A. This complies with the JCAHO criteria for hospitals.
    B. This does not comply with the standards set forth by the Academy of Pediatrics.
    C. This is a higher standard than for 9-1-1 calls.
    D. This complies with all patient situations according to EMTALA rules.
13. Infants and children increase their cardiac output by:
    A. Breathing faster
    B. Allowing their hearts to overfill and pump harder
    C. Increasing their heart rate
    D. Parasympathetic stimulation
14. With regard to congenital heart defects:
    A. An infant with pulmonary stenosis will exhibit cyanosis at rest but will have strong, full pulses
    B. An infant with pulmonary stenosis will not have cyanosis but may have low cardiac output
    C. An infant with hypoplastic left heart will be cyanotic, especially while crying, and high cardiac output
    D. An infant with hypoplastic left heart will be cyanotic only at rest and will have low cardiac output
15. Prostaglandin (PGE_1) is administered to a neonate to keep the ductus arteriosus:
    A. Closed
    B. Open in CHDs such as tetralogy of Fallot
    C. Open in CHDs such as atrial septal defect
    D. Closed and you should be prepared for respiratory depression after the administration
16. In the scenario at the beginning of the Geriatric section, the patient demonstrated an altered mental status and rapidly changing level of consciousness with a recent fall, history of diabetes, and vascular disease. Our list of differential diagnoses must include:
    A. Intracranial incident: ischemic stroke
    B. Subdural hematoma
    C. Hyperglycemia
    D. Acute renal failure
17. The word delirium was used to describe this patient (geriatric scenario). This behavior/sign is always attributed to:
    A. A chronic and natural part of aging of the brain
    B. A side effect of polypharmacy
    C. Psychological issues
    D. An acute event of some sort

18. What information gained from our patient (geriatric scenario) in physical examination and history makes him at risk for rapidly developing bleeding into tissues and organs?
    A. Use of warfarin
    B. Loss of elastin
    C. Falls
    D. All of the above
19. Select the best statement regarding pharmacokinetics and pharmacodynamics in the older adult.
    A. All drug doses should be cut by half for older adults because they absorb drugs so much faster.
    B. Frequency of drug administration may be more important than drug dosing by itself because the older body has difficulty eliminating many medications.
    C. Morphine should never be used because it causes respiratory depression and accumulates rapidly in the fat.
    D. All of the above
20. The older patient is at risk for unrecognized subdural hematoma because:
    A. The brain itself is smaller, allowing more space in the subdural area
    B. There is more tension on the bridging vessels in subdural space
    C. A larger mass of bleeding would need to develop before signs and symptoms of an increase in intracranial pressure would occur
    D. All of the above
21. Airway compromise and aspiration occur easier in the older adult because of:
    A. Presbyesophagus, facial changes, and dysphagia
    B. Presbycusis, presbyopia and osteoporosis
    C. Arthritis, increasing collagen, and loss of hepatocytes
    D. Increasing pH in the stomach, presbyesophagus, and demineralization
22. Select the correct statement regarding renal senescence.
    A. An older adult's kidney will excrete more urine (>0.5/kg/hr) because the ability to save Na^+ and water are diminished through the RAS.
    B. The older patient's kidneys will conserve water adequately while compensating in shock states.
    C. While in shock, the older adult will suffer from more renal damage than the younger patient because of lower blood flow.
    D. The rising GFR will substantially injure the kidney by age 80.
23. While conducting a physical examination on a 90-year-old male, what finding may be a sign of acute disease?
    A. Enlarged heart, especially left ventricle (with corresponding axis deviation)
    B. Room air pulse oximetry levels at 88%
    C. Nonmedicated heart rate of 60 with 8 to 10 PVCs/minute
    D. End-tidal carbon dioxide ($PETCO_2$) of 80 mm Hg
24. You are evaluating an 82-year-old, independent female who was found by her family to be disoriented and weak. They don't think she has eaten for 1 or 2 days and has been sleeping most of the time. She has no obvious clinical signs or symptoms. This patient normally walks 1 to 2 miles per day, swims, and is active in her church and as a volunteer in the community. What differential diagnoses must be ruled out?
    A. Infection/sepsis
    B. Psychoses
    C. Alzheimer's disease
    D. Emphysema
25. You have placed 1 gm of phenytoin into 250 mg of NS. Your patient is an 81-year-old motor vehicle crash patient with head trauma. What rate should be dialed into the IV pump?
    A. 2.5 mL/hr
    B. 5 mL/hr
    C. 150 mL/hr
    D. 300 mL/hr

CHAPTER 10

Special Considerations in Critical Care Transport

OBJECTIVES

1. Identify drug overdoses through toxidromes and chemical toxins common to health care and then discuss the unique management principles for these conditions.
2. Assess for clinical and behavioral pain indicators, apply diagnostic scales and scores, describe the physiologic response seen with different types of pain, and discuss management strategies.
3. Discuss the indications for hyperbaric treatment, its safety, and the therapeutic effects.
4. Describe the gas laws that apply in illnesses involving submersion and altitude.
5. Discuss the assessment for and clinical signs and management of submersion and altitude illnesses.
6. Describe the physical stressors of air medical transport; also describe crew resource management and personal and passenger safety in both air and ground transport.
7. Identify a potential organ or tissue donor patient and discuss the initiation of the process of organ donation, with emphasis on medical management and documentation.

The topics discussed in this chapter deserve special consideration during critical care management and transport; they are toxicology, pain management, hyperbaric medicine, tissue and organ procurement, flight physiology, and flight and ground safety.

TOXICOLOGY IN CRITICAL CARE

Scenario

Your team has been dispatched to a hospital 20 minutes away to transport a 22-year-old female to a tertiary care hospital an additional 90 minutes from there. The staff reports that this patient was anonymously dropped off at the hospital entrance 2 hours ago in an unconscious state from unknown cause.

On arrival, you find that the patient, who weighs 154 pounds (70 kg), has been intubated with a 7.5 mm endotracheal tube inserted to 22 cm at the lip, and she has equal, bilateral breath sounds. Capnography shows a good waveform and an end-tidal carbon dioxide ($PETCO_2$) of 36 mm Hg. The patient has no spontaneous respirations.

The current ventilator settings are: assist-control (tidal volume, 500 mL; rate, 11 breaths/min) positive end-expiratory pressure (PEEP), 5 cm H_2O; and 100% oxygen.

Vital signs are: heart rate, 140 beats/min; BP, 78/40 mm Hg; pulse oximetry, 100%; temperature, 35° C (95° F). The skin is cool and dry.

Thus far, 1 L of crystalloids has been given, and the patient is receiving dopamine by infusion at the rate of 5 mcg/kg/min. A Foley catheter bag shows approximately 20 mL of clear urine.

The patient history is unobtainable. The patient has a strong odor of alcohol. When she was found at the front entrance, her pupils were 2 mm bilaterally, and her initial Glasgow Coma Scale (GCS) score was 7; she also had a low BP, tachycardia, and poor respiratory effort.

Anatomy and Physiology in Toxicology

Most toxicologic emergencies are the result of acute oral overdose of prescription medications. Toxins may enter the body through various routes, and their effects on the body are related to many factors. Treatment for each poisoned patient begins with generic supportive care, but each toxin may have unique antidotes and require management principles that are case based. Your knowledge of the anatomy and physiology described in chapters 3 through 6 will help you understand how these poisons can create certain pathophysiologic presentations.

This section discusses toxins common to the domestic healthcare system, poisons associated with everyday life.

Assessment and Recognition of Toxicity

The priorities of assessment and care for a poisoned patient are the usual ABCDs, with one notable exception—you must first protect yourself. Some patients present with external contamination, and special decontamination procedures are required before or during assessment of the ABCs while rescuers use special barrier protection.

Table 10-1 Common Toxidromes

Sources	Examples	Toxidrome	Mnemonic
Anticholinergics	TCAs, diphenhydramine, scopolamine, jimson weed, some poisonous mushrooms	Tachycardia, flushing, dilated pupils (mydriasis), low-grade fever, dry mucous membranes, dry skin, confusion	Dry as a bone, red as a beet, mad as a hatter, blind as a bat
Opiates	Morphine, heroin, codeine, oxycodone	Pinpoint pupils, hypotension, bradypnea, coma, hypothermia	None
Cholinergics	Organophosphate or carbamate pesticides, some mushrooms, nerve gas	Lacrimation, salivation, muscle weakness, diarrhea, vomiting, miosis	SLUDGE*
Sympathomimetics	Cocaine, Ecstasy, methamphetamine, caffeine and related drugs	Tachycardia, hypertension, elevated temperature, dilated pupils (mydriasis)	None
Serotonergics	Lithium, MAOIs, SSRIs, tramadol, linezolid	Rapid onset after starting or changing drugs: Hyperthermia, myoclonus, diaphoresis, hyperreflexia, rigidity, tremor, agitation, coma, confusion	None
Gamma hydroxybutyrate	GHB, liquid Ecstasy	Coma alternating with agitation, bradypnea, bradycardia, and myoclonus	None

MAOIs, Monoamine oxidase inhibitors; *SSRIs,* selective serotonin reuptake inhibitors; *TCAs,* tricyclic antidepressants.
*SLUDGE stands for *s*alivation, *l*acrimation, *u*rination, *d*efecation, *g*astrointestinal upset, and *e*mesis.

The first step in the assessment and treatment of any poisoned patient is to identify the underlying disorder based on signs and symptoms. Certain patterns should suggest the diagnosis; these symptom complexes are called **toxidromes,** a shortened term for toxic syndromes (Table 10-1).

It is important to note that urine drug screening is notoriously inaccurate, does not include most drugs of abuse, and should not be used to guide diagnosis and treatment. For example, sesame seeds and **fluoroquinolones** may give a false-positive result on urinalysis for opiates. At any rate, in a true emergency you must act without waiting for laboratory results.

Obtaining an overdose history, when possible, is essential to the assessment. As you stabilize the patient's ABCDs, other members of the critical care team should investigate the possible cause of the patient's presentation. This involves checking the patient care record, interviewing family members or friends, and obtaining a medication history from the patient's pharmacy (if time allows). Information about the amount of the substance ingested and the time of ingestion, along with any other toxins consumed (e.g., alcohol), is important. Hazardous material information must be obtained from first response agencies.

Critical care monitoring is vital, and a good primary and a focused secondary assessment should be performed and repeated often.

Diagnostics in the Poisoned Patient

Toxicology screening (urine, blood, gastric contents) rarely helps identify ingested toxins. A comprehensive toxicology screen, as described by the laboratory, does not include the toxins that are life-threatening in the first few hours after ingestion. You may have access to individual drug levels, such as acetaminophen, or a urine screen for drugs of abuse. However, as was stated previously, evaluating for toxidromes is more reliable than waiting for results that are not reliable.

For a critical care patient with a toxicologic presentation, laboratory tests that are appropriate for a patient with hemodynamic or neurologic instability should be done. These tests include electrolytes, coagulation panels, complete blood cell (CBC) count, blood gases, and renal and liver function studies. Radiographs rarely are helpful, unless the clinician is tracking the decontamination of lead, iron, or body packets, which are illegal drugs, packaged for sale, and ingested by those wishing to hide evidence.

Safe Transport for a Poisoned Patient

The overriding issue in transportation of a poisoned patient is the safety of the crew and other emergency personnel. "Conventional" poisonings (e.g., acetaminophen, alcohol) present little risk of contamination of other personnel. However, toxicologic poisonings include volatile substances such as central nervous system (CNS) toxins (organophosphates), organic solvents (gasoline), and radioactive agents, all of which may contaminate the work environment and those attending to the patient. Ideally, the patient will have been decontaminated before transport; when possible, make every effort to decontaminate the person before patient contact. Decontamination should include removal of contaminated clothing and decontamination of the skin. Any equipment or other personnel should be decontaminated as appropriate.

Specific Toxins

Organophosphates

Organophosphates (OPs) are a group of pesticides that account for approximately 38% of the pesticides used worldwide. OPs kill insects by disrupting impulses to the brain and nervous system. Humans also can be harmed by OPs, which are used in nerve gas and chemical weapons. Some OPs, such as malathion (and also sarin, which was used in the 1995 Tokyo subway attacks), can be absorbed through the skin, by inhalation, and through contact with mucous membranes; therefore, direct contact should be avoided.

OPs cause a chemical dysfunction that results in longer nerve impulse activation. They block cholinesterase, which allows acetylcholine levels to rise and causes nerve impulses to remain active longer. *Latex gloves may not be effective in preventing contact with an OP—nitrile gloves are preferred.* With a contaminated patient, contaminated clothing first should be removed safely. The skin then can be decontaminated with soap and water and then washed again with ethanol.

Use the mnemonic SLUDGE to remember the clinical effects of organophosphates and other toxic cholinergic agents: *s*alivation, *l*acrimation, *u*rination, *d*efecation, *g*astrointestinal cramping and *e*mesis. Patients may also develop bradycardia, bronchorrhea, bronchospasm, muscle weakness, and decreased ability to move air. An important point is that these patients may need massive doses of atropine to prevent them from drowning in their own secretions. Starting with a 1 mg dose, administer atropine every 5 minutes until secretions diminish. Remember that atropine is used in both bradycardia *and* tachycardia in organophosphate poisoning.

Because of respiratory muscle weakness (and increased secretions), intubation may be required. If the patient needs to be paralyzed, use a nondepolarizing agent such as rocuronium or vecuronium. *Do not use succinylcholine.* Succinylcholine is metabolized by the same cholinesterase that metabolizes organophosphates; therefore, it may lead to prolonged paralysis. Seizures can be treated with benzodiazepines.

Volatile Hydrocarbons (Volatile Organic Solvents)

Although some differences exist, the terms *volatile organic solvents* (VOS) and *volatile organic compounds* (VOC) are used in this section to include both solvents and other volatile hydrocarbons.

VOS, which are widely used in industry, include compounds such as gasoline, benzene, carbon tetrachloride, and toluene. They are found in a diverse group of products, such as paints, dyes, glues, varnishes, degreasing agents, lamp oil, and other petroleum products. Most VOS are petroleum distillates. Wood distillates, which are made primarily from pine (turpentine, pine oil), are another class of volatile hydrocarbons.

Patients may be exposed to VOS accidentally, such as at work or when siphoning gasoline, or purposely, through inhalant abuse (huffing). Petroleum distillates and wood distillates have different routes of maximum toxicity. Petroleum distillates generally evaporate readily, are easily inhaled, and cause pulmonary toxicity. Pulmonary exposure frequently occurs during ingestion when small amounts are aspirated. The exceptions are diesel fuel and kerosene, which are less volatile and therefore less likely to enter the pulmonary tree. Wood distillates tend to be less volatile, and absorption generally occurs after ingestion. Decontamination should be done at the scene. The patient's VOS-contaminated clothing should be removed to prevent transdermal and pulmonary absorption. Also, the skin should be washed with saline to help reduce further absorption.

Patients with a significant exposure (even recreational) may have arrhythmias and therefore should be placed on a cardiac monitor. For safety reasons, remember that most of these agents are flammable. This may seem obvious, but do not use the defibrillator on a patient who has not yet been decontaminated and whose clothing or body are soaked with hydrocarbons (e.g., gasoline). Even routine use of supplemental oxygen is questioned for safety. Defibrillation may initiate a fire, and oxygen feeds it.

In general, transport teams are concerned with three types of toxicity from petroleum distillates: pulmonary toxicity, CNS toxicity, and cardiac toxicity.

- Pulmonary toxicity occurs as a result of abuse or during purposeful or accidental ingestion. Early signs of inhalation injury (e.g., cough, tachypnea) should be noted, because they may indicate a course of treatment that includes intubation. Patients exposed to even small amounts of inhaled VOS may develop pulmonary injury, including pneumonitis, pulmonary edema, and acute respiratory distress syndrome (ARDS). Therefore, preventing aspiration is important. This includes not using a nasogastric (NG) tube to remove swallowed hydrocarbons unless specifically instructed to do so by poison control. In some cases gastrointestinal (GI) decontamination is desirable (e.g., with chloroform or benzene ingestion). However, for most ingestions (e.g., gasoline, lamp oil, kerosene), gastric decontamination is not particularly helpful and may be counterproductive.
- CNS toxicity may occur as a result of hypoxia that develops secondary to pulmonary injury or as a result of systemic absorption through the GI or respiratory tract. CNS toxicity ranges from euphoria to confusion, hallucinations, and coma. Long-term toxicity may include encephalopathy, ataxia, and tremors. From a transport perspective, keep in mind that the full CNS toxicity of ingested hydrocarbons may not be evident immediately. The patient may become progressively less responsive and require intubation during transport.
- With cardiac toxicity, hydrocarbons may cause dysrhythmias even in doses used for abuse. These arrhythmias seem to be the result of catecholamine release. For this reason, epinephrine and other catecholamines are contraindicated in a patient poisoned or intoxicated with VOS, *except* when the patient does not respond to good cardiopulmonary resuscitation (CPR) during the management of cardiac arrest. Blood pressure should be maintained with IV fluids if possible.

Iatrogenic Problems

Some of the problems the critical care team encounters during transport are **iatrogenic**; that is, they are caused by medical care. Many of these cases are related to decontamination of the GI tract. Traditionally, gastric lavage was performed with a large-bore orogastric tube and followed by the administration of charcoal. Both of these modalities have fallen out of favor among toxicologists. It is clear that except in exceptional circumstances, gastric lavage is not indicated if more than 1 hour has elapsed since the ingestion. The same holds true for administration of charcoal; it has limited efficacy after the first hour. However, it takes time for changes to trickle down, therefore, you may see both of these modalities used. Charcoal is the easiest challenge with which to deal; however, charcoal administration significantly increases the risk of aspiration (as does gastric lavage), so be aware that this may occur. One of the more worrisome complications of a toxicologic emergency is esophageal injury. This may occur as a result of repeated retching (Boerhaave's tear or Mallory-Weiss injury), or it may be caused by gastric lavage.

At least 50% of esophageal injuries are the result of medical instrumentation (not all from gastric lavage). Obvious esophageal perforation may present at the time of gastric lavage, making the diagnosis easy; the patient may have chest pain and a pneumomediastinum on radiographs. However, this tear may not become evident until you are en route. The symptoms and signs of **occult** esophageal rupture overlap significantly with those of other diseases; they include chest pain, especially with swallowing; fever; tachycardia; dyspnea (40% of cases); and sepsis and shock (33% of cases). This is a true emergency, and the patient's condition can deteriorate rapidly.

Did You Know?

Keep in mind the following key points when attempting to prevent further drug absorption in an overdose event:

1. **Ipecac routinely causes vomiting, but no drug is removed.**
2. **Gastric lavage is an invasive procedure that may cause esophageal perforation and rarely removes much drug from the stomach.**
3. **Activated charcoal absorbs most drugs, but to be beneficial, it must be given very soon after the overdose.**
4. **Whole bowel irrigation (GoLYTELY, Colyte) and cathartics generally are of little or no value.**

Table 10-2 Manifestations and Treatment of Selected Drug Toxicities

Drug	Symptoms and Possible Treatment	Symptom and Treatment	Symptom and Treatment	Symptom and Treatment
Benzodiazepines (flumazenil [Romazicon]*)	Central nervous system depression → Flumazenil if no contraindications	Respiratory depression → Support ABCs		
Methamphetamine/cocaine/ other sympathomimetics (e.g., Ecstasy)	Hypertension, tachycardia → phentolamine (alpha blocker)† Benzodiazepines followed by beta blocker	Seizures → lorazepam	Agitation → lorazepam	
Opiates	All symptoms: naloxone (Narcan)‡			
Anticholinergics (e.g., TCAs, diphenhydramine) SNRI antidepressants§ (e.g., duloxetine [Cymbalta], venlafaxine [Effexor])	Arrhythmia (monomorphic ventricular tachycardia or torsades de pointes) → sodium bicarbonate, magnesium sulfate	Seizure → lorazepam	Hypotension → fluid, norepinephrine *(not dopamine)*	Agitation → lorazepam

**Flumazenil should not be used except in extraordinary circumstances; it can induce intractable seizures.* As with opiates, the preferred option is to intubate and allow the patient to remain comatose during transport.

†Using a beta blocker first causes the sympathetic nervous system's alpha receptor sites to be unopposed, which worsens hypertension and tachycardia. The practice of using an alpha blocker first has been called into question but currently is the standard of care.

‡It may be preferable to intubate the patient and allow the person to remain sedated from the narcotics during transport. Smaller doses of naloxone (0.4 mg) may prevent intubation. Remember, administering naloxone puts the patient into withdrawal.

§Data are limited, but overdose with an SNRI seems to produce the same toxicity and to respond to the same treatments as overdose with a tricyclic antidepressant.

SNRI, Serotonin-norepinephrine reuptake inhibitor; *TCAs*, tricyclic antidepressants.

The most important aspect of treating an esophageal tear is recognition. If the injury goes unrecognized, it often is fatal. Do not assume that physiologic changes are strictly the result of an overdose; maintain a high clinical index of suspicion, especially with patients who have had gastric lavage. Antibiotics, fluid, intubation, and pressors all may play a role in treatment, depending on the clinical situation.

Treatment of Toxicologic Emergencies

Table 10-2 reviews some important manifestations of common overdoses and the treatment of these emergencies.

Chemical Toxicity

More than 60,000 new chemicals are produced each year. Most of these, if mishandled, can damage the skin. Factors to consider when treating patients who have been involved in a chemical incident include the concentration of the agent, the duration of contact, and whether a systemic toxicity results. Treatment depends on the agent.

In a chemical hazardous materials (HAZMAT) incident, there are two goals: containment (fire, materials, and cleanup) and treatment of exposed individuals. Most of your involvement with these patients is in a third or fourth layer of response, as you are asked to transport those with systemic toxicity to tertiary care centers. Because of this focus, this section discusses the treatment of exposed individuals.

Chemical Agents

Chemical agents are categorized by their physiologic effects and composition. Table 10-3 lists several of the more common agents and the management of emergencies involving these substances.

Scenario Conclusion

As you review your hand-off report from the local hospital and note the patient's presentation, you recognize the toxidrome associated with opiates. The patient shows no signs of chronic IV drug abuse. The local clinician did not administer any antidotes. According to your protocol, you administer 2 mg of naloxone; the patient immediately begins to awaken and grasp for the tracheal tube. Wrist restraints are applied as you evaluate the patient for the complication of pulmonary edema.

The ongoing evaluation by the local physician and a consultation with a toxicologist result in the decision to abort the critical care transport, extubate the patient, and monitor her condition locally.

PAIN MANAGEMENT

Scenario

A 45-year-old man comes to the emergency department (ED) complaining of sharp posterior-lateral chest pain that increases with breathing and coughing. He reports that he was at a party the previous evening and stepped back into a hot tub, striking the right posterior ribs on the seat. He states that initially the pain "wasn't too bad"; however, this morning he has severe, sharp pain, which he rates as 9 on a 1 to 10 numeric pain scale. The patient took ibuprofen (800 mg PO) every 4 to 6 hours through the night.

The patient weighs 352 pounds (160 kg), and the history shows type 2 diabetes, hyperlipidemia, hypertension, peripheral vascular disease, and sleep apnea.

The physician orders 4 mg of morphine to be given intravenously (IV). After 5 minutes of treatment, the patient reports no relief; the pain remains a 9 on a 1 to 10 scale. The physician repeats the dose (4 mg morphine IV), and 5 minutes later, the patient rates the pain as 8 on a 1 to 10 scale. A third dose of morphine (4 mg IV) is administered but has little or no effect.

The physician then orders 100 mcg of fentanyl to be given IV. Within 5 minutes, the patient reports the pain level as 4 on a 1 to 10 scale; 5 minutes after that, the patient is resting with his eyes closed, and the pulse oximetry reading drops into the 80s. The patient has no respiratory distress, and lung sounds are clear and equal.

The identification and management of pain often are overlooked; however, these skills are crucial for critical care practitioners. Pain is the defense system the body uses to minimize further damage, a process that occurs as part of a negative feedback loop. The more intense the pain, the more the body sends messages to remove itself from the pain. Pain can be difficult to manage, depending on its origin and the variations in presentation. A successful management strategy, therefore, depends on two equal and important factors: a knowledge of the type of pain stimulus and an understanding of the pharmacologic agents used to deal with it.

Assessment for Pain

The best indicator of pain, and most valid means of measuring it, is the patient's description of the pain, along with the associated history. However, critical care patients usually are unable to voice these complaints. Often you must rely on observation, changes in vital signs, and assumptions to note that the patient is experiencing pain. Untreated pain leads to poor treatment. Untreated pain may also lead to serious complications.

Physiologic Response to Pain

Acute pain is associated with an inflammatory response caused by surgery, an acute illness, or trauma. Untreated acute pain, along with the healing process, may lead to chronic pain. Somatic pain involves superficial tissues and usually can be identified as localized. Visceral pain involves organs and usually is identified as diffuse.

Table 10-3 Common Chemical Agents

Category	Signs and Symptoms	Treatment
Pulmonary agents • Phosgene • Chlorine	Respiratory irritation Coughing and sneezing Watery eyes Dyspnea, tachypnea	Decontamination A, B, C support No specific antidote
Blood agents • Cyanide	Cellular anoxia Tachypnea Restlessness, anxiety Weakness Headache, N and V Tachycardia Apnea, cardiac arrest	Decontamination A, B, C support Cyanide kit (amyl nitrate, then Na thiosulfate, then Na nitrate [Old Rx]) Hydroxocobalamin (Cyanokit ®) (new)
Vesicants • Mustard gas • Lewisite	Rhinorrhea Blepharospasm Pruritus Blisters to skin Hoarseness, cough, dyspnea	Decontaminate A, B, C support Dimercaprol (BAL) (antidote for Lewisite)
Nerve agents • Tabun (GA) • Sarin (GB)	Miosis Rhinorrhea Lacrimation (SLUDGE) N and V Fasciculations, seizures Death	Decontaminate A, B, C support Atropine, 2 PAM Cl
Incapacitating agents • BZ	Hallucinations Illusions	Decontaminate
Riot-control agents • CS (mace)	Respiratory irritation Lacrimation	Decontaminate

Modified from Emergency Nurses Association: *Trauma nursing core course provider manual (TNCC)*, ed 6, Des Plaines, Ill, 2007, The Association.

The biologic response to pain can be measured. The sympathetic nervous system reacts by releasing epinephrine and norepinephrine, which results in tachycardia, tachypnea, and elevated blood pressure. If the pain is visceral, especially in the GI system, the parasympathetic system response may trigger a reverse effect (i.e., bradycardia and hypotension).

Behavioral Indicators of Pain

Facial expressions in adults have been studied extensively with regard to pain. The frequency of the patient's facial movements and the appearance of a grimace have become fairly reliable behavioral indicators of pain. Three primary facial movements indicate moderate pain:

- Brow lowering
- Orbit tightening
- Levator contraction (deepening of the nasolabial furrow)

The addition of eye closing to these three facial movements indicates severe pain.

Some body movements also have been observed to be associated with pain. In a sedated patient or in one with altered mental status, pain indicators include touching pain sites or tubes (especially when the person is moved) or moving the arms and legs restlessly. General body tenseness also is interpreted as a behavioral indicator of pain. If the patient has been intubated and is being ventilated, dyssynchrony is an indirect indicator.

Diagnostic Indicators of Pain

Once the assessment for verbal, behavioral, or physiologic indicators of pain is complete, the critical care team should measure those specific indicators for ongoing assessment and comparison during management. Some pain scales and scores are described in Figure 10-1 and Table 10-4.

Pain

According to Merriam-Webster, **pain** is defined as "an unpleasant sensory and emotional experience associated with actual or potential tissue damage, or described in terms of such damage." The difficulty in treatment can be attributed to differences in presentation and intensity, which vary from person to person. The type of pain is another factor that affects treatment.

Types of Pain

Pain generally is classified as one of two major types, neuropathic pain or nociceptive pain. Nociceptive pain is acute and associated with the inflammatory process, which can be

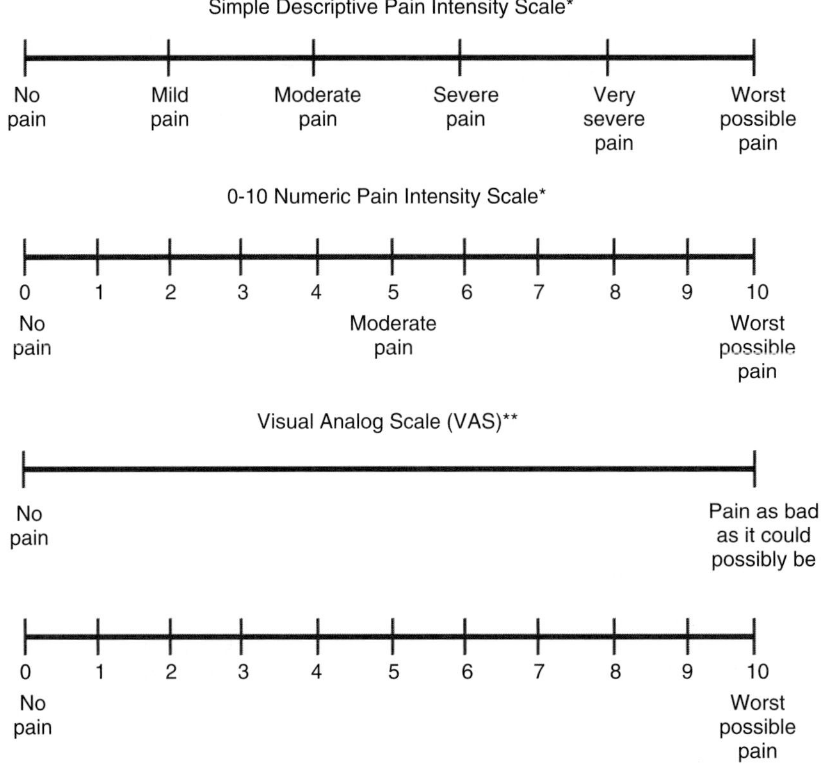

Figure 10-1

Pain intensity scales. **A,** Simple descriptive pain intensity scale. **B,** Numeric pain intensity scale. **C,** Visual analog scale. **D,** Simple descriptive pain intensity scale. **E,** Wong-Baker FACES Pain Rating Sale. (From Wong DL: *Whaley and Wong's essentials of pediatric nursing*, ed 6, St Louis, 2001, Mosby.)

caused by surgery, illness, or trauma. If acute pain is undertreated, it could eventually become chronic pain. Any pain lasting longer than 6 month is defined as chronic pain. Chronic pain usually develops as a result of an incomplete healing process or when the nervous system develops permanent damage. It is important to distinguish between the two types to determine the cause of the pain and, eventually, the treatment.

Neuropathic Pain

Neuropathic pain indicates direct damage to or dysfunction of the structures of the peripheral or central nervous system. Pain most often is triggered by an injury; however, it also may occur after the injury as a result of strangulation of nerves by scar tissue or compression by tumors. Neuropathic pain can occur outside the CNS (peripheral), or it can be central in nature. It usually is chronic and usually responds better to antidepressant sodium channel blockers or antiseizure medications than to opioids. Some components of cancer, carpal tunnel syndrome, phantom limb pain, and **peripheral neuropathy** are examples of neuropathic pain. Diabetes is the most common cause of peripheral neuropathy.

Patients usually describe neuropathic pain as a burning or an electrical shock sensation. Sometimes the patient describes a tingling feeling or a strange sensation; this is described as **dysesthesia**. Patients with diabetic neuropathy frequently experience this feeling.

Did You Know?

Some common causes of neuropathic pain include alcoholism; amputation; back, leg, and hip problems; and chemotherapy.[1]

Nociception

Nociception (or *nociperception*) is the perception of physical pain. It occurs through the stimulation of nociceptors, which are sensory receptors around neurons that react to harmful stimuli and are specifically responsible for notifying the nervous system that an injury has occurred. Nociception consists of four processes: transduction, transmission, perception, and modulation.

Transduction

Transduction is the process by which noxious stimuli are converted to electrical signals in the nociceptors. Unlike other

Table 10-4 Critical Care Pain Observation Tool (CPOT)

Indicator	Description	Rating (Points)
Facial expression	No muscular tension observed	Relaxed, neutral (0)
	Frowning, brow lowering, orbit tightening, and levator (mouth) contraction	Tense (1)
	All previous facial movements plus tightly closed eyelids	Grimacing (2)
Body movements	Does not move at all (does not necessarily indicate absence of pain)	Absence of movements (0)
	Slow, cautious movements; touching or rubbing the pain site; seeking attention through movements	Protection (1)
	Pulling tube, attempting to sit up, moving limbs/thrashing, not following commands, striking out at staff, trying to climb out of bed	Restlessness (2)
Muscular tension	No resistance to passive movements	Relaxed (0)
Evaluation by passive flexion and extension of upper limbs	Resistance to passive movements	Tense, rigid (1)
	Strong resistance to passive movements, unable to complete them	Very tense or rigid (2)
Compliance with the ventilator (intubated patients)	Alarms not activated, easy ventilation	Tolerating movements (0)
	Alarms stop spontaneously	Coughing but tolerating (1)
	Asynchrony (blocking ventilation, alarms frequently activated)	Fighting ventilator (2)
Vocalization (extubated patients)	Talking in normal tone or no sound	Talking in normal tone or no sound (0)
	Sighing, moaning	Sighing, moaning (1)
	Crying out, sobbing	Crying out, sobbing (2)

Courtesy Celine Gelinas, School of Nursing, McGill University, Montreal, Canada.

sensory receptors, nociceptors are not structurally specialized, but rather exist as free nerve endings. They can be mechanical (e.g., surgical incisions), thermal (e.g., burns), or chemical (e.g., toxic substances) receptors.

Transmission

In the transmission process, the electrical signals in the nociceptors are sent from the periphery to the spinal cord, to the thalamus, and then on to the cerebral cortex. Noxious information is relayed via specialized nociceptive fibers. As mentioned, nociceptors are free nerve endings that transmit responses to the brain by means of specialized fibers, A-delta fibers and C-fibers. These fibers innervate the system by way of the dorsal horn of the spinal column and synapse with dendrites of the spinal cord. They transmit stimuli from the extremities to the core of the brain.

Did You Know?

The three major classes of nociceptors in the skin are A-delta mechanosensitive nociceptors, A-delta mechanothermal nociceptors, and polymodal nociceptors.[1]

A-delta fibers are large, myelinated axons that transmit messages rapidly. This network of fibers extends from the distal extremities, connects to the **neospinothalamic tract** via the dorsal root ganglion, and terminates at the **somatosensory cortex**. A-delta fibers transmit well-localized, sharp pain.

C-fibers are smaller diameter axons that lack a myelin sheath and therefore transmit impulses much more slowly. They transmit impulses to the **paleospinothalamic tract** via the dorsal horn of the spinal cord, relaying messages to the area of the midbrain and surrounding tissues. C-fibers diffusely transmit dull and aching pain.

Did You Know?

After the nerve fibers enter the spinal cord, they travel up several ascending pathways on the opposite side of the spinal cord. A pain sensation is routed to two different tracts: the paleospinothalamic tract, which produces a diffuse ache that is difficult to localize, or the neospinothalamic tract, which allows perception of different degrees of pain and permits localization.[2]

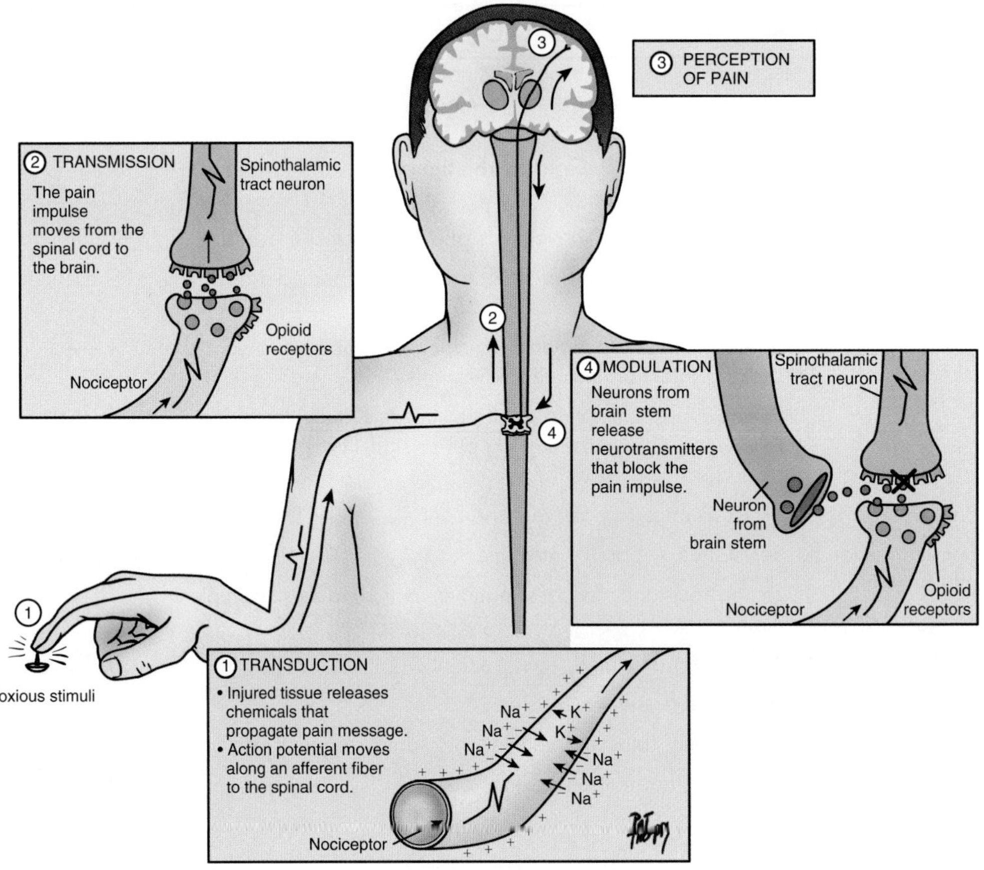

Figure 10-2

The four processes of nociception. (From Jarvis C: *Physical examination and health assessment*, ed 4, Philadelphia, 2004, Saunders.)

Perception

Messages are sent to the nerves by means of *neurotransmitters,* which are chemicals that carry nerve impulses across a synapse. Neurotransmitters bridge the synaptic gap and ferry messages from the dendrites of the sending neurons to the dendrites of the receiver. They work either by blocking the actions between neurons (**inhibitory neurotransmitters**) or by promoting the actions of neurons (**stimulatory neurotransmitters**).

Modulation

Modulation is the release of endogenous opioids that prevent the transmission of the pain sensation in the spinal cord. This process produces analgesia through the descending pathways of the spinal cord.

Pain Assessment

The assessment of pain is an important component of any critical care assessment. To relieve or control pain adequately, you must perform a thorough pain assessment. The two components of the assessment of pain are observable (objective) factors and nonobservable (subjective) factors.

Management of Pain

In acute and critical care, pain is managed with medications, which commonly are administered to reduce the effects of the many causes of pain (Table 10-5). Medications also help stabilize the internal environment, allowing for a more predictable pattern of response in both conscious and unconscious patients. Three types of medications are commonly used in the management of pain: opioid agonists, nonopiods such as nonsteroidal anti-inflammatory drugs, and synthetics.

Opioid

The opioids that are recommended for first-line analgesics are the agonists. These drugs inhibit the delivery of pain impulses to nociceptors by blocking the mu receptors in the brain and spinal cord. The activation of these receptors lessens the pain response and causes analgesia, sedation, and respiratory depression. Morphine is the most frequently used opioid in the prehospital setting. Due to the fact of its water solubility, morphine has a slower onset of action but will have a longer duration. Morphine is indicated when the patient is

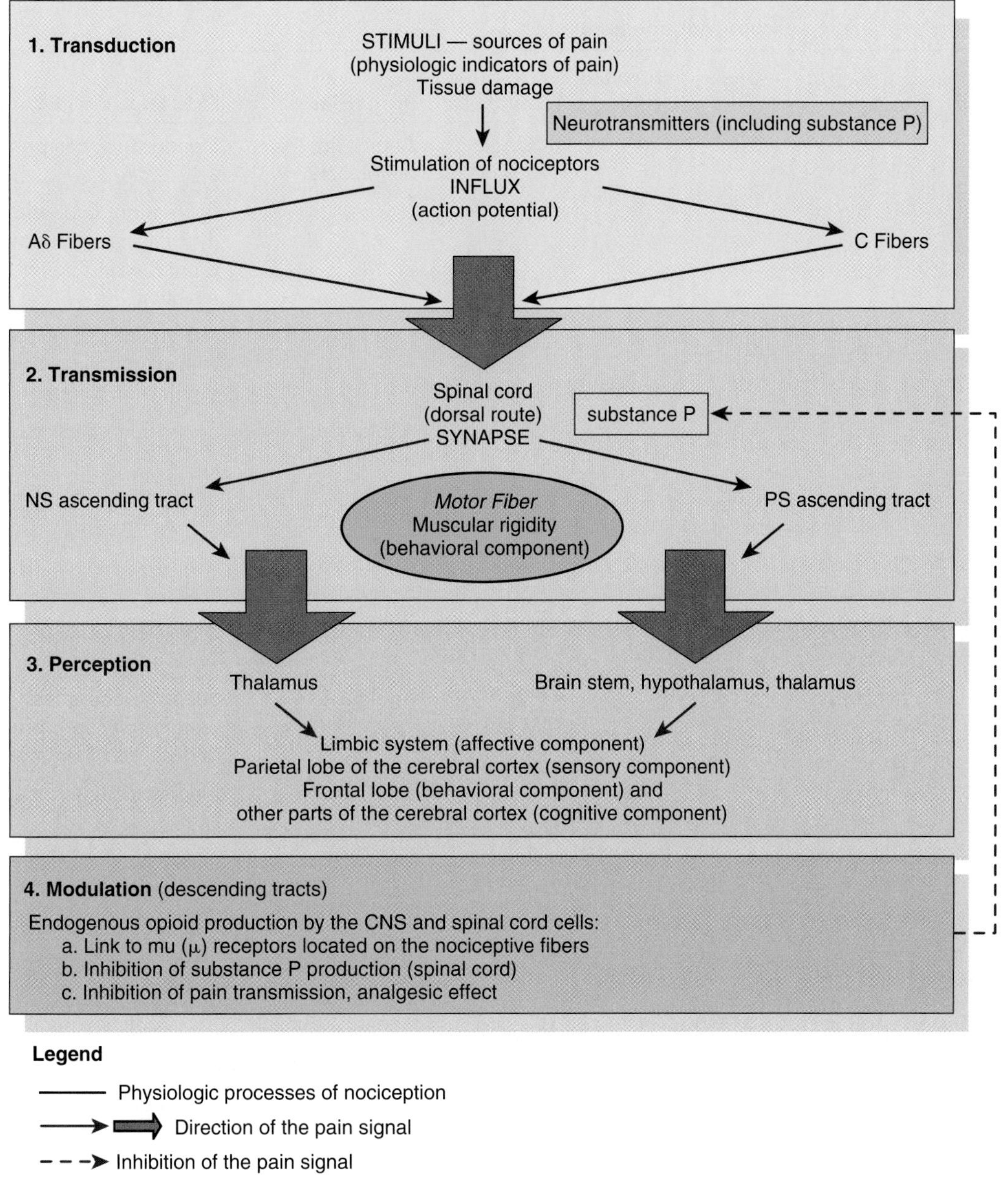

Figure 10-3

Integration of pain assessment in the four processes of nociception. (Courtesy Celine Gelinas, School of Nursing, McGill University, Montreal, Canada.)

experiencing severe pain. Fentanyl is a synthetic opioid most commonly used with patients with an allergy to morphine or who have hemodynamic instability.

Nonopioid Analgesics

Nonopioids are also known as **nonsteroidal antiinflammatory drugs (NSAIDs)**, which help interfere with the mediated process by which pain is relayed to nociceptors. As pain is interpreted by the body, prostaglandin and bradykinin are released at the exposed nerve endings, increasing the intensity and duration of the pain response. NSAIDs interfere with this inflammatory response by inhibiting the formation of prostaglandin and bradykinin in the GI tract. When the catalysis of **cyclooxygenase** (COX-1 and COX-2) is prevented, prostaglandin and thromboxane are not formed. NSAIDs also have antipyretic and analgesic properties that help reduce the duration and extent of inflammation.

Most NSAIDs are weak acids and have some negative effects on the GI system. Hepatic injury, ulcers, and bleeding are relative but common side effects. Acetaminophen is most commonly used to treat mild to moderate pain. Other nonopioids include aspirin, naproxen, and diclofenac and are NSAIDs that are commonly used in treatment plans.

Table 10-5 Pharmacologic Pain Management

Drug	Dosage	Onset (Min)	Duration (Hours)	Available Routes	Properties	Side Effects and Comments
Morphine	1-4 mg IV bolus 1-10 mg IV infusion	5-10	3-4	PO, SL, R, IV, IM, SC, EA, IA	Analgesia, antianxiety	Standard for comparison Side effects: Sedation, respiratory depression, euphoria/dysphoria, hypotension, nausea, vomiting, pruritus, constipation, urinary retention M6G can accumulate in patients with renal failure or hepatic dysfunction
Fentanyl	25-100 mcg IV bolus 25-200 mcg IV infusion	1-5	0.3-4	OTFC, IV, IM, TD, EA, IA	Analgesia, antianxiety	Same side effects as morphine Rigidity with high doses
Hydromorphone (Dilaudid)	0.2-1 mg IV bolus 0.2-2 mg IV infusion	5	3-4	PO, R, IV, IM, SC, EA, IA	Analgesia, antianxiety	Same side effects as morphine
Meperidine (Demerol)	75-100 mg IM	5-10	2-4	PO, IV, IM, SC, EA, IA	Analgesia	Seems to cause less constipation, urinary retention, pruritus, sedation, and nausea than morphine Neurotoxicity (normeperidine) High doses may cause agitation, muscle jerking, seizures, or hypotension Use with care in patients with renal failure, convulsive disorders, or dysrhythmias
Codeine	15-30 mg IM, SC	10-20	3-4	PO, IM, SC	Analgesia (mild to moderate pain)	Lacks potency (unpredictable absorption; not all patients convert drug to active form to achieve analgesia) Most common side effects: Lightheadedness, dizziness, shortness of breath, sedation, nausea and vomiting
Methadone (Dolophine)	5-10 mg IV	10	4-8	PO, SL, R, IV, SC, IM, EA, IA	Analgesia	Usually less sedating than morphine but can accumulate with repeated doses, resulting in serious sedation (2-5 days)
Acetaminophen	650 mg, maximum 4 g/day	20-30	4-6	PO, R	Analgesia, antipyresis	Side effects rare; hepatotoxicity
Ketorolac (Toradol)	15-30 mg IV	<10	6-8	PO, IM, IV	Analgesia, minimal antiinflammatory effect	Only for short-term use (<5 days) Side effects: Gastric ulceration, bleeding, exacerbation of renal insufficiency Use with care in elderly and patients with renal failure

EA, Epidural analgesia; *IA*, intrathecal analgesia; *IM*, intramuscular; *IV*, intravenous, *M6G*, morphine-6-glucuronide; *OTFC*, oral transmucosal fentanyl citrate; *PO*, oral; *R*, rectal; *SC*, subcutaneous; *SL, sublingual; TD*, transdermal.

Synthetics

Synthetic analgesics are a group of drugs made artificially by chemical synthesis, especially so as to resemble a natural product. These drugs have been designed to achieve a greater potency or have a more desirable side effect profile than those that naturally occur. A majority of these drugs are opiate agonists and are made to mimic the drug morphine. Fentanyl is considered the most potent narcotic in clinical use today. It is 80 times more potent than morphine and dosed in micrograms due to this fact. Demerol and methadone are commonly used synthetics. Figure 10-4 illustrates nociception and analgesic action sites.

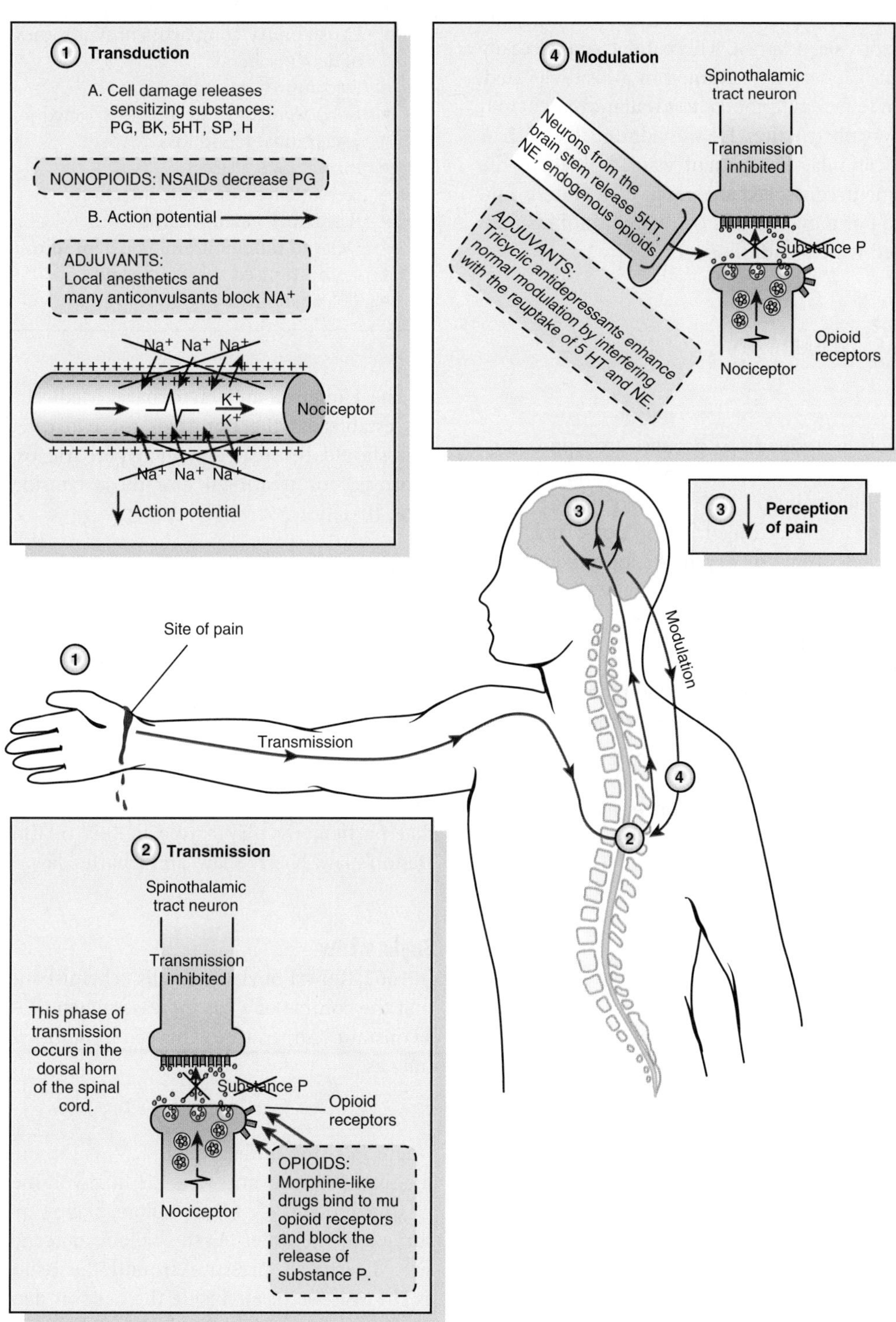

Figure 10-4

Nociception and sites of analgesic action. (From Marx JA, Hockberger R, Walls R: *Rosen's emergency medicine: concepts and clinical practice*, ed 6, St Louis, 2006, Mosby.)

Scenario Conclusion

A 352-pound (160 kg) patient with diabetes complained of severe somatic pain and was treated with a total of 12 mg of morphine over 15 minutes, along with 100 mcg of fentanyl. The cumulative effects of these narcotics were respiratory depression and documented hypoxia.

The physician determined that, besides experiencing the cumulative effect of an opiate and a synthetic narcotic, the patient suffered from sleep apnea. The patient roused easily with verbal stimuli. He was repositioned in a head-elevated, side-lying position to facilitate good chest wall movement and to ease upper airway obstruction. He was administered 2 L of oxygen via nasal cannula. The patient was admitted to the hospital with a patient-controlled analgesia (PCA) pump, and intermittent dosing of narcotics was continued until his pain could be controlled with Vicodin.

HYPERBARIC MEDICINE

Scenario

A local hospital is requesting ground transport for a patient believed to have some type of diving-related problem. The patient is an 18-year-old male who was diving with friends. The friends state that he suddenly ascended from a depth of approximately 45 feet. They add that he is a relatively new diver, and he apparently had had an upper respiratory infection lately.

His symptoms include complaints of chest pain on the left side, vertigo, poor coordination, disorientation, and labored, fast breathing. His vital signs are: pulse, 130 beats/min; respiration, 30 breaths/min; BP, 110/80 mm Hg; pulse oximetry, 88% on 15 L/nonrebreather mask. He has one peripheral IV line infusing normal saline at 125 mL/hour.

Most people associate hyperbaric medicine only with the treatment of diving-related disorders. However, it also is used for many other illnesses encountered by critical care teams. As long ago as the mid-1600s, physicians discovered that placing a patient inside a pressurized chamber improved oxygenation.

Did You Know?

The first hyperbaric chamber was built in 1662, and compression was provided by an organ bellows.[3]

Box 10-1 Indications for Hyperbaric Oxygen Treatment

Fourteen indications for hyperbaric oxygen (HBO) therapy have been recognized:

- Air or gas embolism
- Carbon monoxide poisoning
- Carbon monoxide poisoning complicated by cyanide poisoning
- Clostridial myositis and myonecrosis
- Crush injury, compartment syndromes, and other types of acute ischemia
- Decompression sickness
- Enhancement of healing in selected problem wounds
- Exceptional blood loss
- Intracranial abscess
- Necrotizing soft tissue infections
- Refractory **osteomyelitis**
- Delayed radiation injury, **osteoradionecrosis**
- Compromised skin grafts and flaps
- Thermal burns

The Undersea and Hyperbaric Medical Society (UHMS) has established the standards for two categories of disease that should be treated with hyperbaric oxygenation: those approved for treatment and those considered investigative (Box 10-1).

Hyperbaric Oxygen Therapy

Hyperbaric oxygen (HBO) therapy has two primary effects: (1) it affects all tissues of the body by increasing the partial pressures of oxygen, and (2) it mechanically reduces the size of intravascular and intracompartmental bubbles. HBO simulates the depth of seawater and the pressure exerted there; this is the key factor in HBO as a therapy for critical care patients. As you explore the uses of HBO, keep in mind four gas laws that particularly play a role in this treatment: Boyle's law, Dalton's law, Henry's law, and Charles' law.

Boyle's Law

In 1662, Robert Boyle, an English chemist and physicist, found that the volume of a gas increases when pressure decreases at a constant temperature. This can be summarized mathematically as:

$$P_1V_1 = P_2V_2$$

where P_1 is the initial pressure, V_1 is the initial volume, P_2 is the final pressure, and V_2 is the final volume.

Imagine an air-filled balloon being pulled below the surface of the water. As the balloon descends, it decreases in size. The water pressure around the balloon is increasing as the volume of air inside the balloon decreases. The same is also true in reverse; if the same balloon were taken to a higher altitude, it would increase in size. Boyle's law is the reason people's ears pop and click when they fly (Figure 10-5).

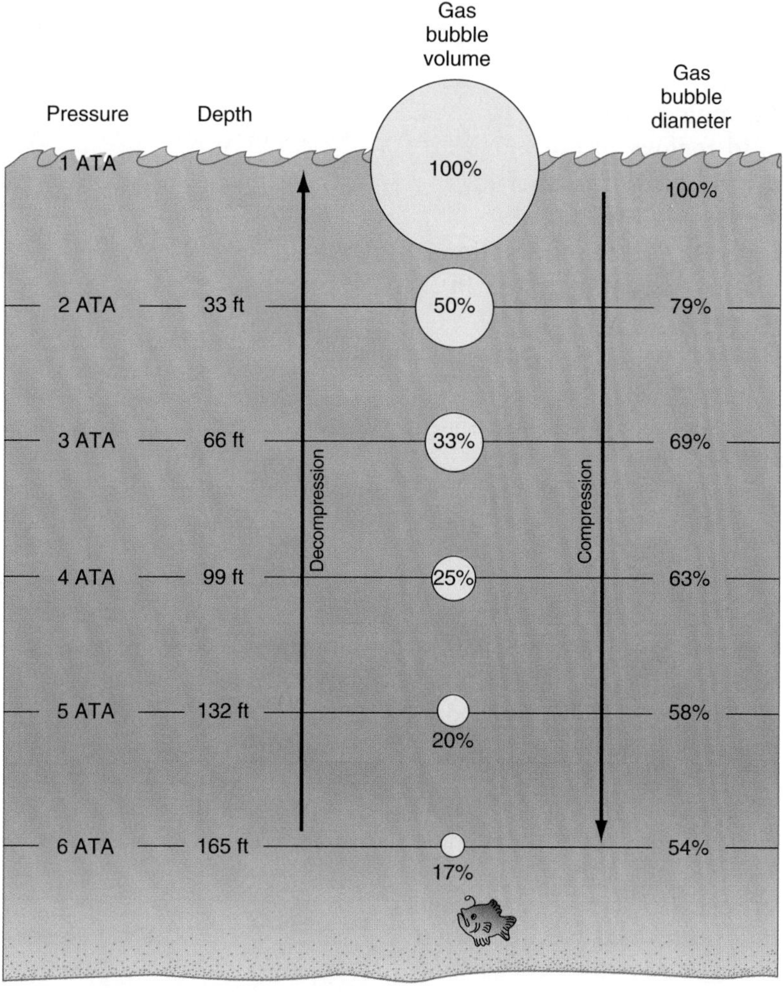

Figure 10-5

Boyle's law: the volume (V) of a given quantity of gas at constant temperature varies inversely with pressure (P): $P_1V_1 = P_2V_2$.

Did You Know?

Once you enter the water, the pressure is determined by the weight of the atmosphere and the water above. Water is about 1000 times denser than air at the sea surface; therefore, a depth of only 33 feet is equivalent to two times normal atmospheric pressure. Every 33 feet thereafter adds another 1 atm of pressure.[4]

Dalton's Law

Also known as Dalton's law of partial pressures, this gas law was described in 1801 by John Dalton, an English chemist and physicist. It states that the total pressure exerted by a gaseous mixture is equal to the sum of the partial pressures of each individual component in the mixture. This can be summarized mathematically as:

$$P_t = P_1 + P_2 + P_3...$$

where P_t is the total pressure and P_1, P_2, P_3, and so on are the partial pressures of the individual components.

For example, air is composed roughly of 21% oxygen and 79% nitrogen. The partial pressure of each gas, which is normal at sea level, can become hazardous as the pressure is increased during HBO therapy. To further explain this, the standard nonrebreather mask used in emergency medical services (EMS) normally delivers up to 15 LPM of 100% oxygen. If that same amount of 100% oxygen that we administer in the back of our ambulance is administered a hyperbaric chamber with 2.4 atmospheres absolute (ATA), or 45 feet of seawater, that oxygen would be equivalent to giving a patient 240% oxygen. This higher concentration of oxygen assists with some great benefits to patients in several treatable indications. (ATA is discussed later in the chapter.)

Did You Know?

The equation for determining how much oxygen a patient should receive at the treatment depth in a hyperbaric chamber is $PaO_2 = FO_2 \times P$, where PaO_2 is the partial pressure of arterial oxygen; FO_2 is the fraction of oxygen; and *P* is the treatment pressure in atmospheres absolute (ATA).[4]

Henry's Law

William Henry, an English physician and chemist, stated that at a constant temperature, the amount of a given gas dissolved in a given type and volume of liquid is directly proportional to the partial pressure of that gas in equilibrium with that liquid. This law is best exemplified by imagining a capped bottle of carbonated soda. The gas has achieved an equilibrium with the soda in this state. When the cap is removed, the pressure of the gas above the soda is reduced, and the gas in the soda (which is seen as bubbles) is released. When a diver ascends too rapidly, nitrogen comes out of solution and lodges in the joints, causing decompression sickness.

Charles' Law

Initially described by Jacques Charles, a French inventor, scientist, and balloonist, this law states that at constant pressure, the volume of a given mass of an ideal gas increases or decreases by the same factor as its temperature (in Kelvin) increases or decreases. An example would be if you were to imagine a balloon filled with helium on a cold winter day. While you are inside, the balloon is normal. As you step outside, the balloon begins to shrivel up. This happens because the temperature of the helium in the balloon deceases and becomes less dense. The helium particles lose energy and become more concentrated, decreasing the volume. However, when you put the balloon in a warm area, it goes back to its original size.

Hyperbarics is successful during hyperoxygenation therapy because (according to Boyle's law) bubbles shrink at treatment depth (e.g., which aids treatment of decompression sickness and carbon dioxide poisoning) and (according to Dalton's law) gas, particularly oxygen, increases under pressure, which promotes new tissue growth and supports healing. This is the combination that makes HBO therapy successful.

"Illnesses with Bubbles"

Diving Injuries

Although problems can arise for a diver using self-contained underwater breathing apparatus (SCUBA) equipment in any phase of the dive, two types of injuries occur during the ascent phase: arterial gas embolism (AGE) and decompression sickness (DCS). It is important to note that these disorders may occur concurrently, complicating the diver's recovery.

Arterial Gas Embolism

Extraalveolar air syndrome occurs when alveoli rupture and air enters other body tissue and cavities. The most serious complication is arterial gas embolism (Box 10-2). As a diver ascends, the gases in the lungs comply with Boyle's law; that is, as the pressure decreases during ascent, the gases in the lungs expand. As long as the diver continues to exhale, this is not a problem. However, if the diver holds the breath or has some sort of mucous plug (such as from a cold or chest congestion), air becomes trapped in the lungs. As this air expands, it can rupture the lung. If the rupture is severe or involves the adjacent blood vessels, free air can enter the pulmonary circulation and be carried to the left side of the heart, where it is pumped into the arterial circulation. This can have catastrophic consequences. The air forms emboli, which can be too large to pass through small blood vessels.

Box 10-2 Symptoms of Arterial Gas Embolism (AGE)

- Weakness
- Paralysis
- Loss of speech
- Convulsions
- Acute myocardial infarction
- Pain
- Swelling
- Death
- Organ problems with a delayed onset
- Cardiac arrhythmia
- Frothy, bloody secretions
- Marbling of the skin

Did You Know?

An AGE can occur in as little as 4 feet of water.[4]

Decompression Sickness

When a diver using SCUBA equipment is at depth and breathing compressed air, the body uses oxygen for metabolism, but the nitrogen is dissolved into the plasma. According to Henry's law, the solubility of a gas depends on the partial pressure of the gas. As a diver ascends, the pressure decreases; therefore, less gas can be dissolved in the plasma. As long as the diver ascends slowly and makes the appropriate decompression stops, the nitrogen is eliminated through normal respiration. However, if the diver panics or has an equipment failure and ascends too rapidly, the dissolved nitrogen comes out of solution in a fashion that resembles a soda being opened after being shaken. This results in intravascular bubbles, which essentially are emboli, that can obstruct the circulation and cause varying symptoms, including death. Six types of DCS have been described (Box 10-3).

DCS and AGE create bubbles that usually are located in the vascular system. Remember, according to Henry's law, blood can carry only a finite amount of gas in solution. Once that point has been reached, excess gas is pushed into the vascular system as bubbles. Once the bubble stage has been reached, larger amounts of gas can be carried. However, the bubbles can become so large that they block blood flow and interrupt

Box 10-3 Classification of Decompression Sickness

Type 1	*Local effects*—joints or limb pain, skin rash or itch, lymphatic obstruction
Type 2	*Cerebral effects*—fatigue, malaise, visual disturbances, headache, impaired coordination, motor and sensory disturbances (e.g., paraplegia, quadriplegia, drowsiness, coma, convulsions, death)
Type 3	*Spinal effects*—weakness and numbness of lower limbs with bladder and sphincter involvement; can involve any degree of motor and sensory symptoms
Type 4	*Pulmonary effects*—may include dyspnea, pain, cough, or altered gas exchange
Type 5	*Stagger*—mild to severe impairment of balance and coordination
Type 6	*Dysbaric osteonecrosis*—bone lesions resulting from long-term participation in diving

the diffusion of oxygen, causing distributive shock, a cerebral vascular accident, or cardiac arrest.

Atmosphere Absolute

Treatment with HBO compression in a specialized chamber can shrink bubbles, allowing better perfusion and alleviating pain. In DCS and AGE, the gas is allowed to be eliminated through respiration. To understand how HBO works in the areas of DCS and AGE, you must understand the concept of atmosphere absolute (ATA).

For example, at sea level a diver is at 1 atmosphere, which is equal to 14.7 psi (760 mm Hg). For every 33 feet of seawater (FSW) the diver descends, another 1 atmosphere is gained (adding another 14.7 psi). Therefore, a diver at 33 FSW is at 2 ATA (29.4 psi), and so on. The term *atmosphere absolute* is used to distinguish between gauge pressure and absolute depth. On hyperbaric chamber gauges at ground level, the reading is 0 psi (which is actually 14.7 psi). As descent proceeds to 33 FSW, the gauge pressure reads 14.7 psig (pounds per square inch gauge). This would actually be 29.4 psi absolute, because sea level is 1 atmosphere and 33 FSW is an additional atmosphere.

At 6 ATA, or 165 FSW (the normal depth of hyperbaric treatment for AGE), a nonspheric bubble can be reduced to 16% of its surface size. This reduction may allow the bubble to continue in circulation until it reaches the lungs, where it can be eliminated.

Other Illnesses That Benefit from Hyperbaric Oxygen Therapy

Thermal Burns

In burn patients, hyperbaric therapy has been shown to limit the amount of lung damage, reduce swelling, and shorten the term of hospitalization. It also can be beneficial for reducing complications (e.g., infection) and the need for surgery and can significantly reduce costs compared to treatment without hyperbaric therapy.

Did You Know?

Treating burns in a hyperbaric chamber has a number of advantages. It reduces fluid requirements, decreases the conversion of partial-thickness to full-thickness injury, preserves marginally viable tissue, improves microcirculation, reduces edema, promotes faster epithelialization, lessens the intensity of the inflammatory response, enhances the activity of polymorphonuclear neutrophils (PMNs), and preserves tissue creatine phosphate and adenosine triphosphate.[4]

Crush Injuries

HBO therapy has proved to be a valuable adjunctive treatment for crush injuries, including compartment syndrome. It not only increases oxygen delivery to compromised tissue, but also reduces swelling, provides an improved environment for healing, and reduces the rate of complications such as infection.

Carbon Monoxide Inhalation

HBO therapy has always been considered standard treatment for carbon monoxide (CO) toxicity, although several recent studies have questioned this standard. Most experts agree that HBO therapy reduces the half-life of carboxyhemoglobin (COHb) in less than 30 minutes at 3 ATA but that it should not be used routinely. The UHMS recommends HBO therapy for CO toxicity in patients with a history of unconsciousness, hemodynamic instability, neurologic signs, or severe acidosis (Box 10-4).

Did You Know?

A patient treated in a hyperbaric chamber for CO poisoning needs two 23-minute periods of breathing oxygen to reduce the carboxyhemoglobin level. After each 23-minute period, the patient should be given a break to breathe chamber air to reduce the onset of oxygen toxicity.[4]

Exceptional Blood Loss Anemia

Cases occur in which a patient loses enough blood to compromise tissue oxygenation, but transfusion is not possible because of religious beliefs or for medical reasons (e.g., incompatibility of available blood products, concern about transmissible disease).

In the average person, each 100 mL of blood carries 20 mL of oxygen. Plasma alone can carry only 0.3 mL of oxygen. The

Box 10-4 Classification and Treatment of Carbon Monoxide Poisoning

Classification

Mild: Carbon monoxide (CO) level below 30% with no signs or symptoms of impaired cardiovascular or neurologic function

Moderate: CO level of 30% to 40% with no signs or symptoms of impaired cardiovascular or neurologic function

Severe: CO level above 40% *or* cardiovascular and/or neurologic impairment at any CO level

Treatment

- Patients with mild to moderate CO poisoning are treated with normobaric oxygen therapy. The patient is given high-flow oxygen by nonrebreather mask (10 to 15 LPM) until the CO level drops below 5%. The level need not be rechecked. Assume that the half-life of CO is about 90 minutes on high-flow oxygen and treat for 4 half-lives (360 minutes, or 6 hours). Very mild symptoms *may* be treated for a shorter time. If a patient is still symptomatic after 6 hours, hyperbaric oxygen (HBO) treatment should be considered.
- The patient should be transferred immediately to a hyperbaric facility, if possible, for any of the following:
    - Neurologic dysfunction, such as a history of syncope (even if the patient currently is awake), current unconsciousness or altered level of consciousness (Glasgow Coma Scale score below 15), or evidence of cognitive impairment
    - Cardiovascular dysfunction, such as anginal chest pain, ischemia (as indicated by ECG changes), or dysrhythmia
    - Metabolic acidosis with a pH below 7.1
    - Pregnant patient whose CO level is above 15%, regardless of symptoms, or if any fetal distress is detected, regardless of the mother's CO level
- All patients with severe CO poisoning should be treated with HBO and admitted to the hospital.

heart, brain, and kidneys require a total of approximately 19 mL of oxygen for every 100 mL of blood. Pressurization enables the plasma to hold enough dissolved oxygen to sustain tissue oxygenation. In fact, one of the original proponents of the concept of pressurized oxygenation showed that he could substitute simulated plasma (without hemoglobin) for the blood in a piglet and maintain respirations with 100% oxygen under pressure, providing enough tissue oxygenation to sustain life.

Did You Know?

Intermittent use of hyperbaric oxygen therapy provides enough oxygen to a severely anemic patient to support the basic metabolic needs of the body's tissues until red blood cells have been restored.[4]

Wound Healing and Treatment of Infections Caused by Anaerobic Bacteria

The main focus of most HBO therapy has become wound healing. The first benefit of hyperbaric oxygen is that it floods all the tissues of the body with oxygen.

Clostridial Myositis and Myonecrosis (Gas Gangrene)

Clostridia bacteria are considered normal flora of the GI tract. However, if clostridia contaminate a wound, they can cause a severe and rapidly advancing infection of the soft tissues, commonly known as gas gangrene. Although more than 150 species of *Clostridia* organisms have been identified, only a few commonly cause gas gangrene.

Gas gangrene has several complicating factors. It is severe and advances quickly as a result of the production of endotoxins. Endotoxins are poisons that basically liquefy healthy tissue and seem to inhibit the normal immune system defenses. Consequently, the bacteria can replicate rapidly, allowing the gas gangrene to migrate quickly and spread within just a few hours, destroying healthy tissue.

Did You Know?

Clostridia are *anaerobic* organisms; that is, they prefer low oxygen concentrations to grow. Exposure of these bacteria to high oxygen levels in a hyperbaric chamber inhibits their replication, migration, and production of exotoxin.

Necrotizing Soft Tissue Infection

Anaerobes can cause several types of severe wound infections, including **necrotizing fasciitis, nonclostridial myonecrosis**, progressive bacterial gangrene, and **crepitant anaerobic cellulitis**. Whether these infections are caused by a single or a mixed strain of bacteria, they are treated much the same way, with antibiotics and surgical excision of infected tissue.

Intracranial Abscess

Certain sinus or bone infections of the skull can result in brain abscesses. The natural protective mechanism of the blood-brain barrier prevents many antibiotics from reaching a brain abscess, and high-risk surgical drainage often is required. Most intracranial abscesses are caused by anaerobic bacteria.

All of the conditions that involve anaerobic bacteria benefit from HBO therapy. Flushing the tissues with oxygen impairs or kills the bacteria, slowing the spread of the infection so that antibiotic or surgical therapy can provide final control.

Side Effects of Hyperbaric Oxygen Therapy

Oxygen Toxicity

The clinical use of oxygen is limited to a maximum partial pressure of 3 ATA (66 FSW). Exceeding this pressure increases the effects of oxygen toxicity but does not increase the

Box 10-5 Symptoms of Central Nervous System Toxicity

- Sweating
- Auditory hallucinations
- Syncope
- Bradycardia
- Nausea
- Depression
- Visual changes
- Pallor
- Anxiety
- Tinnitus
- Facial twitching
- Convulsions

effectiveness of treatment. Above 3 ATA, the oxygen content is so high it causes generalized seizures.

In HBO treatments, oxygen is never used below 3 ATA. Remember that, under pressure, oxygen is no longer a simple oxidizer; it is a drug with a clear therapeutic range. CNS oxygen toxicity can occur in patients breathing oxygen at 2 ATA or higher. This is why HBO treatments for wound healing usually are given 5 days a week, and during daily treatments the patient is given "air" breaks (i.e., allowed to breathe chamber air) to reduce the risk of oxygen toxicity (Box 10-5). Any indication of oxygen toxicity is treated by immediately switching the patient from oxygen to the chamber's ambient air. Reversal of symptoms indicates recovery from oxygen toxicity.

Generally, oxygen toxicity has no long-term effects other than secondary trauma from convulsion. Treatment with HBO for prolonged periods at pressures greater than 0.5 ATA also is associated with other effects, such as bronchial irritation, cough, chest tightness, shortness of breath, progressive myopia, and contraction of visual fields. Some patients report that they have better vision during HBO treatment; however, they are cautioned not to get their eyeglass prescription changed, because after treatment is finished, vision usually reverts to baseline.

Transport Considerations

Keep in mind that any diving accident may involve associated trauma. If possible, rule out a cervical spine injury or transport the patient in spinal immobilization, if needed.

Unless otherwise ordered, a patient with DCS or AGE should be transported on 100% oxygen. Simple administration of 100% oxygen has been shown to eliminate symptoms in 50% of patients. Patients should be transported supine. Although it may seem to be common sense that head-down or Trendelenburg positioning would limit bubbles traveling to the brain, evidence shows that head-down positioning can contribute to cerebral edema.

Depending on the local protocol, IV fluid with normal saline (NS) or lactated Ringer's solution (LRS) should be administered. Analgesic therapy also should be instituted.

Scenario Conclusion

The 18-year-old male seems to have a "bubble illness" with a history of recent upper respiratory infection and a fast ascent during a dive. He is tachypneic, dyspneic, and tachycardic with left chest pain; he also has vertigo and hypoxia, his movements are uncoordinated, and he is disoriented. You prepare the patient for transport to a facility that can provide HBO therapy. He is quickly packaged for ground transport with monitors, supplemental oxygen, IV fluids, and a combination of midazolam and morphine for pain and anxiety. The transport time should be less than 45 minutes.

TISSUE AND ORGAN PROCUREMENT

Scenario

Your team is called to transport a patient with a self-inflicted gunshot wound (GSW) to the head from a very small outside hospital (no operating room) back to your facility. When you arrive, the local physician tells you that, after consultation with the neurosurgical intensive care unit (ICU) physician at your facility, the patient was declared brain dead. The patient has a bulky dressing with pressure around his head. He is intubated with an 8.0 mm endotracheal tube, and correct positioning of the tube has been confirmed. You transfer him to your ventilator and your stretcher. Bleeding from the scalp wound has been controlled.

The GCS score is 3, and the pupils are equal and fixed at 6 mm. There are no other signs of trauma. The pulse is 82 beats/min, pulse oximetry is 100%, BP is 90/60 mm Hg, and capnography shows a good waveform with a $PETCO_2$ of 44 mm Hg. The patient has received 2 L of lactated Ringer's solution and has 1500 mL of clear urine in the Foley bag.

As you make the final arrangements to leave, the patient's mother enters the room crying. She says to you, "Do you think you can save him?" Further consultation with the transferring physician confirms that the patient's prognosis has not been discussed with the family.

Through hard work, the personnel who provide emergency and critical care resuscitation can have a profound effect on the organ and tissue donation process. To understand how your work can affect the process, let's discuss how the actual donation process works and the types of organs and/or tissues that can be transplanted.

Tissue and Organ Donation

In tissue donation, 80 to 100 recipients can be helped by a single donor. Tissues that can be recovered include long bones of the arm and legs, associated soft tendons from the leg (e.g., the anterior cruciate ligament), veins, skin, heart valves, and corneas. These gifts can be lifesaving.

In organ donation, as many as eight people can be helped by one donor. The organs that can be transplanted include the heart, lungs, liver, kidneys, pancreas, and intestine. These organs are recovered and quickly transplanted into the recipient. A crucial consideration is time; time is extremely important in the organ donation process.

Donation Process

The tissue or organ donation process actually begins with the entry of a potential donor into the healthcare system. This is the first and usually most important time the critical care team may be involved in the donation process.

Documentation

During the initial resuscitation, donation usually is not even considered; however, the events documented in the transport record subsequently are very important. All organ procurement organizations (OPOs) and tissue recovery staff members look for that documentation after the donation process has started. OPO personnel look at the documentation for a number of reasons. First, they want to know the injuries involved. This gives them a good picture of everything that has happened to the patient leading up to the donation. Documentation of drugs given, fluids infused, and medical interventions is very important (e.g., insertion of endotracheal tubes and subglottic airways, IV punctures). If high-risk behavior (e.g., IV drug use) might be suspected, it is important to know whether a puncture site was made by medical personnel or by the individual. An unexplained puncture site or scarring in those areas may give insight into the individual's personal choices.

Hemodilution History in the Documentation

Documentation also is important to determine whether hemodilution of the patient's blood has occurred. All tissue recovery agencies are required by the U.S. Food and Drug Administration (FDA) to proceed through an algorithm that is designed to ensure that the patient's blood has not been overly diluted by fluids and blood products given by medical personnel.

Documenting the amount of fluids given is important because blood is collected and used for infectious disease testing (e.g., human immunodeficiency virus [HIV] infection, hepatitis). Large amounts of infused fluids can dilute antibodies to infectious diseases to the point that the required tests are not sensitive enough to detect the disease. This is not to suggest that fluids should be withheld. At that point, the only concern is treating the patient appropriately; in that context, documentation of the fluids and amounts given is important. If hemodilution has occurred, consideration of the person as a potential tissue donor is deferred. If documentation has been less than thorough, extra efforts must be made to contact the EMS agency or ED staff for clarification of the amounts actually infused. This can be difficult and very time-consuming. The overarching goal is to protect the intended recipient.

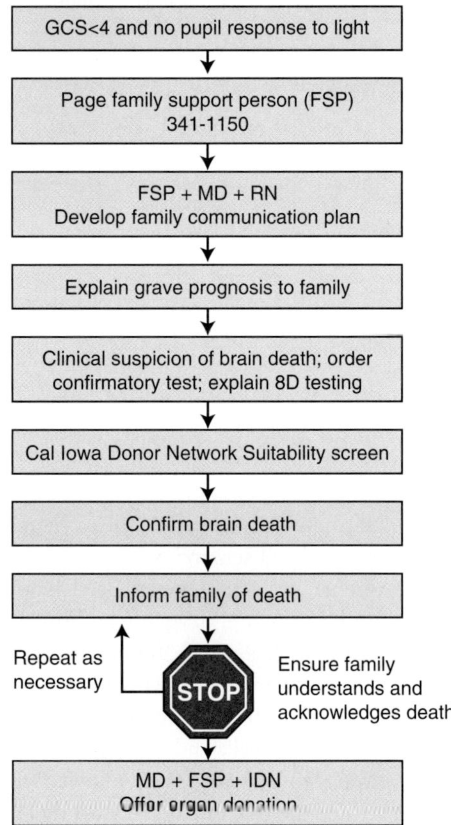

Figure 10-6

Clinical trigger card.

Initiating the Process of Organ Donation

Patients likely to become organ donation candidates usually have either traumatic or anoxic brain injuries. About 90% of organ donation cases in the United States involve patients in whom brain death has occurred. A referral to the OPO starts this evaluation.

The Centers for Medicare and Medicaid Services (CMS) require all hospitals to refer patients to OPOs at the time of death or when death is imminent (in the case of potentially brain-dead patients). Most critical care units have determined effective ways to remind staff members to refer these patients. Many hospitals use a clinical trigger card (Figure 10-6), which provides clinical conditions that guide staff members on when and how to refer patients to the OPO.

OPO Arrival, Assessment, and Consultation

When a patient is referred to the OPO, the organization sends a representative to begin the initial evaluation of the potential donor. Few absolute contraindications to donation exist, although active cancer, HIV infection, and a few other deadly infectious diseases may preclude it. The OPO team's involvement varies from case to case. Often the OPO staff is in the background, working with the hospital's ICU staff. In other cases, the OPO team may be directly involved and have open discussions with the patient's family about the possibility of donation.

Assessing for Brain Death

By this time, the healthcare team most likely is working on diagnosing brain death. Under the Uniform Determination of Death Act of 1982, brain death is defined as the total absence of all neurologic function, including respiratory function. Physicians begin a series of tests to determine this state (Boxes 10-6 and 10-7).

Communicating with the Family

Once brain death has been determined, the family is approached about donation in a collaborative manner by the OPO and members of the healthcare team. This team can be made up of all the key people involved in the care of the patient, including attending physicians, bedside nurses, social workers, chaplains, and OPO staff members. The primary purpose of this discussion is to allow families to state their loved one's wishes or to have the team explain the importance of the decision and how many people can be helped by this process.

Box 10-6 Clinical Determination of Brain Death

The criteria for clinical determination of brain death are:

- Clinical or radiologic evidence indicates a catastrophic cerebral event consistent with brain death.
- Conditions that may confound the clinical assessment of brain death have been ruled out (e.g., metabolic derangements).
- The absence of drugs, intoxication, or poisoning has been confirmed.
- The core body temperature is above 32° C (90° F).

From Urden L, Stacy K, Lough M: *Thelan's critical care nursing: diagnosis and management,* ed 5, St Louis, 2005, Mosby.

Box 10-7 Apnea Testing for Brain Death

If the patient has a core body temperature of 36.5° C (97.7° F) or higher, a systolic blood pressure (BP) of 90 mm Hg or higher, and is euvolemic and eucapnic (partial pressure of arterial carbon dioxide [$Paco_2$] of 40 mm Hg), follow these steps:

1. Disconnect the patient from the ventilator or ventilation system.
2. Deliver 100% oxygen at a rate of 6 L/min via the endotracheal tube.
3. Observe the patient for spontaneous respiratory effort (adequate tidal volume).
4. Measure the partial pressure of arterial oxygen (Pao_2), $Paco_2$, and pH after approximately 8 minutes. Resume ventilations immediately if the patient's condition becomes unstable, as indicated by oxygen desaturation, a drop in the systolic BP below 90 mm Hg, or dysrhythmia.
5. When the apnea test is finished, reconnect the patient to the standard ventilation parameters.

If, during the apneic period, the $Paco_2$ is lower than 60 mm Hg and no respiratory effort is seen, brain death is confirmed. If respiratory effort is seen during the apneic period, regardless of the $Paco_2$ level, brain death is *not* confirmed. If no respiratory effort is seen during the apneic period but the $Paco_2$ is lower than 60 mm Hg with no cardiovascular instability, the test is inconclusive.

From Urden L, Stacy K, Lough M: *Thelan's critical care nursing: diagnosis and management,* ed 5, St Louis, 2005, Mosby.

Obtaining Consent and the Patient History

The method by which personnel obtain consent varies from region to region and may have quite an effect on whether the family signs the consent. Consent rates are still only 55% throughout the nation. The real work of donation starts at the time of consent, when the family and the OPO team work together to create a very detailed medical and social history of the patient. This is a very important step in the process. For tissue donation, many points on this history may rule out a patient as a donor. The past history does not rule out a patient for organ donation, but it does provide valuable information to transplant centers considering accepting organs from a donor.

Medical Management of the Donor Patient

The goal of management in a donor patient is to optimize oxygenation and perfusion. The ultimate goal is transplantation of every organ from every donor; therefore, each organ must be evaluated. Laboratory and radiographic tests are done to evaluate organ function (these tests include the infectious disease testing discussed previously). If organ dysfunction is noted, specific management techniques are implemented to increase their function.

The effects of brain death on the body include profound changes in the ability to regulate vascular size and compliance due to low levels of certain thyroid hormones. Replacement of both triiodothyronine (T_3) and thyroxine (T_4) may significantly reduce the need for vasopressor support for the donor patient.

In addition to just thyroid hormone replacement therapy, many donors require vasopressor support (epinephrine, dopamine) to maintain the mean arterial pressure and end-organ perfusion. When the patient requires a combined vasopressor of greater than 10 mcg/kg/min (either drug or both) the T_4 protocol is administered. This protocol usually consists of 50% dextrose, 1-2 g of methylprednisolone (Solu-Medrol), 10-20 units of regular insulin, and 20 mcg of thyroxone (T_4), followed by a continuous infusion of T_4.

Diabetes insipidus (DI) is very common in potential donors, because this complication frequently occurs with severe brain injury (see Chapter 5). Aqueous vasopressin or desmopressin may be used to control DI.

Maintenance of a normal blood pressure with a limited fluid intake may be initiated. Vasopressin or dopamine (or both) may be used to regulate BP. Central venous pressure (CVP) and hemodynamic monitoring (invasive or noninvasive) may be implemented to monitor the resuscitation carefully.

Optimum oxygenation and ventilation are planned and monitored with the ICU staff. The goal is to maintain the tidal volume at 8 to 10 mL/kg and the peak inspiratory pressure (PIP) below 30 mm Hg. Atelectasis is very common in potential organ donors, so efforts are made to choose the best ventilation techniques that recruit good lung tissue for oxygenation.

Management of the donor patient in the ICU is time-consuming and demanding for all the ICU staff members involved in assisting the OPO. However, the importance of this management period is clear in light of the number of lives that may be saved as a result. This is not a quick process. Many OPOs average 24 to 36 hours in the ICU before actual recovery of the organs.

Organ Allocation

When organ function is optimal, the OPO begins the period of organ allocation. This is the process of offering the organ to a transplant center for a specific recipient. The process can take many hours for each organ offered. Organ information is sent electronically to the transplant centers. The transplant center professional reviews the specific data and either accepts or turns down the offer. If it is turned down, the offer goes to the next center. Up to five offers can be made simultaneously to facilitate the placement of organs. This process is repeated until all transplantable organs have been placed with recipients or a determination has been made that a specific organ is not transplantable.

Most families hope that every organ for which they have given consent can be successfully transplanted. However, this usually is not realistic. Chronic disease processes, traumatic injuries, age, and overall poor function all are reasons an organ may be considered nontransplantable.

Organ Recovery

Once all organs have been allocated, the organ recovery process starts. Transplant surgeons travel to the donor hospital, and the organs are surgically recovered. The recovery surgery allows the surgeons to inspect the organs and make a final decision on whether to accept and transplant the organ in their recipient. Occasionally, the visual findings during surgery preclude an accepted organ from being transplanted.

As the organs are recovered, an intense period of preparation begins at all the accepting transplant centers. In most cases surgeons prepare the recipients for transplantation as the recovery surgery is going on. The preparatory surgery continues as the organ is transported to the hospital, and final excision of the native organ is not performed until the donated organ arrives. Most transplantations are done within 6 to 8 hours after recovery of the organ. Because of the relative durability of the kidneys and some advances in the storage of recovered kidneys, transplantation of these organs can be delayed as long as 48 hours.

As organ and tissue transplantation becomes more widespread, all healthcare personnel involved in the care and transport of a critical care patient will become involved in discussion, referral, and care of the patient within the process.

Scenario Conclusion

Through knowledge and experience, your team recognizes the patient with the GSW to the head as a potential donor. Every effort is made to provide excellent trauma care at the local hospital and while en route, with emphasis on the ABCDs and good end-organ perfusion. Meticulous documentation is completed during transport, including accurate intake and output measurements. The local clinician spends some time speaking with the family about the grave prognosis and the receiving ICU team is prepared to do the same.

FLIGHT PHYSIOLOGY

Scenario

A 36-year-old construction worker falls from a considerable height and is transported to the local trauma center for resuscitation and initial care. Five days later, he requests transport back to his home state for continued care and rehabilitation for the orthopedic injuries. The initial nurse to nurse report states that a pneumothorax on the left side has nearly resolved, but a chest tube remains for pleural drainage. The patient is receiving 1 L/hr of oxygen by cannula; in addition, he has one peripheral IV line that is saline locked; a vertebral brace on the torso; and an external fixator for the femoral and lower leg fractures. His vital signs have been stable. Your colleagues are going to undertake this mission in a fixed wing jet accompanied by a new flight nurse and a critical care paramedic.

When the crew returns from the transport, they report that personnel at the receiving hospital were irate about the patient's condition on arrival. About halfway through the flight, the patient became restless, so the nurse administered 50 mcg of fentanyl and 1 mg of midazolam IV for pain and anxiety. About 30 minutes later, the patient was vomiting and restless, so the nurse administered 4 mg of ondansetron (Zofran) IV. The patient then was restless, pale, disoriented, and difficult to control. The nurse administered another 2 mg of midazolam IV.

The crew quietly admits that they clamped the chest tube before departure, because they did not want to deal with the pleural drainage unit. They also admit that the patient had a tension pneumothorax upon arrival and had to be emergently intubated. He now is in the ICU.

Air medical transport of a critically ill patient requires a thorough working knowledge of flight physiology and the transport stressors that affect not only the patient, but also the medical crew. Whether a rotor wing or fixed wing aircraft is used, the critical care provider must factor in transport physiology variables to provide optimum care for the patient, because failure to do so may further compromise the person's clinical condition.

Atmosphere

The atmosphere is a fairly constant mixture of gases up to a height of 70,000 feet (21,336 meters), at which point the composition changes. The main components of our atmosphere are nitrogen (78.08%) and oxygen (20.95%), and argon, helium, carbon dioxide, hydrogen, neon, and helium make up the remainder of the gases.

The atmosphere weighs more than 5600 trillion tons and is prevented from escaping into space by the Earth's strong gravitational pull. An important concept in this regard is *barometric pressure,* which is the force or weight exerted by the atmosphere at a given point.

Gas Laws

To understand flight physiology, you must understand the gas laws that describe relationships between the temperature, pressure, volume, and mass of the various gases (see the earlier section on hyperbaric medicine). Although they often are thought to be difficult to understand, the gas laws form the foundation of the air medical provider's knowledge of how the environment may affect the physiology of the patient and the provider.

Physiologic Stresses of Air Medical Transport

Several unique physiologic and environmental factors influence the crew and patient aboard a medical transport aircraft. Each crew member is responsible for learning the signs of and recognizing the potential for these stressors and their effects on the patient and co-workers (Table 10-6). These factors include hypoxia; changes in the barometric pressure, temperature, and humidity, noise, vibration, gravitational forces, fatigue, spatial disorientation, and flicker vertigo.

Hypoxia

Hypoxia is a state in which a reduced amount of oxygen is available to the tissues to carry out their cellular processes. The causes of hypoxia are generally broken down into four categories, each of which can contribute to a lack of oxygen available for physiologic function.

Causes of Hypoxia

Hypoxic Hypoxia

Hypoxic hypoxia occurs when oxygen exchange at the alveolar level is insufficient, which in turn means that less oxygen is available in the blood for the tissues to use. This phenomenon can be caused by a number of factors, such as a drop in the barometric pressure, which reduces the alveolar partial pressure of oxygen. For example, a blood oxygen saturation of 98% at sea level drops to 87% at 10,000 feet and 60% at 22,000 feet. Other causes of hypoxic hypoxia are ventilation-perfusion defect caused by a pulmonary embolism and disease states such as asthma, chronic obstructive pulmonary disease (COPD), airway obstruction, pneumothorax, and fulminant pulmonary edema.

Anemic Hypoxia

Anemic hypoxia is a state of reduced oxygen-carrying capacity of the blood, which can be seen with severe anemia (e.g., massive hemorrhage or hypovolemic shock). It also can be the result of hemoglobin abnormalities, drugs (e.g., agents that contain sulfa), and gas poisoning, such as with carbon monoxide, which reduces the oxygen-carrying capacity of hemoglobin by displacing the oxygen molecules.

Stagnant Hypoxia

Stagnant hypoxia can occur in low flow states, such as are seen with depressed cardiac output (possibly as a result of cardiac illness or sepsis), pooling of blood in certain areas of the body, massive pulmonary embolism, and rapid acceleration (G forces).

Histotoxic Hypoxia

Histotoxic hypoxia is hypoxia caused by an inability of the body to use the oxygen available to it. It most often is seen in cyanide and CO poisoning. Often a derangement at the cellular level leads to this condition, which can be missed by medical care providers because it frequently is innocuous.

Effects of Hypoxia

The effects of hypoxia on the human body differ based on the altitude of travel. For discussion's sake, they can be broken into four distinct stages.

- The *indifferent stage* is seen from sea level to approximately 10,000 feet, where oxygen saturations may range from 90% to 98% and the provider and patient may be unaware of and unimpaired by the effects of the hypoxia. As the aircraft ascends beyond 5000 feet, changes in vision may occur, and the heart rate and respiratory rate may rise.
- The *compensatory stage* occurs at 10,000 to 15,000 feet and is characterized by a noticeable increase in the heart rate and respiratory rate and by increased cardiac output. Night vision is reduced, and headaches, nausea,

Table 10-6 Effects of Altitude on the Body's Ability to Function

Physiologic Zone	Physiologic	Physiologic deficient	Space equivalent	Space
Altitude	Sea level to 10,000 feet	10,000 to 50,000 feet	50,000 to 250,000 feet	Beyond 250,000 feet
Physiologic Functioning	Normal function	Severely impaired without proper environmental support	Severely impaired without pressurized environment	Weightlessness

dizziness, and air hunger may occur. At this stage, mental tasks, such as drip calculations and critical thinking, may start to become impaired as a result of the hypoxia.

- At 15,000 to 20,000 feet, providers and the patient experience the *disturbance stage,* which is characterized by the body's inability to compensate for hypoxia. This is manifested by cyanosis, air hunger, agitation or somnolence, nausea, vomiting, decreased visual acuity, weakness, decreased critical thinking skills, decreased coordination, and alteration in personality. It should be noted that aircraft that fly at this altitude are pressurized unless mechanical failure occurs.
- The *critical stage* occurs at 20,000 to 25,000 feet; this is a critical stage, because the previous symptoms can escalate to seizures, coma, and death.

Treatment of Hypoxia

Fortunately, the treatment of hypoxia in the air medical environment is straightforward. The first step is proper evaluation and monitoring of the patient to assess for the cause of hypoxia (e.g., pneumothorax, severe anemia, depressed cardiac output, CO poisoning). Next, supplemental oxygen is provided, which can be done by noninvasive methods such as a nasal cannula or face mask, rather than by invasive endotracheal intubation, depending on the patient's condition. Other methods that may help correct hypoxia include reducing the altitude of the aircraft below 10,000 feet, if possible, and/or adjusting the cabin pressurization to meet the oxygen needs of the patient and providers.

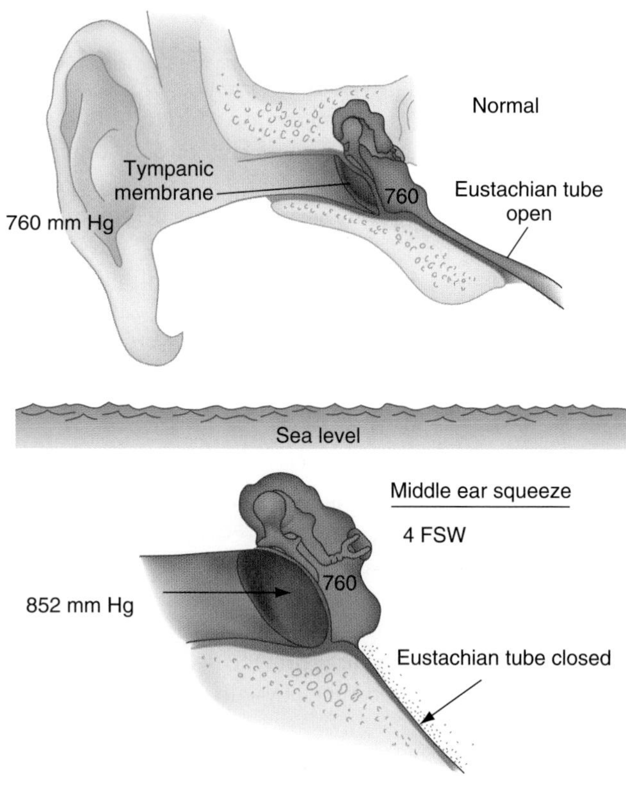

Figure 10-7

Anatomy of the ear and effect of middle ear trauma. *FSW,* Feet of seawater. (From Marx JA, Hockberger R, Walls R: *Rosen's emergency medicine: concepts and clinical practice,* ed 6, St Louis, 2006, Mosby.)

Barometric Pressure Changes

As discussed earlier, gases tend to expand as barometric pressure decreases, which can lead to some physiologic challenges in the air medical environment.

Barotitis Media

Barotitis media is a well-described condition that arises from the middle ear's inability to ventilate when moving from a low to a high atmospheric pressure (descent). It is characterized by severe pain, ringing in the ear, dizziness, and nausea. Normally, during ascent the eustachian tube ventilates expanding gas from the middle ear cavity into the throat by means of a passive process mediated by pressure differences between the middle ear and the throat. However, during descent, the eustachian tube remains closed until an active process such as yawning, the Valsalva maneuver, or swallowing equalizes pressures. If the eustachian tube is not opened during descent, a significant pressure gradient builds between the middle ear and the throat, causing the tympanic membrane to be depressed inward; this in turn causes inflammation and creates the potential for rupture. Any condition that interferes with proper eustachian tube function, such as an upper respiratory infection or a middle ear infection, puts an individual at risk for barotitis media.

Besides the maneuvers already described, a nasal vasoconstrictor can be used approximately 15 minutes before descent; a slow descent can be made (or an ascent if the symptoms are too painful); and crew members with severe middle ear problems can be put on limited duty (Figure 10-7).

Barosinusitis

Barosinusitis is severe pain that occurs during ascent caused by expanding gases in the sinus cavity. These gases normally are ventilated without difficulty. However, a sinus infection or sinus inflammation can interfere with this ventilatory process, and the trapped gases expand, leading to severe sinus pain, pressure, and possible epistaxis. The treatment for barosinusitis is use of nasal vasoconstrictors or a gradual descent.

Barodentalgia

Barodentalgia is dental pain caused by expanding gases, mainly within the tooth pulp, and is worst during ascent. Steps for reducing the possibility of barodentalgia include avoiding flying soon after dental treatment and keeping the teeth in good repair. For acute cases, a gradual descent is helpful.

Temperature Changes

Hyperthermia and hypothermia have significant effects on the human body. The ambient temperature drops with increasing altitude; a drop of 3.5° F (-15.8 C) occurs for every 1000 feet ascended. This becomes especially important in fixed wing transport, in which the crew and patient may be exposed to high altitudes and cold temperatures for an extended period. With rotor wing transports, both hyperthermia and hypothermia may be factors, depending on the weather in the area.

Extremes in temperature increase the body's metabolic demands, resulting in an increase in oxygen consumption and possibly headache, motion sickness, disorientation, and inability to cope with the current critical illness. Confounding factors such as alcohol, dehydration, vibration, and medical use of sedatives and paralytics all affect the body's ability to regulate temperature. Techniques to prevent temperature extremes include adjusting the cabin temperature, adding or removing clothing, and ensuring proper hydration.

Humidity Changes

As altitude increases, the amount of moisture in the air decreases. As fixed wing and rotor wing aircraft fly at high altitudes and draw in fresh air from the outside, they are subjected to low humidity levels. In addition, medical oxygen (unless humidified) is known to be quite dry and predisposes the patient to dry nasal passages, chapped lips, a sore throat, and dry mucous membranes. Both the medical crew and patient are at risk for dehydration in this low humidity environment, and great care must be taken to maintain hydration by using oral or IV fluids and, for extended transports, humidified oxygen.

Noise

Noise is common in the air medical environment, and it may contribute to a stressful setting for the provider and patient. For the provider, loud noise can hamper clear communication with the patient or other medical providers and also verbal and auscultative assessment of the patient. In such situations, the provider must rely on visual cues, monitoring equipment, and sound clinical judgment in caring for the patient. The patient may be unable to communicate clearly with the air medical provider and may feel helpless and frightened. Physiologic changes that can occur in all those exposed to prolonged, loud noise include nausea, fatigue, loss of appetite, headache, temporary or permanent hearing damage, and vertigo. It is very important that the air medical providers and patient wear hearing protection in the form of ear plugs, headsets, or helmets.

Vibration

Transport in either a rotor wing or fixed wing aircraft exposes the provider and patient to vibration. In a rotor wing aircraft, the vibration is caused mainly by the power plant and by the air turbulence encountered during flight. It is most severe when the helicopter transitions to the hover position. In a fixed wing aircraft, vibration is caused to a lesser degree by the power plant and more by flight in turbulent weather or by high-speed, low-level flight. When exposed to moderate vibration, the body reacts as it does when performing mild exercise by increasing the heart rate and metabolic rate. Continued exposure to low level vibration may cause fatigue, motion sickness, blurred vision, and abdominal pain.

Vibration also interferes with the body's ability to regulate its temperature (vibration causes vasoconstriction), which can be problematic in patients with hyperthermia. Medical equipment such as BP monitors can be affected by the vibratory motion of the aircraft. Unfortunately, little can be done to prevent the vibration of vehicles used in air medical transport. Suggestions for dampening the effects include avoiding prolonged contact with the airframe and using padding to lessen the consequences of vibration.

Gravitational Forces

The force a person exerts when seated is in direct response to the gravitational force (G) imposed on the body. This force is equal to weight and is known as 1 G. Whether "G forces" affect the patient and provider during rotor wing and fixed wing transport is the subject of debate. G forces are not a significant factor during air medical transport, but it is important to understand that they are applied to the body on ascent and descent and during changes in speed or direction. The main effects of G forces on the body are the pooling of blood or areas of increased blood flow, depending on the part of the body to which the G forces are applied. They can become a factor in patients with severe heart disease or a significant head injury.

Fatigue

Fatigue is both a stressor of flight in itself and the culmination of all the stressors of flight. Techniques for reducing fatigue include avoiding the use of stimulants or illicit drugs, getting rest at regular intervals, avoiding alcohol consumption, avoiding tobacco use, and eating at regular intervals. Recognizing and addressing fatigue allow the air medical provider to function at the highest level in a very stressful environment.

Did You Know?

The mnemonic DEATH can be used to summarize the factors that affect tolerance to the stressors of flight:

D Drugs. **Many over-the-counter medications (e.g., antihistamines) and stimulants (e.g., caffeine), as well as misuse of prescribed medications, can cause tremors, sleep deprivation, and gastrointestinal (GI) symptoms.**

E Exhaustion. **Fatigue or sleep deprivation (or both) can cause errors in judgment, poor eye-hand coordination, poor attention span, and a detrimental change in the circadian rhythm.**

Continued

Did You Know?—cont'd

A Alcohol. **Histoxic hypoxia may occur with overuse of alcohol, and hangovers are enhanced.**

T Tobacco. **Nicotine and tar, the known carcinogens in cigarettes, have serious consequences for the body. With a two-pack-a-day habit, 8% to 10% of the body's hemoglobin is saturated with carbon monoxide, which displaces oxygen from the compound.**

H Hypoglycemia. **A poor dietary intake can result in GI disturbances, poor attention span, errors in judgment, headache, and vertigo.**

Spatial Disorientation

Spatial disorientation can occur when a person has inaccurate perceptions of his or her own position, altitude, and motion in relation to the center of the Earth. The body relies on the visual system, vestibular system, and **proprioceptive system** to maintain equilibrium, but derangements in the processing of this information lead to spatial disorientation. The pilot or providers may have trouble distinguishing the horizon from the ground, problems judging distance from oncoming terrain, and significant difficulty in the perception of other aircraft and buildings during night flying. Prevention is the key; the pilot and providers should scan the horizon, avoid staring at lights, and get adequate rest and nutrition. All medical personnel trained to fly must be educated in the assessment of the pilot during night flight or special meteorologic conditions.

Did You Know?

***Spatial disorientation* is a condition in which a pilot's perception of direction does not reflect reality. It can be brought on by disturbances in or disease of the vestibular system, but more often it is a temporary condition resulting from flight into poor weather conditions with low or no visibility.[5]**

Flicker Vertigo

Air medical providers or patients staring at rapidly flashing lights (at flash rates of 8 to 60 per minute) may experience nausea, vomiting and even seizures (photoconvulsive response) and unconsciousness. This often is caused by staring at light streaming through rotor blades or an airplane propeller. As with spatial disorientation, prevention is the key. Providers should avoid staring at the flickering light, wear sunglasses, get appropriate rest, and ensure good hydration. If problems with this malady continue, flight personnel may discuss the use of antiemetics or benzodiazepines with the medical director.

Cabin Pressurization

Pressurization of the cabin allows the occupants to be comfortable and protects them against hypoxia and changes in the barometric pressure. A constant pressure is maintained by introducing compressed air into the cabin while allowing leakage of air at a fixed rate with controlled outflow. This environment is called *cabin altitude,* and most pressurized airplanes can create a cabin altitude of 8000 feet while flying above 35,000 feet (10,668 meters). Obviously, helicopters are not pressurized; therefore, their cabin altitude is the same as the actual altitude.

Cabin Depressurization and Decompression Sickness

Cabin depressurization can occur as a result of mechanical failure in the compression apparatus or structural damage to the aircraft. With structural damage, a loud explosion often is followed by a drop in the cabin pressure, an acute drop in temperature, fogging, and sucking out of debris, equipment, and even people through the structural defect. Hypoxia is a major problem with cabin decompression, and it can be addressed with supplemental oxygen for the air medical crew and patient.

DCS may occur with loss of cabin pressure, although it rarely develops below 25,000 feet (7,620 meters). As explained previously, this physiologic phenomenon involves the bubbling out of nitrogen dissolved in tissue fluids under reduced atmospheric pressure. Four main areas are involved: the joints, lungs, skin, and brain.

The "bends" refers to nitrogen bubbles in the joints, a condition that can cause severe pain and disability. The lungs can be affected with the "chokes," which is the formation of nitrogen bubbles in the vessels of the lungs, leading to severe chest pain, shortness of breath, feelings of suffocation, and cough. The skin can be involved as nitrogen bubbles accumulate and cause **paresthesia,** which manifests as tingling and numbness. Nitrogen bubbles that form in blood vessels leading to the brain may cause diminished blood flow, resulting in headache, visual disturbances, confusion, seizures, and even loss of consciousness.

Risk factors for DCS include advanced age, obesity, fatigue, alcohol use, and SCUBA diving 24 to 48 hours before flying (especially if the person dives below 30 feet (9.14 meters) or requires a staged ascent). Acute treatment for DCS involves breathing 100% oxygen and rapid descent; hyperbaric oxygen may be needed if symptoms continue despite initial treatment measures.

Scenario Conclusion

Your program's flight crew was scheduled for a medical debriefing after this event. The medical director and the program manager gathered all the information about the event and had the crew analyze it. Then, a summary that included follow-up and corrective action was mapped out. The physiology and pathophysiology of the thorax were reviewed, along with the gas laws, altitude physiology, and the recognition and treatment of hypoxia.

FLIGHT AND GROUND SAFETY

Scenario

Your crew is being launched by rotor wing aircraft to a trauma scene in a rural setting approximately 15 minutes away. A new crew member is being oriented for a part-time job today. The pilot, flight nurse, and flight paramedic enter the aircraft at various times during the launch procedure, and the new guy piles in last. The pilot hears the doors close and begins his engine start. As the engine begins its startup, the pilot turns around and asks why there are so many on board. A heated discussion begins, and the pilot is totally distracted. A "hot start" occurs, and the engine is shut down. The pilot notes that the engine's internal temperature has exceeded the manufacturer's recommendations. The aircraft is considered disabled until a new engine can be installed. The mission is aborted, and your program is out of service for a week.

Providing critical care in the air medical environment without regard to safety is dangerous and contrary to the very principles of the air medical industry. Providers spend a great deal of time learning about disease processes, the dosages and actions of drugs, and procedural skills; yet frequently they do not think of safety training and education as part of their profession. Sound medical judgment and attention to safety are two crucial attributes of any air medical provider.

Did You Know?

Helicopter operations pose special safety challenges, especially at relatively low altitudes near busy airports and cities where air traffic is dense. Some operations are conducted at such low altitudes that collisions with trees, towers, tall buildings, and power lines are not uncommon. Emergency medical service (EMS) flights have the added pressure of off-airport landing operations, often at night and/or in poor weather.[6]

Importance of Flight Safety

Safety around rotor wing and fixed wing aircraft is important for many reasons. These are complicated machines with many moving parts that can severely injure or kill a person who is not vigilant around them. Often, providers are delivering patient care under stressful circumstances, and they may unknowingly engage in unsafe practices that may jeopardize their own and the patient's safety. Between 1972 and 2006, 230 helicopter EMS incidents occurred, 86 of them resulting in at least one fatality. Those accidents involved 667 individuals, and 226 of them were killed; they included pilots, paramedics, nurses, physicians, respiratory therapists, police officers, firefighters, observers, family members, and patients. In addition, there were 72 serious injuries and 91 minor injuries (278 people were uninjured). A casual attitude toward safety in the air medical environment is a serious error in judgment.

Air Medical Resource Management

The term air medical resource management (AMRM) (formerly cockpit resource management and then crew resource management) recognizes the close working relationship among pilots, mechanics, communications specialists, and medical providers in the transport environment. The origins of crew resource management training in the United States are attributed to a workshop titled "Resource Management on the Flight Deck," sponsored by the National Aeronautic and Space Administration (NASA) in 1979. The workshop was the result of NASA's research into the causes of air transport accidents.

"The research presented at this meeting identified the human error aspects of the majority of air crashes as failures of interpersonal communications, decision making, and leadership. At this meeting, the label cockpit resource management was applied to the process of training crews to reduce 'pilot error' by making better use of the human resources on the flight deck."

The key aspects of AMRM are communication, countering strategies (against failed communication), situational awareness, decision making, leadership, and use of resources.

A simple example of AMRM is the decision to accept a transport request. This decision should be based on a favorable weather forecast, the comfort of the crew, and the airworthiness of the aircraft; also, all crew members must be in agreement on accepting the request. This is communicated clearly and freely among the crew, and any single crew member who is uncomfortable with the idea can deny the request with no backlash or retaliation from the others.

The hope is that applying the principles of AMRM to the air medical setting will reduce the incidence and impact of human error and the rate of accidents in the transport industry.

Did You Know?

Of the 934 helicopter accidents that occurred between 1996 and 2000, 50 were caused by wire strikes. Of those 50, the helicopter was damaged substantially in 33 cases and was destroyed in the remaining 17.[6]

Personal Safety

It is difficult to provide critical care for a patient if the providers are injured or become ill during the transport. Personal safety must be a top priority. It starts with proper nutrition, rest, and physical wellness. The air medical environment can be physically taxing, and people unprepared for such rigors are at risk of making mistakes that could endanger their safety. It is important to take care of yourself so that you can take care of others.

Always use personal protective equipment (PPE), including gloves, masks (if needed), and eye protection. Also, keep up-to-date on immunizations, including hepatitis B, and have regular tuberculosis (TB) tests.

Medical and trauma cases in the critical care environment often can expose the provider to significant biohazards; therefore, vigilance is essential. Head and face protection, in the form of a helmet, is becoming the industry standard, a welcome development considering the potential for head and facial injuries in a rotor wing or fixed wing aircraft. These aircraft have multiple strike surfaces, including knobs, hooks, and medical equipment, which can cause injury if the provider is not properly protected. Bird strikes, in which debris may enter the cabin, are another risk. In addition, helmets provide much-needed hearing protection.

Fire- and heat-resistant material (e.g., Nomex, which allows for about 20 to 30 seconds of high-temperature resistance) may allow the provider to escape a fire and may reduce the chances of severe burns and tissue damage. The provider should make an effort to wear this type of flame-resistant material, as well as fabrics such as cotton, silk, or a wool/cotton blend, to limit the tissue damage done by burning synthetic fibers. Appropriate footwear includes leather boots that are cut to at least above the ankle and have safety toes. These provide protection against hazards on the ground, blood, and sharp objects, which often are found at accident scenes.

Paying close attention to oneself allows for a safer and more productive critical care experience for the air medical provider.

Aircraft Safety

As stated earlier, rotor wing and fixed wing aircraft pose significant safety hazards that must be fully appreciated. A full preflight walk-around and safety checklist should be completed before each departure. The main dangers are the main and tail rotor blades in a helicopter and the propellers of an airplane. Care must be exercised around these blades, especially if they are running, because a single careless move can lead to significant head or bodily injury and probable death (Figure 10-8).

The helicopter should be parked on an even surface that prevents the blades from tilting to one side, possibly striking a provider or the terrain when turning. Always approach the helicopter from the front or the sides (in view of the pilot); *never* approach it from the rear. Running into exposed tail rotor blades have claimed the lives of many people, and great care must be taken to avoid this dangerous piece of equipment. The helicopter should be shut down when patients are loaded or unloaded; if that is not feasible, a safety officer should be appointed to monitor people near the running rotor blades.

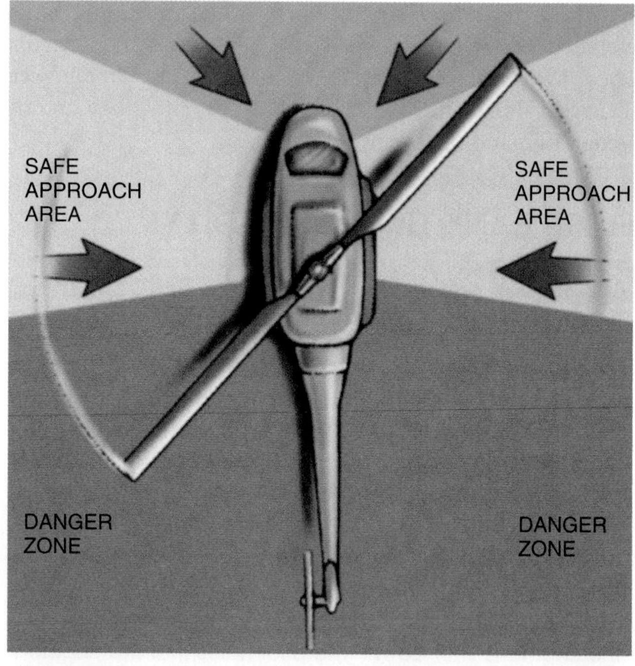

Figure 10-8

Safe approach zones. (From Sanders M: *Mosby's paramedic textbook*, ed 3, St Louis, 2007, Mosby.)

The landing zone for a helicopter (other than an official helipad) should be chosen carefully for safety purposes. Ideally, the area is 75 × 75 feet (22.9 × 22.9 meters) for a daytime landing and 100 × 100 feet (30.5 × 30.5 meters) for a night landing. It should be a flat surface free of loose gravel, shrubs, dirt, large amounts of snow, and any other material that could be propelled by the *rotor wash,* the wind created by the turning helicopter blades. This wind can reach 50 mph in a running helicopter and 25 mph in one that is spooling down. A significant threat to the helicopter is materials on the ground being sucked into the engine because of the rotor wash, resulting in engine failure and other damage.

Helipad Safety

The helipad should be a secure environment free of hazards such as trees, loose gravel, and other obstacles that may impede helicopter function. In addition, it should be secured with either fencing or a large sign designating it as a helipad to deter unauthorized interactions with the helicopter by the public. It should be well lit and should have the appropriate fire safety equipment, including fire hoses and emergency fuel shut-off and alarm boxes. Maintenance of the helipad should be a priority of the air medical program.

In-Flight Safety

Safety on board starts before commencement of the flight, with proper securement of the patient and crew. Equipment also should be secured to prevent it from coming loose during transport and injuring the cabin occupants. During take-off, the medical crew and pilot should scan the surrounding area and the skies to locate potential hazards, such as other aircraft, trees, light poles, buildings, and birds. "Sterile cockpit" conditions must be observed during taxi, take-off, and landing. "Sterile cockpit" means that the medical crew must remain silent unless warning the pilot of hazards. Any conversation at this time must be related to the flight and any urgent or emergent information that must be conveyed. All other conversation must wait until another time. During the flight, medical crew members must balance caring for the patient with scanning the surrounding area for hazards. This occurs to a lesser degree in a fixed wing operation, but vigilance is never wasted when it comes to safety.

In-Flight Emergencies

Even when the best safety procedures are followed, an in-flight emergency may occur, and the medical crew must be prepared to assist. In case of fire, heat and smoke can prove significant obstacles in an enclosed environment; therefore, accessibility and use of a fire extinguisher is essential. All electrical equipment should be unplugged, and the inverter and oxygen should be turned off. Windows or doors may need to be opened to allow the smoke and heat to ventilate.

In case of a forced landing, the medical crew should secure the patient and bring the person out of the helicopter (being careful of turning rotor blades, debris, and foliage) from the nose and proceed to a site away from the aircraft. If the pilot is incapacitated, crew members may need to turn off the fuel and master switch upon landing. Therefore, it is important that medical crew members know about these buttons. In a water landing, the crew should be careful in exiting the helicopter and should attempt to orient themselves in the water and swim to the surface. Services that routinely fly over bodies of water have flotation devices on board, and these should be put on if a water landing seems imminent.

One crash position is to place the arms across the chest and grasp the shoulder harness, place the knees together with the feet slightly apart, and keep the chin slightly tucked. This should provide some protection if the aircraft is forced to make an emergency landing. Follow your service's policies on the recommended crash position, which may be adapted for your height and the type and model of the aircraft.

Post Accident Incident Plan

Every air ambulance should maintain a post accident incident plan (PAIP), which is a framework and action guide for air medical providers, pilots, communications specialists, mechanics, and management to follow in the event of an in-flight emergency or other incident. It includes plans of action, phone numbers for people to be contacted, procedures for dealing with the media, and so on.

In any incident involving an air ambulance, fear, panic, and uncertainty can arise, and the PAIP serves as a roadmap for caring for the medical crew, the patient, and the aircraft during such a situation. Ideally, the PAIP should be clearly written and should specify well-defined roles for the various team members. It should emphasize the importance of following the PAIP implicitly during an actual incident and resisting the common temptation to mount a freelance response. The PAIP should be kept in a prominent location where several people have access to it. The plan should be practiced at least once a year, because executing a PAIP during an actual situation, without having run a practice scenario, is difficult.

The goal is to ensure that no program will have to use its PAIP; however, failure to have one is unacceptable in the air medical environment.

Emergency Survival

It is important for the air medical provider to have basic survival skills in case of an emergency landing with minimal chance of immediate discovery. At the very least, the provider should have access to a survival kit, either in the aircraft or on his or her person, that contains essentials, such as waterproof matches, a flashlight, compass, and a whistle. Priority should be given to finding shelter in extreme environments and locating safe drinking water; these are much more important than food in a survival situation. The air medical provider also should have some skill in building a basic shelter; starting a fire; and basic signaling by smoke, mirror, or flares. Some nourishment will be needed, which will depend on what is available. Transport services should provide formal education and training in survival techniques for their employees.

Ground Safety

Safety is an important factor in ensuring that the patient and crew get to the intended location successfully. Preparation of the patient before transport to your ambulance is important. Usually critical care patients are hooked up to numerous pieces of equipment, including multiple IV drips and pumps, a cardiac monitor with telemetry, a ventilator, hemodynamic monitoring, and other drainage tubes. The critical care practitioner should make sure the team brings to the patient's bedside all equipment and drugs necessary to stabilize the patient's condition during the transition from the hospital to the ambulance.

Once the patient has been secured to your stretcher and all equipment is operating properly, you can transition the patient to your ambulance (Figure 10-9). The trip to the ambulance should be made carefully; many companies have specific policies and procedures regarding safe practice in transporting patients (e.g., no walking backward). Monitor the patient continually, and once inside the ambulance, set up and secure all equipment. Make sure the patient is as comfortable as possible but well secured. All resource personnel who are not part of your crew must have a safety briefing before departing. You are now ready for transport. Critical care ground transport opens up a number of safety concerns for the patient, crew, and bystanders.

Equipment

All equipment must be secured and locked down before the patient is transported. If the ambulance comes to an abrupt stop, any unsecured equipment could move and become

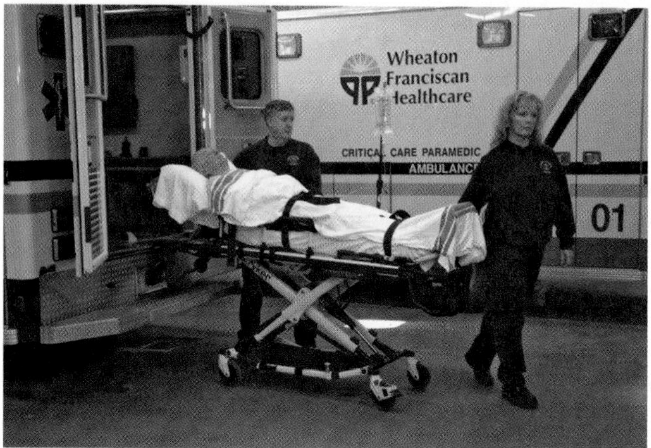

Figure 10-9

Ground critical care transport. (Courtesy Wheaton Franciscan Healthcare, Waterloo, Iowa.)

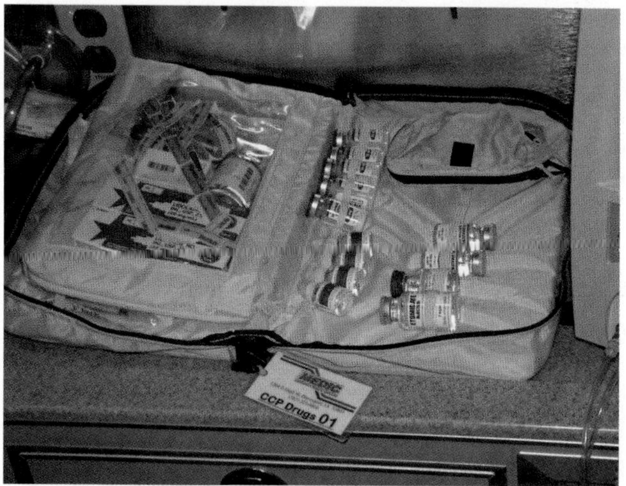

Figure 10-10

Drug kit for ground critical care transport. (Courtesy MEDIC EMS, Davenport, Iowa.)

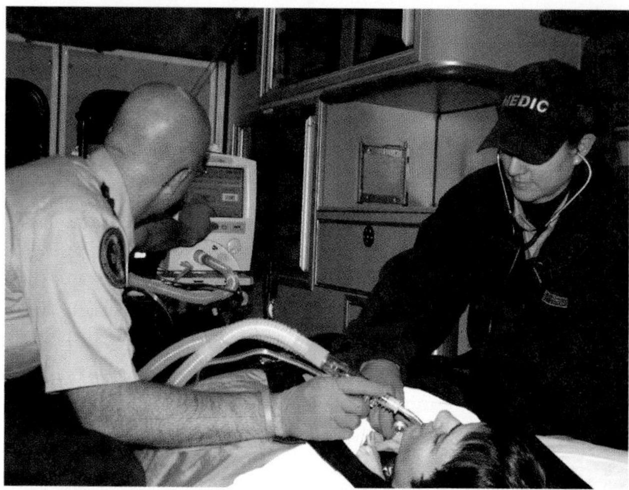

Figure 10-11

Equipment and safety for ground critical care transport. (Courtesy MEDIC EMS, Davenport, Iowa.)

detached from the patient. In the event of a motor vehicle crash involving the ambulance, any unsecured equipment becomes a projectile that can seriously injure all in the ambulance. When an organization decides to begin critical care transports, ambulances must be set up to handle all the additional equipment needed (Figure 10-10). Those setting up transports should determine the type of equipment that may be transported. Crew members then should rehearse where the extra equipment will be placed in the ambulance and how it will be secured. All team members should practice moving and securing equipment for safe transport. This is especially important with large balloon pump consoles (Figure 10-11).

Passengers

It is imperative that all passengers wear the appropriate restraint devices for their positions in the ambulance. Patients on the stretcher should be restrained by a minimum of three straps across the chest, pelvis, and leg area. Shoulder restraints also are recommended. The safety of crew members moving around the patient compartment when providing care also is important. All personnel in the patient compartment should be secured with belts while stationary. All individuals in the cab of the ambulance should be restrained at all times.

Scenario Conclusion

While the flight program is shut down for engine repairs, the entire crew gathers for special education related to flight safety and crew resource management. A safety consultant presents a standard AMRM program, and the crew then assembles privately for a debriefing. Preflight meetings were emphasized, along with sterile cockpit policies.

SUMMARY

A thorough assessment while obtaining the toxicology history aids identification of a toxidrome and the correct treatment plan. A general knowledge of chemical agents, access to resources, and continuation of decontamination procedures instituted by the first and second response during a HAZMAT incident provide critical care guidelines for proper treatment.

During the treatment of a critical care patient, pain management is essential for patient comfort. Pain is an intricate biochemical and neurologic process developed to reduce exposure to and damage caused by noxious stimuli. Successful pain management requires an understanding of the physiologic process of pain transmission and an ability to select the proper medication based on effects and duration of action. This knowledge aids overall patient management and stabilization of the body's systems.

An important mission of the critical care transport team is identification, referral, communication, and assistance with organ and tissue procurement. Critical care health professionals play an integral role in this process.

In every type of mission, safety is an essential component of air and ground transport by the critical care team. The hallmarks of an excellent transport program are superb clinical care and a culture of safety that encompasses the principles of AMRM, scene safety, helicopter safety, and ground safety and that does not tolerate unsafe behavior. The concept of safety is summarized well in this way: "Safety is simply about coming home, and that does not happen by accident!"

KEY TERMS

anemic hypoxia A type of hypoxia that results from a decrease in the concentration of functional hemoglobin or a reduction in the number of erythrocytes.

barodentalgia Sudden, sharp tooth pain that may occur in response to a decrease in atmospheric pressure, such as may occur during flight at high altitudes or ascent during a dive.

barosinusitis Painful symptoms of the maxillary sinus resulting from a change in the barometric pressure.

barotitis media Pain in the ear caused by pressure differences, such as occur during air travel or while diving.

bradykinin A peptide released in response to painful stimuli that increases inflammation around nociceptors, causing an amplified pain response.

crepitant anaerobic cellulitis A necrotic soft tissue infection that occurs with abundant connective tissue gas. It usually develops after local trauma in patients with vascular insufficiency of the lower extremities.

cyclooxygenase An enzyme found in most tissues that helps convert some fatty acids into prostaglandins.

dynorphin A peptide that targets kappa opioid receptors, reducing dopamine levels in the brain and thereby counteracting the addictive effects of opiates.

dysbaric osteonecrosis A condition marked by necrotic lesions in the ball-and-socket joints (hips and shoulders) and in the fatty marrow–containing shafts of the long bones; it is associated with exposure to large ambient pressure changes.

dysesthesia An unpleasant, abnormal sensation, caused by lesions of the peripheral or central nervous system, that is described as burning, wetness, itching, tingling, or "pins and needles."

endorphins Long chains of amino acids that interact with opiate receptor neurons to reduce the body's sensitivity to pain.

enkephalins Neurotransmitters that regulate pain by blocking receptors through action identical to that of endorphins.

fluoroquinolones Antibacterial drugs that interfere with the bacterial gyrase-DNA complex, causing cell death.

histotoxic hypoxia A type of hypoxia that results when tissue cells are unable to use oxygen that may be present at a normal amount and tension.

iatrogenic A descriptive term for a symptom or illness brought on unintentionally by a healthcare provider.

inhibitory neurotransmitters Neurotransmitters that block the actions between neurons.

narcotic A descriptive term referring to opium, opiate derivatives, and their synthetic substitutes.

necrotizing fasciitis A condition marked by death of the fascial tissue, often as a result of overwhelming bacterial infection.

neospinothalamic tract Spinothalmic nerve tracts convey pain, temperature, coarse touch and pressure information to the somatosensory region of the thalamus. The neospinothalamic tract runs directly to the thalamus without any modulation or other input and allows the person to distinguish different levels of pain.

neuropathic pain Chronic pain that occurs or persists after a primary lesion or dysfunction of the peripheral or central nervous system has resolved.

nociception The perception of physical pain.

nonclostridial myonecrosis A particularly aggressive soft tissue infection that is similar to clostridial myonecrosis in that it shows widespread involvement of soft tissue with necrosis of muscle tissue and fascia.

nonsteroidal antiinflammatory drugs (NSAIDs) Drugs that interfere with the mediated process by which pain is relayed to nociceptors.

occult With reference to disease, a condition that is hidden or difficult to detect with the naked eye.

organophosphates (OPs) A class of anticholinesterase chemicals used in certain pesticides and in gases used in warfare.

osteomyelitis Inflammation and infection of the bone and bone marrow.

osteoradionecrosis Necrosis of bone following irradiation.

pain An unpleasant sensory and emotional experience that is associated with actual or potential tissue damage or that is described in terms of such damage.

paleospinothalamic tract The pain tract that runs, via the dorsal horn of the spinal column, first to the medulla, as it receives input from other areas of the brain, then to the pons nuclei, and then to the thalamus.

paresthesia An altered sensation reported by the patient in an area where the sensory nerve has been afflicted by disease or injury. The patient may report burning, prickling, formication, or other sensations.

peripheral neuropathy a functional disturbance or pathological change in the peripheral nervous system, many times as a complication of other diseases. In diabetics, this is a sequential demyelination of peripheral nerves that may cause severe pain, weakness and wasting of the muscles and tendons. Sometimes called *polyneuropathy*.

proprioceptive system The system by which the body senses the relative position of neighboring parts.

prostaglandin A hormone-like substance that mediates the inflammatory response and sensitizes spinal neurons to painful stimuli.

psychogenic pain Pain that originates in mental or emotional rather than physiologic processes.

somatosensory cortex primary afferent fibers carry pain, temperature and coarse touch/pressure information from the trunk and extremities that ascend in the dorsal horn of the gray matter and terminate in the internal capsule of the cortex.

stagnant hypoxia Hypoxia characterized by failure to transport sufficient oxygen as a result of inadequate blood flow secondary to blood pooling.

stimulatory neurotransmitters Neurotransmitters that promote the actions of neurons.

substance P The pain transmitter of the dorsal horn of the spinal cord.

synthetic analgesics Pain-relieving drugs that are produced artificially through chemical synthesis.

toxidromes A set of clinical signs and symptoms that suggest a specific class of toxin or poison.

REFERENCES

1. Urden L, Stacy K, Lough M: *Thelan's critical care nursing: diagnosis and management*, ed 5, St Louis, 2005, Mosby.
2. Vanderhoff TW: Pathophysiology of pain (handout), Department of Pharmacology and Anesthesiology, University of Arizona College of Medicine, Tucson, Arizona.
3. Workman WT, Haux GFK: *History of hyperbaric chambers*, Flagstaff, Arizona, 2000, Best Publishing.
4. Heimbach RD, Sheffield PJ: Protection in the pressure environment: cabin pressurization and oxygen equipment. In Delhart RL, editor: *Fundamentals of aerospace medicine*, Philadelphia, 1985, Lea & Febiger.
5. Holleran RS, editor: *Air and surface patient transport: principles and practice*, ed 3, St Louis, 2003, Mosby.
6. Association of Air Medical Services: *Post accident resources document: a special resource for air medical transport leaders in times of crisis,* 1999, The Association.

Bibliography

Anderson CE: Recognition and prevention of inhalant abuse, *Am Fam Physician* 68:869-874, 2003.

Auerbach PS: *Wilderness medicine*, ed 5, Philadelphia, 2007, Mosby.

Barthold CL, Schier JG: Organic phosphorus compounds: nerve agents, *Crit Care Clin* 21:673-689, v-vi, 2005.

Bateman DN: Gastric decontamination: a view for the millennium, *J Accid Emerg Med* 16:84-86, 1999.

Blumen IJ: Program safety (lecture). Air Medical Physician Association (AMPA) Medical Director Core Curriculum, Part III. Tampa, September, 2007.

Blumen IJ, Abernathy MK, Dunne MJ: Flight physiology: clinical considerations, *Crit Care Clin* 8:597-618, 1992.

Blumen IJ, Callejas S: Transport physiology: a reference for air medical personnel. In Blumen IJ, editor: *Principles and direction of air medical transport*, Salt Lake City, 2006, Air Medical Physician Association.

Blumen IJ, Rinnert KJ: Altitude physiology and the stresses of flight, *Air Med J* 14:2, 1995.

Cannard K: The acute treatment of nerve agent exposure, *J Neurol Sci* 249:86-94, 2006.

Caravati EM, Knight HH, Linscott MS Jr et al: Esophageal laceration and charcoal mediastinum complicating gastric lavage, *J Emerg Med* 20:273-276, 2001.

Chatman TL: Post accident-incident planning. In Blumen IJ, editor: *Principles and direction of air medical transport*, Salt Lake City, 2006, Air Medical Physician Association.

Chyka PA, Seger D, Krenzelok EP et al: Position paper: single-dose activated charcoal. American Academy of Clinical Toxicology, European Association of Poison Centres and Clinical Toxicologists, *Clin Toxicol* 43:61-87, 2005.

Cobb N, Etzel R: Unintentional carbon monoxide–related deaths in the United States, 1979-1988, *JAMA* 266:659-663, 1991.

Ducasse JL, Celsis P, Marc-Nergnes JP: Noncomatose patients with acute carbon monoxide poisoning: hyperbaric or normobaric oxygenation? *Undersea Hyperb Med* 22:9-15, 1995.

Dynorphin: Nature's own antidote to cocaine (and pleasure?) www.dynorphin.com. Accessed March 16, 2010.

Ellis D: From the air to the ground: air medical safety practices applied to ground critical care, *Air Med J* 25:158-159, 2006.

Emergency Nurses Association: *Trauma nursing core course*, ed 6, Philadelphia, 2007, Saunders.

Erickson TB: The approach to the patient with an unknown overdose, *Emerg Med Clin North Am* 25:249-281, 2007.

Feldmeier JJ: *Hyperbaric oxygen 2003—indications and results: the Hyperbaric Oxygen Therapy Committee report*, Kensington, Md, 2003, Undersea and Hyperbaric Medical Society.

Flanagan RJ, Ruprah M, Meredith TJ et al: An introduction to the clinical toxicology of volatile substances, *Drug Saf* 5:359-383, 1990.

Grissom CK: Survival for air medical transport crews. In Blumen IJ, editor: *Principles and direction of air medical transport*, Salt Lake City, 2006, Air Medical Physician Association.

Hawkins MR: Personal protective equipment in helicopter EMS, *Air Med J* 13:123-126, 1994.

Heimbach RD, Sheffield PJ: Decompression sickness and pulmonary overpressure accidents. In Dehart RL, editor: *Fundamentals of aerospace medicine*, Philadelphia, 1985, Lea & Febiger.

Heimbach RD, Sheffield PJ: Protection in the pressure environment: cabin pressurization and oxygen equipment. In Dehart RL, editor: *Fundamentals of aerospace medicine*, Philadelphia, 1985, Lea & Febiger.

Helmreich RL, Merritt AC, Wilhelm JA: The evolution of crew resource management training in commercial aviation, *Int J Aviat Psychol* 9:19-32, 1999.

Hick JL: Protective equipment for health care facility decontamination personnel: regulations, risks, and recommendations, *Ann Emerg Med* 42:370-380, 2003.

Holleran RS, editor: *Air and surface patient transport: principles and practice*, ed 3, St Louis, 2003, Mosby.

Howell C, Wilson AD, Waring WS: Cardiovascular toxicity due to venlafaxine poisoning in adults: a review of 235 consecutive cases, *Br J Clin Pharmacol* 64:192-197, 2007.

Hunter SE, Farmer JC: Ear and sinus problems in diving. In Bove AA, editor: *Bove and Davis' diving medicine*, ed 4, Philadelphia, 2004, Saunders.

Kamin R: Flight physiology (lecture). Air Medical Physician Association (AMPA) Medical Director Core Curriculum, Part I. Austin, October, 2005.

MacDonald E: Safety is about coming home, *Air Med J* 26:198, 2007.

Marx JA, Hockberger R, Walls R: *Rosen's emergency medicine: concepts and clinical practice*, ed 6, Philadelphia, 2006, Mosby.

Mason RJ, Broaddus VC, Murray JF et al: *Murray and Nadel's textbook of respiratory medicine*, ed 4, Philadelphia, 2005, Saunders.

Mathieu D, Wattel F, Mathieu-Nolf M et al: Randomized prospective study comparing the effect of HBO versus 12 hours of NBO in non-comatose CO poisoned patients (abstract), *Undersea Hyperb Med* 23(Suppl):7-8, 1996.

Medline Plus: Anti-inflammatory drugs nonsteroidal (systemic). www.nim.nih.gov/medlineplus/druginfo/meds/a682159.html. Accessed May 5, 2010.

Miller K: Acute inhalation injury, *Emerg Med Clin North Am* 21:533-557, 2003.

Mokhlesi B, Leiken JB, Murray P, Corbridge TC: Adult toxicology in critical care. I. General approach to the intoxicated patient, *Chest* 123:577-592, 2003.

Pyles M, Pringle RP, Hawkins M: Helicopter scene landings: a guide for ground personnel, *J Emerg Nurs* 22:234-236, 1996.

Raphael JC, Elkharrat D, Jars-Guincestre MC et al: Trial of normobaric and hyperbaric oxygen for acute carbon monoxide intoxication, *Lancet* 2:414-419, 1989.

Rayman RB: Aircrew health care maintenance. In Dehart RL, editor: *Fundamentals of aerospace medicine*, Philadelphia, 1985, Lea & Febiger.

Rayman RB: *Clinical aviation medicine*, ed 2, Philadelphia, 1990, Lea & Febiger.

Read K: *Aeromedicine for aviators*, Chatham, 1971, W & J Mackay.

Scheinkestel CD, Bailey M, Myles PS et al: Hyperbaric or normobaric oxygen for acute carbon monoxide poisoning: a randomized controlled clinical trial, *Med J Aust* 170:203-210, 1999.

Seibert JW, Danne C: Eustachian tube function and the middle ear, *Otolaryngol Clin North Am* 39:1221-1235, 2006.

Simpson W Jr: Recognition and management of acute pesticide poisoning, *Am Fam Physician* 65:1599-1604, 2002.

Sumwalt RL: The sterile cockpit. NASA ASRS Directline, June 1993. http://asrs.arc.nasa.gov/publications/directline/dl4_sterile.htm. Accessed March 17, 2010.

Thom SR, Taber RL, Mendiguren II et al: Delayed neuropsychologic sequela after carbon monoxide poisoning: prevention by treatment with hyperbaric oxygen, *Ann Emerg Med* 25:474-480, 1995.

Urden LD, Stacy KM, Lough ME: *Thelan's critical care nursing: diagnosis and management*, ed 5, St Louis, 2006, Mosby.

Vanderah TW: Pathophysiology of pain, *Med Clin North Am* 91:1-12, 2007.

von Mach MA, Weber C, Meyer MR et al: Comparison of urinary on-site immunoassay screening and gas chromatography–mass spectrometry results of 111 patients with suspected poisoning presenting at an emergency department, *Ther Drug Monit* 29:27, 2007.

Yules R: *The pilot's complete medical guide*, New York, 1983, Jason Aronson.

Zacher JL, Givone DM: False-positive urine opiate screening associated with fluoroquinolone use, *Ann Pharmacother* 38:1525-1528, 2004.

Zaidi SA, Shaw AN, Patel MN et al: Multi-organ toxicity and death following acute unintentional inhalation of paint thinner fumes, *Clin Toxicol* 45:287-289, 2007.

REVIEW QUESTIONS

Questions 1 through 3 apply to the scenario described under Toxicology in Critical Care.

1. Based on the patient's presenting signs and symptoms (toxidrome), what toxins may be present?
   A. Alcohol and a sedative
   B. Alcohol and a cocaine like substance
   C. Alcohol alone
   D. Alcohol and a heroin-like substance
2. What treatment should be initiated for this toxidrome?
   A. IV fluids and flumazenil
   B. IV fluids and benzodiazepines
   C. IV fluids and dialysis
   D. IV fluids and naloxone
3. Before transport you should:
   A. Draw blood for a drug screen
   B. Increase the amount of dopamine the patient is receiving
   C. Give the antidote and extubate the patient
   D. Perform gastric lavage to clear the stomach of toxins

4. A patient presents to the local hospital leaning forward in obvious respiratory distress with mucus dripping from his nose, eyes, and mouth. He has been incontinent of urine and feces. Family members report that he is a farm worker, and they do not know what is wrong. What toxidrome likely is present?
   A. Dry as a bone, red as a beet, mad as a hatter, blind as a bat: Anticholinergics
   B. Opiates
   C. SLUDGE: Cholinergics
   D. No toxidrome is present; this may be influenza.
5. What treatment is necessary in the scenario presented in question 4?
   A. Lorazepam, 1 to 2 mg given IV
   B. Immediate intubation and administration of benzodiazepines and succinylcholine
   C. Atropine, possibly in large quantities
   D. IV fluids and rest
6. When transporting a poisoned patient, the overriding concern should be:
   A. Identifying the poison
   B. Ensuring the patient's comfort
   C. Communicating with the flight crew
   D. Safety with the crew
7. Why is succinylcholine contraindicated in organophosphate poisoning?
   A. Five times the normal dose is needed.
   B. It may lead to prolonged paralysis.
   C. Succinylcholine is short acting.
   D. It will not affect the patient.
8. Hydrocarbons may cause a patient to develop dysrhythmias. These seem to occur secondary to:
   A. Catecholamine release
   B. Lack of oxygen to the lungs
   C. Decreased preload
   D. Histamine release
9. Neuropathic pain occurs secondary to damage or dysfunction of the structures of the:
   A. Affected organs or vessels
   B. Skin and muscles
   C. Peripheral or central nervous system
   D. Tissues and ligaments
10. Psychogenic pain may be associated with mental illness; centralized pain commonly is the result of:
    A. Neuropathy
    B. Brain lesion
    C. Psychosis
    D. Paranoia
11. Which of the following is the best definition of transduction?
    A. Transmission of a signal to the spinal cord
    B. Release of endogenous opioids
    C. Conversion of noxious stimuli to electrical signals
    D. Bridging of the synaptic gaps by peptides
12. Prostaglandin is a hormone that sensitizes spinal neurons to painful stimuli and mediates:
    A. Bradykinin
    B. Substance P
    C. Kappa opioid receptors
    D. Inflammatory response
13. Delta opioid receptors are located throughout the:
    A. Brain and spinal cord
    B. Cardiovascular system
    C. Lymphatic system
    D. Respiratory system
14. Which drug is considered the most potent narcotic in clinical use today?
    A. Morphine
    B. Demerol
    C. Methadone
    D. Fentanyl
15. Which of these conditions is not approved by the Undersea and Hyperbaric Medical Society for treatment in a hyperbaric chamber?
    A. Exceptional blood loss
    B. Osteoradionecrosis
    C. Alzheimer's disease
    D. Intracranial abscess
16. Which gas law describes the increase in gas volume in relation to a decrease in pressure?
    A. Dalton's law
    B. Henry's law
    C. Charles' law
    D. Boyle's law
17. Which gas law is described using the example of a carbonated beverage?
    A. Dalton's law
    B. Henry's law
    C. Charles' law
    D. Boyle's law
18. During a wound healing treatment in a hyperbaric chamber, what percentage of oxygen will a patient receive at 45 FSW?
    A. 100%
    B. 21%
    C. 240%
    D. 50%

19. An AGE can occur in as little as ______ feet of water.
    A. 10
    B. 4
    C. 20
    D. 15
20. Which type of DCS may result in altered gas exchange?
    A. Type 4
    B. Type 6
    C. Type 2
    D. Type 3
21. Six atmospheres absolute is equivalent to how many feet of seawater?
    A. 66
    B. 165
    C. 33
    D. 99
22. Pooling of blood may cause which type of hypoxia?
    A. Hypoxic hypoxia
    B. Histotoxic hypoxia
    C. Anemic hypoxia
    D. Stagnant hypoxia
23. The force a person exerts when seated is a direct response to:
    A. G forces
    B. Spatial disorientation
    C. Flicker vertigo
    D. Body fatigue

APPENDIX A

Normal Laboratory Values

PART I. HEMATOLOGY

		Conventional Units	SI Units*
Acid hemolysis test (Ham)		No hemolysis	No hemolysis
Alkaline phosphatase, leukocyte		Total score 14-100	Total score 14-100
Cell counts			
Erythrocytes			
Males		4.6-6.2 million/mm^3	4.6-6.2 × 10^{12}/L
Females		4.2-5.4 million/mm^3	4.2-5.4 × 10^{12}/L
Children (varies with age)		4.5-5.1 million/mm^3	4.5-5.1 × 10^{12}/L
Leukocytes			
Total		4500-11,000 mm^3	4.5-11.0 × 10^9/L
Differential	*Percentage*	*Absolute*	*Absolute*
Myelocytes	0	0/mm^3	0/L
Band neutrophils	3-5	150-400/mm^3	150-400 × 10^6/L
Segmented neutrophils	54-62	3000-5800/mm^3	3000-5800 × 10^6/L
Lymphocytes	25-33	1500-3000/mm^3	1500-3000 × 10^6/L
Monocytes	3-7	300-500/mm^3	300-500 × 10^6/L
Eosinophils	1-3	50-250/mm^3	50-250 × 10^6/L
Basophils	0-1	15-50/mm^3	15-50 × 10^6/L
Platelets		150,000-400,000/mm^3	150-400 × 10^9/L
Reticulocytes		25,000-75,000/mm^3 (0.5%-1.5% of erythrocytes)	25-75 × 10^9/L
Coagulation tests			
Bleeding time (template)		2.75-8.0 min	2.75-8.0 min
Coagulation time (glass tubes)		5-15 min	5-15 min
D-dimer		<0.5 mcg/mL	<0.5 mg/L
Factor VIII and other coagulation factors		50%-150% of normal	0.5-1.5 of normal
Fibrin split products (Thrombo-Welco test)		<10 mcg/mL	<10 mg/L
Fibrinogen		200-400 mg/dL	2.0-4.0 g/L
Partial thromboplastin time (PTT)		20-35 sec	20-35 sec
Prothrombin time (PT)		12.0-14.0 sec	12.0-14.0 sec

	Conventional Units	SI Units*
Coombs test		
Direct	Negative	Negative
Indirect	Negative	Negative
Corpuscular values of erythrocytes		
Mean corpuscular hemoglobin (MCH)	26-34 pg/cell	26-34 pg/cell
Mean corpuscular volume (MCV)	80-96 micrometer^3	80-96 fL
Mean corpuscular hemoglobin concentration (MCHC)	32-36 gm/dL	320-360 g/L
Erythrocyte sedimentation rate (ESR)		
Wintrobe		
Males	0-5 mm/hr	0-5 mm/hr
Females	0-15 mm/hr	0-15 mm/hr
Westergren		
Males	0-15 mm/hr	0-15 mm/hr
Females	0-20 mm/hr	0-20 mm/hr
	20-165 mg/dL	0.20-1.65 g/L
Haptoglobin	26-185 mg/dL	260-1850 mg/L
Hematocrit		
Males	40-54 mL/dL	0.40-0.54 volume fraction
Females	37-47 mL/dL	0.37-0.47 volume fraction
Newborns	49-54 mL/dL	0.49-0.54 volume fraction
Children (varies with age)	35-49 mL/dL	0.35-0.49 volume fraction
Hemoglobin		
Males	14.0-18.0 gm/dL	2.17-2.79 mmol/L
Females	12.0-16.0 gm/dL	1.86-2.48 mmol/L
Newborns	16.5-19.5 gm/dL	2.56-3.02 mmol/L
Children (varies with age)	11.2-16.5 gm/dL	1.74-2.56 mmol/L
Hemoglobin, fetal	<1% of total	<0.01 of total
Hemoglobin A_{1c}	3%-5% of total	0.03-0.05 of total
Hemoglobin A_2	1.5%-3.0% of total	0.015-0.03 of total
Hemoglobin, plasma	0.0-5.0 mg/dL	0-0.8 micromole/L
Methemoglobin	30-130 mg/dL	4.7-20 micromole/L

*Système International d'Unités (International System of Units).

PART II. BLOOD CHEMISTRY

For some procedures, the reference values may vary depending on the method used.

	Conventional Units	**SI Units***
Alanine aminotransferase (ALT, SGPT), serum	1-45 U/L	1-45 U/L
Aspartate aminotransferase (AST, SGOT), serum	1-36 U/L	1-36 U/L
Base excess, arterial blood, calculated	0 ± 2 mEq/L	0 ± 2 mmol/L
Beta-carotene, serum	60-260 mcg/dL	1.1-8.6 micromole/L
Bicarbonate		
Venous plasma	23-29 mEq/L	23-39 mmol/L
Arterial blood	18-23 mEq/L	18-23 mmol/L
Bile acids, serum	0.3-3.0 mg/dL	3-30 mg/L
Bilirubin, serum		
Conjugated	0.1-0.4 mg/dL	1.7-6.8 micromole/L
Total	0.3-1.1 mg/dL	5.1-19 micromole/L
Calcium, serum	9.0-11.0 mg/dL	2.25-2.75 mmol/L
Calcium, ionized, serum	4.25-5.25 mg/dL	1.05-1.30 mmol/L
Carbon dioxide, total, serum or plasma	24-30 mEq/L	24-30 mmol/L
Carbon dioxide tension (PCO_2), blood	35-45 mm Hg	35-45 mm Hg
Ceruloplasmin, serum	23-44 mg/dL	230-440 mg/L
Chloride, serum or plasma	96-106 mEq/L	96-106 mmol/L
Cholesterol, serum or EDTA plasma		
Desirable range	<200 mg/dL	<5.18 mmol/L
LDL cholesterol (optimal)	<100 mg/dL	<1000 mg/L
HDL cholesterol (optimal)	≥60 mg/dL	≥600 mg/L
Copper	70-140 mcg/dL	11-22 micromole/L
Corticotropin (ACTH), plasma, 8:00 AM	10-80 pg/mL	2-18 pmol/L
Cortisol, plasma		
8:00 AM	6-23 mcg/dL	170-635 nmol/L
4:00 PM	3-15 mcg/dL	82-413 nmol/L
10:00 PM	<50% of 8:00 AM value	<0.5 of 8:00 AM value
Creatine, serum		
Males	0.2-0.5 mg/dL	15-40 micromole/L
Females	0.3-0.9 mg/dL	25-70 micromole/L
Creatine kinase (CK), serum		
Males	55-170 U/L	55-170 U/L
Females	30-135 U/L	30-135 U/L
Creatine kinase MB isoenzyme, serum	0-4.7 ng/mL	0-4.7 mcg/L
Creatinine, serum	0.6-1.2 mg/dL	50-110 micromole/L
Estradiol-17-beta, adult		
Males	10-65 pg/mL	35-240 pmol/L
Females		
Follicular phase	30-100 pg/mL	110-370 pmol/L
Ovulatory phase	200-400 pg/mL	730-1470 pmol/L
Luteal phase	50-140 pg/mL	180-510 pmol/L

	Conventional Units	SI Units*
Ferritin, serum	20-200 ng/mL	20-200 mcg/L
Fibrinogen, plasma	200-400 mg/dL	2.0-4.0 g/L
Folate, serum	1.8-9.0 ng/mL	4.1-20.4 nmol/L
Erythrocytes	150-450 ng/mL	340-1020 nmol/L
Follicle-stimulating hormone (FSH), plasma		
Males	4-25 mU/mL	4-25 U/L
Females	4-30 mU/mL	4-30 U/L
Postmenopausal	40-250 mU/mL	40-250 U/L
Gamma-glutamyltransferase (GGT), serum	5-40 U/L	5-40 U/L
Gastrin, fasting, serum	0-110 pg/mL	0-110 ng/L
Glucose, fasting, plasma or serum	70-115 mg/dL	3.9-6.4 mmol/L
Growth hormone (hGH), plasma, adult, fasting	0-6 ng/mL	0-6 mcg/L
Haptoglobin, serum	20-165 mg/dL	0.20-1.65 g/L
Insulin, fasting, plasma	5-25 microU/mL	36-179 pmol/L
Iron, serum	75-175 mcg/dL	13-31 micromole/L
Iron binding capacity, serum		
Total	250-410 mcg/dL	45-73 micromole/L
Saturation	20%-55%	0.20-0.55
Lactate		
Venous whole blood	5.0-20.0 mg/dL	0.6-2.2 mmol/L
Arterial whole blood	5.0-15.0 mg/dL	0.6-1.7 mmol/L
Lactate dehydrogenase (LDH), serum	110-220 U/L	110-220 U/L
Lipase, serum	10-140 U/L	10-140 U/L
Lutropin (LH), serum		
Males	1-9 U/L	1-9 U/L
Females		
Follicular phase	2-10 U/L	2-10 U/L
Midcycle peak	15-65 U/L	15-65 U/L
Luteal phase	1-12 U/L	1-12 U/L
Postmenopausal	12-65 U/L	12-65 U/L
Magnesium, serum	1.8-3.0 mg/dL	0.75-1.25 mmol/L
Osmolality	286-295 mOsm/kg water	285-295 mmol/kg water
Oxygen, blood, arterial, room air		
Partial pressure (PaO_2)	80-100 mm Hg	80-100 mm Hg
Saturation (SaO_2)	95%-98%	95%-98%
pH, arterial blood	7.35-7.45	7.35-7.45
Phosphate, inorganic, serum		
Adult	3.0-4.5 mg/dL	1.0-1.5 mmol/L
Child	4.0-7.0 mg/dL	1.3-2.3 mmol/L
Potassium		
Serum	3.5-5.0 mEq/L	3.5-5.0 mmol/L
Plasma	3.5-4.5 mEq/L	3.5-4.5 mmol/L
Progesterone, serum, adult		

Continued

	Conventional Units	SI Units*
Males	0.0-0.4 ng/mL	0.0-1.3 mmol/L
Females		
Follicular phase	0.1-1.5 ng/mL	0.3-4.8 mmol/L
Luteal phase	2.5-28.0 ng/mL	8.0-89.0 mmol/L
Prolactin, serum		
Males	1.0-15.0 ng/mL	1.0-15.0 mcg/L
Females	1.0-20.0 ng/mL	1.0-20.0 mcg/L
Protein, serum, electrophoresis		
Total	6.0-8.0 gm/dL	60-80 g/L
Albumin	3.5-5.5 gm/dL	35-55 g/L
$Alpha_1$ globulin	0.2-0.4 gm/dL	2-4 g/L
$Alpha_2$ globulin	0.5-0.9 gm/dL	5-9 g/L
Beta globulin	0.6-1.1 gm/dL	6-11 g/L
Gamma globulin	0.7-1.7 gm/dL	7-15 g/L
Pyruvate, blood	0.3-0.9 gm/dL	0.03-0.10 mmol/L
Rheumatoid factor	0.0-30.0 IU/mL	0.0-30.0 KIU/ml
Sodium, serum or plasma	135-145 mEq/L	135-145 mmol/L
Testosterone, plasma		
Males, adult	300-1200 ng/dL	10.4-41.6 nmol/L
Females, adult	20-75 ng/dL	0.7-2.6 nmol/L
Pregnant females	40-200 ng/dL	1.4-6.9 nmol/L
Thyroglobulin	3-42 ng/mL	3-42 mcg/L
Thyrotropin (hTSH), serum	0.4-4.8 microIU/mL	0.4-4.8 mIU/L
Thyrotropin-releasing hormone (TRH)	5-60 pg/mL	5-60 ng/L
Thyroxine, free (FT_4), serum	0.9-2.1 ng/dL	12-27 pmol/L
Thyroxine (T_4), serum	4.5-12.0 mcg/dL	58-154 nmol/L
Thyroxine-binding globulin (TBG)	15.0-34.0 mcg/mL	15.0-34.0 mg/L
Transferrin	250-430 mg/dL	2.5-4.3 g/L
Triglycerides, serum, after 12-hr fast	40-150 mg/dL	0.4-1.5 g/L
Triiodothyronine (T_3), serum	70-190 ng/dL	1.1-2.9 nmol/L
Triiodothyronine uptake, resin (T_3RU)	25%-38% uptake	0.25-0.38 uptake
Urate		
Males	2.5-8.0 mg/dL	150-480 micromole/L
Females	2.2-7.0 mg/dL	130-420 micromole/L
Urea, serum or plasma	24-49 mg/dL	4.0-8.2 nmol/L
Urea nitrogen, serum or plasma	11-23 mg/dL	8.0-16.4 nmol/L
Viscosity, serum	1.4-1.8 times water	1.4-1.8 times water
Vitamin A, serum	20-80 mcg/dL	0.70-2.80 micromole/L
Vitamin B_{12}, serum	180-900 pg/mL	133-664 pmol/L

IU = international unit, U = unit.
*Système International d'Unités (International System of Units).

PART III. URINE CHEMISTRY

For some procedures, the reference values may vary depending on the method used.

	Conventional Units	SI Units*
Acetone and acetoacetate, qualitative	Negative	Negative
Albumin		
Qualitative	Negative	Negative
Quantitative	10-100 mg/24 hr	0.15-1.5 micromole/day
Aldosterone	3-20 mcg/24 hr	8.3-55 nmol/day
Delta-aminolevulinic acid (delta-ALA)	1.3-7.0 mg/24 hr	10-53 micromole/day
Amylase	<17 U/hr	<17 U/hr
Amylase/creatinine clearance ratio	0.01-0.04	0.01-0.04
Bilirubin, qualitative	Negative	Negative
Calcium (regular diet)	<250 mg/24 hr	<6.3 mmol/day
Catecholamines		
Epinephrine	<10 mcg/24 hr	<55 nmol/day
Norepinephrine	<100 mcg/24 hr	<590 nmol/day
Total free catecholamines	4-126 mcg/24 hr	24-745 nmol/day
Total metanephrines	0.1-1.6 mg/24 hr	0.5-8.1 micromole/day
Chloride (varies with intake)	110-250 mEq/24 hr	110-250 mmol/day
Copper	0-50 mcg/24 hr	0.0-0.80 micromole/day
Cortisol, free	10-100 mcg/24 hr	27.6-276 nmol/day
Creatine		
Males	0-40 mg/24 hr	0.0-0.30 mmol/day
Females	0-80 mg/24 hr	0.0-0.60 mmol/day
Creatinine	15-25 mg/kg/24 hr	0.13-0.22 mmol/kg/day
Creatinine clearance (endogenous)		
Males	110-150 mL/min/1.73 m^2	110-150 mL/min/1.73 m^2
Females	105-132 mL/min/1.73 m^2	105-132 mL/min/1.73 m^2
Cystine or cysteine	Negative	Negative
Dehydroepiandrosterone		
Males	0.2-2.0 mg/24 hr	0.7-6.9 micromole/day
Females	0.2-1.8 mg/24 hr	0.7-6.2 micromole/day
Estrogens, total		
Males	4-25 mcg/24 hr	14-90 nmol/day
Females	5-100 mcg/24 hr	18-360 nmol/day
Glucose (as reducing substance)	<250 mg/24 hr	<250 mg/day
Hemoglobin and myoglobin, qualitative	Negative	Negative
Homogentisic acid, qualitative	Negative	Negative
17-Hydroxycorticosteroids		
Males	3-9 mg/24 hr	8.3-25 micromole/day
Females	2-8 mg/24 hr	5.5-22 micromole/day
5-Hydroxyindoleacetic acid		
Qualitative	Negative	Negative
Quantitative	2-6 mg/24 hr	10-31 micromole/day

Continued

	Conventional Units	SI Units*
17-Ketogenic steroids		
Males	5-23 mg/24 hr	17-80 micromole/day
Females	3-15 mg/24 hr	10-52 micromole/day
17-Ketosteroids		
Males	8-22 mg/24 hr	28-76 micromole/day
Females	6-15 mg/24 hr	21-52 micromole/day
Magnesium	6-10 mEq/24 hr	3-5 mmol/day
Metanephrines	0.05-1.2 ng/mg creatinine	0.03-0.70 mmol/mmol creatinine
Osmolality	38-1400 mOsm/kg water	38-1400 mOsm/kg water
pH	4.6-8.0	4.6-8.0
Phenylpyruvic acid, qualitative	Negative	Negative
Phosphate	0.4-1.3 gm/24 hr	13-42 mmol/day
Porphobilinogen		
Qualitative	Negative	Negative
Quantitative	<2.0 mg/24 hr	<9 micromole/day
Porphyrins		
Coproporphyrin	50-250 mcg/24 hr	77-380 nmol/day
Uroporphyrin	10-30 mcg/24 hr	12-36 nmol/day
Potassium	25-125 mEq/24 hr	25-125 mmol/day
Pregnanediol		
Males	0.0-1.9 mg/24 hr	0.0-6.0 micromole/day
Females		
Proliferative phase	0.0-2.6 mg/24 hr	0.0-8.0 micromole/day
Luteal phase	2.6-10.6 mg/24 hr	8-33 micromole/day
Postmenopausal	0.2-1 mg/24 hr	0.6-3.1 micromole/day
Pregnanetriol	0.0-2.5 mg/24 hr	0.0-7.4 micromole/day
Protein, total		
Qualitative	Negative	Negative
Quantitative	10-150 mg/24 hr	10-150 mg/day
Protein/creatinine ratio	<0.2	<0.2
Sodium (regular diet)	60-260 mEq/24 hr	60-260 mmol/day
Specific gravity	1.003-1.030	1.003-1.030
Random specimen	1.003-1.030	1.003-1.030
24-hour collection	1.015-1.025	1.015-1.025
Urate (regular diet)	250-750 mg/24 hr	1.5-4.4 mmol/day
Urobilinogen	0.5-4.0 mg/24 hr	0.6-6.8 micromole/day
Vanillylmandelic acid (VMA)	1-8 mg/24 hr	5-40 micromole/24 hr

*Système International d'Unités (International System of Units).

Adapted from O'Toole MT, editor: *Miller-Keane encyclopedia and dictionary of medicine, nursing, and allied health*, ed 6, Philadelphia, 1997, WB Saunders, pp.1843-1845, 1847-1848.

Glossary

A

abandonment Abandoning, without adequate warning, of a patient needing further medical care by the person responsible for that care.

ablation Removal or destruction of a part, especially by cutting.

accommodation In the eye, adjustment of the lens of the eye for various distances, separately or both.

acetylcholinesterase (AChE) An enzyme of the hydrolase class that catalyzes the cleavage of acetylcholine to choline and acetate.

activated partial thromboplastin time (aPTT or APTT) A performance indicator that measures the efficacy of both the *intrinsic* (contact activation pathway and common coagulation pathway; also used to monitor the treatment effects with heparin.

acute inflammatory demyelinating polyradiculoneuropathy (AIDP) Acute idiopathic polyneuritis; inflammation of several peripheral nerves at once.

acute liver failure (ALF) Liver failure identified by presenting symptoms of jaundice and mental alteration in patients with an illness of less than 26 weeks with massive necrosis of the liver cells and no preexisting liver disease.

acute lung injury (ALI) A systemic process considered to be the pulmonary phase of multiple organ dysfunction syndrome, characterized by noncardiogenic pulmonary edema; acute respiratory distress syndrome (ARDS) is the most severe form of ALI.

acute respiratory distress syndrome (ARDS) Fulminant pulmonary interstitial and alveolar edema, usually developing within a few days after the initiating trauma; thought to result from alveolar injury that has led to increased capillary permeability; also called *adult respiratory distress syndrome* and *shock lung.*

acute tubular necrosis (ATN) Acute renal failure with mild to severe damage or necrosis of tubule cells, usually secondary to either nephrotoxicity, ischemia after major surgery, trauma (crush syndrome), severe hypovolemia, sepsis, or burns.

Adams syndrome Episodic cardiac arrest and syncope due to failure of normal and escape pacemakers, with or without ventricular fibrillation; the principal clinical manifestation of severe heart block.

adaptive immunity Passive immunity of the cell-mediated type conferred by the administration of sensitized lymphocytes from an immune donor.

adhesion Stable joining of parts to each other, as in wound healing or some pathologic process; sometimes done artificially, such as in bonding materials to a tooth; a fibrous band or structure by which parts abnormally adhere.

adventitious Accidental or acquired; not natural or hereditary; in relation to lung or breath sounds, refers to abnormal sounds.

afferent Conveying toward a center; something that so conducts.

afterload In cardiac physiology, the force against which cardiac muscle shortens; in isolated muscle, the force resisting shortening after the muscle is stimulated to contract; in the intact heart, the pressure against which the ventricle ejects blood, as measured by the stress acting on the ventricular wall after the onset of contraction, determined largely by the peripheral vascular resistance and by the physical characteristics of and blood volume in the arterial system.

air trapping A condition in which the lungs do not or are not allowed to completely exhale.

airway resistance Increased turbulence that occurs when high inspiratory airflow is required from positive-pressure ventilation and is passed through the tracheal tube; this creates an overall effect of a small airway diameter and increases the resistance to breathing.

airways Route for passage of air into and out of the lungs.

aldosterone Major mineralocorticoid secreted by the adrenal cortex; promotes retention of sodium and bicarbonate, excretion of potassium and hydrogen ions, and secondary retention of water: large excesses can invoke plasma volume expansion, edema, and hypertension; secretion is stimulated by low plasma potassium concentration and angiotensin II.

aminoglycosides Any of a group of antibiotics (e.g., amikacin, gentamicin, streptomycin) derived from various species of *Streptomyces* or produced synthetically; antibiotics that inhibit bacterial protein synthesis by binding with the 30S ribosomal subunit.

aminotransferase A sub-subclass of enzymes of the transferase class that catalyze the transfer of an amino group from a donor to an acceptor; also called *transaminase.*

amygdala An almond-shaped structure that is a portion of the limbic system that mediates emotion; involved in primitive behavioral responses.

amyloid angiopathy A vascular amyloidosis in the cerebrum that affects small and medium-sized arteries of the leptomeninges and cerebral cortex, resulting in microinfarcts or in hemorrhage; may be asymptomatic or may result in hemorrhagic stroke or dementia.

anatomic dead space Volume of air that remains in the conducting airways and does not contribute to gas exchange.

anemic hypoxia Hypoxia resulting from a decreased concentration of functional hemoglobin or a reduced number of erythrocytes.

angiodysplasia Small abnormalities of blood or lymphatic vessels.

angiotensin Any of a family of polypeptide vasopressor hormones formed by the catalytic action of renin on angiotensinogen; also called *angiotonin.*

angiotensin I A decapeptide cleaved from angiotensinogen by renin; serves mainly as a precursor to angiotensin II.

angiotensin II An octapeptide hormone formed by the action of angiotensin-converting enzyme (ACE) (peptidyl-dipeptidase A) on angiotensin I, chiefly in the lungs but also at other sites, including the blood vessel walls, uterus, and brain; a powerful vasopressor and stimulator of aldosterone secretion by the adrenal cortex; also functions as a neurotransmitter.

anisocoria Inequality in diameter of the pupils.

antidiuretic hormone (ADH) Suppresses the rate of urine formation; an agent that acts as a vasopressin.

antigen Any substance capable, under appropriate conditions, of inducing a specific immune response and of reacting with the products of that response, that is, with specific antibody or specifically sensitized T lymphocytes, or both; antigens may be soluble or particulate substances.

antigen-antibody complex The complex formed by the noncovalent binding of an antibody and an antigen; complexes of antibodies belonging to certain immunoglobulin classes may activate complement.

antiinflammatory cytokine A type of cytokine that counteracts or suppresses inflammation.

Anti-kickback statute Imposes criminal and civil monetary penalties on any entity or individual that knowingly and willfully pays or offers to pay, solicits, or receives any remuneration in exchange for the referral of patients for any item or service that is covered by a federal healthcare program (i.e., Medicare and Medicaid): also prohibits a person from arranging for or recommending the purchase of goods or services for which payment may be made under a federal healthcare program in exchange for remuneration.

antipruritic Agent that relieves or prevents itching, such as Benadryl or hydroxyzine.

antithrombin III An α_2-globulin of the serpin family synthesized in the liver and found in plasma and various extravascular sites, which inactivates thrombin in a time-dependent irreversible reaction; also inhibits certain other proteinases with serine active sites, including coagulation factors Xa, XIIa, XIa, and IXa, and kallikrein.

anxiolysis Cessation of anxiety; an anxiolytic drug has antianxiety action.

APACHE score (Acute Physiology, Age, and Chronic Health Evaluation) A scoring system for classifying patients in the intensive care unit; patients are evaluated by physiologic scores in 8 classes (Cardiovascular, Respiratory, Renal, GI, Hematologic, Septic, Metabolic, and Neurologic) with 34 variables.

apneustic center One of the respiratory centers located near the pons (brainstem); controls normal respirations.

aqueduct of Sylvius A narrow passage or channel that connects the third and fourth ventricles in the brain; a passageway for cerebrospinal fluid; also called *cerebral aqueduct* or *aqueductus mesencephali.*

arachnoid mater Thin web-like membrane in the brain and spinal cord; also called the *arachnoidea mater encephali* (brain) and *arachnoidea mater spinalis* (spinal cord covering).

arachnoid villi Numerous microscopic projections of the arachnoid into some of the venous sinuses; also called *granulationes arachnoideae.*

arcus senilis Fatty deposits that appear within the iris of the eye in older adults.

aryepiglottic folds Pertains to the arytenoid cartilage and to the epiglottis; also termed *arytenoepiglottic folds.*

asynchronous ventilation Respiratory pattern demonstrated by the inability to synchronize spontaneous ventilation with mechanical ventilation; also called *dyssynchrony.*

atrial natriuretic peptide (ANP) A hormone, usually 28 amino acids in length, that is involved in natriuresis and the regulation of renal and cardiovascular homeostasis; ; also called *atriopeptin* and *atrial natriuretic factor.*

auto-PEEP (positive end-expiratory pressure) Pressure created by a patient's own respiratory system that keeps the distal airways open during exhalation and adds to overall oxygenation; occurs with ventilator use when ventilation rate and tidal volume are set to prevent patient from fully exhaling.

autonomy State of functioning independently, without extraneous influence.

autotransfusion Reinfusion of blood or blood products derived from the patient's own circulation; the collection, processing, and reinfusion of the patient's blood shed from the chest after traumatic hemothorax; also called *autologous transfusion.*

azotemia An excess of urea or other nitrogenous compounds in the blood; also called *uremia.*

B

Babinski's reflex Dorsiflexion of the big toe after the side of the foot is stimulated; normal reflex in infants, but in older age groups a sign of a lesion in the central nervous system, particularly in the pyramidal tract; also called *the Babinski phenomenon* or *Bakinski's sign.*

band A late metamyelocyte in which the nucleus is in the form of a curved or coiled band, not having acquired the typical multilobar shape of the mature polymorphonuclear neutrophil; also called *band form* or *neutrophil, rod neutrophil.*

barotrauma Injury caused by pressure, especially to enclosed cavities of the body such as the lung; traumatic damage to the lung as a result of pressure changes, usually characterized by peribronchial rupture and pneumomediastinum.

Barlow syndrome Mitral valve prolapse.

barodentalgia Sudden, sharp tooth pain that may occur in response to a decrease in atmospheric pressure such as that experienced during flight at high altitudes or diving ascent.

barosinusitis The painful symptoms related to the maxillary sinus resulting from a change in barometric pressure.

barotitis media Pain in the ear caused by pressure differences (e.g., during air travel or diving).

Beck's triad Three symptoms characteristic of cardiac compression from pericardial tamponade: jugular venous distention (JVD), hypotension, and muffled heart tones.

bed-confined A term applied to a beneficiary who meets the following criteria: (1) unable to get up from bed without assistance; (2) unable to ambulate; (3) unable to sit in a chair or wheelchair.

beneficence The quality of being kind or helpful or generous.

beta hCG titer Human chorionic gonadotropin titer; substance tested for in pregnancy testing.

bi-level positive airway pressure (BiPAP) A type of noninvasive positive-pressure ventilation (NPPV); ventilation assistance that provides higher pressures on inhalation and lower pressures on exhalation; allows the patient to get more air into and out of the lungs.

bleb (bulla) A large blister; emphysematous bleb; any space in a distended area of an emphysematous lung.

boggy Soft and watery; describes a uterus that is without tone.

Bowman's capsule pressure The pressure exerted by any filtrate in the epithelial sac known as *Bowman's capsule.*

bradykinin Substance released in response to painful stimuli; increases inflammation around nociceptors, which causes an amplified pain response.

breach A failure to perform some promised act or obligation; transgress: act in disregard of laws, rules, contracts, or promises.

Broca's speech area Region of the brain comprising parts of the opercular portion of the inferior frontal gyrus; injury to this area may result in a minor form of motor aphasia.

bronchoscope An instrument for inspecting the interior of the tracheobronchial tree; aids in endobronchial diagnostic and therapeutic maneuvers.

Brudzinski's sign In meningitis, flexion of the neck usually results in flexion of the hip and knee; also called *neck sign*; when passive flexion of the lower limb on one side is made, a similar movement will be seen in the opposite limb; also called *contralateral sign*.

bruit Sound; venous hum.

C

cachexia A profound state of constitutional disorder; general ill health and malnutrition.

cancellous bone Substantia spongiosa ossium; a reticular, spongy, or lattice-like structure; composed mainly of bony tissue.

***Candida* infections** Infections pertaining to or caused by *Candida*, a genus of yeastlike *Fungi imperfecti* of the form-family Cryptococcaceae that produce yeast cells; formerly called *Monilia*, *Mycotoruloides*, and *Oidium*.

canthus The angle at either end of the fissure between the eyelids.

capillary fragility Unusual susceptibility of capillaries under stress to disruption with extravasation, usually with spots visible on the skin, such as ecchymoses, petechiae, or telangiectasias.

capillary hydrostatic pressure The pressure of the blood itself inside the glomerulus.

capnography Monitoring of the concentration of exhaled carbon dioxide; ordered to assess the physiologic status of patients with acute respiratory problems or who are receiving mechanical ventilation and to determine the adequacy of ventilation in anesthetized patients.

capnograph (capnography) Measurement of CO_2 that is placed into a waveform and recorded over time; considered more valuable to the critical care provider than other measures of CO_2.

capnometer (capnometry) A device that measures the amount of CO_2 and projects a number that is not placed in a graph.

carboxy peptidase Any exopeptidase that catalyzes the hydrolytic cleavage of the terminal or penultimate peptide bond at the C-terminal end of a peptide or polypeptide.

cardioesophageal (gastroesophageal) sphincter Lower esophageal sphincter.

catechol-*O*-methyltransferase (COMT) Intracellular enzyme involved in the inactivation of the catecholamine neurotransmitters (dopamine, epinephrine, and norepinephrine); located in the postsynaptic neuron; introduces a methyl group to the catecholamine, which is donated by *S*-adenosyl L-methionine (SAM).

cerebral perfusion pressure (CPP) The difference between the mean arterial pressure and the intracranial pressure, normally 70-95 mm Hg.

chelation Combination with a metal in complexes in which the metal is part of a ring.

cholinergic Term applied to the sympathetic and parasympathetic nerve fibers that liberate acetylcholine at a synapse when a nerve impulse passes.

cholinergic receptor A type of cell-surface receptor that binds the neurotransmitter acetylcholine and mediates its action on postjunctional cells.

choroid plexus Infoldings of blood vessels of the pia mater covered by a thin coat of ependymal cells that form tufted projections into the third, fourth, and lateral ventricles of the brain; supplied by the choroidal arteries and secrete cerebrospinal fluid.

chronic liver failure (CLF) Decreasing liver function that has lasted at least 6 months.

chyme Semifluid, homogeneous, creamy or gruel-like material produced by digestion of food in the stomach; also called *chymus*.

chymotrypsin A serine endopeptidase that preferentially cleaves peptide bonds on the carboxyl side of amino acids with bulky hydrophobic residues, particularly tyrosine, tryptophan, phenylalanine, and leucine; secreted by the pancreas as the inactive proenzyme chymotrypsinogen.

circle of Willis Circulus arteriosus cerebri; union of the anterior and posterior cerebral arteries (branches of the carotid), forming an anastomosis at the base of the brain.

circumferential burns Pertaining to a circumference; encircling; peripheral; burns that encircle an area.

cistern A closed space serving as a reservoir for lymph or other body fluid, especially one of the enlarged subarachnoid spaces containing cerebrospinal fluid.

civil law The body of laws established by a state or nation for its own regulation; refers to that branch of law dealing with disputes between individuals and/or organizations.

clopidogrel An inhibitor of platelet aggregation used as an antithrombotic; administered orally.

clubbing A digital deformity produced by proliferation of the soft tissues about the terminal phalanges of the fingers or toes, with no constant osseous changes; as in *clubbed finger*.

coagulation cascade The series of steps beginning with activation of the intrinsic or extrinsic pathways of coagulation, or of one of the related alternative pathways, and proceeding through the common pathway of coagulation to the formation of the fibrin clot; each step involves the activate zymogen, which catalyzes activation of the subsequent step.

coagulopathy Any disorder of blood coagulation; may refer to diffuse intravascular coagulation or disseminated intravascular coagulation; also called *bleeding disorder*.

coclooxygenase An enzyme, found in most tissues, that helps turn some fatty acids into prostaglandins.

cold caloric examination Tests cranial nerves III, VI, and VIII and brainstem integrity by injecting water into each ear canal and noting any subsequent eye movement; also referred to as *oculovestibular response*.

collagen Any of a family of extracellular, closely related proteins occurring as a major component of connective tissue, giving it strength and flexibility;

colloid solution A substance composed of very small, insoluble particles, usually 1 to 1000 nm in diameter, that are uniformly dispersed or suspended in a finely divided state throughout a continuous dispersion medium, not settling readily; either phase can be solid, liquid, or gas.

compensatory To compensate or make up for a loss or lack of some capability or for an injury.

competent Properly or sufficiently qualified or capable or efficient.

competitive NMBA (neuromuscular blocking agent) agent that competes with and blocks the action of acetylcholine at the neuromuscular junction receptor site, thereby causing paralysis.

complement A term originally used to refer to the heat-labile factor in serum that causes immune cytolysis, the lysis of antibody-coated cells.

complement cascade Activation of a series of events that occur by two different sequences, classic and alternative pathways, with cell lysis as the goal.

complement system The functionally related system of complement, comprising at least 20 distinct serum proteins (C1 through C9 with fragments), their cellular receptors, and related regulatory proteins, that is the effector not only of immune cytolysis but also of other biologic functions including anaphylaxis, phagocytosis, opsonization, and hemolysis.

conducting To serve as a medium for conveying; transmitting. In respirations, this refers to the airways that conduct air from the nares to the terminal bronchioles.

condyloma acuminatum A warty growth on the skin or a mucous membrane; a type of papilloma usually found on the mucous membrane or skin of the external genitals or in the perianal region; a growth caused by the human papillomavirus that is infectious and autoinoculable; also called *acuminatum*, *genital* or *venereal wart*.

confidentiality The principle in medical ethics that the information a patient reveals to a healthcare provider is private and has limits on how and when it can be disclosed to a third party; usually the provider must obtain permission from the patient to make such a disclosure.

conjugate Paired, or equally coupled; working in unison.

consent To assent or approve; to grant permission.

continuous positive airway pressure (CPAP) Ventilation assistance that provides a single continuous level of pressure; also termed *noninvasive positive pressure ventilation (NPPV)*.

CO-oximetry (carbon monoxide oximetry) A measurement of hemoglobin and oxygen gas exchange, including oxyhemoglobin and oxygen saturation; also concerned with the so-called dyshemoglobins, carboxyhemoglobin, and methahemaoglobin.

contralateral Situated on, pertaining to, or affecting the opposite side, as opposed to ipsilateral.

conus medullaris A structure resembling a cone in shape; the lower end of the spinal cord, at the level of the upper lumbar vertebrae.

convergence Coordinated inclination of the two lines of sight toward their common point of fixation, or the point of fixation itself.

corneal reflexes Irritation of the cornea that results in reflex closure of the eyelids; also called *blink* or *lid reflex*.

corpus callosum An arched mass of white matter, found in the depths of the longitudinal fissure, composed of three layers of fibers, the central layer consisting primarily of transverse fibers connecting the cerebral hemispheres; its subsections, from anterior to posterior, are called rostrum, genu, trunk, and splenium.

cortisol A major natural glucocorticoid synthesized in the zona fasciculata of the adrenal cortex; affects the metabolism of glucose, protein, and fats and has appreciable mineralocorticoid activity; also regulates the immune system and affects many other functions; when used as a pharmaceutical, usually referred to as *hydrocortisone*.

coude tip *Coude,* French term for elbow; coude tip applies to a catheter or device that has a firm tip that is bent like an elbow.

C reactive protein A globulin that forms a precipitate with the somatic C polysaccharide of the pneumococcus in vitro; the most predominant of the acute phase proteins.

crepitant anerobic cellulitis A necrotic soft tissue infection with abundant connective tissue gas.

criminal law Any of various bodies of rules in different jurisdictions whose common characteristic is the potential for unique and often severe impositions; sometimes called *penal law*.

Crohn's disease One of the principal forms of inflammatory bowel disease, a chronic granulomatous disease of the gastrointestinal tract of unknown etiology; most often found in the terminal ileum; also called *Crohn colitis* and *regional* or *segmental enteritis*; when confined to the ileum, also called *regional* or *terminal ileitis*.

Cullen's sign A bluish discoloration of the skin around the umbilicus, indicative of intraperitoneal hemorrhage.

culpability To find fault if a wrong has been committed.

Cushing's triad A rise in systemic blood pressure as a result of an increase in intracranial pressure; refers to a set of three signs that includes bradycardia, systolic hypertension, and irregular respirations; seen with elevated intracranial pressure and may indicate herniation syndrome; also called *Cushing's phenomenon*.

cytochrome P450 2D6 (CYP2D6) One of the most important enzymes involved in the metabolism of xenobiotics in the body; involved in the oxidation of a wide range of substrates of all the CYPs; expression in the liver has considerable variability.

cytokines A generic term for nonantibody proteins released by one cell population (primed T lymphocytes) on contact with specific antigen, which act as intercellular mediators, as in the generation of an immune response (e.g., lymphokines and monokines).

cytotoxic T-cells (CTLs) Differentiated T lymphocytes that can recognize and lyse target cells bearing specific antigens recognized by their antigen receptors.

D

damages A sum of money paid in compensation for loss or injury.

dead space The amount of respiratory system in contact with ventilating gases but not in contact with pulmonary blood flow; this air does not contribute to the oxygen–carbon dioxide exchange.

debulking Removal of a major portion of the material that composes a lesion; also called *cytoreduction* and *cytoreductive surgery*.

defamation A false accusation of an offense or a malicious misrepresentation of someone's words or actions.

defasciculation Treatment given to prevent a fasciculation.

defensive medicine The practice of diagnostic or therapeutic measures conducted primarily not to ensure the health of the patient, but as a safeguard against possible malpractice liability.

degranulate Release of the contents of secretory granules from the cell by fusion with the plasma membrane.

dehiscence A splitting open; wound dehiscence is a separation of the layers of a surgical wound; may be partial and superficial only, or complete, with disruption of all layers.

delegation of authority A statement of instruction given to a care provider by the medical director delegating authority and assigning responsibility.

delirium An acute, transient disturbance of consciousness accompanied by a change in cognition and having a fluctuating course.

demineralization Excessive elimination of mineral or inorganic salts, as in pulmonary tuberculosis, cancer, and osteomalacia (inadequate mineralization of osteoid into mature bone).

denervation Resection or removal of the nerves to an organ or part.

denudement Pulmonary hemorrhage or bleeding.

depolarizing paralytics Neuromuscular blocking agents (NMBAs) that compete at the motor end plate by simulating acetylcholine and creating an impulse (depolarize) but then blocking its ability to be reset for subsequent stimulation, first creating fasciculations, then paralysis.

dermatome The area of skin supplied with afferent nerve fibers by a single posterior spinal root.

descending transtentorial hernation Most common kind of transtentorial herniation, with downward displacement of the most medially placed cerebral structures through the tentorial notch, compressing parts of the cerebrum, and structures below the notch; caused by a supratentorial mass.

deterrence Act or process of discouraging actions or preventing occurrences by instilling fear or doubt or anxiety.

diabetes insipidus (DI) Any of several types of polyuria in which the volume of urine exceeds 3 liters per day, causing dehydration and great thirst, as well as sometimes emaciation and great hunger.

dicrotic notch A small downward deflection in the arterial pulse or pressure contour immediately after the closure of the semilunar valves and preceding the dicrotic wave; sometimes used as a marker for the end of systole or the ejection period.

diencephalon The caudal part of the prosencephalon, which largely bounds the third ventricle and connects the mesencephalon to the cerebral hemispheres; each lateral half is divided by the hypothalamic sulcus into a dorsal part, comprising the epithalamus, dorsal thalamus, and metathalamus, and a ventral part, comprising the ventral thalamus and hypothalamus; also called the *interbrain.*

diffuse Not localized; widely distributed.

diffuse brain injury Refers to an injury that spreads throughout the brain.

dilutional hyponatremia Condition in which there is a low plasma concentration of sodium resulting from loss of sodium from the body with nonosmotic retention of water, such as that induced by vasopressin; there may also be hypovolemia.

disseminated intravascular coagulation (DIC) A bleeding disorder characterized by abnormal reduction in the elements involved in blood clotting due to their use in widespread intravascular clotting; also known as *diffuse intravascular coagulation.*

distal Away from or the farthest from a point of origin or attachment. In anatomy this refers to tissue or organs farthest away from midline or another point of origin. As opposed to proximal

diversionary status Refers to a situation in which a hospital may divert individuals to other facilities because the staff or the hospital are overloaded and not able to accept any additional emergency patients at that time.

doll's eyes response When the head is rotated laterally, the eyes deviate synergistically in the opposite direction; assessed in premature infants and the comatose to test for integrity of function of the oculomotor nerves and brainstem; also referred to as the *oculocephalic reflex* or *oculocephalogyric reflex.*

dura mater The outermost, toughest, and most fibrous of the three membranes (meninges) covering the brain and spinal cord; also called *pachymeninx.*

duty The social force that binds one to the courses of action demanded by that force; work that one is obliged to perform for moral or legal reasons.

E

ethics The rules or principles that govern right conduct; clinical ethics is the application of ethical analysis to decision making in the care of individual patients; medical ethics are the values and guidelines that should govern decisions in medicine.

DVT prophylaxis (deep vein thrombosis or deep venous thrombosis) Therapy aimed at the prevention of DVT.

dyesthesia An unpleasant, abnormal sensation caused by lesions of the peripheral or central nervous system that create a sensation described as burning, wetness, itching, tingling, or "pins and needles."

dynorphin A peptide that targets kappa opioid receptors, reducing dopamine levels in the brain, thereby counteracting the addictive effects of opiates.

dysbaric osteonecrosis Condition associated with exposure to large ambient pressure changes; composed of necrotic lesions in the fatty marrow-containing shafts of the long bone, and in the ball and socket joints.

dysconjugate Related to eye gaze; refers to the eyes not working in unison; opposite of conjugate.

dysoxia Difficulty oxygenating cells, tissues, and organs.

dyssynchrony Respiratory pattern demonstrated by the inability to synchronize spontaneous ventilation with mechanical ventilation; also called *asynchronous.*

echocardiogram A method of graphically recording the position and motion of the heart walls, internal structures of the heart, and neighboring tissue by the echo obtained from beams of ultrasonic waves directed through the chest wall.

efferent Conveying away from a center; something that so conducts.

ejection fraction Proportion of the volume of blood in the ventricles at the end of diastole that is ejected during systole; the stroke volume divided by the end-diastolic volume, often expressed as a percentage.

embolization Therapeutic introduction of a substance into a vessel in order to occlude it.

empyema Abscess; a pleural effusion containing pus; also called *thoracic empyema, purulent* or *suppurative pleurisy,* and pyothorax.

encephalopathy Any degenerative disease of the brain.

endorphins Long chains of amino acids that interact with opiate receptor neurons to reduce the sensitivity of pain.

endothelium The layer of epithelial cells that lines the cavities of the heart, the lumina of blood and lymph vessels, and the serous cavities of the body; originates from the mesoderm.

endotoxins Heat-stable toxins associated with the outer membranes of certain gram-negative bacteria, including brucellae, the enterobacteria, neisseriae, and vibrios; are not secreted but instead are released only when the cells are disrupted.

enkephalins Neurotransmitters that regulate pain by blocking receptors in identical fashion to endorphins.

enteral Within the small intestine.

epidural space Situated upon or outside the dura mater.

epoprostenol A prostaglandin used to reduce pulmonary artery pressure.

esophagogastroduodenoscopy (EGD) Endoscopic examination of the esophagus, stomach, and duodenum.

erythematous Characterized by erythema.

erythema Redness of the skin caused by capillary congestion; a common side effect of radiotherapy treatment due to patient exposure to ionizing radiation.

E time (T_E) Expiratory phase time or exhalation time; the time required to exhale in one respiratory cycle.

euthermic Normothermic; a normal temperature.

euvolemic Normal water volume; referred to as *normovolemia.*

excursion Movements that emanate from a normal, or resting, position of a movable part in performance of a function, as those of the mandible to attain functional contact between the cusps of the mandibular and maxillary teeth in mastication, or of the chest wall in respiration.

exotoxins Toxic substances formed by species of certain bacteria (e.g., *Bacillus, Bordetella, Clostridium, Corynebacterium, Escherichia, Pseudomonas, Salmonella, Shigella, Staphylococcus, Streptococcus, Vibrio, Yersinia*) found outside the bacterial cell, or free in the culture medium; protein in nature and heat-labile; become detoxified with retention of antigenicity by treatment with formaldehyde (formol toxoid); are the most poisonous substances known to humans.

expiratory reserve volume A pulmonary function test in which the maximum volume of air that can be exhaled from the end of a normal breath is measured.

exteroception Perception of stimuli originating outside or at a distance from the body.

extracorporeal membrane oxygenation (ECMO) Oxygenation that occurs outside the body, as when a patient's blood is moved through a mechanical pump, where it is oxygenated and sent back into the body.

extrapyramidal Outside of the pyramidal tracts; an imprecise term referring to a functional rather than an anatomic part of the central nervous system that controls motor activities and is not part of the pyramidal tract.

extrinsic PEEP Positive end-expiratory pressure (PEEP) applied by positive pressure ventilation.

F

factor II Prothrombin; a plasma protein that is converted to the active form thrombin (factor IIa) by cleavage by activated factor X (Xa) in the common pathway of blood coagulation.

factor VII Proconvertin; a heat-and storage-stable factor participating in the extrinsic pathway of coagulation; also called *serum prothrombin conversion accelerator (SPCA)* and *stable f*; activated form is also called *convertin.*

factor X Stuart factor; a storage-stable factor that participates in both the intrinsic and extrinsic pathways of blood coagulation, uniting them to begin the common pathway of coagulation; also called *autoprothrombin C, Prower factor,* and *Stuart-Prower factor;* activated form is also called *thrombokinase.*

falx cerebri A fold of dura mater that extends downward in the longitudinal cerebral fissure and separates the two cerebral hemispheres.

fasciculation An uncoordinated, uncontrollable twitching of a muscle group that occurs when a depolarizing neuromuscular blocking agent (NMBA) is administered; represents a spontaneous discharge of a number of fibers innervated by motor nerve filaments.

feedback loop Control system of sensors and effectors that respond to disturbances; the body's sensors feed information back to a control center where effectors make changes.

fiberoptic bronchofiberscope A flexible bronchoscope that uses fiberoptics.

fiberoptic bronchoscope (FOB) A bronchoscope equipped with fiberoptics.

fidelity A principle that forbids misleading or deceiving any creature capable of being misled or deceived.

fluoroquinolones Important antibacterial drugs found to interfere with the gyrase-DNA complex which causes cell death.

focal Pertaining to a focus; the chief center of a morbid process.

focal brain injury The center or focus of a morbid process or injury to the brain (e.g., epidural hematoma).

fontanelle A soft spot, such as one of the membrane-covered open spaces in an incompletely ossified skull of a fetus or infant.

foramen magnum The large opening in the anterior and inferior part of the occipital bone, interconnecting the vertebral canal and the cranial cavity.

fossa A trench, channel, or hollow place.

fremitus A palpable vibration; a thrill.

frequency The number of occurrences of a process per unit of time; a rate.

functional When pertaining to respiratory function, refers to airways involved in the act of respiration: oxygen and carbon dioxide exchange.

functional residual capacity Volume of air in the lungs after a normal tidal volume exhalation.

G

galea aponeurotica A helmet like structure or part; the aponeurotic structure of the scalp, connecting the frontal and occipital bellies of the occipitofrontalis muscle.

gametogenesis The development of the male and female sex cells, or gametes.

ganglion A knot or knotlike mass; refers to a group of nerve cell bodies located outside the central nervous system; occasionally applied to certain nuclear groups within the brain or spinal cord such as the basal ganglia.

gastrin Any of the several polypeptide hormones released from peptidergic fibers in the vagus nerve and from G cells in the pyloric glands of the gastric antrum; stimulates secretion of gastric acid, causing contraction of the lower esophageal sphincter and modification of gastric and esophageal motility; increases growth of acid-secreting mucosa cells; and weakly stimulates secretion of pancreatic enzymes and gallbladder contraction.

gastroduodenal muscosal defense mechanism An immune or defense mechanism arising from the communication between the stomach and the duodenum.

glia "Glue"; a word termination denoting the neuroglia.

glomerular filtration rate (GFR) A laboratory analysis calculated from the serum creatinine, age, race, and gender of a patient; best overall index of kidney function.

glucuronidation Detoxification pathway that occurs in the liver; glucuronate, a salt, ester, or anionic form of glucuronic acid derived from glucose, forms conjugates with drugs and toxins in their biotransformation.

G protein Any of a family of similar heterotrimeric proteins of the intracellular portion of the plasma membrane that bind activated receptor complexes and, through conformational changes and cyclic binding and hydrolysis of glutamyl transpeptidase (GTP), directly or indirectly effect alterations in channel gating and so couple cell surface receptors to intracellular responses.

gram negative Denotes loss or decolorization of the stain by alcohol in the Gram's method of staining; a primary characteristic of bacteria having a cell wall composed of a thin layer of peptidoglycan covered by an outer membrane of lipoprotein and lipopolysaccharide.

gram positive Denotes retention of stain or resisting decolorization by alcohol in the Gram's method of staining; a primary characteristic of bacteria whose cell wall is composed of a thick layer of peptidoglycan with attached teichoic acids.

grasp reflex A reflex consisting of a grasping motion of the fingers or toes in response to stimulation; normal reflex in infancy, but in later life is pathologic.

Grey Turner's sign (or Turner's sign) Discoloration (bruising) and induration of the skin of the costovertebral angle caused by extravasation of blood in acute hemorrhagic pancreatitis.

gross negligence Fault characterized by extreme carelessness showing willful or reckless disregard for the consequences to the safety or property of another.

H

***Helicobactor pylori* (*H. pylori*)** A genus of gram-negative, microaerophilic bacteria of the family Helicobacteraceae, consisting of motile, spinal organisms with multiple sheathed flagella; the *H. pylori* species causes gastritic and pyloric ulcers, associated with stomach cancer.

helper T cells Major regulatory cells that secrete interleukin-2 (IL-2), which stimulates the activity of B cells and other T lymphocytes; also called *helper T- 1, T-4 (CD4).*

hemoglobin-based oxygen carriers (HBOCs) Human or bovine hemoglobin manufactured without a cell membrane to eliminate the need for a specific type because the antigen has been removed..

hemostatic Causing hemostasis; an agent that arrests the flow of blood.

hepatocyte A parenchymal liver cell that performs all the functions ascribed to the liver.

hepatopulmonary syndrome Arterial hypoxemia caused by pulmonary vasodilation in conjunction with chronic liver disease, usually a result of portal hypertension in cirrhosis.

hepatorenal syndrome Functional renal failure, oliguria, and low urinary sodium concentration, without pathologic renal changes; associated with cirrhosis and ascites or with obstructive jaundice.

herniation The abnormal protrusion of an organ or other body structure through a defect or natural opening in a covering membrane, muscle, or bone; also called *herniation syndrome.*

hippocampus A curved elevation of gray matter extending the entire length of the floor of the temporal horn of the lateral ventricle.

hippus phenomenon Abnormally exaggerated rhythmic contraction and dilation of the pupil, independent of changes in illumination or in fixation of the eyes; also called *papillary athetosis.*

histotoxic hypoxia Condition that results from the inability of the tissue cells to use the oxygen that may be present in normal amount and tension.

Horner's syndrome Sinking in of the eyeball, ptosis of the upper eyelid, slight elevation of the lower lid, constriction of the pupil, narrowing of the palpebral fissure, and anhidrosis and flushing of the affected side of the face; caused by a brainstem lesion on the ipsilateral side that interrupts sympathetic nerve fibers; also called *Horner-Bernard syndrome.*

humoral Pertaining to elements dissolved in the blood or body fluids (e.g., humoral immunity from antibodies in the blood as opposed to cellular immunity); pertaining to one of the humors of the body or to humoralism.

hydramnios Excess of amniotic fluid, usually exceeding 2000 mL; also referred to as *polyhydramnios.*

hydrothorax A pleural effusion containing serous fluid; *see also* **pleural effusion.**

hyperbilirubinemia Excessive bilirubin in the blood, which may lead to jaundice; classified as either *conjugated* or *unconjugated,* according to the predominant form of bilirubin involved.

hypercirculatory Characterized by elevated rate, pressure, pumping functions of the circulatory system.

hyperdynamic Pertaining to or characterized by hyperdynamia; hyperactivity.

hyperresonance An exaggerated resonance; resonance is the prolongation and intensification of sound produced by transmission of its vibrations to a cavity, especially a sound elicited by percussion.

hypopharyngeal sphincter Upper esophageal sphincter.

I

iatrogenic Describes a symptom or illness brought on unintentionally by something that a medical provider does or says.

ideal (optimal) PEEP (positive end-expiratory pressure) Minimum amount of pressure necessary to provide oxygenation but avoid the complications of high intrathoracic pressures.

ileus Intestinal obstruction due to a nonmechanical cause, such as paralysis and failure of peristalsis.

immune system A system designed to protect against infectious diseases.

immunoglobulins Any of the structurally related glycoproteins that function as antibodies, divided into five classes (IgM, IgG, IgA, IgD, and IgE) on the basis of structure and biologic activity.

implanted port Catheter tunneled beneath the skin; has a subcutaneous port attached to a reservoir with a self-sealing septum, implanted subcutaneously and accessed with a noncoring needle.

inflammation A localized protective response elicited as a result of injury or destruction of tissues, which serves to destroy, dilute, or wall off both the injurious agent and the injured tissue; characterized in the acute form by classic signs of pain, heat, redness, swelling, and loss of function.

informed consent Voluntary permission given by a subject or guardian for participation in a study or investigation, or for medical care, after having been informed of the purpose, methods, procedures, benefits, and risks.

inhibitory Refers to neurotransmitters that block the actions between neurons.

innate immunity Immunity based on the genetic constitution of the individual (e.g., immunity of humans to canine distemper); also called *familial i., genetic i., inherent i., inherited i.,* and *native i.*

inspiratory/expiratory ratio (I:E ratio) A proportion of time it takes to inhale and exhale in a given time unit; normal human I:E ratio is 1:2 or 1:3.

inspiratory reserve volume (IRV) A pulmonary function test in which the maximum volume of air that can be inhaled above the standard inhalation in a normal breath is measured.

inspiratory time (I time) (T_I) Pertaining to the time it takes to inhale; the inspiratory portion of the I:E ratio.

Interferon (IFN) Any of a family of glycoproteins that exert virus-nonspecific but host-specific antiviral activity by inducing the transcription of cellular genes coding for antiviral proteins that selectively inhibit the synthesis of viral RNA and proteins.

interleukin-1-beta (IL-1-β; i.-4 [IL-4]) A lymphokine produced by antigen- or mitogen-activated T cells; principal role is regulation of IgE- and eosinophil-mediated immune reactions; formerly called *B lymphocyte stimulatory factor 1.*

interleukins A generic term for a group of multifunctional cytokines that are produced by a variety of lymphoid and nonlymphoid cells and have effects at least partly within the lymphopoietic system; originally believed to be produced chiefly by and to act chiefly upon leukocytes.

international normalized ratio (INR) Developed by the World Health Organization in 1982 to standardize PT (prothrombin time) results among clinical laboratories; used to guide anticoagulation therapy with Warfarin.

intrinsic PEEP *See* **auto-PEEP.**

inverse I:E ratio (inspiration/expiration ratio) Prolonged or sustained inspiration time that reduces mean airway pressure while increasing the PO_2, but can be uncomfortable for the conscious patient.

involuntary consent Refers to the patient who is unable to give consent because of a physical or mental impairment.

ipsilateral Situated on, pertaining to, or affecting the same side, as opposed to contralateral.

ischemic cascade A series of steps or stages (physiologic process) that once initiated continues to the final step by virtue of each step being triggered by the preceding one, sometimes with cumulative effect; in this process, a deficiency of blood flow is caused by an obstruction of a vessel in an organ or the body.

isovolumetric period The interval of the cardiac cycle during which the cardiac muscle fibers are contracting or relaxing but the valves remain closed, anchored by the chordae tendineae.

J

Jackson-Pratt drain A closed wound drainage system comprising a drainage tube and collection vessel.

jet ventilation Refers to insufflation of gas (air) with high velocity into the airway with a catheter; used during a failed airway protocol; high-frequency jet ventilation (HFV) refers to delivering high-flow, short-duration pulses of pressurized gas, usually to a patient with pulmonary hypertension.

justice The quality of being just or fair; judgment involved in the determination of rights and the assignment of rewards and punishments.

K

Kernig sign A sign of meningitis; the patient can easily and completely extend the lower limb when in dorsal decubitus position but not when in the sitting posture or when lying with the thigh flexed upon the abdomen.

kinesthetic sense A muscular sense; an awareness of movement, weight, tension, and position of body parts, which depends upon input from joint and muscle receptors and hair cells.

Kupffer cell A type of stellate cell found in the sinusoids of the liver, having intense phagocytic activity and forming part of the reticuloendothelial system.

Kussmaul's sign Distention of the jugular veins during inhalation, seen in constrictive pericarditis and mediastinal tumor; paradoxical pulse.

L

lacrimal Pertaining to tears.

lactulose A synthetic disaccharide used as a cathartic and to enhance excretion or formation of ammonia in the treatment of portosystemic encephalopathy, including the stages of hepatic precoma and coma.

lanugo The fine hair on the body of the fetus; also called *down, downy hair,* and *primary hair.*

lecithin Phosphatidylcholine; a phospholipid in which choline is attached to the phosphate group of phosphatidic acid by an ester linkage; a major component of cell membranes that is localized preferentially in the outer surface of the plasma membrane.

Leopold maneuver Four maneuvers in palpating the abdomen for ascertaining the position and presentation of the fetus; may include manipulation of malposition.

leukocytosis A transient increase in the number of leukocytes in the blood; seen normally with strenuous exercise and pathologically accompanying hemorrhage, fever, infection, or inflammation.

leukocytosis with left shift Laboratory report of leukocytosis with greater than 10% *bands* (immature neutrophil cells); demonstrates a left shift; indicates that the bone marrow is generating many neutrophils in the setting of an acute infection.

leukopenia Reduction in the number of leukocytes in the blood below about 4000 per mm^3; types of leukopenia named for the type of cell, such as *agranulocytosis* and *neutropenia*; also may be called *aleukia, aleukocytosis,* and *leukocytopenia.*

ligament of Treitz Musculus suspensorius duodeni; ligament that suspends the fourth part of the duodenum from the retroperitoneal cavity.

ligamentum arteriosum A short, thick, strong fibromuscular cord extending from the pulmonary artery to the arch of the aorta; the remains of the ductus arteriosus; also called the *ligament of Botallo.*

local inflammation Focal; an infection confined to a single spot or to a few limited spots.

lymphocyte Any of the mononuclear, nonphagocytic leukocytes, found in the blood, lymph, and lymphoid tissues, that are the body's immunologically competent cells and their precursors.

M

macrophages Any of the many forms of mononuclear phagocytes found in tissues; two types, *fixed macrophages* and *free macrophages* are distinguished.

macrosomia Abnormally large size; also called *macrosomatia.*

magnetic resonance cholangiopancreatography (MRCP) Radiographic examination of the bile ducts and pancreas after administration of contrast dye; obtained through magnetic resonance imaging (MRI).

Mallampati score Derived from the Mallampati classification system that creates a score that predicts easy intubation based on the anatomy of the oral cavity, from base of uvula, faucial pillars to soft palate.

Mallory-Weiss tears Hematemesis or melena that typically follows many hours or days of severe vomiting and retching, traceable to one or several slitlike lacerations of the gastric mucosa, longitudinally placed at or slightly below the esophagogastric junction; also called *Mallory-Weiss syndrome.*

mandatory reporter Professionals who, in the ordinary course of their work and because they have regular contact with children, disabled persons, senior citizens, or other identified vulnerable populations, are required to report whenever financial, physical, sexual, or other types of abuse have been observed or is suspected, or when there is evidence of neglect, knowledge of an incident, or an imminent risk of serious harm.

Marfan syndrome One of the manifestations of abnormal fibrillin metabolism, a congenital disorder of connective tissue characterized by abnormal length of extremities, especially fingers and toes, subluxation of the lens, cardiovascular abnormalities (commonly dilation of the ascending aorta) and other deformities.

mastication Chewing.

maximum occlusion technique Involves air being injected into the tracheal tube cuff until no leak is heard, then withdrawal of the air until a small leak is heard on inspiration, then addition of more air until no leak is heard on inspiration; technique that decreases the risk of aspiration.

mean airway pressure (MAP) The average pressure over one inspiration/exhalation cycle; the value displayed on a ventilator is the average of this calculation over 1 minute.

medullary respiratory center The part of the respiratory center that is in the medulla oblongata, divided between the dorsal respiratory group and the ventral respiratory group.

melanocyte A type of dendritic clear cell found in the stratum basale of the epidermis; synthesizes tyrosinase and contains melanosomes that produce melanin that can be transferred from melanocytes to nearby keratinocytes.

menopause The cessation of menstruation in the human female, usually around the age of 50.

methemoglobinemia The presence of excessive methemoglobin in the blood, resulting in cyanosis and headache, dizziness, fatigue, ataxia, dyspnea, tachycardia, nausea, vomiting, and drowsiness, which can progress to stupor, coma, and occasionally death; may be caused by toxic exposure to a chemical or drug including nitrates, sulfonamides, and aniline dyes.

minimal leak technique Technique that decreases mucosal injury; performed by slowly inflating tracheal tube cuff until all leaks stop, then removing a small amount of air slowly until a small leak may be heard on inspiration.

minute volume The capacity of gas exhaled from the lungs per minute; tidal volume multiplied by respiratory rate.

miotic pupil A pupil that is constricted or contracted.

monoamine oxidase (MAO) A mitochondrial enzyme present in many tissues including nerve endings; has a vital role in regulating catecholamines in peripheral sympathetic nerve endings.

morality Concern with the distinction between good and evil or right and wrong.

Moro reflex Flexion of an infant's thighs and knees, fanning and then clenching of the fingers, with arms first thrown outward then brought together as if in an embrace; produced by a sudden stimulus such as the table being struck next to the child, or by sudden extension of the neck when the head is allowed to fall backward or the child is pulled up by both hands from a lying position and then let go; normally seen in infants up to 4 months of age; also called *embrace reflex* or *startle reflex*.

multiorgan dysfunction syndrome (MODS) Clinical syndrome of progressive dysfunction of organ systems; progressive physiologic failure (absolute or relative) of two or more separate organ systems in an acutely ill patient such that homeostasis cannot be maintained without medical support; also known as *systemic inflammatory response syndrome (SIRS)*.

muscarinic Denoting the effects of muscarine or acetylcholine at muscarinic receptors.

muscarinic cholinergic receptors A type of cholinergic receptor that is stimulated by the alkaloid muscarine and blocked by atropine; found on autonomic effector cells and central neurons in the thalamus and cerebral cortex; three types may be distinguished on the basis of pharmacologic specificity and five types on the basis of molecular structure.

muscularis layer Pertaining to a muscle layer or coat.

myasthenia gravis A disorder of neuromuscular function due to the presence of antibodies to acetylcholine receptors at the neuromuscular junction; characteristics include muscular fatigue and exhaustion tending to fluctuate in severity, without sensory disturbance or atrophy; also called *Erb-Goldflam, Goldflam's,* or *Goldflam-Erb disease.*

mydriatic pupil A pupil that is dilated.

myelin sheath A cylindrical covering on the axons of some neurons; consists of concentric layers of myelin, formed in the peripheral nervous system by the plasma membrane of Schwann cells, and in the central nervous system by oligodendrocytes.

myotomes A group of muscles innervated from a single spinal segment.

myocardial infarction Condition in which heart cells are not getting enough perfusion.

myoclonic movement (myoclonus) Shocklike contractions of a portion of a muscle, an entire muscle, or a group of muscles, restricted to one area of the body or appearing synchronously or asynchronously in several areas.

myoglobin The oxygen-transporting pigment of muscle, a type of hemoprotein resembling a single subunit of hemoglobin, composed of one globin polypeptide chain and one heme group (containing one iron atom); combines with oxygen released by erythrocytes, stores it, and transports it to the mitochondria of muscle cells, where it generates energy by combustion of glucose to carbon dioxide and water.

N

N-acetylcysteine An antidote that interferes with the metabolic process that results in the formation of hepatotoxic metabolite of acetaminophen during overdose.

narcotic Refers to opium, opiate derivatives, and their synthetic substitutes.

nasal turbinates Any of the nasal conchae; concha nasalis, or turbinal; bony plates that project from the nasal walls, shaped like shells.

necrotizing fasciitis A process in which fascia tissue is dying, many times resulting from overwhelming bacterial infections that cause cell death or necrosis.

negative feedback loop Those communication loops that oppose or negate a change in conditions, hopefully back to normal.

negligence The failure to act as a reasonably prudent person with the same knowledge, experience, and background would do under similar circumstances, which causes injury or damage to a person.

neoplasms Any new or abnormal growth; specifically a new growth of tissue in which the growth is uncontrolled and progressive; also called *tumor.*

neospinothalamic tracts Tracts that run directly to the thalamus without any modulation or other input.

neurites Axis cylinder process of a neuron; includes both axons and dendrites.

neurogenic shock A condition of profound hemodynamic and metabolic disturbance characterized by failure of the circulatory system to maintain adequate perfusion of vital organs, resulting from inadequate vasomotor tone.

neuroglia Supporting structure of nervous tissue; consists of a fine web of tissue made up of modified ectodermal elements in which are enclosed peculiar branched cells known as *neuroglial cells* or *glial cells.*

neuroinhibitor transmitter Any of a group of substances that are released upon excitation from the axon terminal of a presynaptic neuron of the central or peripheral nervous system and travel across the synaptic cleft to inhibit the target cells.

neuromuscular blocking agent (NMBA) A chemical substance that interferes locally with the transmission or reception of impulses from motor nerves to skeletal muscles.

neuron Any of the conducting cells of the nervous system; a typical neuron consists of a cell body, containing the nucleus and the surrounding cytoplasm; several short radiating processes (dendrites); and one long process (the axon), which terminates in twiglike branches and may have branches projecting along its course.

neuropathic pain A chronic pain condition that occurs or persists after a primary lesion or dysfunction of the peripheral or central nervous system.

neurotransmitter Any of a group of substances that are released upon excitation from the axon terminal of a presynaptic neuron of the central or peripheral nervous system and travel across the synaptic cleft to either excite or inhibit the target cell.

neutropenic Refers to a decrease in the number of neutrophils in the blood.

neutrophil A mature granular leukocyte that is polymorphonuclear; neutrophils have the properties of chemotaxis, adherence to immune complexes, and phagocytosis; also called *neutrocyte* and *neutrophilic leukocyte.*

nicotinic receptor A type of cholinergic receptor that is stimulated initially and blocked at high doses by the alkaloid nicotine and blocked by turbocurarine.

nitric oxide Gas that in combination with oxygen reduces pulmonary hypertension.

nociception The perception of physical pain.

nodes of Ranvier Constrictions occurring on myelinated nerve fibers at regular intervals of about 1 mm; at these sites the myelin sheath is absent and the axon is enclosed only by Schwann cell processes.

nonclostridial myonecrosis A particularly aggressive soft tissue infection; Similar to clostridial myonecrosis in that there is widespread involvement of soft tissue with necrosis of muscle tissue and fascia.

noncompetitive NMBA (neuromuscular blocking agent) Agent that simulates the appearance of acetylcholine at the motor end plate and stimulates (depolarizes) activity, then blocks its ability to reset for subsequent stimulation, thereby causing first fasciculations, then paralysis; also called *depolarizing agent.*

nondepolarizing paralytics Competitive, nondepolarizing neuromuscular blocking agents (NMBAs); drugs that compete with and block the action of acetylcholine at the neuromuscular junction receptor site, thereby causing paralysis.

noninvasive positive-pressure ventilation (NPPV) Ventilation support that does not require an advanced airway, such as BiPAP and CPAP.

nonmaleficence The ethical principle of doing no harm, based on the Hippocratic maxim, *primum non nocere,* first do no harm.

nonthrombogenic An agent or item that prevents the production of a thrombus or blood clot.

nontunneled central venous catheter Noncuffed catheter placed by a cutdown or percutaneous approach and secured by sutures or an intact dressing.

normocarbia Normal PCO_2.

nosocomial Pertaining to or originating in the hospital, usually referring to a disease or other pathologic condition; a nosocomial infection is one acquired in the hospital.

NSAIDs Nonsteroidal antiinflammatory drugs that interfere with the mediated process by which pain is relayed to nocirceceptors.

nucleoside A heterocyclic nitrogenous base, particularly a purine or pyrimidine, in *N*-glycosidic linkage with a sugar, particularly a pentose; often used specifically to denote a compound obtained by hydrolysis of nucleic acids; a purine or pyrimidine linked to ribose or deoxyribose (e.g., adenosine or cytidine).

nystagmus An involuntary, rapid, rhythmic movement of the eyeball, which may be horizontal, vertical, rotatory, or mixed.

O

occlusion technique A technique that allows minimal cuff pressure in tracheal tubes.

occult Refers to a disease condition that is hidden or difficult to detect with the naked eye.

oculocephalic response Doll's eyes phenomenon or response; *see also* **doll's eyes response**.

oculovestibular response Response elicited during the cold caloric examination.

oliguria Diminishing urinary output.

open-book pelvic fracture An anterior-posterior compression fracture that includes the pelvic ring and occurs in about 15% of pelvic fractures.

ophthalmia neonatorum Severe inflammation of the eye or of the conjunctiva or deeper structures of the eye; any hyperacute purulent conjunctivitis occurring during the first 10 days of life, usually contracted during birth from infected vaginal discharge of the mother; formerly referred only to gonorrheal infections; an iatrogenic form sometimes occurs after administration of silver nitrate; also called *neonatal conjunctivitis.*

ordinary negligence Failure to do what a reasonable person would do or would not do under the circumstances.

organophosphates Any class of anticholinesterase chemicals used in certain pesticides and military gases.

osteomyelitis Inflammation and infection of bone and bone marrow, caused by infection.

osteoporosis Reduction in bone mineral density, leading to fractures after minimal trauma.

osteoradionecrosis (ORN) Condition that may occur after tooth extraction in patients who have had their jaws irradiated as part of management of head and neck malignancy.

P

pain An unpleasant sensory and emotional experience associated with actual or potential tissue damage, or described in terms of such damage.

paleospinothalamic tract Pain tract that transmits to the medulla via the dorsal horn of the spinal column, first as it receives input from other areas of the brain, then to the pons nuclei, then to the thalamus.

pancytopenia Condition that may be induced by the use of heparin, which stimulates formation of antibody to the person's own platelets and creates intravascular clots composed of platelet aggregation.

paracentesis Surgical puncture of a cavity with a needle or other hollow instrument for diagnostic or therapeutic aspiration of fluid; in the abdomen, a trocar is inserted through an incision into the peritoneal cavity to inject a therapeutic agent or remove ascitic fluid.

paralytic Affected with or pertaining to paralysis; a person affected with paralysis.
paratonia Gegenhalten; involuntary resistance to passive movement, as may occur in cerebral cortical disorders.
parenchyma Functional part of an organ in the body (e.g., lungs).
parenteral Pertains to entry route other than through the alimentary canal (GI tract) (e.g., injection through subcutaneous, intramuscular, intraorbital, intracapsular, intraspinal, intrasternal, or intravenous).
paresthesia An abnormal touch sensation, such as burning, prickling, or formication (tactile hallucination: "bugs crawling"), often in the absence of an external stimulus.
pathogen Any disease-producing agent or microorganism, such as a bacterium, fungus, protozoan, or virus.
Penrose drain A thin rubber tube, usually 0.5 to 1 inch in diameter.
penumbra Area of a shadow where there is partial illumination; surrounds the umbra; ischemic penumbra is an area of moderately ischemic brain tissue surrounding an area of more severe ischemia; blood flow to this area may be enhanced to prevent the spread of a cerebral infarction.
pepsinogen A proenzyme secreted by chief cells, mucous neck cells, and pyloric gland cells, which is converted into pepsin in the presence of gastric acid or of pepsin itself.
percutaneous cricothyrotomy Percutaneous refers to being performed through the skin with a needle; introduction of a needle through the cricothyroid membrane to create an airway in an emergency.
percutaneous endoscopic gastrostomy (PEG) A method used for long-term tube feeding in which a tube is inserted through the chest wall into the stomach under endoscopic guidance.
percutaneous endoscopic jejunostomy (PEJ) A method used for long-term tube feeding in which a tube is inserted through the abdominal wall into the jejunum under endoscopic guidance.
perfluorocarbons (PFCs) Synthetic compounds (free of biologic materials) that have high oxygen solubility vs. blood products.
pericardiocentesis Surgical puncture of the pericardial cavity for the aspiration of fluid.
periosteum A specialized connective tissue covering all bones of the body and possessing bone-forming potentialities.
peripheral neuropathy A disease or disorder, especially a degenerative one, that affects the nervous system.
permissive hypercapnea Condition that occurs when clinicians decrease alveolar ventilation and allow the $Pa{CO_2}$ to rise.
$PETco_2$ Pressure of CO_2 near the end of exhalation; synonymous with end-tidal CO_2.
pharmacodynamics The study of the biochemical and physiologic effects of drugs and the mechanisms of their actions, including the correlation of actions and effects of drugs with their chemical structure; also refers to such effects on the actions of a particular drug or drugs.
pharmacokinetics The activity or fate of drugs in the body over a period of time, including the processes of absorption, distribution, location in tissues, biotransformation, and excretion.
phenylephrine A direct-acting sympathomimetic amine that stimulates α-adrenergic receptors and is a powerful vasoconstrictor.
pheochromocytoma A usually benign, well-encapsulated, lobular, vascular tumor of chromaffin tissue of the adrenal medulla or sympathetic paraganglia; also called *medullary chromaffinoma, medullary paraganglioma, chromaffin cell tumor,* and *pheochromoblastoma.*
photophobia Abnormal visual intolerance of light.
physiologic dead space Those portions of the airway, from the nose and mouth to the terminal bronchioles, in which exchange of oxygen and carbon dioxide does not occur.
pia mater Tender or soft; the innermost layer of the meninges.
plantar reflex *See* **Babinski's reflex.**
plasma colloid oncotic pressure The pressure or the osmotic pull of the plasma proteins in the bloodstream.
plasmapheresis The removal of plasma from withdrawn blood, with retransfusion of the formed elements into the donor; generally, type-specific fresh frozen plasma or albumin is used to replace the withdrawn plasma.
plateau pressure A pressure value that is maintained constantly during a portion of the inspiratory phase of the breath; represents the pressure at the alveolus and therefore is the best predictor of barotraumas.
pleural effusion The presence of fluid in the pleural space .
pneumotaxic center A center in the upper part of the pons that rhythmically inhibits inhalation independently of the vagus nerve; also called *Lumsden.*
poikilothermy Body temperature that varies with the environmental temperature.
polypharmacy Administration of many drugs together; administration of excessive medication.
portal hypertension Increased pressure in the portal vein caused by obstruction of flow of blood through the liver.
positive end-expiratory pressure (PEEP) Pressure that is maintained above the level of atmospheric pressure at the end of exhalation; achieved by preventing the complete release of gas during exhalation, usually by means of a valve within the circuit.
positive feedback loop Those loops of communication that enhance a process or stimulate; an ever-increasing rate of events that occur until something stops the process (e.g., the clotting process with platelet aggregation and labor contractions).
postprandial After a meal.
preganglionic fibers Fibers situated anterior or proximal to a ganglion; said especially of autonomic nerve fibers so located.
presbycusis A progressive, bilaterally symmetric sensorineural hearing loss occurring with age.
presbyesophagus Alteration in motor function of the esophagus as a result of degenerative changes occurring with advancing age.
presynaptically Before the synapse.
primary MODS (primary multiorgan dysfunction syndrome) Direct trauma to the organ system that causes progressive dysfunction (e.g., pulmonary contusion that creates acute respiratory dysfunction syndrome [ARDS] or acute lung injury [ALI]).
proinflammatory cytokine A type of cytokine that is capable of stimulating inflammation.
pronation sign Pronation of the forearm caused by passive flexion, seen in hemiplegia.
proprioception Perception mediated by proprioceptors (sensory nerve terminals) or proprioceptive tissues found in muscles, tendons, and joint capsules that give information concerning movements and position of the body.
proprioceptive The sense of the relative position of neighboring parts of the body.
prostaglandin A hormone-like substance that mediates inflammatory response and sensitizes spinal neurons to painful stimuli.
proteinuria Excessive serum proteins in the urine, such as in renal disease, after strenuous exercise, and with dehydration; also called *albuminuria.*

proximate causation An event that is *closest*, or immediately responsible, for causing some observed result.

psychogenic pain Originating in mental or emotional rather than in physiologic processes.

ptosis Drooping of the upper eyelid from paralysis of the third nerve or from sympathetic innervation; also called *blepharoptosis*; *Horner's syndrome*.

punitive Inflicting punishment; "punitive justice"; "punitive damages."

pyloric sphincter Sphincter of the pylorus, which is located in the most distal part of the stomach, helps move chyme through to the duodenum.

pyramidal Shaped like a pyramid.

Q

quiet tachypnea Refers to a rapid rate of breathing that does not involve accessory muscle use.

R

radiopaque Not penetrable by x-rays or other forms of radiant energy; radiopaque areas appear light or white on exposed film.

recombinant Refers to a new entity (gene, protein, cell, individual) that results from genetic recombination.

recombinant factor VIIa A man-made factor that is heat- and storage-stable and that participates in the extrinsic pathway of coagulation and is activated by contact with calcium, and in concert with factor III activates factor X; also called *proconvertin*..

recombinant human activated protein C (rhAPC) An activated protein that exerts an antithrombotic effect by inhibiting factors Va and VIIIa; may have indirect profibrinolytic activity through its ability to inhibit plasminogen activator inhibitor-1 and may exert an antiinflammatory effect by limiting the chemotactic response of leukocytes to inflammatory cytokines.

renin angiotensin aldosterone system (RAAS) System that regulates sodium balance, fluid volume, and blood pressure by renal secretions: in response to reduced perfusion, renin is secreted, which hydrolyzes a plasma globulin to convert angiotensin to angiotensin I; angiotensin then converts from I to II; this in turn stimulates aldosterone secretion, which brings about sodium retention, increase in blood pressure, and restoration of renal perfusion, which snuffs out the signal for renin release.

resistance Refers to opposition of the tracheobronchial tree to air flow; the mouth-to-alveoli pressure difference divided by the air flow; opposition or counteracting force.

respiration The cellular metabolic process by which oxygen is taken in, substances are oxidized, energy is released, and carbon dioxide and oxidized products are given off.

reticular activating system (RAS) The system of cells of the reticular formation of the medulla oblongata that receive collaterals from the ascending sensory pathways and project to higher centers; they control the overall degree of central nervous system activity, including wakefulness, attentiveness, and sleep.

reversible ischemic neurologic deficit (RIND) Any focal neurologic deficit that resolves completely within 24 hours; previously called *transient ischemic attack (TIA)*.

rhabdomyolysis Disintegration or dissolution of muscle, associated with excretion of myoglobin in the urine.

rhodanase A mitochondrial enzyme that detoxifies cyanide (CN^-) by converting it to thiocyanate (SCN).

roving eye movements Spontaneous, slow, and random eye deviation that moves in the horizontal plane similar to the slow eye movements of sleep.

S

SCIWORA (spinal cord injury without radiographic abnormality) A syndrome in children usually less than 8 years of age in which the spinal cord is injured but the bony vertebrae show no evidence of fracture or trauma.

sclerosing agent An agent administered to sclerose or harden, as in sclerosing of spider veins in the leg.

secondary MODS (secondary multiorgan dysfunction syndrome) A latent development of organ dysfunction caused by a systemic inflammatory response; the organs affected are not involved in the initial insult to the body.

Seldinger technique A method for introducing a catheter into a hollow lumen structure or body cavity; a narrow needle is used to enter the structure, a guidewire is passed through the needle, the needle is removed, and the catheter is advanced over the wire.

Sellick maneuver A maneuver in which pressure is applied to the cricoid cartilage to compress the esophagus and prevent passive regurgitation during endotracheal intubation.

senescence The process or condition of growing old.

Sengstaken-Blakemore tube A multilumen esophageal tube used for the tamponade of bleeding esophageal varices.

sepsis The presence in the blood or other tissues of pathogenic microorganisms or their toxins; also referred to as *septicemia*.

septicemia Systemic disease associated with the presence and persistence of pathogenic microorganisms or their toxins in the blood; also called *blood poisoning* and *sepsis*.

shunting To turn to one side; to divert or bypass.

slander Words falsely spoken that damage the reputation of another.

somatosensory cortex Describes sensory stimuli coming from the skin and internal organs and the perception of those stimuli.

somatostatin Any of several cyclic tetradecapeptides elaborated primarily by the median eminence of the hypothalamus and by the delta cells of the pancreatic islets; they inhibit release of growth hormone, thyrotropin, and corticotrophin by the adenohypophysis, of insulin and glucagon by the pancreas, of gastrin by the gastric mucosa, of secretin by the intestinal mucosa, and of renin by the kidney.

sphincter Ringlike band of muscle fibers that constricts a passage or closes a natural orifice.

spinal shock A variable state of paralysis after a spinal cord injury.

spirometry Measurement of the breathing capacity of the lungs, such as in pulmonary function tests.

splanchnic Visceral; pertaining to one of the splanchnic nerves.

squamous bone Flattened or platelike bone; scalelike.

squamous cells Epithelial cells described as scaly; resembling a squama; flattened or platelike.

stagnant hypoxia Failure to transport sufficient oxygen because of inadequate blood flow secondary to blood pooling.

standard of care In medicine, treatment that experts agree is appropriate, accepted, and widely used; healthcare providers are obligated to provide patients with the standard of care; also called *standard therapy* or *best practice*.

stimulatory Neurotransmitters that promote the actions of neurons.

strabismus Deviation of the eye that the patient cannot overcome in which the visual axes assume a position relative to each other

that is different from that required by the physiologic conditions.
striatum. In anatomy, a sheetlike mass or substance.
subarachnoid space The potential space between the arachnoid and the pia mater of the meninges, covering the brain.
subdural space The potential space between the dura mater and the arachnoid layers of the meninges.
substance P The pain transmitter of the dorsal horn of the spinal cord.
sulfation The addition of a sulfate group to a molecule.
suppressor T-cells Cells that stop a specific immune response after several days and create memory cells; also called *T-8 cells (CD8).*
surgical cricothyrotomy A tracheotomy involving incision through the skin and cricothyroid membrane to secure a patent airway for emergency relief of upper airway obstruction.
sutures Suturae cranii; the sutures between the various bones of the skull, named generally for the specific components participating in their formation.
syndrome A set of symptoms that occur together; the sum of signs of any morbid state; a symptom complex.
syndrome of inappropriate antidiuretic hormone (SIADH) Persistent hyponatremia, hypovolemia, and inappropriately elevated urine osmolality, associated with the release of vasopressin (antidiuretic hormone) in amounts excessive for the state of hydration; causes include vasopressin-secreting tumor cells, neoplasms, pulmonary disorders, and central nervous system diseases, including head trauma.
synthetic Drugs that are made artificially by chemical synthesis.
systemic inflammation Diffuse inflammation; an infection spread over a large area.
systemic inflammatory response syndrome (SIRS) A syndrome of symptoms related to a response of the immune system to an antigenic stimulus, including antibody production, cell-mediated immunity, and immunologic tolerance.

T

tactile sense Pertaining to the sense of touch.
T cells Cells primarily responsible for cell-mediated immunity; originate from lymphoid stem cells that migrate from the bone marrow to the thymus and differentiate under the influence of the thymic hormones thymopoietin and thymosin.
temporomandibular ankylosis Condition in which the temporomandibular joint becomes immobile and consolidated due to disease, injury, or surgical procedure.
tentorial herniation Protrusion of the brain structures through the tentorial notch.
tentorium cerebelli The process of dura mater that supports the occipital lobes and covers the cerebellum.
teratogen Any agent or factor that induces or increases the incidence of abnormal prenatal development.
tet spell An acute onset of symptoms when cardiac output falls and hypoxia occurs in a child with the congenital heart defect called *tetralogy of Fallot.*
thiocyanate Substance produced in the metabolism of cysteine and detoxification of cyanide and excreted in the urine.
thoracentesis Surgical puncture of the thoracic cavity with a needle or catheter over a needle for aspiration of fluids; also called *pleurocentesis.*
thoracostomy (tube and needle) Surgical creation of an opening in the wall of the chest for the purpose of drainage; tube thoracostomy refers to insertion of a chest tube for the purposes of draining fluid and air from the pleural space; needle thoracostomy refers to drainage of air from the pleural space.
thrill A sensation of vibration felt by the examiner on palpation of the body, such as a murmur or aneurysm felt over the heart.
thrombocytopenia Decrease in the number of platelets, such as in thrombocytopenic purpura.
thymus A bilaterally symmetric lymphoid organ consisting of two pyramidal lobes situated in the anterior superior mediastinum.
tidaling The rise and fall of fluid in a chest tube that is synchronized with the respiratory cycle.
tissue factor Tissue thromboplastin: a lipoprotein functioning in the extrinsic pathway of coagulation, activating factor X; also called *coagulation factor III.*
tocolytic Refers to tocolysis, inhibition of uterine contractions, or the agent that causes inhibition of such contractions.
toilette French term that refers to cleansing; respiratory toilette refers to the action of a healthcare provider who cleanses the upper airway by instilling saline and then suctioning the respiratory secretions.
tonsillar herniation Protrusion of the cerebellar tonsils through the foramen magnum, exerting pressure on the medulla oblongata.
tort (law) Any wrongdoing for which an action for damages may be brought.
toxidrome A set of clinical signs and symptoms that suggest a specific class of toxin or poison.
tracheostomy/tracheotomy Creation of an opening in the anterior trachea for insertion of a tube to relieve upper airway obstruction and facilitate ventilation.
transcranial Refers to a procedure performed through the cranium.
transjugular intrahepatic portosystemic shunt (TIPS) An artificial percutaneous shunt between the hepatic and portal veins within the liver with placement of an expandable stent in the tract created; performed by way of a transjugular route under radiologic guidance for treatment of bleeding esophageal varices.
transsphenoidal Refers to a procedure performed through the sphenoid bone.
trichomoniasis Infection with protozoa of the genus *Trichomonas.*
trypsin A serine endopeptidase that catalyzes cleavage of peptide bonds on the carboxyl side of either arginine or lysine; secreted by the pancreas as the proenzyme trypsinogen and converted to the active form in the small intestine by enteropeptidase; the active enzyme catalyzes the cleavage and activation of additional trypsinogen and other pancreatic proenzymes important to protein digestion.
trypsinogen The inactive proenzyme of trypsin secreted by the pancreas, activated in the duodenum via cleavage by enteropeptidase.
T tube A self-retaining drainage tube in the shape of a T; often used in the common bile duct.
tumor necrosis factor (TNF) A cytokine produced primarily by macrophages in response to infection with gram-negative bacteria; facilitates inflammation by causing the vascular endothelium to become stickier, which results in increased adherence of neutrophils from the vessels; acts directly on the brain to induce fever, on the liver to produce plasma proteins
tunneled cuffed Catheter implanted into subclavian, internal jugular, or femoral vein with a cuff that inhibits migration of organisms into the tract.
turgor Condition of being turgid; normal or other fullness; in reference to the skin, a reflection of the skin's elasticity, measured by monitoring the time it takes for the skin of the forearm to return

to position after it is lightly pinched between the examiner's thumb and forefinger.

tympany A tympanic, or bell-like, percussion note; ruminal tympany is a kind of indigestion or bloat.

U

uncal herniation Descending transtentorial herniation in which the uncus protrudes through the notch.

unifascicular block An impairment of conduction in the right bundle branch or in either the anterior or posterior limb of the left bundle branch.

V

values Beliefs of a person or social group in which they have an emotional investment (either for or against something).

ventilation A passive activity in which air is moved into or out of the lungs for the purpose of exchanging oxygen for carbon dioxide.

ventilator-assisted pneumonia (VAP) A nosocomial pneumonia acquired while undergoing mechanical ventilation; also known as *ventilator-associated pneumonia.*

ventriculostomy The operation of establishing a free communication or shunt between the floor of the third ventricle and the underlying cisterna interpeduncularis; for the treatment of hydrocephalus.

veracity Unwillingness to tell lies.

vernix caseosa An unctuous substance composed of sebum and desquamated epithelial cells that covers the skin of the fetus.

$\dot{V}/\dot{Q}$ The ratio of ventilation to perfusion.

$\dot{V}/\dot{Q}$ mismatch Anatomic or physiologic shunt indicative of impaired gas exchange.

W

Wernicke's speech area A term originally denoting a language center in the brain thought to be confined to the posterior part of the superior temporal gyrus adjacent to the transverse temporal gyri; the term now includes a wider zone that encompasses the supramarginal and angular gyri as well; also called *Wernicke area* and *Wernicke second motor speech area.*

Wilson's disease A rare, progressive, autosomal recessive disease due to a defect in metabolism of copper; a characteristic feature is a pigmented ring at the outer margin of the cornea.

work of breathing Use of accessory muscles of respiration; an indicator of respiratory muscle fatigue and impending ventilatory failure.

Answers to Review Questions

CHAPTER 1

1. A
2. B
3. C
4. C
5. C
6. A
7. A
8. A
9. D
10. D
11. D
12. D
13. B
14. C
15. A
16. A
17. C
18. C
19. A
20. A

CHAPTER 2

1. A
2. C
3. C
4. D
5. C
6. B
7. D
8. B
9. B
10. A

CHAPTER 3

1. A
2. A
3. C
4. A
5. D
6. C
7. A
8. D
9. A
10. C
11. A
12. C
13. A
14. A
15. D
16. B
17. C
18. B
19. A
20. D

CHAPTER 4

1. 20
2. Myogenic theory
3. Coronary sulcus
4. Thorel's pathway
5. S3, S4
6. Prinzmetals
7. MVP
8. 60%
9. Sanford; DeBakey; descriptive proximal and distal
10. Primary
11. C
12. D
13. D
14. A
15. B
16. D
17. A
18. B
19. A
20. B
21. D
22. A

CHAPTER 5

1. The MAP for a BP of 92/60:
   [(2 X Diastolic) + Systolic]/3
   Answer: 70.7 mmHg

2. A. CPP = MAP – ICP
   70.7 – 42.0
   Answer: 26.7
   B. Barely any perfusion is occurring in the brain. Blood flow is passive. Ischemia is present.
   C. Treatment in the initial scenario asked for an additional fluid bolus to improve perfusion and overall blood pressure. That is appropriate. Oxygenation, ventilation, and perfusion must be optimized to improve this patient's CPP and reduce secondary brain injury.
   D. The MAP is outside the range for autoregulation by the patient. Noncompliant.
3. ICP measurement devices are leveled to the reference point of the foramen of Monro, which correlates to the top of the external auditory canal.
4. A. To accurately assess for mental status, the patient must be able to understand the commands. If possible, a Spanish-to-English translator should be used. The GCS may be untestable in the verbal response category, a "V" entered, and *1* used as that section's total.
   B. Spinal immobilization will need to be applied due to the mechanism of injury and potential for spinal injury. The patient cannot answer questions nor follow commands from the English language to meet the protocol standards for not applying neutral immobilization.
5. True. Anisocoria is a normal variant in about 20% of the population.
6. Herniation syndrome.
7. Position patient to facilitate venous return and good blood flow. Reduce environmental stimulation. Reduce this patient's body temperature aggressively without causing shivering. Maintain PaCO2 at normal levels and follow orders for use of diuretic agents and/or vasoactive agents to reduce ICP. Assess for and treat any signs of pain.
8. The blood gas shows respiratory alkalosis with complete compensation. The patient is showing signs of neurogenic hyperventilation in his attempt to blow off CO2 to reduce blood flow to the brain – autoregulation mechanism.
9. The limbic system may have been injured. This area includes the hippocampus, and amygdala and is responsible for keeping you safe.
10. Oculocephalic reflex is performed on an unconscious patient who has had his spine cleared from injury. With the eyelids held open, the patient's head is turned to the side, and the observer watches for eyeball movement.
    A. The patient described is considered negative. The patient does not have the response.
    B. Commonly termed "doll's eye response"
    C. When the eyes stay midpoint or drop to the dependent side, the patient is said to have a non-intact brainstem.
11. Epidural hematoma forms 80% of the time in the temporal lobe from a tear in the middle meningeal artery.
12. Usually found in children and adolescents because the dura is less firmly attached to the bone in this location versus older adults.
13. Those at risk for chronic subdural hematoma formation are the elderly, those on antiplatelet therapy, and those with clotting disorders.
14. A. 70% of patients suffering from a subarachnoid hemorrhage from aneurysm will incur post-event vasospasm that will cause a worsened neurologic result.
    B. To try to prevent this, three types of therapy were discussed in the chapter: Hypertensive/Hypervolemic/Hemodilution (HHH) therapy, use of Nimodipine, and cerebral angioplasty.
15. The patient appears to be suffering from diabetes insipidus due to a decrease in the secretion of antidiuretic hormone (ADH) from the posterior pituitary gland. The patient may have injury to his hypothalamic or pituitary area. Treatment may include Desmopressin or Vasopressin.

CHAPTER 6

1. A
2. A
3. D
4. C
5. D
6. A
7. D
8. B
9. C
10. B

CHAPTER 7

1. C
2. C
3. A
4. B
5. B
6. C
7. A
8. B
9. B
10. A
11. B
12. A
13. A
14. B
15. D
16. C
17. A
18. A
19. B
20. B

CHAPTER 8

1. B
2. C
3. A
4. D
5. B
6. C
7. D
8. D
9. C
10. B
11. D
12. D
13. B
14. B
15. B
16. C
17. B
18. D
19. A
20. C

CHAPTER 9

Obstetric Section

1. A
2. C
3. B
4. D
5. C

Pediatric Section

6. A
7. D
8. B
9. B
10. C
11. A
12. B
13. C
14. B
15. B

Geriatric Section

16. B
17. D
18. D
19. B
20. D
21. A
22. C
23. D
24. A
25. A

CHAPTER 10

1. D
2. D
3. B
4. C
5. C
6. D
7. B
8. A
9. C
10. B
11. C
12. D
13. A
14. D
15. C
16. D
17. B
18. C
19. B
20. A
21. B
22. D
23. A

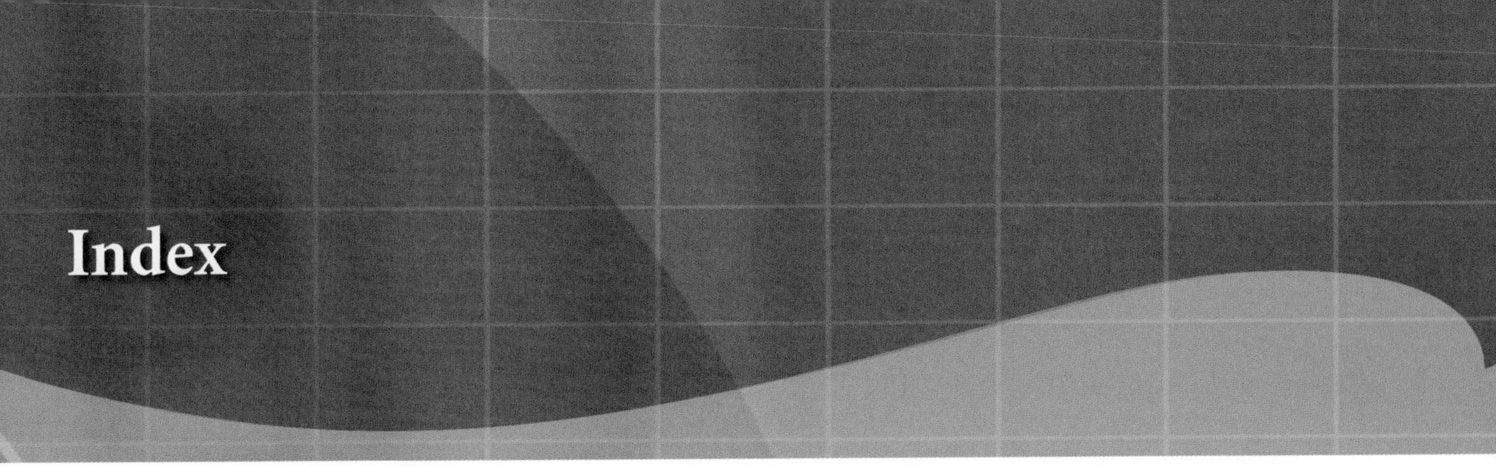

Index

The letter *t* indicates a table, *b* indicates a box, and *f* indicates a figure.

M